C-reactive protein, CRP

Calcium (total)

Glucose, fasting

Prostate-specific antigen,

T_4 (total thyroxine)

Thyroid stimulating hormo

T0177469

Biochemistry refere___ ...ervals

HbAc1	
Normal	<42mmol/ml (<6%)
Pre-diabetes	42–47mmol/ml (6–6.4%)
Diabetes	≥48mmol/ml (≥6.5%)

Reproduced with permission from Longmore M, Wilkinson IB, Baldwin, A, and Wallin, E (2014). *Oxford Handbook of Clinical Medicine* (9th edn). Oxford: Oxford University Press.

UKMI specialist centres

Specialist topic	Centre	Contact number
Drugs in pregnancy	Regional Drug & Therapeutics Centre, Newcastle Upon Tyne	0191 282 4631
Drugs in lactation	UK Drugs in Lactation Advisory Service (UKDILAS)	0116 258 6491
Complementary medicine	Welsh Medicines Information Service	029 2074 2251
Drugs in cardiothoracics	Royal Brompton and Harefield NHS Foundation Trust	0207 351 8901
Drugs in dentistry	North West Medicines Information Centre	0151 794 8206
Drugs in renal impairment	South West Medicines Information	0117 342 2867
Drugs in porphyria	Welsh Medicines Information Service	029 2074 2251
Drugs in psychiatry	The Maudsley Hospital	0203 228 2317
Drugs in HIV	Chelsea and Westminster NHS Trust	0208 746 8398

UK National Poisons Information Service (NPIS)

NPIS is comprised of four individual units (Birmingham, Cardiff, Edinburgh, and Newcastle) with a single national telephone number: 0844 892 0111.

OXFORD MEDICAL PUBLICATIONS

Oxford Handbook of
Clinical Pharmacy

Published and forthcoming Oxford Handbooks

Oxford Handbook of
Clinical
Pharmacy

Third Edition

Edited by

Philip Wiffen

Editor in Chief, European Journal of Hospital Pharmacy;
Visiting Professor, Dept of Pharmacy and Pharmacology,
University of Bath, UK

Marc Mitchell

Divisional Lead Pharmacist, Oxford University
Hospitals NHS Foundation Trust, UK

Melanie Snelling

Lead HIV/Infectious Diseases Pharmacist,
Oxford University Hospitals NHS Foundation Trust, UK

Nicola Stoner

Cancer Consultant Pharmacist, Oxford Cancer and
Haematology Centre and Oxford Cancer Research
Centre, Churchill Hospital, Oxford University
Hospitals NHS Foundation Trust, UK;
Visiting Professor, School of Chemistry, Food and
Pharmacy, University of Reading, UK

OXFORD
UNIVERSITY PRESS

Great Clarendon Street, Oxford, OX2 6DP,
United Kingdom

Oxford University Press is a department of the University of Oxford.
It furthers the University's objective of excellence in research, scholarship,
and education by publishing worldwide. Oxford is a registered trade mark of
Oxford University Press in the UK and in certain other countries

© Oxford University Press 2017

The moral rights of the authors have been asserted

First Edition published in 2007
Second Edition published in 2012
Third Edition published in 2017

All rights reserved. No part of this publication may be reproduced, stored in
a retrieval system, or transmitted, in any form or by any means, without the
prior permission in writing of Oxford University Press, or as expressly permitted
by law, by licence or under terms agreed with the appropriate reprographics
rights organization. Enquiries concerning reproduction outside the scope of the
above should be sent to the Rights Department, Oxford University Press, at the
address above

You must not circulate this work in any other form
and you must impose this same condition on any acquirer

Published in the United States of America by Oxford University Press
198 Madison Avenue, New York, NY 10016, United States of America

British Library Cataloguing in Publication Data
Data available

Library of Congress Control Number: 2016945512

ISBN 978–0–19–873582–3

Printed and bound in China by
C&C Offset Printing Co., Ltd.

Oxford University Press makes no representation, express or implied, that the
drug dosages in this book are correct. Readers must therefore always check
the product information and clinical procedures with the most up-to-date
published product information and data sheets provided by the manufacturers
and the most recent codes of conduct and safety regulations. The authors and
the publishers do not accept responsibility or legal liability for any errors in the
text or for the misuse or misapplication of material in this work. Except where
otherwise stated, drug dosages and recommendations are for the non-pregnant
adult who is not breast-feeding

Links to third party websites are provided by Oxford in good faith and
for information only. Oxford disclaims any responsibility for the materials
contained in any third party website referenced in this work.

Preface to the third edition

When we embarked on the first edition almost 10 years ago we did not envisage the enthusiasm that has developed for the *Oxford Handbook of Clinical Pharmacy*. We are very happy to launch the third edition. This edition has some 25 or so new topics and most of the existing topics have been revised or reworked in some way. We have widened the number of authors to bring new skills and knowledge into this edition.

Clinical pharmacy has undergone rapid development during the lifetime of this little book. In the UK, a hospital pharmacy without clinical services now seems strange but the battle to establish clinical pharmacy is still not won in parts of Europe, particularly in Eastern Europe. The last 10 years have also seen rapid development around the appointment and role of consultant pharmacists, who are making major contributions in improving patient outcomes and raising the research agenda within pharmacy. We have sections in this edition on annotating medicine charts and writing in patients' notes. We suspect the life of these topics is limited as we progress rapidly into electronic patient records. Finally, we are encouraged to see the concept of evidence-based practice permeating the whole of hospital pharmacy activities.

We would remind you that this handbook was never perceived as a formulary but sits alongside such texts to provide evidence and hopefully wisdom for clinical pharmacists.

PW
MM
MS
NS

Acknowledgements

We are grateful to the following people who provided comments and help: Jen Weston, Janice Craig, David Hutchings, Rhiannon Thomas, Eunice Morley, Emma Pullan, Sarah Cripps, Charlotte Harris, Jo Coleman, Vicky Price, Yovana Sooriakumaran, and Hannah Hunter.

Contents

Contributors

Judith Bailey
Oxford University Hospitals
NHS Foundation Trust,
Oxford, UK

Nina Barnett
Pharmacy, London Northwest
Healthcare NHS Trust & NHS
Specialist Pharmacy Service, UK

Rachel Brown
Oxford Health
NHS Foundation Trust,
Oxford, UK

Fearn Davies
Oxford University Hospitals
NHS Foundation Trust,
Oxford, UK

Louise Dunsmure
Oxford University Hospitals
NHS Foundation Trust,
Oxford, UK

Clare Faulkner
Oxford University Hospitals
NHS Foundation Trust,
Oxford, UK

Janet Hemingway
Oxford University Hospitals
NHS Foundation Trust,
Oxford, UK

Gwen Klepping
Oxford University Hospitals
NHS Foundation Trust,
Oxford, UK

Katie McDonald
Oxford University Hospitals
NHS Foundation Trust,
Oxford, UK

Olivia Moswela
Oxford University Hospitals
NHS Foundation Trust,
Oxford, UK

Bernard Naughton
Formerly Oxford University
Hospitals, NHS Foundation
Trust, Oxford, UK

Sarah Poole
Oxford University Hospitals
NHS Foundation Trust,
Oxford, UK

Jas Sagoo
Medicines Management
Lead, Oxfordshire Clinical
Commissioning Group, UK

Aarti Shah
Formerly Oxford University
Hospitals, NHS Foundation
Trust, Oxford, UK

Laura Smith
Oxford University Hospitals
NHS Foundation Trust,
Oxford, UK

Amy Tse
Oxford University Hospitals
NHS Foundation Trust,
Oxford, UK

Laura Watson
Formerly Oxford University
Hospitals, NHS Foundation
Trust, Oxford, UK

Symbols and abbreviations

↑	increased
↓	decreased
>	greater than
<	less than
♂	male
♀	female
°	degrees
5-HT	5-hydroxytryptamine (serotonin)
A&E	accident and emergency
A&W	alive and well
AAA	abdominal aortic aneurysm
ABC	airway, breathing, and circulation
abdo	abdominal
ABPI	Association of the British Pharmaceutical Industry
ACE	angiotensin-converting enzyme
ACV	assist-control ventilation
ADR	adverse drug reaction
AF	atrial fibrillation
AFB	acid-fast bacilli
ALP	alkaline phosphatase
ALT	alanine aminotransferase
APPT	activated partial thrombin time
ARB	angiotensin receptor blocker
ASCO	American Society of Clinical Oncology
AS	ankylosing spondylitis
AST	aspartate aminotransferase
AUC	area under the plasma concentration curve
AV	arteriovenous
BDP	beclometasone dipropionate
BiPAP	bi-level positive airway pressure
BMI	body mass index
BMR	basal metabolic rate
BNF	British National Formulary
BP	blood pressure
BPH	benign prostatic hyperplasia
BSA	body surface area

CAD	coronary artery disease
CAPD	continuous ambulatory peritoneal dialysis
CAVD	continuous arteriovenous haemodialysis
CAVH	continuous arteriovenous haemofiltration
CD	controlled drug
CHF	congestive heart failure
CMV	continuous mandatory ventilation
CNS	central nervous system
C/O	complaining of
CO_2	carbon dioxide
COC	combined oral contraceptive
COPD	chronic obstructive pulmonary disease
COSHH	Control of Substances Hazardous to Health
COX	cyclooxygenase
CPAP	continuous positive airway pressure
CrCl	creatinine clearance
CRP	C-reactive protein
CSF	cerebrospinal fluid
CTC	common toxicity criteria
CVC	central venous catheter
CVP	central venous pressure
CVS	cardiovascular system
CVVHDF	continuous venovenous haemodiafiltration
CXR	chest X-ray
CYP450	cytochrome P450
Da	dalton
DDx, ZZ	differential diagnosis
DHx	drug history
DIC	disseminated intravascular coagulation
DM	diabetes mellitus
DOE	disease-orientated evidence
DTI	direct thrombin inhibitor
DUE	drug-use evaluation
DVT	deep vein thrombosis
Dx, Z	diagnosis
E/C	enteric-coated
EBM	evidence-based medicine
ECF	extracellular fluid
ECG	electrocardiogram
eGFR	estimated glomerular filtration rate

ESBL	extended-spectrum B-lactamases
ESR	erythrocyte sedimentation rate
EU	European Union
FBC	full blood count
FH	family history
G6PD	glucose-6-phosphate dehydrogenase
GABA	gamma-aminobutyric acid
GCP	good clinical practice
GFR	glomerular filtration rate
GI	gastrointestinal
GIT	gastrointestinal tract
GMP	good manufacturing practice
GOR	glucose oxidation rate
GORD	gastro-oesophageal reflux disease
GP	general practitioner
GSL	general sales list
GTN	glyceryl trinitrate
HbA_{1c}	glycosylated haemoglobin
HCP	healthcare professional
HD	haemodialysis
HDF	haemodiafiltration
HDL	high-density lipid
HF	haemofiltration
HIT	heparin-induced thrombocytopenia
HIV	human immunodeficiency virus
HPA	Health Protection Agency
HPC	history of presenting complaint
HR	heart rate
HRS	hepatorenal syndrome
HRT	hormone replacement therapy
IA	intra-articular
ICF	intracellular fluid
ICS	inhaled corticosteroid
IM	intramuscular(ly)
IMP	investigational medicinal product
IMV	intermittent mandatory ventilation
INR	international normalized ratio
IO	intra-osseous
IPS	Institute of Purchasing Supply
ITU	intensive therapy unit

IV	intravenous(ly)
Ix	investigations
JVP	jugular venous pressure
K$^+$	potassium
KCCT	kaolin cephalin clotting time
LABA	long-acting beta-2-agonist
LFT	liver function test
LMWH	low-molecular-weight heparin
LTOT	long-term oxygen therapy
M/R	modified-release
MAOI	monoamine oxidase inhibitor
MARS	molecular absorbent recirculating system
MCH	mean corpuscular haemoglobin
MCHC	mean corpuscular haemoglobin concentration
MCV	mean cell volume
MDA	Medical Devices Agency
MDI	metered-dose inhaler
MDS	monitored dose system
MHRA	Medicines and Healthcare products Regulatory Agency
MI	myocardial infarction
MIC	minimum inhibitory concentration
MOAI	monoamine oxidase inhibitor
MRSA	meticillin-resistant *Staphylococcus aureus*
MSSA	meticillin-susceptible *Staphylococcus aureus*
NBM	nil by mouth
ng	nanogram
NG	nasogastric
NGT	nasogastric tube
NHS	National Health Service
NICE	National Institute for Health and Care Excellence
NNH	number needed to harm
NNRTI	non-nucleoside reverse transcriptase inhibitor
NNT	number needed to treat
NPSA	National Patient Safety Agency
NSAID	non-steroidal anti-inflammatory drug
NSF	National Service Framework
NSTEMI	non-ST-segment elevation myocardial infarction
NYHA	New York Heart Association
O/E	on examination
O$_2$	oxygen

ortho	bones and joints
PA	psoriatic arthritis
PABA	para-amino benzoic acid
$Paco_2$	partial pressure of carbon dioxide in arterial blood
Pao_2	partial pressure of oxygen in arterial blood
PC	presenting complaint
PCC	prothrombin complex concentrate
PCI	percutaneous coronary intervention
PE	pulmonary embolism
PEEP	positive end-expiratory pressure
PEG	percutaneous endoscopic gastroscopy
PGD	patient group direction
PICC	peripherally inserted central catheter
PMCPA	Prescription Medicines Code of Practice Authority
pMDI	pressurized metered-dose inhaler
PMH	past medical history
PMR	prescription medication records
PMS	pre-menstrual syndrome
PNS	peripheral nervous system
PO	*per os* (by mouth)
POD	patient's own drug
POEM	patient-orientated evidence that matters
POM	prescription-only medicine
PONV	postoperative nausea and vomiting
POP	progestogen-only pill
PPI	proton pump inhibitor
ppm	parts per million
PR	*per rectum* (by the rectum)
PRN	*pro re nata* (as required)
PSV	pressure support ventilation
PT	prothrombin time
PUD	peptic ulcer disease
QP	qualified person
R&D	research and development
RA	rheumatoid arthritis
RBC	red blood cell
Resp	respiratory system
SABA	short-acting beta-2-agonist
SBOT	short-burst oxygen therapy

SC	subcutaneous/ly
S/R	systems review
SH	social history
SIMV	synchronous intermittent mandatory ventilation
SOB	short of breath
SPC	summary of product characteristics
SR	sinus rhythm
SSRI	selective serotonin re-uptake inhibitor
stat	at once
STEMI	ST-segment elevation myocardial infarction
T_3	tri-iodothyronine
T_4	thyroxine
T_{max}	time to maximum drug concentration
TB	tuberculosis
TBC	to be confirmed/awaiting confirmation
TBG	thyroid-binding globulin
TDM	therapeutic drug monitoring
TENS	transcutaneous electronic nerve stimulation
TG	triglyceride
TIA	transient ischaemic attack
TNF	tumour necrosis factor
t-PA	tissue plasminogen activator
TPN	total parenteral nutrition
TPO	thyroid peroxidase
TRH	thyrotropin-releasing hormone
TSH	thyroid-stimulating hormone
TTO	to take out
U&Es	urea and electrolytes
UFH	unfractionated heparin
UKMI	UK Medicines Information
UV	ultraviolet
v/v	volume in volume
v/w	volume in weight
VAC	vacuum-assisted closure
VAS	visual analogue scale
VAT	value added tax
VF	ventricular fibrillation
VRE	vancomycin resistant enterococci
VRSA	vancomycin resistant MRSA

VT	ventricular tachycardia
VTE	venous thromboembolism
VV	venovenous
WCC	white cell count
w/v	weight in volume
w/w	weight in weight
WHO	World Health Organization

Adherence

Introduction to adherence

What is adherence?

It is estimated that 30–50% of prescribed medicines for long-term conditions are not taken as recommended. This represents a cost both in physical (ill health) and economic terms.

'Compliance' is defined as the extent to which the patient's behaviour matches the prescriber's recommendations. It implies that the patient will simply follow the recommendations of the doctor (or other healthcare professional) with little, if any, discussion or negotiation.

'Concordance' is a two-way exchange between the healthcare professional and the patient whereby the prescriber and the patient agree therapeutic decisions that incorporate their respective views. The patient participates in both the consultation and the decision-making process, and the patient's preferences and beliefs are taken into account.

'Adherence' is somewhere between compliance and concordance. It is the extent to which the patient's actions meet the prescriber's recommendations or expectations. Ideally, the healthcare professional should accept that the patient's beliefs, preferences, and prior knowledge influence medicine-taking and should attempt to address this. However, adherence interventions are often made after the prescription is written and the patient might not have had much influence on the choice of drug. Consequently, pharmacists and other healthcare professionals may have a bigger role in facilitating adherence than doctors.

Adherence support is often a key activity for specialist pharmacists but it can (and should) be carried out to some extent by pharmacists in their everyday practice.

Why is adherence important?

Non-adherence usually limits the benefits of medicines, although occasionally it may be beneficial, e.g. if the patient is not taking the medicine because they have read the patient information leaflet and realized a caution or contraindication applies to them. The costs of this non-adherence are potentially significant on both personal and public levels. For the patient, non-adherence could lead to an ↑ in symptoms, a deterioration in health, or onset of disease that might otherwise be prevented. Public health may be affected, e.g. non-adherence to tuberculosis (TB) treatment could lead to the patient infecting others. Economic costs include the cost of wasted medicines and costs resulting from the patient needing ↑ healthcare input if their health deteriorates, possibly requiring alternative, more expensive treatment. It is estimated that up to 30% of drug-related hospital admissions result from non-adherence. In one study, 91% of non-adherent renal transplant patients experienced organ rejection or death compared with 18% of adherent patients.[1]

Why do patients not take their medicines?

Numerous studies have attempted to identify the causes of non-adherence and many factors have been identified (Box 1.1). Different factors are relevant to different diseases and settings; e.g. cost is an issue in the US

Box 1.1 Factors reported to affect adherence
- Ability to attend appointments
- Age
- Beliefs about medicines
- Chaotic lifestyle
- Complexity of regimen
- Concerns about confidentiality
- Cost
- Cultural practices or beliefs
- Depression
- Educational status
- Frequency of doses
- Gender
- Health beliefs and attitudes (towards self and others)
- Impact on daily life
- Language (if the patient's first language is different from that of the healthcare professional)
- Literacy
- Manual dexterity
- Past or current experience of side effects
- Satisfaction with healthcare
- Self-esteem
- Side effects
- Socioeconomic status.

(because patients have to pay for medicines/health insurance) but rarely in the UK. The reasons for non-adherence generally fall into two categories:
- Unintentional (involuntary) or behavioural (e.g. simply forgetting)
- Intentional (voluntary) or cognitive (e.g. concerns about side effects).

Pharmaceutical manufacturers tend to concentrate on behavioural factors, producing combination tablets or once-daily versions of their medicines, which are supposedly easier to take. There is evidence to suggest that adherence is reduced if the dose frequency is more than three times daily, but no data are available to support once-daily over twice-daily dosing. Patients might prefer combination products or once-daily dosing, but preference does not necessarily relate to adherence. Once-daily dosing could, in fact, lead to a worse therapeutic outcome because missing one dose means missing a whole day's therapy.

Many adherence strategies focus on cognitive issues. Intuitively it seems right that if patients do not adhere because of fears or misconceptions about their medicines, addressing these issues should improve adherence. However, it is not clear whether non-adherent patients lack knowledge and understanding or whether these are the patients who fail to seek advice. Ultimately, it is the patient's, not the healthcare professional's, agenda that influences whether or not they take their medicines.

In practice, multiple factors affect behaviour (and ultimately behaviour change). In this instance, the behaviour is whether or not a medicine is taken. These factors interact with each other and can be summed up in the COM-B model (Fig. 1.1).[2]

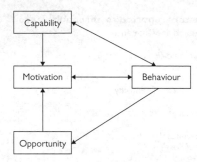

Fig. 1.1 COM-B—a model to understand behaviour.

In this model:
• Capability is the psychological or physical ability to actually perform the activity, e.g. the patient is able to remove the tablet from the container
• Opportunity is the factors that are not specific to the individual which make it possible or otherwise for the person to perform that activity, e.g. lack of transport may mean the patient cannot attend an appointment for monitoring and a new prescription
• Motivation is both the conscious and unconscious processes that direct behaviour, e.g. the patient knows a medicine is preventative rather than active treatment and so tends to forget to take it
• The single- and double-headed arrows in Fig. 1.1 indicate the interactions between these factors and how they might affect each other.

Adherence support strategies need to take these factors and their influence on each other into account. Addressing just one will not produce lasting or effective change.

References

1. De Geest S, Borgermans L, Gemoets H, *et al.* (1995). Incidence, determinants, and consequences of subclinical noncompliance with immunosuppressive therapy in renal transplant patients. *Transplantation* 59: 340–7.
2. Michie S, van Stralen M, West R (2011). The behaviour change wheel: a new method for characterising and designing behaviour. *Implement Sci* 6: 42.

Assessing adherence

In order to identify whether or not a patient is adherent to their treatment—and to assess progress in adherence support—it is important to have a means of assessing adherence. Various strategies have been used but none are entirely satisfactory:

- Treatment response—the most clinically relevant method of assessing adherence. A reasonably non-invasive and simple marker of treatment success is necessary (e.g. measuring blood pressure (BP) or cholesterol levels). However, some markers might only show recent adherence (e.g. blood glucose levels).
- Therapeutic drug monitoring (TDM)—this has limited use for assessing adherence. If serum levels are within the therapeutic range, recent, but not long-term, adherence can be assumed. Sub-therapeutic levels can be an indicator of erratic or recent non-adherence, but could also reflect malabsorption of the drug or a drug interaction.
- Medication event monitoring systems (MEMSs)—these are special bottle caps that record each time the bottle is opened. The information can be downloaded so that each time and date the bottle was opened can be read. However, MEMS caps can only record whether the bottle has been opened, not whether any drug (or how much) was taken out of the bottle. Ideally, they should be used in conjunction with some form of patient diary so that if the bottle is opened or not opened for some reason (e.g. taking out two doses at once), this can be recorded. MEMS caps are expensive and are usually only used in clinical trials.
- Pharmacy records (refills)—these can be used to check whether the patient collects the correct quantity of tablets each time, so that they do not run out if they have been taking their drugs correctly. However, this system cannot determine whether the patient actually takes the tablets.
- Patient self-report—ask the patient (in a non-judgemental way) whether they have missed or delayed any doses, and if so, how many. It is easier for the patient if a timescale is given, e.g. in the last month or since the last appointment. Patients tend to overestimate their level of adherence and could give the answer they feel the enquirer wants to hear rather than a true picture. However, patient self-report correlates well with other measures and is relatively cheap and easy to do.

Adherence support

Various practical strategies have been used in an attempt to improve adherence (Table 1.1).[3] These strategies predominantly address the capability and opportunity aspects of the COM-B model and may help to reduce unintentional non-adherence, but there is limited evidence that any of them will lead to long-term improvement in intentional non-adherence. It is all too easy to assume that if a patient has had their medicines provided in a monitored dosage system (MDS) they will then take their medicines, but this is not necessarily the case.

Comprehensive management

This involves a multidisciplinary approach, which encompasses all the strategies outlined in this section. It is potentially complex, labour-intensive (with associated costs), and not feasible or necessary in many situations. However, it is appropriate for some diseases and treatments (e.g. diabetes mellitus and antiretrovirals). Some schemes can be quite intensive and care must be taken that patients do not lose autonomy as a result of participating in the scheme. Expert patient schemes are a good example of comprehensive disease self-management (alongside conventional care), whereby patients are taught by their peers.[4] These schemes deal with complete management of the disease, not just drug therapy.

Table 1.1 Practical adherence support strategies

Strategy	Advantages	Disadvantages
Monitored dose systems (MDSs)[3]	Potentially useful for patients who: • cannot read or understand labels (e.g. because of language issues or learning difficulties) • are on complex regimens • are usually adherent but sometimes cannot remember whether or not they have taken a dose Provide a visible indication of doses not taken (note empty compartments may not mean dose has been taken)	Unsuitable for patients with limited dexterity Not suitable for PRN or variable-dose drugs Cannot be used for liquids, injections (e.g. insulin), refrigerated medicines Changes in medication regimen require a new MDS to be filled Takes control away from the patient (disempowering) Over-reliance on MDS may give a false impression of the degree of adherence Stability concerns Safety—easier for children to see and access the medicines than original packs Time-consuming to fill
Alarms/apps/text messages	Relatively easy to set up (by patient or healthcare professional) Useful prompt Apps may provide additional medicines information	Potentially intrusive May be ignored
Refills/follow-up reminders	Involves direct engagement with the patient Can be linked to appointments	Could lead to stockpiling
Regimen simplification	Patient preference	Not always feasible May require use of more expensive drugs (e.g. SR formulations)
Written and oral information	Educating and empowering the patient Enables patient to make their own decisions	Information overload Time-consuming Written information needs regular updating

References

3. Royal Pharmaceutical Society (2013). 'Improving patient outcomes: the better use of multi-compartment compliance aids', ℗ www.rpharms.com/support-pdfs/rps-mca-july-2013.pdf
4. NHS Choices (2016). 'NHS general practitioners (GPs) services', ℗ www.nhs.uk/conditions/Expert-patients-programme-/Pages/Introduction.aspx

Adherence consultations

Pharmacists involved in adherence counselling should ideally use the communication skills discussed in Chapter 4 (see ➲ 'Communication skills', pp. 86–9). It is important that the consultation is not just about imparting information to the patient but about empowering them to make their own decisions. The four E's system (Fig. 1.2) can be used to guide the consultation.

When discussing treatment with the patient for the first time, it is important to establish what they already know and any beliefs they hold. Possible questions to ask the patient include the following:
- Tell me anything you already know about the disease/treatment
- What have the doctors already told you?
- Have you read/found any information about the disease/treatment (e.g. on the Internet)?

Having established baseline knowledge, the pharmacist can then proceed to fill in gaps and attempt to correct any misconceptions. The latter must be done tactfully, in order not to undermine patient self-confidence and their confidence in others (bear in mind that the most cited sources of information about medicines are family and friends). A checklist of information that could be provided is shown in Box 1.2, but this should be tailored according to the setting and the patient's needs. It must be borne in mind that sometimes patients will not be ready to receive such information so the pharmacist should be sensitive to any indication of this and tailor the session accordingly.

Sometimes it is useful to provide written information (to complement verbal information) at the beginning of the session so that you can go through the information with the patient, but sometimes it is better to supply written information at the end so that the patient is not distracted by what they have in their hand. Suggest other sources of information, such as self-help organizations and suitable websites, and provide your contact details for further questions that may arise.

When questioning the patient about their level of adherence, it is important to do so in a non-judgemental way. A reasonably accurate picture of adherence, and whether the patient's lifestyle affects it, can be obtained if the patient is asked how many doses they have missed or delayed:
- in the past month
- in the past week
- over a weekend.

This method tends to give a more realistic idea of adherence, but patients tend to underestimate how many doses they have missed. It is also important to confirm that the correct dose (e.g. number of tablets) has been taken and that any food restrictions have also been adhered to.

If the patient has been non-adherent, ask them why they think they missed doses and if they can think of ways to overcome this. Work together with the patient to find strategies to overcome non-adherence. Ask the patient to tell you in their own words why adherence is important and reflect this

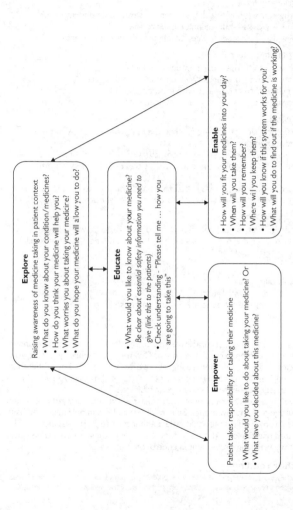

Explore

Raising awareness of medicine taking in patient context
- What do you know about your condition/medicines?
- How do you think your medicine will help you?
- What worries you about taking your medicine?
- What do you hope your medicine will allow you to do?

Educate
- What would you like to know about your medicine? *Be clear about essential safety information you need to give (link this to the patients)*
- Check understanding – "Please tell me … how you are going to take this"

Empower

Patient takes responsibility for taking their medicine
- What would you like to do about taking your medicine? Or
- What have you decided about this medicine?

Enable
- How will you fit your medicines into your day?
- When will you take them?
- How will you remember?
- Where will you keep them?
- How will you know if this system works for you?
- What will you do to find out if the medicine is working?

Fig. 1.2 The four E's triangle. Reproduced with permission from Barnett, N.L. & Sanghani, P. (2013). A coaching approach to improving concordance. *IJPP.* 21(4): 270–272, Wiley.

Box 1.2 Checklist of medication information for patients

Basic information
- Drug name (generic and trade name), strength, and formulation
- How it works—non-technical explanation
- Why it is important to keep taking the treatment correctly.

Using the treatment
- How much to use—e.g. number of tablets
- How often to use—e.g. twice daily, about 12h apart
- Special information—e.g. with food or drink plenty of water
- Storage—e.g. in the original container, in the fridge, or expiry date.

Side effects
- Common side effects—e.g. when they might occur and what to do about them
- Managing side effects—e.g. taking drugs with food might reduce nausea or using over-the-counter drug treatments for symptom control
- Serious side effects—e.g. what to do and whether to contact the clinic (provide a phone number, if appropriate), local doctor, or hospital.

Drug interactions
Any drugs that the patient should avoid/be cautious with—in particular, mention over-the-counter medicines, herbal and traditional medicines, and recreational drugs.

Other
- Availability
- Cost—per month/year
- Monitoring—e.g. frequency of tests and costs of tests.

back, correcting any inaccuracies as you do so. Verify that the patient understands the regimen, e.g. ask the patient 'Tell me exactly how you take your medicines'. Try to find something positive to say about their adherence, even if this is saying something along the lines of 'I'm glad you've told me about these problems with taking your tablets …'.

Give positive reinforcement to patients who are fully adherent and encourage any improvements. Be careful not to be patronizing! If you have access to any results that could reflect adherence (e.g. BP readings and glycosylated haemoglobin (HbA_{1c})), show the patient these results, and explain how they reflect improvement in control of the disease.

Further reading

National Institute for Health and Care Excellence (2009). 'Medicines adherence: involving patients in decisions about prescribed medicines and supporting adherence', ℘ www.nice.org.uk/guidance/cg76

Writing patient information leaflets

Written information is an important supplement to the verbal information on medicines and disease that pharmacists provide. Patient information leaflets help patients retain the information discussed and provide a source of information for future reference. In the European Union, pharmacists are required to distribute patient information leaflets supplied by the pharmaceutical industry with each drug when it is dispensed, but additional information might also be required.

Pharmacy-generated patient information leaflets can be used to describe the following:

- The disease and how it could affect the patient's daily life
- Disease prevention—e.g. stopping smoking
- Treatment or treatment options if there is more than one
- Details of drug therapy, including the following:
  - Dose and regimen
  - The importance of continuing chronic therapy even if the patient feels well
  - Side effects—e.g. risks and benefits, and what to do if they occur
  - Drug interactions—e.g. over-the-counter and herbal medicines, food, alcohol, and recreational drugs
  - Other special considerations—e.g. use in pregnancy and lactation
  - Further sources of information and support—e.g. pharmacy contact details, self-help organizations, and websites.

Before you start

- Discuss the following with patients:
  - Do they feel they need additional information? What information would they like?
  - What are they worried about?
  - What type of leaflet design do they prefer?
- Don't reinvent the wheel! Check whether a leaflet covering the topic you intend to write about is already available—useful sources are the pharmaceutical industry and patient organizations (although watch out for bias in industry-produced leaflets and some patient organizations have significant industry sponsorship).
- Look at other leaflets and see how they have been written:
  - Does the style and layout fit what you want to do?
  - Do you find them easy to read and understand?
  - What good/bad aspects of design and content can you learn from these?
- Check whether your hospital or Clinical Commissioning Group has guidelines on writing patient information leaflets. Some organizations require leaflets to be written in a standard format and the final version to be formally approved.
- Check what facilities there are for printing and distribution and what funding is available. There is no point spending hours producing a full-colour leaflet that requires professional printing if the funds will only stretch to a black and white photocopy.
- Talk to your organization's information technology adviser/medical illustration department—they might have access to computer programs that will make designing the leaflet much easier.

Content

- State the aim of the leaflet at the beginning—e.g. 'This leaflet is for people starting treatment for …'.
- Be relevant—decide on the scope of the information you are providing and stick to that. Don't get sidetracked into providing information that is not directly relevant to the aim. The leaflet should provide sufficient detail that the reader can understand the main points but not so much that it becomes confusing and the main points are lost.
- Be accurate—the leaflet must include the most up-to-date information available and should also address the following points:
  - Be consistent with current guidelines or best practice
  - Give an honest description of risks and benefits
  - Where there is a lack of clear evidence, explain that this is the case
  - Be updated as new information becomes available or guidelines are updated.
- Be understandable, acceptable, and accessible to the audience:
  - Apply the rules for clear writing discussed in Chapter 4 (see ➔ 'Writing reports', pp. 77–80).
  - Consider the target group—are there any religious or cultural issues that could influence the content? How can you make the leaflet accessible to patients with visual impairment or who do not speak English? Be careful about getting leaflets translated because sometimes the meaning can be inadvertently changed.
  - Get patients' opinions on the content—check that they understand/ interpret the information correctly, tone and style are acceptable (see Table 1.2), layout and presentation are easy to follow, and they think that it covers all the relevant issues.

Table 1.2 Patient preferences for tone and style of written information

Likes	Dislikes
• Positive tone	• Negative tone
• Friendly	• Stress on what could go wrong
• Encouraging	• Unrealistic
• Reassuring	• Over-optimistic
• Non-alarmist	• Misleading
• Honest	• Patronizing
• Practical	• Childish
• Understanding	• Cold
• Not condescending	
• Talking to you personally	
• Using 'you' a lot	
• Warm	

Design and layout

Once you have drafted the text, think about how best it can be presented (Fig. 1.3). Use the guidance in Chapter 4 (see ➜ 'Writing reports', pp. 77–80, on font type and basic layout).

A large amount of type on an A4-size sheet of paper is hard work for anyone to read. A5 size (ideally a single side) is the maximum size that should be used. If you have a lot of information to present, use an A5 or smaller booklet format or a three-fold A4 leaflet.

Graphics can be helpful to break up the text and 'signpost' new ideas, but be careful not to overdo it so that the graphics overwhelm the text. Graphics must be relevant to the text. Ensure that graphics are culturally acceptable and bear in mind that some stylized pictures or icons could be interpreted differently by people of different cultures (e.g. a crescent moon to indicate night time might be interpreted as a religious symbol).

Review and update regularly

The leaflet should state the author's name and job title, the date of production, and a future review date. Depending on what new information becomes available, it might be necessary to update the leaflet sooner than the planned review date. If the information is significantly out of date, the leaflet should be withdrawn from use until an updated version is available.

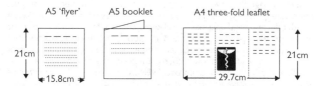

Fig. 1.3 Patient information leaflets: design and layout.

Health coaching to support adherence

What is health coaching?

Health coaching is a patient-centred consultation method which supports shared decision-making, self-care, and self-management through raising patients' awareness of their health issue and increasing their responsibility for managing it. Traditionally, pharmacists' consultations with patients are mostly about giving advice and educating patients about their medicines. While this is a key aspect of safe medicines use, it assumes that the patient will take the advice given. However, evidence suggests that up to 50% of patients don't take their medicines as intended. Both practical and perceptual issues affect adherence and many practical issues have perceptual basis. Therefore, pharmacists can better support patients by using behavioural techniques, together with patient education, to optimize adherence.

Health coaching acknowledges that it is the patient who has to live with their condition and the consequences of the health-related outcomes, and uses behavioural techniques to give patients a choice about how to manage optimizing health outcomes that are within their control.

How does it work?

Health coaching requires the development of new ways of thinking for patients and clinicians—an attitude that sees the patient as resourceful and able to manage their own health and solve their own problems. It sees the healthcare professional's (HCP's) role as supportive through provision of health education and pharmaceutical knowledge together, while helping the patient to think positively and creatively about their medicines adherence issues. For example, when patients bring information about medicines or therapies into a consultation, rather than seeing this as a challenge to the HCP's authority, a coaching approach welcomes it, recognizing it for what it is: a desire to engage and improve their own health. In order to use health coaching, HCPs need to develop their skills around active listening, creating rapport and trust as well as challenging limiting beliefs to help patients find solutions. For example, patients may say that remembering to take a medicine regularly is impossible for them. Health coaching uses specific behavioural techniques to work with limiting beliefs, resistance to change, and ambivalence and includes aspects of motivational interviewing, cognitive behavioural therapy, and other techniques developed from psychology.

The application of health coaching in a pharmacy consultation was developed from the GROW coaching model[1] (Fig. 1.4) and adapted for pharmacy. Pharmacists can successfully use the GROW model in short (10min) consultations to work with patients:

- *Goal*: agreeing an agenda for the consultation (rather than having the agenda led by the clinician)
- *Reality*: working through the current situation around the patient's issues or concerns
- *Options*: generating solutions or a strategy
- *Will*: working towards a plan for implementation of the patient's preferred solution.

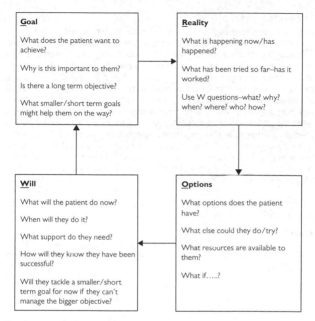

Goal

What does the patient want to achieve?

Why is this important to them?

Is there a long term objective?

What smaller/short term goals might help them on the way?

Reality

What is happening now/has happened?

What has been tried so far–has it worked?

Use W questions–what? why? when? where? who? how?

Will

What will the patient do now?

When will they do it?

What support do they need?

How will they know they have been successful?

Will they tackle a smaller/short term goal for now if they can't manage the bigger objective?

Options

What options does the patient have?

What else could they do/try?

What resources are available to them?

What if.....?

Fig. 1.4 The GROW model. Reproduced from Whitmore, Sir John (2009). *Coaching for performance: GROWing human potential and purpose: the principles and practice of coaching and leadership*. People skills for professionals (4th ed.). Boston, with permission from Nicholas Brealey Publishing.

While learning health coaching techniques requires formal skill development, practice, and support, the four E's triangle (see ➲ Fig. 1.2, p. 9) gives an outline structure to a consultation, based on GROW. To be effective, it requires the HCP to actively engage with patients in an empathic way.

Why is it useful?

The health coaching approach centres around the concept that people are more likely to implement ideas if they have come up with the ideas themselves and this is inherent in all health coaching conversations. Patients should have a choice about what aspect of their health they want to manage, and in their own way. It relies on the HCP giving the patient the space to find their own solution rather than taking the traditional route of providing solutions to the patient. As a wider public health issue, the health economy benefits from motivated patients who manage their own care, reducing utilization of scarce health resources.

When to do it?

It is important to recognize that not all patients require health coaching—remember that at least 50% of patients do take their medicines as intended. The four E's structure can be used when consulting with a patient as part of medicines reconciliation, medication review and discharge consultations in a hospital setting, in any clinic setting, and as a Medicines Use Review or New Medicines Service consultation in community settings. If the HCP becomes aware of an adherence issue as part of a consultation, a health coaching approach will help to open a non-judgemental discussion about what the patient wants to do about managing their health and how they see medicines fitting in to their health management and their lives. It may transpire that a patient wishes to manage their health without taking medicines and a health coaching approach encourages engagement with the patient in working on their own solutions (even if the HCP doesn't agree with them). The relationship with the patient is maintained and the 'door left open', recognizing that patients have choice and exercise this choice anyway. The HCP's role is to stay engaged with the patient and be available to offer support according to the patient's agenda.

Reference

5. Whitmore J (2009). *Coaching For Performance: GROWing Human Potential and Purpose—The Principles and Practice of Coaching and Leadership* (4th ed). Boston, MA: Nicholas Brealey Publishing.

Adverse drug reactions and drug interactions

Introduction to adverse drug reactions (ADRs)

ADRs, also known as 'side effects', 'adverse drug events', or 'drug misadventures', are a frequent cause of morbidity in hospital and the community. They have a significant cost both financially and in terms of quality of life. Few studies of ADRs have been carried out in the community so the effect on primary care is harder to assess, but studies in the hospital environment have shown the following:

- ADRs occur in 10–20% of patients in hospital.
- ADRs are responsible for 5% of admissions to hospital.
- ADRs might be responsible for 1 in 1000 deaths in medical wards.
- ADRs are the most common cause of iatrogenic injury in hospital patients.

The World Health Organization (WHO) defines an ADR as follows:
'a drug-related event that is noxious and unintended and occurs at doses used in humans for prophylaxis, diagnosis or therapy of disease or for the modification of physiological function.'

However, this definition does not take into account the following scenarios, all of which can also cause ADRs:

- Overdose (including prescribing or administration errors)
- Therapeutic failure
- Drug interactions
- Drug withdrawal.

Pharmacists have an important role in identifying, reporting, and preventing ADRs.

Classification of ADRs

A number of classification systems exist, but the most widely accepted is to group ADRs as either type A (augmented or predictable) or type B (bizarre or unpredictable) reactions. This system is not ideal because some types of reaction (e.g. teratogenic effects) do not fit easily into either category. However, it is a useful system in most cases because immediate management of the ADR and future drug choices can usually be guided by the ADR type.

Type A reactions

An exaggerated, but otherwise normal, pharmacological action. Type A reactions have the following characteristics:
• Largely predictable
• Usually dose dependent
• Incidence and morbidity high
• Mortality low.

Examples of type A reactions include respiratory depression with opioid analgesia, cough with angiotensin-converting enzyme (ACE) inhibitors, and withdrawal effects with benzodiazepines or alcohol.

Type B reactions

Idiosyncratic, aberrant, or bizarre drug effects that are unrelated to the pharmacology of the drug. Type B reactions have the following characteristics:
• Usually unpredictable
• Might not be picked up by toxicological screening
• Not necessarily dose related
• Incidence and morbidity low
• Mortality high.

Type B reactions are most commonly immunological (e.g. penicillin allergy).
   Some sources add three further classifications. These are not related to the mechanism of the ADR but to characteristics of its manifestation.

Type C (chronic or continuing) reactions

These ADRs persist for a relatively long time after the drug has been stopped, e.g. bisphosphonate-induced osteonecrosis of the jaw.

Type D (delayed) reactions

ADRs that can become apparent some time after the drug has been used. This can make it difficult to determine whether or not the drug caused the reaction.

Type E (end-of-use) reactions

These are ADRs which occur as a result of the drug being stopped. This might include withdrawal effects on stopping benzodiazepines or reflex hyperacidity after stopping proton pump inhibitors.

Adverse reactions: drug or disease?

Determining whether or not a symptom is an ADR can be difficult, especially if the patient has multiple pathologies. Experience has shown that pharmacists tend to blame the drug and doctors tend to blame the disease. Questions to ask are as follows:

- Is there another explanation for the symptom (e.g. disease related)?
- Is this a previously reported side effect of this drug? How common is it? This is harder to assess for new drugs because there is less information available.
- Is the timing right? Most ADRs occur soon after starting a drug, although some ADRs (e.g. hepatotoxicity) might be delayed. The onset of some hypersensitivity reactions (e.g. penicillin rash) can be delayed for up to 10 days after starting the drug. This can cause confusion, especially if the antibiotic course has been completed before the rash appears.
- Is the dose excessive? Check serum levels if available. Check renal function—was the dose too high if renal function is impaired? If the symptom can be explained as a type A reaction and the dose is high for whatever reason, it is more probable that the reaction is drug induced.
- Does the symptom resolve on stopping the drug or reducing the dose (de-challenge)? Type A reactions are usually dose dependent and so will worsen on dose increase, but rapidly resolve or improve on dose reduction or drug withdrawal. Type B reactions are dose independent and will rarely resolve with dose reduction. Drug withdrawal is necessary, but if symptoms are caused by immunological effects (rather than direct drug action) it could take some days or weeks for symptoms to resolve. Note some drugs may cause the same ADR by both type A and B mechanisms, e.g. bone marrow suppression due to carbimazole may be direct toxicity or immunologically mediated.
- Does the symptom recur on restarting the drug (re-challenge)? Remember that re-challenge can be especially hazardous for type B reactions and is usually not advised.

If the answer to the first question is 'no' and the answer to (most of) the other questions is 'yes', it is highly probable that the event is an ADR.

Factors predisposing to ADRs

Factors that predispose to ADRs are many and varied, and some are related only to specific disease–drug interactions, such as rash with amoxicillin in patients with glandular fever. However, the following factors are generally considered to ↑ patient risk:

- Age
- Renal impairment
- Hepatic impairment
- 'Frailty'
- Polypharmacy
- ♀
- Previous history of ADRs
- Genetics.

The first four factors predispose to type A reactions because they are determinants of drug toxicity, but the remaining factors predispose to type A or type B reactions.

Helping patients understand the risk of ADRs

Terms such as 'common' and 'uncommon' are used to describe levels of risk of ADRs in patient information leaflets and summaries of product characteristics (SPCs). The terms are standardized by the European Union (EU) according to the reported frequency found in clinical trials for example (Table 2.1), but patients routinely overestimate the level of risk that these terms are intended to imply.

The following strategies should help in communicating levels of risk to patients:
- Avoid using verbal descriptors such as 'common'.
- Use frequencies rather than percentages—e.g. 1 person in every 1000 rather than 0.1%.
- Use the same denominator throughout—i.e. 1 in 1000 and 10 in 1000 rather than 1 in 1000 and 1 in 100.
- Give both positive and negative information—e.g. 95 out of 100 patients did not get the side effect and 5 patients did.
- Give information about baseline risk—e.g.:
  - The risk of deep vein thrombosis (DVT) in non-pregnant women who are not taking the combined oral contraceptive (COC) is 5 cases per 100 000 women per year.
  - The risk of DVT in pregnancy is 60 cases per 100 000 pregnancies.
  - The risk of DVT in women taking the COC is 15–25 cases per 100 000 per year.

Table 2.1 Terminology as standardized by the European Union according to reported frequency in clinical trials

EU terminology	Level of risk
Very common	>10% (≥1/10)
Common	1–10% (≥1/100 to <1/10)
Uncommon	0.1–1% (≥1/1000 to <1/100)
Rare	0.01–0.1% (≥1/10 000 to <1/1000)
Very rare	<0.01% (≥1/100 000 to <1/10 000)

Reporting ADRs

Most ADRs are not reported and this can lead to delays in identifying important reactions. The reasons for failure to report ADRs have been called the 'seven deadly sins' (Box 2.1). Pharmacists should attempt to address these and encourage their medical and nursing colleagues to report ADRs, in addition to sending in their own reports.

The regulatory authorities in many countries have systems for reporting ADRs, and it is important to find out how ADRs are reported and whether pharmacists can submit reports. In the UK, doctors, dentists, pharmacists, nurses, and patients can report ADRs to the Medicines and Healthcare products Regulatory Agency (MHRA) through the Yellow Card Scheme. New drugs are labelled with a black inverted triangle in the *British National Formulary* (*BNF*), and the MHRA requests that all ADRs to these drugs are reported. For established drugs, unusual or significant reactions should be reported. Yellow Card data can be accessed online.[1]

Box 2.1 Failure to report ADRs: the 'seven deadly sins'

1. *Complacency*—a mistaken belief that only safe drugs are allowed onto the market and that these will not cause serious ADRs
2. *Fear* of involvement in litigation, or of a loss of patient confidence
3. *Guilt* that a patient has been harmed by a prescribed treatment
4. *Ambition*—to collect and publish a personal series of cases
5. *Ignorance* of what should be reported or how to make a report
6. *Diffidence*—a reluctance to report an effect for which there is only a suspicion that it is drug related
7. *Lethargy*—this may include a lack of time or interest, inability to find a report card, etc.

Reference

1. 'Yellow Card' website: ⅌ https://yellowcard.mhra.gov.uk

Drug interactions

Drug interactions occur when the effect of a drug is altered by the co-administration of any of the following:
- Another drug
- Food
- Drink.

The outcome of this is as follows:
- Frequently clinically insignificant
- Sometimes beneficial
- Occasionally potentially harmful.

Mechanisms of drug interactions

Interactions can be caused by pharmacokinetic mechanisms (i.e. the handling of the drug in the body is affected) or pharmacodynamic mechanisms (i.e. related to the pharmacology of the drug). Sometimes the interaction can be caused by more than one mechanism, although usually one mechanism is more significant. The majority of interactions are caused by the following mechanisms.

Pharmacokinetic mechanisms

Absorption

One drug will ↑ or ↓ the absorption of another. This is most frequently due to one drug or compound interacting with another—by adsorption, chelation, or complexing—to form a product that is poorly absorbed. This can be beneficial (e.g. activated charcoal adsorbs certain poisons) or problematic (e.g. antacids and tetracyclines).

Changes in gastric pH affect the absorption of certain drugs, e.g. itraconazole requires an acidic environment to be absorbed; thus proton pump inhibitors can ↓ absorption and an acidic drink such as fruit juice or soft drinks (especially Coca Cola®) will ↑ absorption.

Most drugs are absorbed from the upper part of the small intestine. Thus changes in gut motility potentially affect absorption. Usually the total amount absorbed is unaffected, but the rate of absorption might be altered. This effect is used in some combination migraine products, e.g. including metoclopramide as the antiemetic also speeds up the rate of absorption of the analgesic.

Distribution

Some drugs are bound to proteins in the serum. Only free (unbound) drug is active. Protein binding is a competitive effect, so one drug can displace the other from protein binding sites. This interaction is only an issue with highly protein-bound drugs and is only significant if most of the drug remains in the plasma rather than being distributed into tissues (i.e. a low volume of distribution). Displacement of drug from protein binding sites often only causes a small 'blip' in drug levels before equilibrium is restored (because the free drug is also now available for metabolism and excretion), but it could be significant for drugs with a narrow therapeutic index (e.g. warfarin).

Metabolism

Accounts for the majority of clinically significant pharmacokinetic interactions. Induction or inhibition of the cytochrome P450 (CYP450) system leads to changes in drug levels. CYP450 represents a large group of iso-enzymes; drugs are rarely metabolized by a single enzyme, although one usually predominates. Equally, drugs can induce or inhibit several enzymes and some drugs (e.g. efavirenz) can induce some enzymes and inhibit others. In addition, some (but not all) enzyme inhibitors or inducers can induce or inhibit their own metabolism.

When only two drugs are involved, the effect is fairly easy to predict, even if each drug is likely to affect the metabolism of the other. However, if three or more drugs, all of which are inducers or inhibitors, are involved, the effect is almost impossible to predict, and this type of combination should be avoided if possible.

The full effects of enzyme induction and inhibition do not occur immediately:

• Enzyme induction takes about 2–3wks to develop and wear off
• Enzyme inhibition takes only a few days.

Thus, it might be necessary to delay dose adjustment or TDM until a few days (inhibition) or at least a week (induction) after starting or stopping the offending drug(s).

Drug interactions involving induction or inhibition of P-glycoprotein are also potentially significant. This can be protective, e.g. loperamide has negligible CNS effects despite being opioid related as P-glycoprotein prevents its transport across the blood–brain barrier. However, it can also be problematic such as rapid metabolism in the gut wall of certain drugs, e.g. protease inhibitors. Frequently (but not always) a drug will be a substrate of or affect P-glycoprotein and CYP450 and it is important to check for both. However, P-glycoprotein metabolism is less well elucidated so it cannot be ruled out even if it is not listed in sources such as the SPC.

Uridine 5'-diphospho-glucuronosyltransferase (UGT) catalyses the glucuronidation of some drugs. Few clinically significant interactions have been documented. However, it does account for the interaction of rifampicin with some drugs which are not CYP450 metabolized. Variability in the production of UGT enzymes accounts for interindividual susceptibility to paracetamol overdose.

Excretion

Some drugs interfere with excretion (usually renal) of other drugs. If both drugs are excreted by the same active transport system in the kidney tubule, the excretion of each drug is ↓ by the other. This might be used as a beneficial effect—e.g. probenecid has been used to prolong the half-life of penicillin—or be problematic—e.g. methotrexate and non-steroidal anti-inflammatory drugs (NSAIDs).

Pharmacodynamic interactions

These occur if the pharmacological effects of two drugs are additive or opposing.

- Additive—the desired or adverse effects of the two drugs are the same. This can be beneficial or potentially harmful (e.g. ↑ sedation with alcohol plus hypnotics).
- Synergism—which is a form of additive effect. In this instance, the combination of the two drugs has a greater effect than just an additive effect (e.g. ethambutol ↑ the effectiveness of other anti-tubercular drugs).
- Antagonism—at receptor level (e.g. a β-blocker should be prescribed with caution to an asthmatic patient who uses a β-agonist inhaler) or because of opposing effects (e.g. the desired effects of diuretics could be, at least partly, opposed by fluid retention caused by NSAIDs).

Predicting drug interactions

- Are the desired or adverse effects of the two drugs similar or opposing?
- If there is no information available for the drugs in question, are there reports of drug interactions for other drugs in the same class?
- Are both drugs metabolized by the liver and, if so, by which enzymes? Information on which drugs are metabolized by which CYP450 enzymes or P-glycoprotein might be listed in the SPC and can also be found on the following websites:
  - ℘ www.hiv-druginteractions.org
  - ℘ www.medicine.iupui.edu/clinpharm/ddis/clinical-table/
  - ℘ www.pharmacytimes.com/publications/issue/2008/2008-12/2008-12-8474
- Drugs that are predominantly renally cleared are unlikely to interact with CYP450 enzyme inducers and inhibitors but may still have P-glycoprotein-mediated interactions.

Managing drug interactions

- Check whether or not the drug combination is new.
- If the patient has already been taking the drug combination, have they tolerated it? If yes, there is probably no need to change therapy, although monitoring might be required.
- Is the interaction potentially serious (e.g. significant risk of toxicity or ↓ drug effect)? If so, seek alternatives.
- Is the interaction potentially of low to moderate significance? If so, it might only be necessary to monitor side effects and therapeutic effect, or arrange TDM.
- Remember that some drugs in the same class can have different potentials to cause interactions (e.g. ranitidine versus cimetidine).
- Remember that not only do interactions occur when a drug is started, but unwanted effects can also occur when a drug is stopped.
- The elderly are at greater risk of drug interactions, because of polypharmacy and impaired metabolism and excretion. Additive side effects can be a particular problem.
- Be aware of high-risk drugs and always check for potential interactions with these drugs:
  - Enzyme inhibitors and inducers (e.g. erythromycin, rifampicin, pheny-toin, and protease inhibitors)
  - Drugs with a narrow therapeutic index (e.g. warfarin, digoxin, lithium, phenytoin, theophylline, and gentamicin).
- Remember that interactions can occur with non-prescription drugs, which the patient might not tell you about:
  - Herbal or traditional medicines
  - Over-the-counter medicines
  - Recreational or party drugs, including alcohol, tobacco, and drugs obtained by other means, such as sildenafil purchased on the Internet.

Anaphylaxis

Symptoms and signs of anaphylaxis

Anaphylaxis is a severe, life-threatening, generalized or systemic hypersensitivity reaction. Rapidly developing airways oedema, bronchospasm, and shock are life-threatening and immediate emergency treatment is usually required.

Theoretically, prior exposure to the agent is required and the reaction is not dose or route related, but in practice, anaphylaxis to injected antigen is more frequent, severe, and rapid in onset than following exposure to oral or topical antigen.

Agents which commonly cause anaphylaxis include:
• drugs—e.g. penicillins, aspirin
• insect stings—e.g. wasp and bee venoms
• food—e.g. nuts.

The onset of symptoms following parenteral antigen (including stings) is usually within 5–30min. With oral antigen, there is often a delay. Symptoms usually occur within 2h, but may be immediate and life-threatening. A late-phase reaction may also occur with recrudescence of symptoms after apparent resolution. Recurrence is a fairly frequent phenomenon and healthcare workers should be aware of this. Anyone who has experienced anaphylaxis symptoms should attend an emergency department even if their symptoms appear to have fully resolved.

End-of-needle reactions

Some patients may experience an anaphylactic-like reaction during rapid intravenous (IV) drug administration. This is known as an end-of-needle reaction. Initial symptoms may suggest anaphylaxis, but in fact this is a vasopressor effect and can be distinguished from anaphylaxis as bradycardia occurs which is rare in anaphylaxis. Skin symptoms are also rare in end-of-needle reactions. Stopping or slowing down the infusion or injection usually leads to resolution of symptoms, and administration at a slower rate usually avoids a repeat event.

Recognition of an anaphylactic reaction

An anaphylactic reaction is likely if the patient develops sudden symptoms of airway and/or breathing difficulty with or without circulatory problems rapidly following exposure to an allergen. Skin changes (e.g. flushing, angio-oedema, urticaria) are usually also present but the absence of skin changes does not rule out anaphylaxis. Gastrointestinal symptoms such as vomiting and abdominal pain may also be present.

Treatment of anaphylaxis

Anaphylaxis is a life-threatening condition, therefore rapid recognition and treatment is essential. The first response is to secure the airway and lay the patient flat to reduce hypotension. If the patient cannot tolerate a supine position (because this can worsen breathing difficulties), a semi-recumbent position is preferable. Basic life support should be started if necessary. Wherever possible, the allergen should be removed or minimized (e.g. stop antibiotic infusion, remove stinger for bee stings).

In hospital and some community settings (e.g. home IV antibacterial therapy), it might be appropriate to keep an 'anaphylaxis box' for emergency use, which contains the following essential drugs:

• Adrenaline (epinephrine)
• An antihistamine (usually chlorphenamine injection)
• A steroid (usually hydrocortisone injection).

Adrenaline

In adults and children >12 years, 500 micrograms of adrenaline (1:1000 solution) should be administered intramuscularly (IM) if the patient is showing clinical signs of shock, airway swelling, or breathing difficulty (stridor, wheezing, and cyanosis). The subcutaneous (SC) route is not used because absorption is too slow. IV adrenaline is hazardous and should only be administered by an appropriately qualified specialist in the hospital setting. The IV route is preferred if there are concerns about IM absorption; however, time should not be wasted looking for IV access in the event of vascular compromise. For IV administration, use a dilution of at least 1:10 000 and administer the injection over several minutes, titrating with 50-microgram boluses according to response. Continuous electrocardiography (ECG), pulse oximetry, and non-invasive BP monitoring should be carried out. The 1:1000 solution is never used IV. See Table 3.1 for doses of adrenaline IM for adults and children.

Adrenaline auto-injectors

Patients at risk of re-exposure to the allergen should be supplied with an adrenaline auto-injector (pen) device, such as an EpiPen® (Meda Pharmaceuticals), Jext® (ALK-Abello), Emerade® (iMed Systems), or AnaPen® (Lincoln Medical[1]). Some of the adult auto-injectors only deliver 300 micrograms of adrenaline, which is less than the recommended adult dose. Ideally, patients (adults and children) should carry two auto-injectors and the second one administered if symptoms persist or recur. Patients should always attend hospital for medical review even if the symptoms have resolved.

Note that the auto-injectors all contain a residual volume after use and patients should be warned about this. Information for patients and HCPs on the different types of auto-injectors can be found on the Anaphylaxis Campaign website (http://www.anaphylaxis.org.uk/hcp/medication/). Trainer auto-injectors can be purchased from the manufacturers and it is recommended that the patient, carer, and others such as teachers, friends, etc. are taught how and when to use the device. The manufacturers of each

---

[1] Anapen® is no longer available in the UK but is available in other countries.

Table 3.1 Dose of IM adrenaline for anaphylaxis (dose can be repeated at 5min intervals, as needed)

Age	Dose	Volume of adrenaline in 1:1000 solution (1mg/mL)
<6yrs	150 micrograms	0.15mL
6–12yrs	300 micrograms	0.3mL
>12yrs*/adult	500 micrograms	0.5mL
* If child is small or prepubertal	300 micrograms	0.3mL

auto-injector have websites providing advice, training videos, and the facility to register for text alerts when the pen is due to go out of date.

Adrenaline Minijets® are no longer recommended for self-administration.

Emergency administration of adrenaline without a prescription

Adrenaline 1:1000 solution for IM use is exempt from prescription-only control if it is used for the purpose of saving a life in an emergency. The Royal Pharmaceutical Society considers that a pharmacist is justified in supplying and administering adrenaline without a prescription in a life-threatening situation.

Chlorphenamine

Chlorphenamine should be given after adrenaline and continued as needed for 24–48h to prevent relapse. It should be administered IM or by slow IV injection to ↓ the risk of exacerbating hypotension.

Hydrocortisone sodium succinate

Hydrocortisone is administered by IM or slow IV injection after severe attacks to help prevent or shorten protracted reactions. The onset of action is delayed for several hours. Asthmatics may especially benefit from treatment with steroids and may benefit from higher doses.[1]

Additional treatment

Symptomatic and supportive care as needed include:
- bronchodilators
- oxygen (O_2) or other respiratory support
- crystalloid infusion (e.g. sodium chloride 0.9%).

Patients already on β-blockers may be refractory to adrenaline and glucagon has been used in this setting.

All patients treated initially in the community should be transferred to hospital for further treatment and observation.

Algorithms for the treatment of anaphylaxis in adults and children in hospital and community settings are available from the Resuscitation Council (UK) website.[2]

Late sequelae

Patients should be warned of the possibility of symptom recurrence, and if necessary kept under observation for up to 24h. This is especially applicable in the following circumstances:

- Past history of a recurrence (biphasic reaction)
- Severe reaction, with slow onset
- Possibility that allergen could still be absorbed (e.g. oral administration)
- Past history of asthma or a severe asthmatic component to the reaction
- Patient unable to recognize or respond to deterioration
- Difficulty accessing emergency care (e.g. patient resides in rural area).

All patients should be assessed by a senior clinician before discharge and as appropriate be:

- given education and advice on managing late sequelae and repeat incidents
- provided with an adrenaline auto-injector
- supplied chlorphenamine tablets and a 3-day course of oral steroids
- have a plan for follow-up including contact with the general practitioner (GP) and potential referral to an allergy clinic.

References

1. The Resuscitation Council (UK). 'Anaphylaxis', ℘ www.resus.org.uk/anaphylaxis/emergency-treatment-of-anaphylactic-reactions/
2. Manser R, Reid D, Abramson M (2001). Corticosteroids for acute severe asthma in hospitalised patients. *Cochrane Database Syst Rev* 1: CD001740.

Prevention of anaphylaxis

The risk of an anaphylactic reaction can be reduced by good history-taking and antigen avoidance:

- Check the patient's drug history for reports of allergy. If necessary, clarify the details of the reaction with the patient, relative, or healthcare provider. A previous history of a mild penicillin-associated rash in infancy might not be a contraindication to future use, but bronchospasm, angio-oedema, or anaphylaxis would be.
- Be aware of cross-sensitivity between drug classes:
  - Up to 7% of people allergic to penicillin are also allergic to cephalosporins
  - Patients allergic to aspirin are frequently also allergic to other prostaglandin inhibitors.
- Advise patients with severe allergies to carry some form of warning information (e.g. MedicAlert® bracelet).
- Some drugs (e.g. NSAIDs and ACE inhibitors) can exacerbate or ↑ the risk of a reaction. Avoid concomitant use of these drugs in situations where the patient could be exposed to the allergen (e.g. desensitization programmes).
- Remember that patients with peanut allergies should avoid pharmaceutical products containing arachis oil (groundnut oil).

Clinical pharmacy skills

Concept and core elements of pharmaceutical care

Pharmaceutical care was probably first defined by Mikeal et al. in 1975 as 'the care that a given patient requires and receives, which assures safe and rational drug use'.[1] Hepler, in 1988, described pharmaceutical care as 'a covenantal relationship between a patient and a practitioner in which the pharmacist performs drug use control functions governed by the awareness of and commitment to the patients' interest'.[2] The widely accepted definition by Hepler and Strand states 'Pharmaceutical care is the responsible provision of drug therapy for the purpose of achieving definite outcomes that improve a patient's quality of life'.[3] This definition built on an earlier one describing pharmaceutical care as 'a practice in which the practitioner takes responsibility for a patients drug-related needs and is held accountable for this commitment'.[4] The term 'patient-centred care' and 'medicines optimization' is gaining wider acceptance and is similar in principle.

Pharmaceutical care differs from traditional drug treatment because it is an explicitly outcome-orientated cooperative systematic approach to providing drug therapy directed not only at clinical outcomes, but also at activities of daily life and other dimensions of health-related quality of life. Historically, pharmacists have used a variety of methods to improve drug therapy, including formularies, drug-use reviews, prescriber education, and clinical pharmacy, but these have all been drug or prescription focused.

Pharmaceutical care involves the process through which a pharmacist cooperates with a patient and other professionals in designing, implementing, and maintaining a therapeutic plan that will produce specific outcomes for the patient. This, in turn, involves three major functions:

- Identifying potential and actual drug-related problems
- Resolving actual drug-related problems
- Preventing drug-related problems.

Core elements of pharmaceutical care

The pharmacist

- Collects and documents relevant information in a systematic, structured manner for the purpose of determining whether the patient is experiencing potential or actual drug-related problems.
- Identifies and lists the drug-related problems the patient is experiencing or is at risk of experiencing.
- Establishes and lists the desired therapeutic outcomes for each drug-related problem identified.
- Considers and ranks all the therapeutic interventions that might be expected to produce the desired therapeutic outcomes for each problem.
- Decides which therapeutic alternative to select and records the dosage regimen for each medication for each patient.
- Formulates and documents a pharmaco-therapeutic monitoring plan to verify that the drug-related decisions implemented have resulted in the outcomes desired and not in undesirable ADRs or toxicities.[5]

All must be in place for a comprehensive pharmaceutical care service. The only variable that affects the level of service is the patient's needs. This is assessed by determining the patient's risk factors. Patients who are considered at low risk might only require minimal intervention, whereas high-risk patients, by definition, require a higher level of pharmaceutical care.

Identifying risk in clinical practice

Risk factors fall into three distinct areas:

- Patients' clinical characteristics—these include physical and readily determined characteristics, such as age, gender, ethnicity, pregnancy status, immune status, kidney, liver, and cardiac functions, nutritional status, and patient expectations.
- The patient's disease—some assessment of the rate and extent of harm caused by the disease and the patient's perception of these factors.
- The patient's pharmacotherapy—the risk is determined by an assessment of the toxicity of the drug therapy, the ADR profile, the route and techniques of administration, and the patient's perception of these three elements.

Medication problem checklist

The following list covers the range of potential medication problems that could be encountered by pharmacists seeking to deliver pharmaceutical care:

- Medications without medical indications.
- Medical conditions for which no medications are prescribed.
- Medications prescribed inappropriately for a particular medical condition.
- Inappropriate medication dose, dosage form, schedule, route of administration, or method of administration.
- Therapeutic duplication.
- Prescribing of medications to which the patient is allergic.
- Actual and potential ADRs.
- Actual and potential adverse clinically significant drug–drug, drug–disease, drug–nutrient, and drug–laboratory test interactions.
- Interference with medical therapy by social or recreational drug use.
- Failure to receive the full benefit of prescribed medication therapy.
- Problems arising from the financial impact of medication therapy on the patient.
- Lack of understanding of the medication therapy by the patient.
- Failure of the patient to adhere to the medication regimen.
- There have been a number of attempts to formulate these problems into an easily remembered checklist. One of these is called PRIME, which is an acronym for Pharmaceutical Risks to patients, Interventions Mismatch between medications and indications, and Efficiency issues (Box 4.1). The key message behind these detailed checklists is that pharmacists must move from a prescription focus to a patient focus.

Box 4.1 PRIME pharmacotherapy problem types

Pharmaceutical

Assess for incorrect factors, as follows:
- Dosage
- Timing
- Form
- Duration
- Route
- Frequency.

Risks to patients

Assess for risks, as follows:
- Known contraindication
- Improper use (i.e. risk if misused)
- Medication allergy
- Common/serious ADRs
- Drug-induced problem
- Medication error considerations.

Interactions

Assess for the following:
- Drug–drug
- Drug–food
- Drug–disease/condition
- Drug–laboratory test

Mismatch between medications and indications/conditions

Assess for the following:
- Medication used without indication
- Indications/condition untreated.

Efficacy issues

Assess for the following:
- Suboptimal selection of pharmacotherapy for indications
- Minimal or no evidence of therapeutic effectiveness
- Suboptimal pharmacotherapy (taking/receiving medications incorrectly)— e.g. patient preference considerations (undesirable prior experiences with medications or does not believe it works)
- Medications availability considerations (e.g. no access to medications)
- Compliance/administration considerations (e.g. inability to pay or unable to administer correctly or at all).

References
1. Mikeal RL, Brown TR, Lazarus HL, *et al*. (1975). Quality of pharmaceutical care in hospitals. *Am J Hosp Pharm* 32: 567–74.
2. Hepler CD (1988). Unresolved issues in the future of pharmacy. *Am J Hosp Pharm* 45: 1071–81.
3. Hepler CD, Strand LM (1990). Opportunities and responsibilities in pharmaceutical care. *Am J Hosp Pharm* A47: 533–43.
4. Strand LM (1984). Re-visioning the professions. *J Am Pharm Assoc* 100–258.
5. Strand LM (1991). Pharmaceutical care: challenge of implementation. *ASHP Annual Meeting* 48: PI–28.

Working in a clinical area

Starting work on a new ward

- If possible, speak to the pharmacist who previously covered that ward. Take a handover of patients and find out anything unusual about how the ward works.
- Introduce yourself to the ward manager, key medical staff, nursing staff, and other relevant staff (e.g. the ward clerk—they usually know everything about the ward including where to find things).
- Check how the ward functions.
- Find out the best time for your visit.
- Establish if there are any handover meetings or ward rounds that would be useful for you to attend, attending these will help you become integrated into the multidisciplinary team.
- Check how pharmacy requests are made—does the ward keep a pharmacy order diary or is another system in place such as electronic prescribing?
- Find out the ward system that the multidisciplinary team use to know which patients are in which beds.
- Explain how much time you can spend on the ward and the degree of pharmaceutical care that you can provide.
- Establish what sort of pharmaceutical care service the ward is expecting from you.
- Be aware of local policies/guidelines that pertain to your ward work.
- Comply with any rules regarding hand-washing and wearing an apron, gloves, and mask.

Each ward visit

- Introduce yourself to the nursing coordinator.
- If the ward uses one, obtain a patient list.
- Check whether there are specific pharmaceutical care issues the nursing coordinator and medical staff would like you to follow up that day.
- Check which patients are new admissions and which patients are being discharged that day to prioritize work so that take-home medication is dispensed on time (especially for patients requiring booked transport).
- If the curtains are around a patient with whom you need to consult, check why.
- If patients in side rooms have their doors shut, knock before entering.
- Make the nursing staff aware when you leave the ward and ensure they know how to contact you for further issues.
- Don't ignore telephone calls to the ward phone if you are the only member of staff by the phone. It could be a concerned relative or urgent message for a member of the ward team. If you do answer the ward telephone, greet the caller, say where you are, and who you are.

Patient etiquette

When delivering pharmaceutical care to patients, it is essential that pharmacists follow an appropriate code of conduct:

- Introduce yourself to the patient, stating your name and job title or role.

- Ask if it is convenient for you to speak to the patient about their medication. Be aware that the patient may not feel well enough to do so.
- It is good practice to draw the curtains around the patient's bed prior to the pharmacy consultation to ensure patient privacy.
- Check the patient's identity against the drug chart/notes.
- In accordance with guidance from the National Patient Safety Agency, before taking a history from any patient, the patient should always be asked to confirm their name, date of birth, and allergy status. This should correspond to what is written on their wrist band. If they have any form of allergy, the patient should have a red wrist band confirming what they are allergic to. The wrist band will also have a hospital number. The name, date of birth, hospital number, and allergy status should then be cross-checked with the details on the drug chart and the patient notes. If any of these details are inaccurate or missing you should not proceed until either you or the nursing staff have made the necessary amendments. Additionally, patients admitted through Accident & Emergency (A&E) will often be admitted under an A&E attendance number. However, as soon as the patient's Medical Records Number (MRN) and/or NHS number is known, the drug chart and wrist band should be amended accordingly. If the patient has multiple MRNs these should be merged into one clinical record by the clinical records team. A large number of clinical incidents and patient deaths have been directly attributed to this check not being properly carried out (e.g. two patients with similar names on the ward have medication for one patient prescribed on the other patient's drug chart; patients are administered penicillin-based antibiotics when they are penicillin allergic because they did not have a wristband or had the wrong coloured wrist band).
- Ask the patient how they would prefer to be addressed—e.g. by first name or Mrs/Mr.
- Explain what you will be doing—e.g. checking the medicine chart, checking the patient's own drugs (PODs), taking a medicines history, counselling patients on their new medicine. If you are using a computer or tablet while talking to the patient, explain why.
- Use the term 'medicine' rather than 'drug' when talking to patients.
- Always check whether the patient has any questions at the end of the consultation.
- If you are sorting out any problems with the medication, ensure that the patient is kept fully informed.
- Avoid consultations while patients are having their meals. If it is essential to speak to the patient at that time, check that it is acceptable with the patient to interrupt their meal.
- If patients have visitors present, check with the patient if it is all right to interrupt. If so, check with the patient whether they are happy for the visitors to be present during the consultation. If the patient does not want the visitors present, ask the visitors to return after a set period of time.
- If the curtains are around the patient's bed or the side-room door is closed, check with the ward staff as to the reason. If necessary, speak to the patient from outside the curtain to check whether it is all right for them to see you or whether you should return later.

- If the patient becomes distressed, or is too unwell, try to sort out the task with the help of the notes/ward staff/relative or return later when the patient can be involved with the consultation.
- Be polite at all times.
- Respect the patient's privacy.

Medical hierarchy

In the UK, doctors must complete a 5yr medical degree (or 6yrs including an intercalated BSc/BMedSci degree) which leads to provisional registration with the General Medical Council. They then undertake a 2yr period of foundation training. During the foundation training, doctors will be known as 'foundation house officer 1' (F1) in year 1 and 'foundation house officer 2' (F2) in year 2. The important distinction within the 2yr foundation pro-gramme is that FY1 doctors are working under direct supervision, whereas FY2 doctors can work without direct supervision. This is important because a number of NHS Trusts now require FY1 doctors to pass a prescribing examination or may have restrictions imposed as to what drugs they can or cannot prescribed, whereas FY2 doctors will not.

Foundation training is almost universally followed by a period of 2–3yrs of core training (the CT1 and CT2 grades) followed by a period of run-through training (starting at ST3 and extending up to ST8 depending on speciality) which leads to a CCT (Certificate of Completion of Training) at which point the doctor is able to apply for consultant posts. Junior doctors are often *not* training to work in the consultant's speciality, but rotate into that speciality for a 3–6-month post as part of their training programme. GP trainees will rotate through hospital medical specialities as part of their Vocational Training Scheme (VTS) training programme (this starts after F2).

A consultant leads a team of junior doctors who are rotating through or training to work in the consultant's specialty. Other doctors who work in the team include clinical assistants, clinical fellows, and staff grade doctors. The specialist registrars often rotate between teams of the same speciality to ↑ their experience.

Approach to working with medical staff

- Deal with the correct team of doctors. Check that they are familiar with the patient before asking about prescribing. If the doctor is on call, they may not know the patient well and you can help by providing a short history.
- Ideally, talk directly to the prescriber if a change in the prescription is required. This also helps the prescriber to learn.
- Be aware of the medical hierarchy, and deal with the appropriate grade of doctor. Be aware that often a junior doctor may wish to refer to a senior colleague for decisions around stopping and starting medicines.
- Be assertive and be confident with your knowledge of the subject. If necessary, do some background reading.
- Try to anticipate questions and have answers ready.
- Explain succinctly.
- Repeat, if necessary.
- Understand and explore their viewpoint.
- Be prepared with alternative suggestions.

- Come to a mutual agreement.
- Remember you are working in the patient's best interest, do not leave points of contention unresolved. Escalate to your seniors if necessary.
- Be honest, acknowledge if you 'don't know', and be prepared to follow up.
- If necessary, walk away from a difficult situation and seek the support of a more experienced colleague.
- Occasionally, you might need a discussion with a more senior grade of doctor if you are unhappy with the response from the junior doctor. This should be approached with tact and diplomacy.
- Seek opportunities to work collaboratively with doctors, e.g. on a guideline, on a ward round, or on an audit. This builds rapport, confidence, and experience.

Understanding medical notes

When a patient is first admitted to hospital, a standard series of questions, investigations, and results relating to their physical examination is recorded in the medical notes. This is known as 'medical clerking' and is essentially the story (history) of the patient's illness to date. After interpretation of the initial clerking is mastered, it is usually easy to understand subsequent entries in the notes because these are mostly brief updates. Notes written by GPs follow a similar format but are generally less detailed.

Medical clerking

Clerking usually uses the following format, although not every history includes every step:

- General information about the patient—name, age, gender, marital status and occupation.
- 'Complaining of' (C/O) or 'presenting complaint' (PC)—a statement of what symptoms or problems have led to the patient's admission or attendance, ideally using the patient's own words.
- 'History of presenting complaint' (HPC)—more detail about the symptoms (e.g. timing, whether they have occurred previously, whether anything improves or worsens them, severity, and character).
- 'Past medical history' (PMH)—does the patient have a past history of any medical complaint, including the following:
  - Previous hospital admission
  - Surgery
  - Chronic disease (e.g. diabetes mellitus or asthma).
- 'Drug history' (DHx)—the patient's current drugs and any drugs stopped recently are listed. Ideally, this should include any frequently used over-the-counter and herbal medicines. ADRs and allergies are also recorded here. Never use this as the sole source for a medicines' reconciliation, it can be used to support or inform what you find from other sources.
- 'Social history' (SH) and 'family history' (FH)—relevant details of the patient's occupation, home circumstances, and alcohol and tobacco consumption are recorded. Significant information about the medical history of close family members is noted:
  - Whether parents and siblings are alive and well (A&W).
  - Does anyone in the family have a medical problem related to the presenting complaint?
  - If close family members have died, at what age and what was the cause of death?

All the information in this section is found by asking the patient questions before the doctor examines the patient. This is known as 'systems review' (S/R). Negative findings are recorded, in addition to positive findings:

- On examination (O/E)—this is a general comment about what the patient looks like (e.g. pale, sweaty, or short of breath (SOB)).
- The doctor examines each body system in turn, recording what they have found by looking, listening, and feeling. They concentrate on any systems that are most relevant to the symptoms described

by the patient (e.g. if the patient has complained of chest pain, the cardiovascular system (CVS) and respiratory system (Resp) are most relevant). The following body systems are usually covered:
- CVS
- Resp
- Gastrointestinal system (GI, GIT, or abdo)
- Central nervous system (CNS)
- Peripheral nervous system (PNS)
- Bones and joints (ortho).
- Much of the information is recorded using abbreviations and medical 'shorthand' (Table 4.1).
- 'Investigations' (Ix)—the results of any investigations, such as chest X-rays (CXRs), are recorded.
- 'Diagnosis' (Dx or Z)—the doctor now draws a conclusion from the history and examination and records the diagnosis. If it is not clear what the diagnosis is, they might record several possibilities. These are known as 'differential diagnoses' (DDx or ZZ).
- The doctor now writes a plan for treatment, care, and further investigations.
- Finally, the doctor signs the report and writes down their bleep number or other contact details.

Other clinical information

Remember that the complete clinical record is much more than the paper medical notes. To obtain a complete picture of the patient's history and progress you might need to use other information. This may include electronic records and paper notes:
- Admission form (includes the patient's address, next of kin, and GP details).
- GP's referral letter.
- Nursing notes.
- Observation charts—e.g. temperature, BP, blood glucose levels, and fluid balance.
- Laboratory data—may be paper copies in notes or on computer.
- Results of investigations, e.g. X-ray, MRI, ECG—may be paper copies in notes or on computer.
- Notes from previous admissions or out-patient attendances (including discharge summaries and clinic letters).
- Old drug charts.
- The current drug chart.

Table 4.1 Abbreviations commonly found in medical notes

+	increased, enlarged, or present (more +s indicates increased severity)
↑	increase
↓	decrease
→	normal
()	represents the thoracic and abdominal areas
↔	normal
♀	female
♂	male
#	fracture
O	normal or none
†	dead or died
ABG	arterial blood gases
ACTH	adrenocorticotrophic hormone
ADH	antidiuretic hormone
AF	atrial fibrillation
AFB	acid-fast bacilli
Ag	antigen
AIDS	acquired immunodeficiency syndrome
ALL	acute lymphoblastic leukaemia
AML	acute myeloid leukaemia
ANF	antinuclear factor
APTT	activated partial thromboplastin time
ARDS	acute respiratory distress syndrome
ASD	atrial septal defect
AST	aspartate transaminase
A&W	alive and well
AXR	abdominal X-ray
Ba	barium
BBB	bundle branch block
BMT	bone marrow transplant
BP	blood pressure
BS	breath sounds or bowel sounds
C/O	complaining of
Ca	carcinoma or cancer

(Continued)

Table 4.1 (*Contd.*)

CABG	coronary artery bypass graft
CAPD	continuous ambulatory peritoneal dialysis
CCF	congestive cardiac failure
CHD	congenital heart disease
CHF	chronic heart failure
CLL	chronic lymphoblastic leukaemia
CML	chronic myeloid leukaemia
CMV	cytomegalovirus
CNS	central nervous system
COPD	chronic obstructive pulmonary disease
CPAP	continuous positive airways pressure
creps	crepitations
CSF	cerebrospinal fluid
CSU	catheter specimen of urine
CT	computed tomography
CVA	cerebrovascular accident
CVP	central venous pressure
CVS	cardiovascular system
CXR	chest X-ray
D&C	dilatation and curettage
D&V	diarrhoea and vomiting
DDx, ΔΔ	differential diagnoses (used if there is more than one possible diagnosis)
DHx	drug history
DIC	disseminated intravascular coagulation
DM	diabetes mellitus
DNA	did not attend or deoxyribose nucleic acid
DVT	deep vein thrombosis
D/W	discussed or discussion with
Dx, Δ	diagnosis
DXT	deep X-ray therapy, i.e. radiotherapy
EBV	Epstein–Barr virus
ECF	extracellular fluid
ECG	electrocardiogram
EEG	electroencephalogram
ELISA	enzyme-linked immunosorbent assay

Table 4.1 (Contd.)

EMU	early morning urine
ENT	ear, nose, and throat
ERCP	endoscopic retrograde cholangiopancreatography
ESR	erythrocyte sedimentation rate
EUA	examination under anaesthesia
FBC	full blood count
FEV_1	forced expiratory volume in 1 second
FFP	fresh frozen plasma
FHx	family history
FSH	follicle-stimulating hormone
FSHx	family and social history
FVC	forced vital capacity
G6PD	glucose-6-phosphate dehydrogenase
GA	general anaesthesia
GABA	γ-aminobutyric acid
GFR	glomerular filtration rate
GGT	γ-glutamyl transpeptidase
GH	growth hormone
GI	gastrointestinal
GU	gastric ulcer or genitourinary
GVHD	graft-versus-host disease
Hb	haemoglobin
HBV	hepatitis B virus
HCV	hepatitis C virus
HIV	human immunodeficiency virus
HLA	human leucocyte antigen
HPC	history of presenting complaint
HRT	hormone replacement therapy
HSV	herpes simplex virus
IBD	inflammatory bowel disease
ICP	intracranial pressure
IDDM	insulin-dependent (type 1) diabetes mellitus
Ig	immunoglobulin
IHD	ischaemic heart disease
IM	intramuscular

(Continued)

Table 4.1 (*Contd.*)

INR	international normalized ratio
ISQ	*idem status quo* (i.e. unchanged)
IT	intrathecal
ITP	idiopathic thrombocytopenic purpura
IUD	intrauterine device
IV	intravenous
IVC	inferior vena cava
Ix	investigations
JVP	jugular venous pressure
KCCT	kaolin cephalin clotting time
LBBB	left bundle branch block
LFT	liver function tests
LH	luteinizing hormone
L°K°S°	liver, kidneys, spleen (° = normal)
LP	lumbar puncture
LVF	left ventricular failure
MC&S	microscopy, culture, and sensitivities
MCHC	mean corpuscular haemoglobin concentration
MCV	mean corpuscular volume
MI	myocardial infarction
MND	motor neurone disease
MSU	midstream urine
N&V	nausea and vomiting
NAD	nothing abnormal detected
NG	nasogastric
NIDDM	non-insulin-dependent (type 2) diabetes mellitus
NKDA	no known drug allergies
NSTEMI	non-ST-elevation myocardial infarction
O/E	on examination
OA	osteoarthritis or on admission
OC&P	ova, cysts, and parasites
OGTT	oral glucose tolerance test
PC	presenting complaint
PCP	*Pneumocystis jirovecii* (previously *carinii*) pneumonia
PCV	packed cell volume

Table 4.1 (*Contd.*)

PDA	patent ductus arteriosus
PE	pulmonary embolism
PEEP	positive end-expiratory pressure
PEFR	peak expiratory flow rate
PERLA	pupils equal reactive to light and accommodation
PID	pelvic inflammatory disease
PM	post-mortem
PMH	past medical history
PR	*per rectum* (through the rectum) or pulse rate
PT	prothromhin time
PTH	parathyroid hormone
PTT	partial thromboplastin time
PUO	pyrexia of unknown origin
PV	*per vaginum* (through the vagina)
RA	rheumatoid arthritis
RAST	radio-allergosorbent test
RBBB	right bundle branch block
RBC	red blood cell
RF	renal function
RIP	rest in peace (i.e. dead or died)
Rh	Rhesus
ROS	rest of systems
RS/RES	respiratory system
RTA	road traffic accident
RTI	respiratory tract infection
RVF	right ventricular failure
$S_1 S_2$	heart sounds (first and second)
SCD/SCA	sickle cell disease/anaemia
SIADH	syndrome of inappropriate diuretic hormone
SLE	systemic lupus erythematosus
SOA	swelling of ankles
SOB	shortness of breath
SOBOE	short of breath on exercise/exertion
ST	sinus tachycardia
STEMI	ST elevation myocardial infarction

(Continued)

Table 4.1 (*Contd.*)

SVC	superior vena cava
SVT	supraventricular tachycardia
TB	tuberculosis
TBG	thyroxine-binding globulin
TFT	thyroid function tests
THR	total hip replacement
TIA	transient ischaemic attack
TIBC	total iron-binding capacity
TLC	tender loving care
TOE	transoesophageal echocardiogram
TOP	termination of pregnancy
TPN	total parenteral nutrition
TRH	thyrotropin-releasing hormone
TSH	thyroid-stimulating hormone
TURP	transurethral resection of the prostate
U&Es	urea and electrolytes
UC	ulcerative colitis
URTI	upper respiratory tract infection
UTI	urinary tract infection
VDRL	Venereal Diseases Research Lab (used to refer to the test for syphilis)
VF	ventricular fibrillation
VRIII	variable rate intravenous insulin infusion
VSD	ventricular septal defect
VT	ventricular tachycardia
W/R	ward round
WBC	white blood count
WCC	white cell count

Guidelines for prescription endorsement of hospital or institutional drug charts by pharmacists

Administration/prescription chart review

- Drug charts are available either electronically or as paper copies. For electronic prescribing systems, pharmacy approval/review of drug charts will be recorded by individual logins and specific processes dependent on the local processes and electronic system.
- Pharmacists should initial and date all sections of drug charts where drugs have been prescribed when reviewing charts on the ward. This includes one-off or stat, PRN, syringe driver, and fluid prescriptions. The 'clinical check' assumes that all patient parameters are available to the pharmacist (i.e. drug history, medical notes, urea and electrolyte (U&E) levels, PODs, etc.).
- If the pharmacist clinically checks the drug chart in the dispensary, the following applies:
  - All drug entries should be clinically checked using the resources available in the dispensary (i.e. no access to patient's notes, limited access to U&E levels); however, if required, the pharmacist should obtain further information, e.g. by contacting the nurse or doctor looking after the patient.
  - All entries should be initialled and dated by the pharmacist, ideally in a different coloured ink to the rest of the prescription (e.g. green ink). Any items supplied should be endorsed with the quantity, strength, and form supplied.
  - The ward pharmacist should then treat the drug chart as for a new patient (i.e. check drug history, PODs, notes, and U&E levels, as appropriate).
- Ideally, a drug history should be taken from the patient by the pharmacist or pharmacy technician. This should be indicated by DHx, date and initial, and should be documented according to local policy.
- All endorsements by pharmacists are ideally made in a different coloured ink to the rest of the prescription (e.g. green ink, to distinguish pharmaceutical input from the prescribing process), although this is not a legal requirement. Ensure that the coloured ink used can be reproduced if photocopied, in line with local policy.
- Pharmacists should check and write any identified drug allergies, sensitivities, intolerances, or ADRs, in the appropriate section on the drug chart, in addition to the reaction, in the appropriate section on the drug chart.
- If the patient's name, consultant, ward name, or hospital number is missing, illegible, or incorrect, this should be added or corrected by the pharmacist. If appropriate and if it is missing from the chart, the patient's weight and/or surface area should be added by the pharmacist.

Drug name section

- All drugs should be endorsed by the pharmacist with their non-proprietary approved names, unless they are combination products with no approved names.

- Brand names should be added for medication where the brands are not interchangeable, such as ciclosporin, theophylline, mesalazine, interferon, and lithium, for example. Brand names should also be added for modified release (M/R) nifedipine, diltiazem, and verapamil. They are also desirable for oral contraceptives, hormone replacement therapy (HRT), multiple-ingredient skin products, and inhalers.
- If M/R or enteric-coated (E/C) formulations are intended but not prescribed, drug names should be endorsed M/R or E/C.
- When liquid formulations are intended but not prescribed, drug names should be endorsed as liquid. The concentration should be specified. The dose in millilitres should be calculated and specified, if possible.
- When a dose is prescribed that requires a combination of strengths, the usual combination should be clarified—e.g. digoxin 187.5 micrograms, 3 × 62.5micrograms, or 62.5 micrograms + 125-microgram tablets.
- All changes agreed with the prescriber should be endorsed 'confirmed with Dr [name]', dated, and initialled. Do not use the abbreviation 'pc'.
- Non-formulary, clinical trial, or 'named-patient' items should be endorsed as such.

Advice for insulins

The source of insulin should be specified (i.e. human, bovine, or porcine) along with the generic, brand, and the word insulin (e.g. Lantus® (glargine) insulin. The device used should also be endorsed (i.e. vial, 1.5mL or 3mL penfill, or disposable pen). Lastly, the mixture of insulin should be specified, if appropriate (e.g. 50/50).

Advice for inhalers

The strength of inhaler and the device (e.g. metered-dose inhaler (MDI), Easi-Breathe®, Accuhaler®, etc.) and whether used via a spacer should be specified.

Dose section

- Doses should be endorsed as whole units when not so prescribed (e.g. 500mg not 0.5g).
- Abbreviations should not be used: doses prescribed as 'micrograms' or 'µg' should be endorsed as 'micrograms', doses prescribed as 'ng' should be endorsed as 'nanograms', and similarly 'IU' or 'U' should be endorsed as 'units'.
- Dose times should be amended, as appropriate:
  - To suit meal times—Calcichew®
  - To avoid drug interactions related to absorption—e.g. ciprofloxacin and antacids
  - Dose interval—antibiotics
  - At night (nocte)—statins (not atorvastatin)
  - In the morning (mane)—fluoxetine/paroxetine
  - At 8am and 2pm to avoid nitrate tolerance—isosorbide mononitrate
  - Note: changes to dose time usually do not need to be referred to the prescriber, dependent on local policy.
- The dose and/or route should be clarified where ambiguous, e.g. 'propranolol 1 tablet' or (sublingual) 'GTN PO'. These details should be confirmed with the patient or their notes, and do not usually have to be referred to the prescriber, dependent on local policy. Endorse that the details were confirmed with patient/GP/notes etc.

- Endorsement of drugs administered weekly (e.g. methotrexate and alendronic acid) must be clear, specifying the day of the week the drug is usually taken. This can be made clearer on the drug chart by crossing out administration tiles for all days except the prescribed day for clarity.
- As required, drugs specifying multiple routes are not encouraged, but if prescribed are endorsed with the appropriate dose for each route—e.g. prochlorperazine buccal/PO/IM 3mg/5mg/12.5mg, respectively.
- As required, drugs should be endorsed with their maximum frequency or dose (e.g. analgesics) and/or instructions for use (e.g. anti-diarrhoeals).
- Prescriptions for IV drugs should be endorsed with injection or infusion rates or special requirements for boluses (e.g. furosemide). High-dependency areas could be exceptions from this requirement.
- The rates of currently running drug-containing infusions should be checked, initialled, and dated (as described on ➔ 'Pharmacy annotation section', p. 51) in the pharmacy box.
- Eye drops and ointments should have left/right/both eye(s) specified.

Pharmacy annotation section

All drugs should be initialled and dated by a pharmacist, constituting the 'clinical check'. Supply endorsements should then be made by the pharmacist:

- Stock items (S)
- One-stop supply (28 days)
- Controlled drugs (CDs)
- Patient's own drugs (PODs), including details of quantity and strength brought in and highlighting the date supplies were checked.

Symbols, such as triangle, circle, and slash, are used to distinguish entries from people's initials:

- Although self-administration should be encouraged, such systems must be supported by specific protocols that have been agreed by your institution.
- 'Non-formulary', 'clinical trial', or 'named patient' should be written in full in the drug name box.
- Prescriptions should be endorsed with the date that a supply is made.
- Prescriptions should be endorsed with the quantity supplied each time a supply is made and the appropriate strength of the product supplied.
- When a chart is rewritten, the ward pharmacist should check each entry against the previous chart, initialling and dating each entry if it is correct. The pharmacist should add the appropriate endorsing information with the date of the last supply (for information).

Further information

- Drugs stored in the refrigerator should be endorsed 'Fridge'.
- Endorse prescriptions with guidance on unusual or complex administration (e.g. disodium etidronate or alendronic acid).
- Administration information to aid the nurses may also be included, such as 'Give one hour before, or two hours after food' for flucloxacillin, or instructions for bisphosphonate administration.
- Clarify bioavailability differences if relevant (e.g. phenytoin capsules and suspension).
- Alert the prescriber to clinically significant drug interactions that are identified. Communicate other potential interactions to the relevant doctor either by telephone or by documentation in the patient's notes.

Writing on drug (medicine) charts

Pharmacists should provide relevant prescription information to medical and nursing staff by writing on the drug chart (see ➔ 'Guidelines for prescription endorsement of hospital or institutional drug charts by pharmacists', pp. 49–51). Information provided on the drug chart will vary according to local practice but should ideally include the following:

- Ensure patient details (e.g. name and ward) are complete and correct.
- Document medicines reconciliation information (see ➔ 'Medicines reconciliation', pp. 57–8) on an appropriate page of the prescription chart. (If current drug chart doesn't have a dedicated area on chart, agree local practice.)
- ADRs/drug and food allergies.
- Additional instructions on administration:
  - IV administration
  - Information about appropriate oral administration (e.g. with or after food)
  - Maximum daily dose
  - 'Not with' (e.g. regular prescription).
- Brand name/form—if different version affects bioavailability (e.g. Sandimmun Neoral®, long-acting/M/R).
- Local formulary restrictions, as appropriate.
- Clarify dose if it is not clear or could cause confusion:
  - Change 0.5g to 500mg
  - Liquid—annotate the concentration and volume required
  - Ensure clarity for unusual frequencies (e.g. weekly or alternate days).
- Clinical information—drug interactions (e.g. drugs affecting warfarin levels).
- Monitoring requests or information:
  - Potassium (K^+) levels for drugs affecting/affected by potassium
  - Creatinine levels for drugs affecting/affected by creatinine
  - Drug levels.
- Requests to doctors to review a prescription plan—length of course of antibiotics.

All information should be set out as follows:
- Written in coloured ink according to local practice (e.g. green ink).
- Clear, legible, and in indelible ink (if handwriting is poor, please print capitals).
- Initialled and dated, including bleep number, as appropriate.
- Use only well-recognized abbreviations.
- Any actions for the doctors, such as amendments to prescriptions should be communication in person (or via phone) if urgent, and documented in the medical notes.
- Remember, a drug chart is a legal document.

Prescription screening and monitoring

In an ideal world, pharmacists would review prescriptions with all relevant patient information to hand and individualize drug therapy accordingly. In reality, time and circumstances do not allow this, and pharmacists must be able to identify problems with only limited information, or be able to identify where more information is required. Time rarely allows for a full examination of all patient data, even if it is available, so pharmacists must learn to determine whether or not this is necessary.

The choice of information sources available could range from just the prescription, the patient or their representative, or, possibly, prescription-medication records (PMRs) in the community pharmacy to full laboratory data and medical and nursing notes in the hospital setting. The following discussion assumes that all information is available but it can be adapted to situations in which there are more limited data.

First impressions

Look at the prescription and patient (if present). This might seem an obvious first step, but these simple observations can tell you a great deal.

What does the prescription or chart tell you about the patient?
- Age—think about special considerations in children (see ➋ 'Medicines for children: introduction', p. 204) and the elderly (see ➋ 'Medicines for older people: introduction', p. 214).
- Weight—is the patient significantly overweight/underweight? Will you need to check doses according to weight?
- Ward name or consultant—may tell you the presenting illness (if this is not already obvious).
- Other charts can also provide important information—e.g. diet sheets, blood glucose monitoring, BP, and temperature.
- What does observation of the patient tell you?
- Old frail patients probably need dose adjustments because of low weight or poor renal function.
- Take extra care checking children's doses; also check that the formulation is appropriate and consider licensing issues (see ➋ 'Medicines for children: licensing', p. 207).
- Unconscious patients cannot take drugs by mouth. Will you need to provide formulations that can be administered through a nasogastric (NG) or gastrostomy tube?
- Do they have IV fluids running? Consider fluid balance if other IV fluids will be used to administer drugs (notably antimicrobials).
- If the patient's weight is not recorded on the prescription, do they look significantly overweight/underweight? If you have concerns, ask the patient if they know their weight or weigh them.
- Is the patient pregnant or breastfeeding?
- Could the patient's racial origin affect drug handling—e.g. there is a higher incidence of glucose-6-phosphate dehydrogenase (G6PD) deficiency in people of African origin (see ➋ 'Glucose 6-phosphate dehydrogenase deficiency', pp. 198–9).

At this point, you might already have decided on points that need to be checked or monitored. Make a note of these as you think of them. In many hospitals, a ward patient list is produced each day, which gives patient names, diagnosis, and basic clinical details. This is a useful source of readily available patient information, and you can make notes and pharmaceutical care points on your copy. Remember that the information on the list is confidential and you should be careful how you handle it. Do not leave it lying around for others to see and dispose of it by shredding or in a confidential waste bin.

Review prescribed drugs

Check each drug on the prescription carefully. Newly prescribed drugs are the highest priority, but it is important to periodically review old drugs.

- Are the dose, frequency and route appropriate for this patient, their weight and their renal function?
- What is the indication for the drug?
  - Is it appropriate for this patient?
  - Does it comply with local or national guidelines or formularies?
  - Could the drug be treating a side effect of another drug—if so, could the first drug be stopped or changed?
- Are there any potential drug interactions (see ➲ 'Drug interactions', pp. 23–5)?
  - Are they clinically significant?
  - Do you need to get the interacting drug stopped or changed, or just monitor for side effects?
- Is therapeutic drug monitoring (TDM) required?
  - Do you need to check levels or advise on dose adjustment?
  - Are levels being taken at the right time?
- Is the drug working?
  - Think about the signs and symptoms (including laboratory data and nursing observations) you should be monitoring to check that the drug is having the desired effect. Are any symptoms due to lack of effect? Talk to the patient!
- Are any signs and symptoms due to side effects?
  - Do you need to advise dose adjustment, a change in therapy, or symptomatic treatment of side effects? Remember that it is some-times appropriate to prescribe symptomatic therapy in anticipation of side effects (e.g. antiemetics and laxatives for patients on opioids).
- Check that the patient is not allergic to or intolerant of any of the prescribed drugs. This is usually recorded on the front of hospital prescription charts or you might need to check the medical notes or talk to the patient. Community pharmacy PMRs often record drug allergies or intolerance.

Ensure that you have looked at all prescribed drugs. Hospital prescription charts usually have different sections for 'as required' and 'once-only' ('stat') drugs and IV infusions. Many patients might have more than one prescription chart, and some might have different charts for certain types of drug (e.g. chemotherapy).

By now, you will probably have added to your list of points to follow up and have some idea of which patients you should focus on.

Check the patient's drug history

When patients are admitted to hospital, it is important that the drugs they normally take at home are continued, unless there is a good reason to omit them. Check that the drugs the patient usually takes are prescribed in the right dose, frequency, and form (see ➔ 'Medicines reconciliation', pp. 57–8).

- Ideally, use a source of information that is different from the admission history (in case the admitting doctor has made any errors):
    - GP's referral letter or computer printout
    - Copy of community or repeat prescription
    - POD supplies.
    - Electronic or faxed record from GP's surgery
    - Talk to the patient/relative/carer
    - Residential home medication administration record (MAR) chart.
- Talking to the patient often reveals drugs that might otherwise be overlooked (e.g. oral contraceptive pill, regular over-the-counter medicines, or herbal medicines).
- If there are any discrepancies between what has been prescribed and what the patient normally takes that you cannot account for, ensure that the doctors are aware of this. Depending on your local practice, it might be appropriate to record discrepancies on the prescription chart or in the medical notes.
- Many patients may not remember the names and doses of medication they are taking, but they will often bring in their current tablets which can be a vital source of information. It is also important to check that they are taking their medications as directed (e.g. with or without food or at the correct time of day) rather than assuming that they are following the instructions given. Additionally, it is now best practice to ask the patient's GP to fax through a list of current medications or access the GP electronic records for all in-patients as an independent cross-check.

Talk to the patient

Patients are an important source of information about their drugs, disease, and symptoms. Talk to them! You might find out important information that is not recorded in the medical notes or prescription chart. If you are reviewing charts at the bedside, always introduce yourself and explain your role and what you are doing. It is a good idea to ask the patient if they have any problems with or questions about their medicines. If the patient is on many drugs or complex therapy, check their adherence by asking if they are managing to take all their medicines at home.

Care plan

You will now have notes of various problems, questions, and monitoring that you need to do. Resolve any problems and form a plan to continue monitoring the patient. Prioritization is important: an elderly patient with renal impairment who is taking multiple drugs is at higher risk of drug-related problems than a young, fit patient who is only taking one or two drugs. If you are short of time, concentrate on the high-risk patients. Check your notes, decide what jobs are essential, and deal with these first.

In some hospitals, a formal pharmaceutical care plan is written for each patient. This can be quite time-consuming, but it is good practice if you can do it (for high-risk patients if not for all).

Screening discharge prescriptions

- Are all regular drugs from all prescription charts prescribed? If not, can you account for any that are omitted?
- Are timings correct and complete (e.g. diuretics to be taken in the morning)?
- Are any 'as required' drugs used frequently and therefore needed on discharge?
- Are all the prescribed drugs actually needed on discharge (e.g. hypnotics)?
- Does the patient actually need a supply? They might have enough of their own supply on the ward or at home.
- Will the GP need to adjust any doses or drugs after discharge? If so, is this clear on the prescription or discharge letter?
- Is there any information that you need to pass on to the patient, carer, or GP (e.g. changes to therapy or monitoring requirements)?
- Does the patient understand how to take the drugs, especially any new ones or those with special instructions—e.g. warfarin (see ➜ 'Heart failure', pp. 328–32)?
- Are adherence aids needed (see ➜ 'Strategies to improve adherence', pp. 6–7)?
- When is the patient being discharged? It is important to identify which patients are being discharged that day.
- If any changes are required to the discharge prescription, the junior doctor needs to be contacted.

Medicines reconciliation

Medicines reconciliation is defined by the National Prescribing Centre as the process of obtaining a current and accurate medication list, including documentation of any discrepancies, changes, additions, or deletions.[6] There are two stages to medicines reconciliation: basic (stage 1) and full (stage 2). Stage 1 involves the identification of a patient's current list of medication, whereas stage 2 includes the comparison of the current list to the most recent available list for the patient, and identifying and acting upon discrepancies.

Guidance issued by NICE[7] states that:

- pharmacists should be involved in medicines reconciliation as soon as possible
- the responsibilities of pharmacists and other staff involved in medicines reconciliation are clearly defined.

Strategies should be incorporated to obtain information from patients with communication difficulties, such as speaking to a parent or carer.

For each medication, documentation of the following information will be required:

- Drug name
- Dose
- Frequency
- Formulation
- Duration of treatment
- Indication
- Any problems with medication, such as with administration (e.g. inhaler), ADRs, or allergies
- Is the patient taking their medication according to the prescribed instructions?

It is essential that details of all types of medication are obtained from a number of sources, including the following:

- Medicines prescribed by the GP.
- Medicines prescribed by the hospital.
- Over-the-counter medicines.
- Alternative (e.g. herbal or homeopathic) medicines or vitamins.
- Recreational drugs—discuss with patient before documenting, as many patients may not want this documented.
- All forms of medicine (e.g. tablets, liquids, suppositories, injections, eye drops/ointments, ear drops, inhalers, nasal sprays, creams, patches, and ointments).
- If a compliance aid (e.g. Dosette® box) is used, who fills it?

Medication will often have to be verified if patients cannot remember the details of their medication and have not brought their medication with them. Local hospital procedures may specify a minimum number of sources that are required and sources may include:

- checking against the POD supply
- checking against GP letters

- checking records of prescriptions used in the community (FP10 prescriptions in UK)
- telephoning the GP's practice, and requesting a faxed copy of the patient's current medication, or checking against electronic patient record.

As part of medicines reconciliation, it is vital that any allergies are established along with the nature of the reaction.

In addition to the above-mentioned information, the following should be documented as part of the medicines reconciliation process:

- Date and time
- Information provided to the patient as a result of this process
- Signature
- Name, profession, and contact information
- If appropriate, any discrepancies or pharmacist recommendations may be documented in the medical notes. See ➔ 'Writing in medical notes', p. 59 for further information.

References

6. National Prescribing Centre. 'Medicines Reconciliation: A Guide to Implementation', ℘ https://www.nicpld.org/courses/fp/assets/MM/NPCMedicinesRecGuideImplementation.pdf
7. NICE (2015). 'Medicines optimisation: the safe and effective use of medicines to enable the best possible outcomes (NG5)', ℘ www.nice.org.uk/guidance/ng5

Writing in medical notes

Pharmacists should write in the medical notes to communicate information relating to the pharmaceutical care of the patient to the medical staff if immediate action is not required. The information should significantly influence the care of the patient, or ensure that information is available to all members of the medical and nursing teams. The notes are a legal document, and if the pharmacist has contributed to, or attempted to contribute to, the patient's care, this should be documented.

The following is appropriate information to write in the medical notes:
• Clinically significant interactions.
• Contraindications to medicine use.
• ADRs.
• Identification of a problem that could be related to medicine use.
• Any history medication from the medicines reconciliation that is not prescribed and where there is no documented reason.
• General medicines information about unusual medicines/conditions.
• Counselling details and outcome.

Pharmacists who are authorized (according to local practice) to make an entry in the patient's notes include the following:
• Registered pharmacists who have received suitable training.
• Junior pharmacists and locums should discuss potential entries with their seniors or clinical supervisor before making the entry.

The pharmacist should ensure that each entry into the notes is as follows:
• Directly relevant to that patient's care.
• At the appropriate point in the notes.
• Succinct and informative.
• Follows a logical sequence.
• Subjective—e.g. records relevant patient details.
• Objective—e.g. records clinical findings.
• An assessment of the situation.
• Recommendations are clearly expressed.
• The entry should follow a standard format, for example:
  • 27/11/16 Pharmacist entry
  • Amiodarone will increase plasma concentration of digoxin. *BNF* states— halve dose of digoxin. Please review current prescription and adjust accordingly. If you require further information please bleep me.
  • Tom Smith (sign) bleep 1178.

Entries in the patient's notes should be as follows:
• Clear, legible, and in indelible ink (many hospital pharmacists use green ink, provided that the ink quality can be photocopied).
• Signed, with printed name, and dated.
• Include a contact number (bleep or extension).
• Use only well-recognized abbreviations.
• Include any discussion of the issue with medical or nursing staff.
• Not be informal.
• Not directly criticize medical/nursing care.

Medication review

Definition of medication review

A structured critical examination of a patient's medicines by a healthcare professional:

- reaching an agreement with the patient about treatment
- optimizing the use of medicines
- minimizing the number of medication-related problems
- avoiding wastage.

Regular medication review maximizes the therapeutic benefit and minimizes the potential harm of drugs. It ensures the safe and effective use of medicines by patients. Medication review provides an opportunity for patients to discuss their medicines with a healthcare professional. Medication review is the cornerstone of medicines management.

What does medication review involve?

- A structured critical examination of a patient's medicines (prescription and other medicines, including alternatives) by a healthcare professional.
- Identification, management, and prevention of ADRs or drug interactions.
- Minimizing the number of medication-related problems.
- Optimizing the use of medicines.
- Simplification of regimen.
- Ensuring all drugs are appropriate and needed.
- Avoiding wastage.
- Medication counselling.
- Adherence counselling—to encourage patients to adhere to their drug regimens.
- Assessment of ability to self-medicate.
- Education of patient or carer—to help them understand their drugs better.
- Education of the patient on safe and effective medication use.
- Forum for suggesting effective treatment alternatives.
- Recommendation of compliance aids.

Principles of medication review

- Patients must be informed that their medication is being reviewed.
- Patients should have the opportunity to ask questions and highlight any problems with their medicines.
- Medication review should improve the impact of treatment for an individual patient.
- A competent person (e.g. pharmacist) should undertake the review in a systematic way.
- Any changes resulting from the review are agreed with the patient.
- The review is documented according to local policy (e.g. in the patient's notes).
- The impact of any change is monitored.

Levels of medicine review

- Level 3 (clinical medication review)—face-to-face review of medication with the patient and their notes, specifically undertaken by a doctor, nurse, or pharmacist. Provides an opportunity to discuss what medication the patient is actually taking and how medicine-taking fits in with the patient's daily life.
- Level 2 (treatment review)—review of medicines, with reference to the patient's full notes, in the absence of the patient and under the direction of a doctor, nurse, or pharmacist.
- Level 1 (prescription review)—technical review of a list of the patient's medicines in the absence of the patient and under the direction of a doctor, nurse, or pharmacist.
- Level 0 (ad hoc review)—unstructured, opportunistic review of medication.

Who to target

- Patients on multiple medications or complicated drug regimens
- Patients experiencing ADRs
- Patients with chronic conditions
- Elderly patients
- Non-adherent patients.

Potential benefits of medication review

- Identification, management, and prevention of ADRs.
- Ensuring patients have maximum benefit from their medicines.
- Improved adherence due to patient involvement, possibly due to clarification of dosing directions, or identification of impractical directions or physical barriers to administering medication (e.g. certain inhalers).
- Reduced risk of drug-related problems and potential interactions between medication and food ↑ appropriate use of medicines.
- Improved clinical outcomes.
- Cost-effectiveness.
- Improve quality of life.
- Optimizing therapy and monitoring.
- Reduce waste of medicines by identifying medication which is no longer required (including medication used to treat the side effects of another)
- Enables patients to maintain their independence.
- Reduces admissions to hospital.
- Reduction in drug-related deaths.

Recording medication reviews

- There is no universally agreed way of documenting medication reviews.
- Local guidance for recording medication reviews needs to be followed.
- The minimum information that should be recorded is as follows:
  - Current medication history
  - Problems identified
  - Advice given
  - Suggested time-frame for the next medication review
  - Date, signature, name, position, and contact details.

Further reading

NICE (2009). 'Medicines adherence: involving patients in decisions about prescribed medicines and supporting adherence (CG76)', ℘ www.nice.org.uk/guidance/cg76

Intervention monitoring

Clinical pharmacists can audit their impact on patient care by intervention monitoring. Some hospitals undertake these audits at regular intervals and present the results internally or to the multidisciplinary team. This information may also be used as evidence for the recruitment of more staff, or to show the benefit of a change to service, such as weekend working.

Data collection forms or electronic hand-held systems are used to collect the relevant data on a pharmacist's interventions to improve patient care. Examples of data collected for this purpose include the following:

- Patient details and demographics.
- Area of work/specialization.
- Written details of the intervention.
- Date of intervention.
- Other healthcare professionals contacted.
- Evidence used to support the intervention.
- Who initiated the intervention—e.g. pharmacist, doctor, nurse, or patient.
- Possible effect the intervention would have on patient care.
- Outcome of the intervention.
- Actual outcome on patient care that the intervention had.
- Significance of intervention (Table 4.2 shows an example of one of the ways for deciding significance of the intervention).
- Category of intervention (examples are given in the section that follows).

Examples of the categories of pharmacist interventions in drug therapy

- ADRs
- Allergy
- Additional drug therapy required
- Medication error
- Medication without indication (especially antibiotics)
- Untreated condition or undertreated condition
- Minimal or no therapeutic effectiveness
- Therapeutic duplication
- Patient adherence, compliance, or drug administration issue
- Patient education
- Communication with prescriber
- Incorrect medication prescribed
- Inappropriate or suboptimal dose, schedule, or route
- Optimization of drug therapy, including improving cost-effectiveness
- Dose advice
- Advice on drug choice
- Drug–drug, drug–food, or drug–disease interaction
- Side effect/toxicity
- Therapeutic monitoring for toxicity or effectiveness
- Formulation
- Compatibility
- Formulary or protocol adherence.

Table 4.2 Example of significance definitions of pharmacist interventions

Significance of intervention	Definition
Minor	Unlikely to have effect on patient outcome
Moderate	Potentially undesirable for patient outcome
Severe	Potentially detrimental for patient outcome (e.g. potentially serious prescribing error)

Further reading

Becker C, Bjornson DC, Kuhle JW (2004). Pharmacist care plans and documentation of follow-up before the Iowa Pharmaceutical Case Management program. *J Am Pharm Assoc* 44: 350–7.

Hoth AB, Carter BL, Ness J, *et al.* (2007). Development and reliability testing of clinical pharmacist recommendation taxonomy. *Pharmaco-therapy* 27: 639–46.

McDonough RP, Doucette WR (2003). Drug therapy management: an empirical report of drug therapy problems, pharmacists' interventions, and results of pharmacists' actions. *J Am Pharm Assoc* 43: 511–18.

References

8. Dean B, Barber N, Schater M. (2000). What is a prescribing error? *Qual Safe Health Care* 9: 232–7.
9. Dodd C (2003). Assessing pharmacy interventions at Salisbury Health Care NHS Trust. *Hosp Pharm* 10: 451–6.

Dealing with mistakes

Medication errors are patient safety incidents involving medicines in which there has been an error in the process of prescribing, dispensing, preparing, administering, monitoring, or providing medicine advice, regardless of whether any harm occurred. Medication errors are associated with significant unexpected drug-related morbidity and mortality.

Medicines management policies and procedures should be in place to minimize the risk of medication errors occurring during the medication process (i.e. for prescribing, dispensing, and administration). Pharmacists can play a prominent role in optimizing safe medication use and preventing errors in all steps of the medication process.

Prescribing
- Adequate knowledge of the patient and their clinical condition.
- Clear multi-professional treatment plans.
- Complex calculations checked by two members of staff.
- Review drug treatments regularly.
- Implement electronic care records and prescribing systems.
- Legible prescriptions.
- Avoiding abbreviations.

Dispensing
- Training and competency assessment for checking prescriptions and dispensing.
- Checking medication with a patient when it is being issued and allowing patients the opportunity to ask questions about their medication.
- Formal dispensary procedures and checking systems.

Administration
- Risk management must be built into the previous steps to ensure that medication is administered safely:
  - Training of staff administering medication.
  - Procedures for drug administration.
  - High-risk areas of administration to have a double check by a second member of staff (e.g. for IV infusions or complex calculations).
  - Involving patients or their carers in the administration process if appropriate.
  - Storage of medication appropriately to minimize errors. Controlling the availability of high-risk drugs (e.g. potassium chloride ampoules).
  - Using information technology to support prescribing, dispensing, and administration of medication.
- Create a culture where staff can learn from their mistakes. Do not have a blame culture:
  - Explore why a mistake has happened.
  - Remain calm.
  - Find out the facts.
  - Focus on the processes that allowed the mistake to happen.
  - Provide support.
  - Assume that the person wants to learn from their mistakes.
  - See mistakes as part of a learning process.

- Harness the power of mistakes:
  - Create mechanisms to provide support when mistakes occur.
  - Learn to question and challenge without antagonism.
  - Create personal learning contracts to promote self-managed learning.
  - Acquire a habit of active reflection.
- Reporting mistakes:
  - Use the appropriate reporting mechanism within your hospital or institution.
  - Inform a more senior member of staff of the mistake.
  - Inform the multidisciplinary team of the mistake.
  - Document the mistake and the steps leading up to the mistake.
- Dealing with mistakes:
  - Dealing with your own feelings, if you are the person who made the mistake—remember that we are all human and can make mistakes. You will probably feel remorse that you have made the mistake. Reflect on how the mistake was made, and plan how you will learn from the mistake to ensure that it isn't repeated.
  - Dealing with people who don't acknowledge their own mistakes or who make repeated mistakes—the person's manager should be involved in dealing with the person who does not acknowledge their mistakes. Evidence must be used to discuss the mistakes, and performance management strategies put in place to ensure that the mistakes are acknowledged and learnt from.
  - Dealing with a more senior member of staff who has made a mistake—it is difficult for a junior member of staff to deal with mistakes made by a more senior member of staff. Whenever possible, it is best to speak directly to the member of staff who has made the mistake, informing them of the outcome and any action you have taken. If necessary, involve another senior member of staff or your manager in the discussion.

Remember

Mistakes can be fatal. Ensure that you are aware of local policies and procedures to minimize the risk of mistakes occurring.

Further reading

Smith J (2004). *Building a Safer NHS for Patients: Improving Medication Safety*. London: Department of Health.
Williams DJP (2007). Medication errors. *J R Coll Physicians Edinb* 37: 343–6.

Dealing with aggressive or violent patients

Many pharmacy staff will experience some form of threatening behaviour from patients at some stage during their working lives. This can range from a patient becoming verbally abusive because of a long wait for medicines to be dispensed to an armed robbery of a community pharmacy. Aggressive behaviour may also be via the telephone or written communication. Even if there is no physical injury, the psychological effect of a violent or aggressive encounter can be significant and could affect the victim's attitude to work, co-workers, and patients. The emotional distress can be ↑ in a healthcare setting because staff might feel unprepared for this type of behaviour from a patient or customer they are trying to help. There could be feelings of guilt, embarrassment, shame, fear of blame, or denial. Incidents should not be accepted as 'part of the job' and should be reported so that appropriate action can be taken to both protect and support the victim and other members of staff. If healthcare teams have strategies to review and discuss incidents of threatening behaviour, staff find this useful for coping and learning.

The NHS has a 'zero tolerance' policy on verbal or physical abuse or aggressive behaviour against staff and it is the employers responsibility to ensure that staff are adequately protected.[10] Staff should raise concerns if they feel they are being expected to work in an unsafe situation, if necessary taking this to a higher authority.

Facing an aggressive or violent patient can be a frightening and shocking experience, and often the response is a 'fight or flight' reaction. Being prepared for this type of incident, and knowing strategies to deal with or defuse such a situation, is of great value.

The safety of staff and other patients/customers is of paramount importance:

- Be aware of and develop systems to avoid vulnerable times and situations—e.g. pharmacy opening and closing times, a lone pharmacist, or dealing with patients with a history of aggressive behaviour.
- Don't attempt any heroics—your personal safety is far more important than the contents of the shop till. Hand over any money or goods demanded, because insurance cover can replace loss but not lives.
- Be aware of 'escape routes' and try not to let the patient get between you and the door.
- Ensure that you are aware of any safety procedures—e.g. panic buttons and how to activate them.
- Aim to avoid situations where you are on your own with a potentially difficult patient. If you have to go into a room alone with them, leave the door open and make sure a colleague is close by to give you back-up if necessary.
- When dealing with an aggressive or verbally abusive patient, good handling of the incident can help defuse the situation, or at least prevent it from escalating.

Don't

- Take the threatening behaviour personally.
- Be defensive or aggressive in return.
- Attempt to appease the patient by giving in to their demands, although be prepared to compromise if appropriate.
- Ignore or tolerate the behaviour.
- Be over-apologetic.
- Argue with the patient.
- Be overly sympathetic and take the patient's side.
- Use defensive or aggressive body language.

Do

- Remain calm and state your case clearly and concisely.
- Be assertive, without being aggressive.
- Maintain eye contact.
- Speak in a manner that is calm, clear, simple, slow, and non-confrontational.
- Listen to the patient and give them a chance to voice their complaints.
- Apologize if there clearly is some justification for the patient's complaint, without being overly apologetic or apportioning blame.
- Explain to the patient how to make a written complaint if they wish (frequently the patient will back down at this point).
- Call a more senior colleague if you feel out of your depth.
- In an extreme situation, it may be necessary to enlist the help of security staff or even call the police.

Limit setting

In some situations, it might not be possible to avoid continued contact with a patient who has been aggressive or violent towards staff. This might be an in-patient who needs further medical care or someone attending for further out-patient appointments or repeat prescriptions (e.g. injecting drug users on opioid replacement therapy). In these cases, it might be possible to avoid further threatening incidents by setting limits.

An effective system is to draw up a contract detailing what is expected of the patient and what behaviour is considered unacceptable, and, in return, what the patient can expect from the healthcare team. The contract should state what will happen if the patient breaks the limits—usually a single warning, followed by withdrawal of services if the limits are broken again. These contracts can be very helpful in controlling patient behaviour, but it must be a two-way process—healthcare staff must also stick to their side of the contract both in terms of providing care and being prepared to carry out the threat of withdrawing care if the limits are broken.

Reference

10. NHS Employers. 'Violence against staff', 🔊 www.nhsemployers.org/~/media/Employers/ Publications/Violence%20against%20staff.pdf

Dealing with distressed patients

Occasionally pharmacists might have to deal with patients who are distressed or agitated for one of the following reasons:
- Their diagnosis
- Difficulty in tolerating side effects
- Witnessing an upsetting event with another patient
- The behaviour of visitors, other staff, or other patients.

If faced with this situation, even the busiest pharmacist should try to spend some time comforting or supporting the patient as best they can. Spending even a little time with the patient can bring considerable relief from distress:
- Do not ignore the patient, even if you are busy or unsure how to deal with the situation. If you feel you cannot deal with the situation yourself, acknowledge the patient's distress and ask if they would like you to call another member of staff.
- Ask the patient if they would like to talk to you about what it is that is upsetting them.
- Listen and don't interrupt.
- Never say 'I know how you feel'. Even if you have had to deal with the same situation yourself, it is presumptuous to state that you know how another person feels.
- If any misunderstandings or misconceptions are contributing to the patient's distress, try to correct these. If necessary, ask the medical team to talk to the patient.
- Answer any questions the patient has as honestly and openly as you can.
- Provide reassurance about symptoms that might be causing anxiety—e.g. pain can be controlled, morphine won't make them an 'addict', and side effects can be managed.
- If the patient's distress is caused by another colleague's behaviour, do not offer any comment or judgement. Listen and make a non-committal comment, such as 'I'm sorry that's how you feel'. As appropriate, suggest that they might like to speak to a senior member of staff—e.g. ward sister or senior doctor.
- Remember that silence is often as helpful as conversation. Just sitting with a patient for a few minutes while they get their emotions under control can be very helpful.
- As appropriate, physical contact, such as holding the patient's hand or touching their arm, can be a source of comfort.
- Offer practical comfort—e.g. tissues, glass of water, a chair, or privacy.
- Don't avoid the patient or the incident next time you see them, but be careful not to become too emotionally involved. A simple question like 'How are you today?' acknowledges the patient's previous distress and allows them to talk further if they wish.

Dealing with dying patients

Death is an almost daily occurrence on most wards. Although in general, patients spend most of their final year of life at home, 90% of patients spend some time in hospital and 55% die there.

As a pharmacist, you might not be as closely involved in the care of a dying patient as the nursing or medical staff, but it is still a situation that affects most pharmacists at some stage. Some pharmacists, such as those working in palliative care, oncology, or intensive care units, may be quite involved in the care of both the dying patient and their family. Learning how to deal with your own feelings, in addition to those of the patient and their family, is important.

The patient

On being told that they are dying, a patient (or their relatives) usually goes through the following stages (although not all people go through every stage):
• Shock/numbness
• Denial
• Anger
• Grief
• Acceptance.

It is important to let these processes happen, while supporting the patient and family sensitively.

Providing information about the illness enables the patient and family to make informed decisions about medical care and personal and social issues, and this is where you can help. Patients and relatives may perceive doctors as being too busy to answer their questions or be embarrassed to ask. A pharmacist might be perceived as having more medical knowledge (and being less busy!) than the nursing staff, but being more approachable than the medical staff.

When talking to dying patients and answering their questions, bear the following points in mind:
• Be honest—don't give the patient false hope. Answer questions as honestly and openly as possible. If the patient asks you directly whether they are dying, it is probably not appropriate for a pharmacist to confirm this. An appropriate response might be to ask why they are asking you this or to enquire what they have been already told and then formulate an appropriate response.
• Be sensitive—some patients might want lots of information about their diagnosis and care, but others might not be interested. Respect the patient's need for privacy at a difficult time but do not be afraid of talking to a dying patient—sometimes patients can feel lonely and isolated, and even a discussion lasting a few minutes can be of real benefit. Remember that different cultures have different responses to death. Whatever your own views, respect patients' religious or secular beliefs.
• Be careful—patients might not wish family or friends to know the diagnosis or that they are dying, so be especially careful what you say if other people are present.

Patients often have questions about treatment:
● Will current treatment be continued or stopped?
● Can pain or other symptoms be controlled?
● Will they become 'addicted' to morphine?
● What happens if they can no longer take medication orally?

Answer these questions as fully as you can, without overloading the patient with information. Be practical with your information and remember that some cautions become irrelevant at this stage—e.g. do not insist on NSAIDs being taken with food if the patient is not eating. If you don't feel that it is appropriate for you to answer a question, tactfully tell the patient that it would be better to ask someone more appropriate—e.g. the doctors. However, you could help the patient to formulate the question so that they feel better able to ask the doctors.

   The information you provide will depend on the situation and your level of expertise. If you feel out of your depth, ask a senior colleague for advice.

Carers and relatives

Carers' and relatives' needs and questions will often be the same as the patient's, and you might need to go over some issues more than once. If the patient is going to be cared for at home, there can be many practical questions and information needs that you can answer:
● A simpler (layman's) explanation of the diagnosis and symptom management.
● Coping with (potentially complex) medication regimens.
● Side effects and what to do about them.
● What to do if the patient vomits soon after taking a dose.
● Medicine storage.
● Obtaining further supplies.
● What to with unused medicines when the patient dies.
● What to do if symptoms are not controlled.
● What to do if the patient becomes too unwell to take oral medicines.

Yourself

It is important to recognize your own emotional needs, especially if your job means that you are frequently involved in the care of dying patients or if a death is especially 'close to home'. The patient or the circumstances of their illness/death might remind you of the death of a close relative or friend. This can 'open up old wounds', which you must come to terms with.
   When a patient dies, you might experience various emotions:
● Sadness—a natural response to any death, but accept that it is a 'hazard' of working in healthcare.
● Relief—a prolonged or distressing illness is over.
● Grief or loss—you might have become quite attached to the patient and/or their family.
● Guilt/inadequacy—if symptoms weren't controlled or the patient's death was unexpected.
● It is important to find ways to cope with this. Talking to a colleague, hospital chaplain, or close friend might help, but bear in mind that you must maintain confidentiality.

- If the patient is well known to the ward/community pharmacy staff, the family might invite them to the funeral or memorial service. Attending the funeral can benefit healthcare workers, in addition to giving the family support. Consider whether your attendance could breach confidentiality. Avoid wearing a uniform, remove identification badges and bleeps, and consider whether wearing a symbol, such as a red or pink ribbon, would be inappropriate. If you are unsure whether it would be appropriate to attend, discuss it with a senior member of staff—e.g. the ward sister or your manager.

Euthanasia

- It is extremely unlikely that a patient would directly ask a pharmacist to assist them to die. However, you might be aware that a patient has expressed this desire to other staff. Whatever your personal view on the morality of euthanasia, you should treat the patient the same as any other.
- Euthanasia is still illegal in most countries. However, it is generally considered acceptable to give treatment that is adequate to control symptoms, even if this could shorten the duration of life, provided that the primary intent is symptom control. If you have any concerns about the appropriateness of therapy/doses in this situation, you should discuss this with the prescriber and/or a senior colleague.

What if your patient is dead in the bed?

Although not a common occurrence, clinical pharmacists can be the first to realize that a patient has died, often quietly in their bed or a chair. Here are some things to bear in mind should this happen on your round:

- Do not panic, but remain calm.
- Withdraw yourself from that patient's area and close the bed curtains, if open.
- Speak to the member of the nursing team responsible for that patient to check that they are aware of the situation.
- Consider what you feel about the incident.
- If necessary, speak to a member of the multidisciplinary team.
- Take a break to recover.
- Speak to a colleague for support.
- Continue with the day's work.
- If a relative is with the patient, they might call the pharmacist to the bed if they are concerned that the patient has died. Inform the relative that you will get a nurse to attend. Find a nurse or a member of the medical team immediately to deal with the patient, as appropriate.

It might be useful, as part of the pharmacist induction, to visit the mortuary, because dealing with death requires professional support.

Ethical dilemmas

Medical ethics deals with situations where there is no clear course of action. This might be because of a lack of scientific evidence, but it is more frequently where moral, religious, or other values have a significant influence on decision-making. Thus, medical ethics differs from research ethics; the latter is concerned with evaluating whether clinical trials are appropriate, safe, and in the best interests of the participants and/or the wider population. Many hospitals have a medical ethics committee in addition to a research ethics committee.

The issues debated by medical ethics committees are many and varied. They might produce guidelines to cover certain issues, but frequently a committee does not give a definite answer and simply provides a forum for debate. Issues debated by medical ethics committees include the following:

- Consent to or refusal of treatment, especially with respect to those unable to make decisions themselves—i.e. children or incapacitated adults.
- End-of-life issues, such as 'do not resuscitate' orders, living wills, and withdrawal of treatment.
- Organ donation and transplantation.
- Contraception and abortion.

Like most other healthcare professionals, pharmacists are expected to conduct their professional (and to a certain extent their personal) lives according to ethical principles. In the UK, the General Pharmaceutical Council (GPhC) gives advice in a code of ethics which covers many areas of pharmacy practice. However, there are occasions where pharmacists are faced with dilemmas for which there is no clear course of action. For example:

- The pharmacist's religious beliefs or moral values are in conflict with what is expected of them—e.g. over-the-counter sale of emergency hormonal contraception.
- There is no clear scientific or evidence-based treatment available—e.g. use of unlicensed or experimental treatments.
- Business or economic issues clash with patient or public interests.

Ethical decision-making attempts to deal with these dilemmas using the following considerations:

- The values or beliefs that lie behind the dilemmas.
- The reasons people give for making a moral choice.
- Duty of care—to the patient, to their family, and to other healthcare professionals or yourself.
- Medical law.

In many instances, there is not a right or wrong answer and different people might make different—but equally justifiable—decisions based on the same set of circumstances.

It is best not to attempt to deal with ethical dilemmas alone. Depending on the situation, it is advisable to discuss the situation with the following people:

- A colleague
- The multidisciplinary team
- Other interested parties, such as management, patient advocates, religious leaders or legal advisers.

Consider the following points:
- What are the patient's wishes? It is good to ask yourself 'Do I know what the patient really wants?'
- What do the patient's relatives or representatives think? Are they adequately informed to make a decision? Do they have the patient's best interests at heart? (Remember that you need to have the patient's permission to discuss the situation with their family.)
- Would you be willing for a member of your own family to be subject to the same decision-making process?
- Could the decision made in this situation adversely affect the treatment of other patients?
- Do issues of public health or interest outweigh the patient's rights?
- Is the decision or course of action legally defensible?
- Is the decision just and fair—e.g. are scarce resources being used appropriately?

It is also important to remember the following points:
- 'Do no harm' is a good basic principle, but sometimes some 'harm' must be done to achieve a greater individual or public good.
- Ensuring patient health should include mental and spiritual health in addition to physical health.
- Acting with compassion is not necessarily the same as acting ethically.
- Slavishly following scientific or evidence-based decision-making could lead to a morally inappropriate action (or lack of action).

Financial reports and budget statements

On the basis of data provided from pharmacy computer systems, pharmacists often take responsibility for providing financial information to their clinical area. Reports are generally monthly or quarterly. At the end of the financial year, an annual finance report is usually produced. Reports are usually sent to the finance manager, clinical director, and manager of a clinical area.

The objectives of a financial report are as follows:
- Relevant and timely information.
- Easy to understand and concise information.
- Verifiable and complete numbers.
- Format enables comparison.
- Reporting is consistent in form and content.
- Reports are adequate for the audience.
- Reports are periodic.
- Data are inclusive, analytical, and comparative.
- Assumptions are attached.

Financial reports should include the following elements:
- Statistical data.
- Financial data.
- Current month.
- Actual versus budgeted.

The type of financial information that a pharmacist supplies is as follows:
- Overall drug expenditure for a financial year by month or quarter.
- Actual drug expenditure to date.
- Projected expenditure for the current financial year and the next financial year.
- Comparison of expenditure with that of the previous financial year (e.g. by month, quarter, or year).
- Analysis of expenditure by clinical areas, in-patient/out-patient/take-home medication.
- The top 20–50 high-expenditure drugs by month, quarter, or year.
- High-expenditure therapeutic areas for a specified period of time (e.g. month, quarter, or year).
- Explanation of any areas of unexpected high expenditure.
- Interpretation of financial information, detailing areas where cost savings can be made.
- Detail where cost savings have already been achieved.
- Interpretation of changes in expenditure or drug use.
- Exceptions to previous trends.

This information can be portrayed in tabular or graphical form but should be presented in ways that are easy to interpret and include a commentary. It is helpful to determine what the recipient actually wants in the report before providing financial reports.

Hospital budget statements

- The finance department often produces budget statements, which it is useful for pharmacists to understand.
- The financial year in the UK NHS runs from April 1 to March 31.
- The budget statement reflects the budget that is available and the financial position at a point in a financial year.
- These budget statements include salary (pay), non-salary (non-pay), and income budgets for a department or group of departments.
- Drug budgets are included in the non-salary budget.
- The drug budget expenditure is based on the cost of drugs issued by pharmacy.
- Budget statements usually include the following information for each of the budgets:
  - The total annual budget.
  - The budget available for the year to date.
  - The actual budget spent for the year to date.
  - The difference between the available budget and the actual budget spent (variance).
  - The percentage of budget spent to date.
  - The forecast spend for the financial year.
  - Total financial position.
- If a budget is overspent, it is usually represented as a positive number.
- If a budget is underspent, it is usually represented as a negative number.
- Finance department budget statements should be linked to financial reports prepared by pharmacy staff (see ➔ 'Financial reports and budget statements', p. 75).
- Pharmacists might be asked for a breakdown of drug expenditure information.

Writing reports

Pharmacists can be required to write reports on a variety of subjects, such as the following:
- Drug expenditure analysis
- Evaluation of a new drug
- Proposal for a new project.

A well-written and well-presented report is more likely to be read and acted on than something that is messy and incoherent. Much of the guidance given here also applies to writing business letters, e-mails, and memos (Box 4.2).

Define the aim
- What is the purpose of the report and what are you trying to achieve? Is it simply to inform the reader or is some course of action expected as a result of the report?
- Use a title that describes the aim or the content. As appropriate, write aims and objectives:
  - Aims describe what you intend to do.
  - Objectives describe how you intend to achieve the aims.

Content
The content should all be relevant to the title/aims. Look through your notes and delete any unnecessary material.
- Ensure that the content is appropriate to the readership:
  - Who are the readers?
  - What do they already know about the subject?
  - How much time will they have to read the report?
  - Might they have certain expectations of the report or preconceptions about the subject?
  - Why are you submitting this report to them?
- What type of information will you be including and how is this best presented?
  - Drug expenditure report—graphs and tables.
  - Review of papers—predominantly text.

Review the information and classify it under headings or sections, following the suggested structure and the rules:
- Headings should follow a logical sequence:
  - Problem/Cause/Solution
  - Chronological Order
  - Priority—By Urgency Or Need
  - Drug review—follow *BNF* headings, i.e. drug, indications, contraindications, and cautions.
- Headings should clearly tell the reader what that section is about.
- Ideally, the maximum number of items in a section is seven; otherwise there is too much information for the reader to take in at once. If necessary, subdivide sections.
- Ensure that the content of each section is relevant to the heading.
- Try not to repeat information in different sections.

Box 4.2 Report structure

The following is a suggested structure. Depending on the type of report, the structure can vary.

- Title
- Identification
- Your name, department and contact details, and the date
- Distribution
- It might be helpful to list the following:
  - Those who need to take action.
  - Those for whom the report is for information only.
- Contents
- Aims and objectives
- Summary or abstract
- Introduction:
  - Provides the background and context of the report
  - Explains why the report was written
  - Gives the terms of reference
- Method/procedure:
  - There should be sufficient information for the reader to under-stand what you did, without giving every detail
- Results/findings
- Discussion
- The main body of the report; use section headings here
- Conclusions
- A re-statement of the main findings:
  - Includes recommendations or proposals for future work
- References:
  - Use a standard system, such as the Harvard style—i.e. author, date in brackets, title of the article, journal title, volume and page numbers
- Appendices:
  - These should include information that informs the reader but not essential on the first reading
- Glossary:
  - Explain any unusual or scientific terms or unavoidable jargon
- Footnotes:
  - Author name, date of preparation, review date, and page numbers.

Layout

Even a well-written report with good content can be overlooked if it is difficult to read. A large amount of type crowded on to a page is difficult to read and the eye soon becomes tired.

- Leave wide margins at both sides and ample space at the top and bottom of each page. This also gives the reader space to write notes and ensures that print on the left-hand side doesn't disappear into the binding.
- Avoid left and right justification. Left justifying creates spaces in the text, which is easier on the eye.
- Use 1.5 or double spacing.

Bullet points and numbering

Putting information into lists using bullet points or numbering has the following benefits:

• Makes it easier to read.
• Has more impact.
• Cuts the number of words (and waffle).

Most word processing programs offer a selection of bullet points. Keep things simple and only use one or two different types of bullet in your report.

Use a straightforward numbering system (e.g. 1, 1.1, 1.2, 1.2.1) and avoid over-numbering (e.g. 1.2.1.1.1!).

Font

Use a font that is clear and easy to read. Use fonts without serifs ('sans serif'; e.g. Arial) and use a 12-point font size for the majority of the text e.g. Gill Sans MT, 12 point is easier to read than Times New Roman, 12 point or Gill Sans MT, 10 point.

Avoid using capitals or underlining to highlight text: **bold** is easier to read than CAPITALS or <u>underlining</u>. People with poor literacy skills find upper-case text especially difficult to read.

For a lesson in how font style and layout affects ease of reading, compare the *Sun* newspaper with *The Times*!

Paragraphs

A paragraph should cover only one point or argument. As a rule, it should be about seven or eight lines long, and certainly no longer than 10 lines. The most important information should be in the first or last sentence of the paragraph.

Charts and tables

These should be used to convey information, usually of numerical origin, which might be too complex to describe in words. However, overuse or inappropriate use can divert the reader from the main message, making your work confusing. When deciding whether to use a chart or table consider the following points:

• Will it save words?
• Will it clarify things for the reader?
• Is the information to be presented quantifiable in some way?
• Will it help the reader to make comparisons?
• Will it help to illustrate a specific point?

In general, bar charts are the simplest charts to produce and suit most data. They are easier to interpret and less prone to be misleading than pie charts, graphs, or pictograms. When using charts, consider the following points:

• Give the chart a title.
• Make sure that bars or axes start at zero.
• If comparing two charts, the axes should have the same scale.
• Label axes and bars.
• Show actual amounts on bars and pie chart slices.
• Use only two-dimensional versions—three-dimensional bars and slices can distort the relative proportions.
• Avoid overuse of colour or hatching, which might not reproduce clearly.
• Keep it simple!

Language

- Keep language simple and to the point.
- Avoid long sentences.
- Avoid foreign language phrases—e.g. *ad hoc* and *pro rata*.
- Use active rather than passive sentences—'Use paracetamol regularly for pain' is preferable to 'Paracetamol is to be used regularly for pain'.
- Avoid double negatives as these can cause confusion—'Paracetamol is not incompatible with breastfeeding' could easily be misinterpreted as 'Paracetamol is not compatible with breastfeeding'.
- Only use common abbreviations, such as 'e.g.', without explanation. Where you wish to use an abbreviation, write in full the first time, followed by the abbreviation—e.g. Royal Pharmaceutical Society (RPS). Thereafter, the abbreviation can be used.
- Avoid jargon and clichés.

Revision and editing

As much as 50% of the time spent writing a report should be devoted to revision and editing (Box 4.3):

- Print the report and check for spelling mistakes and other obvious errors (do not just rely on computer spelling and grammar checks).
- Check punctuation.
- Work through the report using the editing checklist and revise as necessary.
- Ask a colleague to read the report and make comments. Check that they interpret the information as you intended.

Box 4.3 Editing checklist

Aim

- Is the aim clear?
- Is the content at the right level for the reader?
- If action is required as a result of the report, is this clear?

Content

- Is the structure logical?
- Do the conclusions follow the argument?
- Are numerical data accurate and clearly presented?
- Do graphs and tables achieve their aim?
- Have you quoted references and sources appropriately?

Language

- Are paragraphs the right length?
- Have unnecessary words, double negatives, clichés, and jargon been avoided?
- Are spelling and punctuation correct?

Presentation

- Are abbreviations and symbols explained and used consistently throughout?
- Do page breaks fall at natural breaks in the text?
- Are page numbers and footers etc. included, as needed?
- Does any of the text get lost on printing?
- Does the whole report look tidy and professional?

Managing meetings

To manage meetings efficiently, get the best results, and use time effectively, follow the tips:

- Ensure that the agenda is understood in advance. Circulate a written agenda at least a week before the meeting, including the following points for each item to be discussed:
  - Topic
  - Duration
  - Responsibility.
- Circulate any necessary or pertinent materials to be read before the meeting.
- The meeting should have a chairperson who must ensure that it runs smoothly and to time, allowing all participants to be involved.
- Be clear with the participants why the meeting is being held and what it will achieve.
- Ensure that at least two-thirds of the participants have a role in every topic on the agenda. Consider rearranging the agenda so that people do not waste time listening to a topic in which they have no active interest.
- Be clear what preparation is required in advance of the meeting.
- Always start and finish on time.
- Discourage deviations from the agenda and tangential topic discussions.
- Discourage AOB (any other business).
- Consider using a flip chart and record actions on it for all to see.
- Try to ensure that individuals record their actions in their diaries before leaving, and do not wait for the arrival of the 'minutes'.
- Minute-taking depends on the culture of the organization. The material to be recorded, how and by whom it is recorded, may vary between meetings and institutions.
- Minutes should be circulated as soon as possible after the meeting, ideally delaying no longer than 2wks.
- Do not hold meetings that are only for information. Minimize the use of meetings just to distribute information that could be circulated electronically.

Confidentiality

Pharmacists and pharmacy staff are expected to maintain the confidentiality of any patient or customer they have contact with during the course of their professional duties. Information that should remain confidential includes the following:

- Patient's identity and address
- Diagnosis
- Details of prescribed and non-prescribed medicines.

Pharmacists must also ensure that any written or electronic patient information is stored and disposed of securely and that electronic systems are password protected.

To avoid unintentional disclosure, it is important to develop good habits when dealing with patient information:

- Discussing a patient with colleagues is often necessary for patient care or training purposes, but be cautious about revealing names or other patient identifiers.
- Do not discuss patients in public areas—e.g. the lifts or the front of the shop.
- If talking about your work to family or friends, only talk about patients in very general terms.
- Ensure that written information (e.g. patient handover lists and prescriptions) is not left lying where other patients or the public can see it.
- If discussing medication with a patient, try to do this in a reasonably private area. If hospital in-patients have visitors, ask if the patient would like you to return when they have gone.
- Ensure that computers have passwords and always log off at the end of a session.

Remember that information that is not necessarily directly patient related may also be confidential or sensitive and should not be shared with others (e.g. drug costs, media-worthy information, etc.).

Disclosure of information

Sharing of confidential information with other healthcare professionals is often necessary for patient care. However, patients have the right to know that information about them is being shared with colleagues and have the right to refuse that information is disclosed. Frequently, consent to disclose information is taken as implicit—e.g. sending a discharge summary to the patient's GP. However, if the information is potentially sensitive, the patient's formal consent must be sought.

In certain situations, pharmacists might have to disclose confidential information without consent and to non-healthcare professionals. The UK pharmacy code of ethics allows this in the following circumstances:

- With patient consent or parent/guardian/carer consent for a child. Information about adolescent patients should not normally be revealed without their consent.
- If required by law or statute.
- If necessary to prevent serious injury or damage to the health of the patient, a third party, or the public health.

Confidentiality when a friend, relative, or colleague is a patient

- Pharmacists and pharmacy staff can be put in a difficult position in this situation, especially if others know that the patient is in their care. Well-meaning questions about the patient's welfare might be difficult to deal with without causing offence.
- Explain to the patient what level of involvement you have in their care and that you would have access to their medical notes. Ask whether they would prefer that another pharmacist deals with their care (although this might not always be feasible).
- If at all possible, discuss the situation with the patient and ask what they would like you to do if friends, family, or colleagues are enquiring about them.
- If the patient is unwilling for you to reveal any information, or if you are unable to discuss this with the patient, any enquiries should be dealt with by politely explaining that you cannot provide information about the patient. Bear in mind, however, that simply making this statement potentially discloses the fact that the individual is known to you as a patient.
- Try to avoid compromising your integrity by denying all knowledge of the patient, but in some situations this might be necessary.
- Inform the medical team that the patient is known to you socially.
- Personal information known to you because of your relationship to the patient should not be revealed to medical or nursing colleagues without the patient's consent.
- The patient might use your relationship to ask you to provide medical information that you would not normally reveal. Provide only the same information as you would to any other patient.
- If a colleague is a patient, be especially sensitive to any aspect of care that could breach confidentiality. As appropriate, you might need to consider the following:
  - Avoid writing your colleague's name on ward order sheets.
  - Use an agreed alias for labelling of medicines.
  - Label, dispense, and deliver medicines yourself.
  - Keep any written records separate from those to which other pharmacy staff have access.

Further reading

Advice on disclosure of information if necessary to protect children and vulnerable adults: ℘ www. pharmaceutical-journal.com/libres/pdf/society/pj_20050806_childprotectionguidance.pdf

Department of Health (2003). 'Confidentiality: NHS Code of Practice', ℘ www.gov.uk/government/uploads/system/uploads/attachment_data/file/200146/Confidentiality_-_NHS_Code_of_Practice.pdf

Assertiveness

Assertiveness is an essential skill that can be learnt, developed, and practised. Applying assertive strategies enables you to stand up for yourself and express yourself appropriately and constructively.

Definition of assertiveness

- Expressing thoughts, feelings, and beliefs in a direct, honest, and appropriate way.
- Having respect for yourself and others.
- Relating well to people.
- Expressing your needs freely.
- Taking responsibility for your feelings.
- Standing up for yourself if necessary.
- Working towards a 'win–win' solution to problems.
- Ensuring that both parties have their needs met as much as possible.

Assertive people effectively influence, listen, and negotiate so that others choose to cooperate willingly. Assertiveness promotes self-confidence, self-control, and feelings of positive self-worth, and it is the most effective means for solving interpersonal problems.

Assertive behaviour

- When you differ in opinion with someone you respect, you can speak up and share your own viewpoint.
- You stand up for your rights or those of others no matter what the circumstances.
- You have the ability to correct the situation when your rights or those of others are violated.
- You can refuse unreasonable requests made by friends or co-workers.
- You can accept positive criticism and suggestion.
- You ask for assistance when you need it.
- You have confidence in your own judgement.
- If someone else has a better solution, you accept it easily.
- You express your thoughts, feelings, and beliefs in a direct and honest way.
- You try to work for a solution that, as much as possible, benefits all parties.
- You interact in a mature manner with those who are offensive, defensive, aggressive, hostile, blaming, attacking, or otherwise unreceptive.

Non-assertive behaviour

- Aggressive behaviour involves a person trying to impose their views inappropriately on others. It can be accompanied by threatening language and an angry glaring expression, and communicates an impression of disrespect.
- Submissive behaviour is the opposite of aggressive behaviour. The person plays down their own needs and is willing to fit in with the wishes of others to keep the peace. It shows a lack of respect for the

person's own needs and communicates a message of inferiority. It can be accompanied by passivity, nervousness, and lack of eye contact.
- Manipulative behaviour occurs when a person seeks to ingratiate themselves with another through flattery and other forms of deceit. It can be accompanied by over-attention and a simpering smarmy voice.

Strategies for behaving more assertively
- Identify your personal rights, wants, and needs.
- Use 'I' messages to give people complete information to address a problem. 'I' messages are assertions about the feelings, beliefs, and values of the person speaking, and the sentences used begin with 'I'. The 'I' messages should include three parts:
  - Behaviour—what it is that the other person has done or is doing?
  - Effect—what is happening because of their behaviour?
  - Feelings—what effect does their behaviour have on your feelings?
- Be direct and express your request succinctly.
- Choose assertive words.
- Use factual descriptions.
- Avoid exaggerations.
- Express thoughts, feelings, and opinions reflecting ownership.
- Convey a positive assertive attitude using the following communication techniques:
  - Maintain good eye contact.
  - Maintain a firm, factual, but pleasant, voice.
  - Pay attention to your posture and gestures.
  - Stand or sit erect, possibly leaning forwards slightly, at a normal conversational distance.
  - Use relaxed conversational gestures.
  - Listen, to let people know that you have heard what they said.
  - Ask questions for clarification.
  - Look for a win–win approach to problem-solving.
  - Ask for feedback.
- Evaluate your expectations and be willing to compromise.

Examples of assertive language
- I am …
- I think we should …
- I feel bad when …
- That seems unfair to me.
- Can you help me with this?
- I appreciate your help.

Communication skills

Communication is a key skill for pharmacists. Every day pharmacists communicate with a variety of different groups:

- Patients/customers
- Other healthcare professionals
- Drug company representatives
- Managerial staff.

Depending on the audience and circumstances, a different approach might be required, but the core skills are the same (Boxes 4.4 and 4.5).

Planning and preparation

Before any encounter, a certain amount of planning and preparation is required, even if it is just a few words with a counter assistant to establish a customer's requirements:

- Establish the most appropriate means of communication—this might be written, in the form of a letter, email, leaflet, or verbal, such as a conversation, seminar or oral presentation, or both.
- Know the subject—if necessary, do some background reading or research. Even if it means keeping a customer waiting, a quick look in the *BNF* could mean that ultimately your message is accepted more readily because it is well informed.
- Know the audience—understanding their background, knowledge base, and requirements aids effective communication. Communicating with one person requires different strategies compared with communicating with a small or large group.
- Prepare the message—a simple straightforward piece of information, such as dosage instructions, requires little, if any, preparation. However, a more complex message, such as the answer to a medicines information enquiry, might require some preparation:
  - Be clear in your own mind about what message or messages you want to get across.
  - Break the message down into a series of points.
  - Structure the message so that ideas are presented in order of importance.
  - Provide a one- or two-sentence summary/conclusion at the end.
- Think ahead—try to anticipate any questions that might arise and be prepared with the information needed to answer them.
- Use email carefully as it is easy for messages to be forwarded and misunderstood

Delivering the message

Whether communicating in writing or verbally, the same rules apply:

- Use language appropriate to the audience—avoid jargon and complex terms, and use simple direct words.
- Avoid vague terms, e.g. 'occasionally' or 'frequently', because these might mean different things to different people.
- Check understanding by asking for feedback or questions.

Remember that verbal communication is made up of three aspects:
- 55% body language
- 38% tone of voice
- 7% words that make up the communication.

Listening skills

An essential part of communication is listening (see Box 4.6). Not only does this ensure your own understanding, but it shows interest and concern and empowers the respondent by enabling them to participate fully in the communication process. The traditional active/passive roles of healthcare professional talking and patient listening, respectively, are not conducive to good communication. Good listening (by both parties) ensures that the encounter has the mutual participation of healthcare professional and patient, and fits with the current patient-centred care model. This should lead to the information elicited being of more value; any message is more likely to be remembered and acted upon.

- Reflecting back—clarify your understanding by repeating back ('mirroring') information, but in paraphrase.
- Summarizing—'What I think I hear you saying is …'.
- Body language:
  - Use facial expressions and postures to show empathy.
  - Mirror facial expression.
  - Nod encouragingly.
  - Adopt a listening posture—as appropriate, lean towards the speaker while being careful to avoid invading their personal space.
  - Maintain eye contact.
  - Avoid signs of impatience or being in a hurry.
- Ask open-ended questions—e.g. how and why.
- Use closed questions, as appropriate–i.e. those with a 'yes' or 'no' response.
- Use silences appropriately:
  - Allow the speaker to finish what they want to say and avoid the temptation to jump in.
  - Do not interrupt or finish the speaker's sentences.
  - If necessary, allow a short period of silence to elapse, especially if the speaker is slow or hesitant in their speech.
  - Silences can be helpful in giving thinking time.
- Use verbal or non-verbal signals to show that you are listening and encourage the speaker—e.g. nodding and saying 'yes' or 'mm'.
- If necessary, note down key points while the other person is speaking, but avoid scribbling throughout. Warn the speaker that you will be doing this so that they don't find it off-putting.
- In responding, avoid the following:
  - Exclamations of surprise, intolerance, or disgust.
  - Expression of over-concern.
  - Moralistic judgements, criticism, or impatience.
  - Being defensive and getting caught up in arguments.
  - Making false promises, flattery, or undue praise.
  - Personal references to your own difficulties.
  - Changing the subject or interrupting unnecessarily.
  - Speaking too soon, too often, or for too long.

Questioning

Questioning is also an important skill for communicating effectively. As pharmacists, this often involves direct questioning of a colleague regarding a course of action or prescribing decision. However, when dealing with patients, a broader approach might be required to obtain all the information required:

• Use open questions to enable the respondent to elaborate and give new information—e.g. 'How are you getting on with your medications?'.
• Phrasing questions in different ways often elicits different information—e.g. asking 'Do you have any problems with your medicines?' can elicit more information than asking 'Do you have any side effects?'.
• Avoid leading questions, e.g. 'You're not getting any side effects are you?', because usually the respondent will give the answer that they think the questioner wants (in this case, 'No').
• Closed questions can be used to establish specific information—e.g. 'Are you taking this medicine with food?'.
• Be specific because the respondent might interpret certain terms differently to you—e.g. 'Are you taking these medicines regularly?' could mean the respondent is taking them once daily, once weekly, or once monthly!
• Avoid questions that the respondent might interpret as being judgemental or critical.
• As appropriate, ensure that you understand the answer by paraphrasing it back to the respondent—e.g. 'Just to be clear, I think you are saying …'.

Box 4.4 Barriers to good communication

Physical barriers
• Speech problems
• Hearing impairment
• Communicating in a language that is not the audience's first language or through a translator
• Visual impairment
• Learning difficulties
• Noisy or distracting environment.

Emotional barriers
• Preconceptions and prejudice
• Fear
• Aggression.

Box 4.5 Checklist of essential interpersonal skills to improve communication

- Body language:
  - Be aware of body language when interacting with people
  - Mirror body language
  - Ensure that body language, tone, and words are sending out the same messages
- Rapport with people
- Social poise, self-assurance, and confidence
- Tact and diplomacy
- Consideration of others
- Assertiveness and self-control
- High standards
- Ability to analyse facts and solve problems
- Tolerance and patience
- Ability to make good decisions
- Honesty and objectivity
- Organizational skills
- Good listening habits
- Enthusiasm
- Persuasiveness
- Ability to communicate with different types of people.

Box 4.6 Ten ways to become a better listener

- Schedule a time and place to listen
- Create comfort
- Avoid distractions
- State the reasons for the conversation
- Use non-verbal signals
- Use reflection, paraphrasing, and summarizing
- Listen for the message behind the emotions
- Be patient
- Write down any commitments
- Follow up.

Oral presentation skills

Pharmacists often make presentations to a variety of audiences. These can be both formal and informal. Some suggestions on how to prepare and effectively deliver an oral presentation include the following:

- Know the expected duration of the presentation.
- Know the composition and experience of the audience.
- Know the format—e.g. workshop or formal presentation.
- Know about the facilities—e.g. availability of audiovisual aids.
- Prepare approximately one slide per 1–2min of presentation.
- Find out whether you are expected to supply handouts to the audience, how many, and what level they should be aimed at.
- Check whether you are expected to send the presentation slides in advance, and, if so, the timelines for this.
- Plan and prepare your presentation.
- A presentation usually consists of three parts:
  - Tell the audience what you are going to talk about.
  - Talk about it.
  - Tell the audience what you told them.
- Always take a back-up option for the presentation—have the presentation saved on more than one USB stick and take a paper copy to refer to if the technology fails.
- Arrive at the presentation in plenty of time to ensure that the equipment can be tested or your presentation can be downloaded.
- Familiarize yourself with the venue and the equipment available—e.g. pointer or computer equipment.
- Ensure that you are not blocking the audience's view of your slides from where you are standing.
- Check that your slides are in focus.
- Look at the audience and *not* the screen!
- Make sure you look at *all* of the audience, so that they all feel included.
- Minimize how much you move around.
- Ensure that the audience can hear you.
- Introduce yourself, why you are presenting, and your background experience to the subject.
- Use a pointer to highlight points of data; avoid overuse and excessive circling.
- Involve the audience by asking questions or for input, as appropriate.
- Ask if the audience have any questions. Depending on the time and format, invite questions during the presentation and/or at the end.
- When responding to questions, consider repeating the question asked so that all audience members can hear the question and response, and to ensure that the question was understood.

Time management and prioritization

Pharmacists can be called upon to undertake a variety of tasks. Time has to be managed effectively to prioritize work and to complete tasks in a timely manner.

Quick techniques for managing time include the following:
- The four Rs of paperwork:
  - Recycle (bin)
  - Refer (out-tray and delegation)
  - Respond
  - Record (file).
- Invest time, don't spend it.
- De-clutter.
- Use a system for time management:
  - Use a list system to write down ideas, thoughts, and tasks as you think of them.
  - Use a diary system.
  - Use a name and address system.
  - Bracket tasks, appointments, and travel time.
  - Set time limits, with interruptions.
  - Use 'scrap time' wisely.
  - Take frequent quick breaks to ↑ productivity.
  - Do the most important tasks first.
  - Or, do the fastest and easiest tasks first.
  - Demand completed work from your staff.
  - Communicate upwards when you have problems:
    —Description of problem
    —List of possible solutions
    —Recommended solution
    —List of necessary resources
    —Implementation of the solution.

The ability to understand the priorities of others and to prioritize your own work is a very important skill to learn. Some tips on prioritizing:
- When deciding the priority of a particular task, consider both its importance (is it worth doing?) and its urgency (does it need to be done right now?).
- Fig. 4.1 shows a useful tool for prioritizing your work—write tasks in the boxes according to whether they fit the labels:
  - Urgent and important tasks take first priority.
  - Important tasks that are not urgent take second priority.
  - Unimportant tasks that are also not urgent take lowest priority.
- When deciding whether to do a particular task, consider the number of people it affects and the cost of undertaking the task.
- Numbered daily checklists are often helpful.

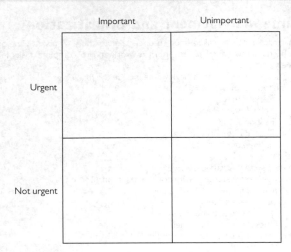

Fig. 4.1 Tool for prioritizing work—write tasks in the boxes according to where they fit the labels.

- To understand the priorities of others requires excellent communication skills, especially the ability to ask good-quality questions, listen to the answers, and notice body language.
- Knowing where your plan fits into the plans of others is useful in predicting problems, solving problems, and influencing solutions.
- Knowing where your plan fits in your own organization's priorities ensures access to and release of resources.

Project planning

The purpose of a project plan is to determine and facilitate the achievement of a set of objectives, i.e. achievement of milestone objectives en route to achievement of goal objectives. Planning is done in the context of the stated mission of the organization and the vision of the organization. Planning is about the following:

- Ensuring that every individual involved knows what to do, when, how, where, and why.
- Communicating the plans to those who need to be confident that the ambitions will be delivered to the specification required, on time, and within budget.
- Forecasting what might occur in order that action can be taken to achieve the desired goal and avoid undesirable outcomes.
- Making decisions about actions that will be taken prior to and during anticipated situations.

A project plan needs to be broken down into tasks that need to be done, and then sequencing the tasks in a logical order. Tasks are actions. Accurate identification of the tasks is essential as they are the basis of:

- developing schedules
- identifying milestones
- implementing change plans
- planning communication
- resource planning: manpower, materials, and machinery
- monitoring
- maintaining records
- managing risk
- measuring progress
- forecasting remaining work.

It can be useful to complete a one-page summary of each task that contains all the information needed to delegate the responsibility for completion of the task to one person, as each task is effectively a 'mini-project'.

The quickest and most effective way to produce outline plans is to do it in five phases:

- Describe the scope of the project.
- Identify the tasks.
- Schedule the tasks into a sensible order that will achieve the outcome of the plan.
- Identify milestones. Milestones are the significant objectives that are to be achieved on the way to completing the project, and serve as visible indications of progress. They enable people to know that the plan is being implemented without having to know the details.
- Implement the plan.

When scoping the project, the questions to be considered are as follows:

- Obtain a simple description.
- Why it is being considered?
- Where does it fit with other projects?

- What are the benefits to the organization?
- What are the downsides or penalties of not doing it?
- What are the major issues?
- What are the risks?
- What are the measures of success?
- What is the return on investment? Obtain a summary for this.
- What are the names of key stakeholders and stakeholder groups?
- Get an indication of whether to invest resources in a project plan.

Software is available to help with project planning and the production of time flowcharts (Gantt charts).

Using Medicines Information services

The Medicines Information (UKMI) service is an NHS countrywide network comprising of one national (Wales), 14 regional, and 220 local MI centres. Local services range from one pharmacist, providing information part-time, to a large centre, with pharmacists, technicians, and administrative staff. Most MI centres provide an information service to hospital-based and community-based enquirers, including members of the public, but some only answer enquiries from within their NHS trust. For both community pharmacists and hospital pharmacists, it is a good idea to check who provides the MI service for your area.

Some centres provide a specialist information service (Table 4.3) but it is usually advisable to contact your local service first. Remember to contact local specialists as well, because advice from another centre might not reflect local practice.

Before contacting your MI centre with an enquiry, do some basic research. Most MI centres expect pharmacist colleagues to have checked basic sources before contacting them—e.g. *BNF*, SPCs, and *Martindale*. Before contacting the MI centre, try to anticipate what background information they might require and have this ready. Depending on the type of enquiry, this might include the following:

- Drug details, including dose, route, formulation, brand, and indication.
- Patient details, including underlying condition, relevant laboratory results, age, weight, and past medical history.
- The identity of the original enquirer.
- Urgency.
- Contact details.
- Whether a written or verbal response is required.
- Any sources already checked for information and what was found.
- ADRs—nature of reaction, timing of the event, other drugs, any de-challenge/re-challenge and the outcome.

Table 4.3 UKMI specialist information centres

Specialist topic	Centre
Drugs in pregnancy	Regional Drugs and Therapeutics Centre (Newcastle)
Drugs in lactation	Trent and West Midlands MIC
Drugs in dentistry	North West MIC
Drugs in renal disease	South West MIC
Alternative medicine/ drugs in porphyria	Welsh MIC
Drugs in oncology	Royal Marsden Hospital MIC
Drugs in psychiatry	Pharmacy Department, Maudsley Hospital
Toxicology and poisoning (not emergency enquiries)	Regional Medicines and Poisons Information Centre, Northern Ireland

Contact details are on the UKMI website: ℘ www.ukmi.nhs.uk

- Pregnancy—number of weeks of gestation, whether or not the drug has already been taken by the mother, and indication.
- Breastfeeding—age, weight, medical status of infant, and whether the treatment is short or long term.
- Drug interactions—which drugs/drug classes are involved and the nature of the event, if a suspected interaction has already occurred.

After the enquiry is complete, it is really helpful if you feed back the outcome to your MI centre. It is rare that they hear what happened as a result of the answer given, and it is useful information to add to their enquiry records. Remember to fill in a yellow card for any significant ADRs and all ADRs occurring with 'black triangle' medicines (see ➔ 'Reporting ADRs', p. 22).

Further reading
NICE. 'Evidence search' website, ℬ www.evidence.nhs.uk
'UK Medicines Information' website, ℬ www.ukmi.nhs.uk

On call/residency

Description

- The provision of a clinical pharmacy service outside normal working hours; to support safe and cost-effective prescribing of time-critical and take-home medicines.
- It is the duty of the resident/on-call pharmacist to prioritize, clinically screen, and supply clinically appropriate time-critical medicines to patients in secondary care. The role involves answering medical/pharmaceutical questions and dispensary management.

Awareness of the environment

Distractions that require action include the following:
- Telephone calls
- Bleeps/radio-page
- Medical/nursing staff at the pharmacy hatch
- Fridge alarms
- Pharmacy colleagues requesting advice
- Doorbells.

Prioritization

- Does the request relate to a time-critical medicine?
- When is the dose due?
- Is it safe?
- It is easy to get carried away with the possible outcomes associated with supplying one prescription medicine before another; it is therefore important to look at your list of tasks broadly. The first question to ask when prioritizing is '*When is this request needed for*'. If you fail to identify the specific time that the task needs to be completed by, it is impossible to appropriately prioritize requests.
- It is frequently the case that a resident pharmacist will have two to three competing requests that are required in the same time frame. When this scenario presents itself it is *then* important to think about the implications of completing one task above another.
- In the case of drug supply, in the UK the NPSA's 'Rapid Response Report' from February 2011 recommends that all hospitals have a local guideline on time-critical medicines. This guideline can be a useful decision tool in this situation.
- Having clinical conversations with medical and nursing staff regarding the pharmaceutical advice or prescription requested will help to identify the true urgency of the request.

Staff management and delegation

- Clinical issues are best dealt with by a pharmacist while system errors, work process issues, and dispensing can be suitably dealt with by a pharmacy technician.
- Most NHS trusts that provide an on-call/residency service also have senior on-call pharmacists who can be utilized for specialist clinical and higher-level decisions.

- Delegate highly specialized clinical questions to a senior pharmacist if available. Spending long periods of time trying to solve a complex question is not efficient in a busy environment when a senior colleague may easily know the answer.

Most useful resources

- Local/national guidelines—e.g. NICE, Department of Health, SIGN, *BNF*
- Local Medicines Information database (e.g. MI database)
- Trust/national IV drug monographs
- Newt Guide/Handbook of drug administration
- SPCs
- Trust subscribed resources (e.g. Up-to-Date®).

Recording calls out of hours

- It is important to keep records of the calls received out of hours to audit and justify the service.
- This lends itself to service improvement—highlighting the busiest working periods and identifying trends that may need to be addressed, e.g. frequent advice about particular medicines, may highlight a learning need for ward staff.

Skills developed

- The pharmacist on-call bleep/radio-page has been described by switchboard staff as the busiest bleep/radio-page in a hospital.
- The role of resident pharmacist can therefore be daunting, but brings with it a wealth of experience and skills, performed under intense pressure.
- Skills such as problem-solving, efficiency, time/personnel management, and most importantly prioritization form a great base for a career as a clinical pharmacist and are highly sought after by employers in all sectors.

Tips for working on call

Supply options

When a request for a time-critical medicine is received out of hours and the resident is not in a position to dispense the item, the following could be considered:

- Emergency drug cupboard.
- Borrow from a ward holding the medicine as stock.
- Has a supply of this medicine been issued to another patient on a nearby ward?
- Has the patient brought a supply into hospital with them?
- Where does the patient live? Could a relative bring the medication in from home?
- Is the drug non-formulary? Is there a local therapeutic substitution guideline which allows for the substitution of the unavailable medicine?
- Is the medication on a local 'Rarely used medicine guide' highlighting a local trust that may stock the product?

Wholesale supply outward
- When asked to supply to a community pharmacy or another hospital, first establish if you have available stock. If so, prioritize the task as usual, however it must be understood that local trust patients are your first priority.
- A written request from a registered pharmacist, with their name, registration number, product details, on company-headed paper is required. The pharmacy purchasing department must be informed, and they can sort out the remaining details during normal working hours.

Wholesale supply inward
- If you require an unusual medicine that is not in stock, suggest changing to an alternative product. Some hospitals have therapeutic substitution lists which allow you to substitute non-formulary medicines for their formulary equivalents.
- If it is a rarely used medicine then check your area's 'rarely used medicine' list. This document will identify which hospitals keep which rarely used medicines. If you do not have access to a 'rarely used medicines' list then contact the on-call pharmacy service at the nearest large NHS teaching hospital. Speak to the on-call pharmacist and ask if they have the medicine available.
- Fax a request to the supplier on headed paper describing the product details, your name, pharmacist registration number, hospital name and address. If you struggle to find a hospital stocking the medicine, you are required to speak to the senior on-call pharmacist.

Medical staff
When alone it is important to avoid answering every question you are asked or to supply against every prescription that is presented to you. Occasionally junior doctors will be hesitant to ask their registrar or consultant clinical medical questions, and instead opt to ask the on-call pharmacist. Please refer junior doctors to their medical team for questions that are unsuitable for a clinical pharmacist to advise on (especially when you do not have access to clinical notes).

Nursing staff
Nurses may ask for your confirmation on prescribing issues, try to avoid feeling pressured into giving them the answer they are looking for, investigate the scenario, and establish the real issues associated with the call.

How to present a patient to another healthcare professional

Clinical pharmacists often have to give oral or written case presentations on patients they come across during their practice, to colleagues as part of postgraduate training, and beyond. They have to present patients to other healthcare professionals on a smaller scale, over the telephone and face to face on the ward, e.g. on ward rounds, in order to ensure pharmaceutical interventions are communicated to the relevant people. This is a platform to demonstrate medication expertise and an understanding of clinical therapeutics applied to the particular patient, where treatment guidelines, co-morbidities, concurrent medication, and the patient's preferences or beliefs, etc. may conflict.

It is best to follow a logical framework to ensure the relevant information is covered so that the audience can easily follow it. Table 4.4 is a suggested presentation framework. It may not be suitable for all presentations and in some cases, the order and/or selection of information may need to be altered to best present the case and interventions. When verbally presented, this can be a teaching aid for colleagues. Individually, the framework itself may help everyday practice to ensure all aspects of the patient and their presenting complaint are considered in the management plan.

Table 4.4 Presentation framework

Introduce the patient	Give their age, sex and occupation Remember to anonymize the patient
Presenting complaint (PC)	Describe the patient's symptoms that made them call an ambulance, come to A&E, be admitted to the ward, or be referred by their GP
History of presenting complaint (HPC)	Explain how long they had those particular symptoms for, and if anything made them better or worse It is also important to include relevant symptoms not experienced by the patient here
Past medical history (PMH)	Give details of any current or previous medical problems and/or surgical procedures Include detail of timing, if relevant
Family history (FH)	If appropriate, give details of immediate family history related to the case
Drug history (DHx)	This is an important section for pharmacists as this is often incomplete on admission clerking List all of the patient's currently prescribed medication, over-the-counter, herbal/alternative medications If relevant, give details of recently issued acute medications or recently stopped medications and a reason why Confirm the patient's drug allergy status. If they have allergies, explain the nature

Table 4.4 (*Contd.*)

Social history	Again, explain the patient's social history if it is relevant, e.g. lives locally with four-times-a-day carer If relevant, state how much the patient: • Smokes in pack years—(number of cigarettes smoked in a day/20) × years smoked[11] • Consumes of alcohol (usually in units per week) Also consider illicit drug-taking if appropriate
Examinations, observations	List any relevant findings: • On general observation—e.g. physical presentation of patient • Of the systems review, e.g. on cardiovascular exam—BP, HR, RR
Investigations	List relevant blood work results—e.g. FBC, LFTs, U&Es Also consider: microbiology, imaging Highlight abnormalities Explain if there are any omissions
Differential diagnoses	Explain if the clinicians are querying any alternative diagnoses If they are, what needs to be performed and the outcome for a positive diagnosis
Summarize the patient and their problem	Here is a good point to quickly summarize the information already conveyed to the audience to ensure understanding and so they can use this as point of reference for the next part of the presentation
Working diagnosis	Briefly explain the working diagnosis
Clinician's medical management plan	Briefly explain the plan outlined by the clinicians on how this patient will be managed, e.g.: • Referrals to specialists • Pharmaceutical intervention (medications being stopped/started) • Surgical intervention
Pharmaceutical issues and management plan	Highlight the presenting condition, clinical therapeutics, pharmacology and apply it to this particular patient. Pharmacists are the experts in medication and can make a valid intervention, no matter how small, in the vast majority of patients' management plans Think about: • Is the main presenting complaint being treated optimally? • Is it following appropriate guidelines? (local/national) • If there is no guideline; what is the available evidence? • Are the doses/route appropriate? • Should any changes be recommended? (If so, why?) • What are the treatment aims? • How can we tell if the presenting complaint is resolving? • How long does treatment take? • If this doesn't work, what are the alternatives? • What happens if we don't treat? Consider the risks vs benefits of treatment.

(*Continued*)

Table 4.4 (*Contd.*)

Does the patient have co-morbidities? If so, are these being managed appropriately? (see above in table)

Are there any interactions with the patient's medications, and if so, are they clinically important?

• How can we manage these?

What are the monitoring parameters?

• Of the condition itself?
• Of the initiated pharmaceutical management?
• How often does this need to be carried out? And by whom?
• What are 'normal' ranges?
• What course of action needs to be taken if outside of these ranges?

Compliance/counselling:

• How does the patient feel about taking these medications?
• What are their beliefs regarding medication?
• Can the patient take the proposed treatment?
• Will they feel any benefit? When should they feel this?
• Are they likely to develop side effects? What are these?
• Are there potential adverse effects that they need to be aware of?
• Do they need help taking their medications?

Discharge process (links to social history)

• Do they need further help at home to take their treatment?
• Where do they get further supplies from?
• Do they have/would they benefit from compliance aids, e.g. MDS, spacers for inhalers?
• Do they have carers?
• If they require further monitoring, who will do this?
• Can the pharmacist aid effective communication to the patient's GP/community pharmacy?

Note this list isn't exhaustive and it may be appropriate to present these issues in a different order, depending on the patient in question

It is worth considering which issue would be most important to the patient, the clinicians and the pharmacist. Pharmacists often have different priorities and it is important to consider what matters most to the patient. This helps to develop rapport and improve adherence, which together can considerably influence clinical outcomes for patients.

Further reading

Olaitan A, Okunade O, Corne J (2010). How to present clinical cases. *Student BMJ* 18: c1539
🔗 http://student.bmj.com/student/view-article.html?id=id:5136

Reference

11. NICE (2011). 'Chronic obstructive pulmonary disease in over 16s: diagnosis and management (CG101)' 🔗 www.nice.org.uk/guidance/cg101

Building a portfolio

The use of portfolios to demonstrate competence and progression is ↑ in pharmacy. This may be in the form of a paper portfolio, or an online record. As well as the piece of evidence, it is useful to include a reflection statement, which will also serve as a reminder should any assessors ask about that particular piece of evidence.

Portfolios may be used for personal documents for review, or to provide evidence for the following:
- Pre-registration
- Diploma
- Continued professional development
- Advanced Pharmacy Framework[12]
- Return to registration application
- Non-medical prescribing course.

Identifying suitable pieces of evidence can be difficult, and will vary depending on experience. A high-quality piece of evidence can be used to demonstrate competency in a number of areas. Your evidence will demonstrate areas of learning, experiences, and achievement, as well as your current knowledge base.[13]

Ideas for evidence
- Policies/procedures that you've implemented
- Ward assessments
- Emails
- Testimonials/peer reviews from colleagues (both pharmacy and other healthcare professionals)
- Continued Professional Development entries
- Presentations and feedback
- Poster presentations
- Actions from meeting agendas
- Achievements.

Organizing a portfolio

The person assessing your portfolio will need to be able to find information quickly, so it is important to label and index evidence. A contents page, CV, and job descriptions are common inclusions. To show which pieces evidence demonstrate a certain area of competence, a matrix such as Table 4.5 might be useful.

Table 4.5 Evidence number

	1	2	3	4
Professional	√	√	√	√
Teamwork	√	√	√	
Knowledge	√	√		√
Research	√			

At a glance, the assessor can see that record number 1 covers numerous areas, and that the area that may require more discussion for proof of competence is the 'Research' component.

References

12. Royal Pharmaceutical Society Faculty, ℘ http://www.rpharms.com/faculty/portfolio.asp
13. Middleton H (2011). How to build your professional portfolio (and why you should). *Clin Pharm* 3: 119.

Clinical trials

Clinical trial regulations

Clinical trials form a fundamental part of the research, development, and licensing of new medicines. Research into how the drug interacts in humans is essential to ensure that safe and effective medicines are licensed as new treatments. It is an exciting and varied role at the cutting edge of modern research with trials ranging across all therapeutic specialities. Clinical trial pharmacists are therefore required to have a broad clinical knowledge and a specialist knowledge of the regulations that clinical trials have to follow.

New regulations were introduced in 2004 to help regulate the field of clinical trials in human subjects. The European Clinical Trials Directive (2001/20/EC) was implemented across the EU in 2004 and transposed into local law (Statutory Instrument (SI)1031 in the UK). Its primary aim is to ensure that patient safety is paramount in all clinical trials. Its secondary aim is to ensure the integrity of the data that is collected so that the decisions that are made based on the outcomes of the trial are representative of the true effects of the medicine and not due to bias in the trial.

All clinical trials involving investigational medicinal products (IMPs—unlicensed drugs in a clinical trial) have to follow the principles outlined as good clinical practice (GCP). This is a defined quality standard devised by the International Conference on Harmonisation which provides guidelines on how clinical trials should be conducted and defines the roles and responsibilities of clinical trial sponsors, clinical research investigators, and monitors. In addition, all medicines used as IMPs in a clinical trial must have been manufactured and released according to good manufacturing practice (GMP).

GCP aims to ensure that the safety of the patient and the integrity of the data collected are paramount at all times. The guidelines include protection of the human rights of subjects in a clinical trial and provide assurance of the safety and efficacy of the newly developed compounds. Everyone involved in running a clinical trial (clinicians, nursing staff, pharmacists, radiologists, etc.) must have GCP training to ensure that they complete their role to the required standard.

A new European Regulation (No 526/2014) has been approved which will repeal both the Clinical Trials Directive and the GCP Directive; however, this is not expected to come into effect until 2017 at the earliest.

Licensing of a clinical trial

Before a clinical trial starts, the following authorizations/approvals must be obtained:

- Clinical trial authorization from a competent authority—in the UK this is the MHRA:
  - The competent authority must consider the application within 60 days (maximum). This application can run in parallel with the ethics opinion.
  - This application outlines the design and outcomes of the trial so that the competent authority can assess whether the trial is safe to conduct.
  - The competent authority must notify the sponsor within 35 days if there are grounds for refusal.
- A favourable opinion from one ethics committee, if the trial is deemed ethical to complete.
- Permission from the NHS trust for the trial to take place within that trust (often called Trust Management Approval (TMA) or Research and Development (R&D) Approval) for each site. This now also includes an opinion on the suitability of the local investigator and facilities (this used to be obtained from the local research ethics committee).
- A EudraCT number must be obtained from the EudraCT database. The EudraCT number is a unique number allocated to each trial by the competent authority. The EudraCT database registers details of all trials approved in the EU.
- The MHRA enforces these standards in the UK by performing inspections of GCP and GMP. The MHRA is also responsible for ensuring that suitable safety monitoring occurs in all clinical trials.
- There is no distinction between commercial and non-commercial trials.
- New guidance has been issued relating to 'Risk-adapted approaches to Clinical Trials'. This is to allow for reduced requirements when certain criteria are known relating to the medication being used in the trial. Any reduction in requirements should be clearly documented in writing to the competent authority with a rationale why they are not required. The sponsor still has a responsibility to show that the medication was suitable for use and only certain adaptations are permitted. These are often called 'type A' trials.
- All clinical trials will follow a protocol which will contain detailed information about the design of the trial and the drugs involved. All processes and requirements outlined in the trial must be followed as the protocol will have been written in compliance with GCP to ensure the study follows the required regulations.

Clinical trial development phases

The development of new drugs has four phases of clinical trials in humans. These trials can only occur following extensive modelling of the effects of drugs and testing in animals.

Phase I trials

- First time that the drug is given to humans.
- Provide data on the safety and tolerability of a range of doses and assess maximum tolerated dose (MTD) and toxicity of a drug used for the first time in humans.
- Provide data on pharmacokinetics and pharmacodynamics of the drug.
- Often designed to start at a single low dose, which is gradually ↑ depending on the side effects until the MTD is reached.
- Usually only involve small numbers of participants (20–100), and are usually undertaken in healthy volunteers unless it is unethical (e.g. cytotoxic drugs must be tested in cancer patients).

Phase II trials

- Usually the first time that the drug is given to a patient with the disease state it is thought to treat (with the exception of anti-cancer drugs). Often called proof-of-concept studies.
- Assess efficacy and define therapeutic dose range and dosing regimen for a specific indication, with minimal side effects.
- Provide further information on safety, pharmacokinetics, and pharmacodynamics in the presence of the disease process.
- Provide information on the doses that should be tested in phase III studies.
- Relatively small numbers of patients (50–300) are studied under close supervision, usually by specialized investigators.
- Phase II studies can be subdivided into phase IIa and phase IIb studies:
  - Phase IIa studies assess the dose required
  - Phase IIb studies assess the efficacy at specific doses.
- Phase I and phase II studies may be combined in one protocol to assess both efficacy and toxicity.

Phase III trials

- Assess treatment outcomes in a variety of patients approximating to the population of patients who will receive the drug once it is launched.
- May compare new treatments with existing treatments.
- May use a placebo arm if there is no current treatment protocol.
- Aim to demonstrate long-term safety, tolerance, and potential superiority to current licensed treatments.
- Undertaken in large numbers of patients (100–<2000), often in multiple centres across the globe.

Phase IV trials

- Performed after a product licence is obtained (i.e. post marketing).
- May be stipulated by the regulatory authority.
- Aim to investigate the incidence of relatively rare ADRs or to compare drugs with comparative treatments, maybe to extend the range of approved indications.

Trial design, randomization, and blinding

- The most robust trials include blinding and randomization.
- Controlled clinical trials compare a test treatment with another treatment or placebo agent. These can be designed as parallel or crossover studies, particularly in relatively stable chronic conditions:
  - Parallel studies assign patients to receive one study treatment only. They do not receive the other agent during the trial, i.e. the two groups of patients continue in the study 'in parallel'.
  - Crossover studies assign patients to receive one study treatment for a set period of time and, following a washout period, the same patients receive the second treatment.
- Randomized trials assign treatments to successive patients in a predetermined random way:
  - Randomized trials aim to show that one treatment is superior to another, and they avoid investigator bias.
  - Patients are randomly allocated to the new drug, or an existing recognized treatment, or a placebo agent, which provides comparisons for treatment outcomes.
- These trials are often blinded:
  - Open-label studies—no one is blinded and everyone is aware of which treatment has been administered.
  - Single-blind study—the investigator or assessor does not know which treatment has been administered but the patient is aware.
  - Double-blind study—neither the subject nor the investigator knows which treatment has been given. This is the preferred type of study. Often the pharmacist is the only person who is aware of which subject is receiving which treatment. ▶ Care must be taken to ensure that participants or investigators in the trial are not inadvertently unblinded as this can introduce bias to the outcomes of the study and invalidate the trial.

Controlled, randomized, double-blind, parallel-group studies are the reference standard for comparing treatments.

- There can be problems with blinding in a clinical trial:
  - If the drugs have obvious differences—e.g. IV versus oral forms, different looking or tasting tablets/capsules
  - When ADRs are associated with only one arm of the trial
  - Ethical issues of withholding information from patients on the exact treatment they are receiving.
- When trials are blinded, mechanisms must be in place (accessible 24h a day if indicated) to ensure that individuals can be unblinded in the case of emergencies.
- If an attending clinician needs information about a patient participating in a clinical trial and needs information about treatment options, for most placebo controlled trials the worst-case scenario is usually to treat as if the patient is on active treatment. The usual advice is to stop the trial drug and treat conventionally.
  - Many clinical trials now have web pages containing information on the treatments involved and contact information for emergencies. There is usually a study identifier (a shortened name of the title) which can be researched through a web search to provide additional information. The information provided may be sufficient to provide suitable treatment options without requiring the patient to be unblinded and potentially have to withdraw from the trial.
  - Patients may also carry information on the trial.

European Clinical Trials Directive

The Clinical Trials Directive provides regulations that need to be followed for all clinical trials to ensure patient safety. The Clinical Trials Directive was first implemented in 2004 and there have been three subsequent amendments to ensure that it covers current requirements and has been expanded to include blood products used in a clinical trial. The latest amendment was completed in 2009 and was transposed in the UK in SI 2009/1164.

There are some specific requirements within the Directive that are particularly relevant to pharmacy or are in areas where pharmacists can help ensure compliance:

- Trials have to be under the control of a named sponsor. The sponsor is the person legally responsible for the conduct of a clinical trial. This is usually the chief executive of the body registered as the sponsor (this can be a pharmaceutical company or a clinician in a hospital trust or university department). This person is responsible for ensuring that the required systems are in place and that all the regulations are complied with.
- All staff involved in clinical trials must have evidence of suitable training, including GCP, in their continuing professional development log.
- All sites that manufacture, label, or assemble clinical trial materials must hold an Investigational Medicinal Product Manufacturing Authorization (MIA(IMP)).
- Hospitals or healthcare centres with patients who are participating in a clinical trial fall under the Section 37 exemption within SI 1030. This allows a pharmacist (or a person under their authorization) to reconstitute, assemble, or label a clinical trial material without this licence. This does not allow pharmacies to manufacture a drug. Definitions of what constitutes manufacture and what is reconstitution are available from the MHRA.
- An individual in the pharmacy department will be named as the responsible pharmacist for clinical trials within that hospital or trust. This pharmacist must liaise with the trust's R&D department to ensure that the trials are valid and acceptable. They are also the contact person for any pharmaceutical company or investigator who wishes to run a clinical trial within that hospital.
- Clinical trial protocols must be made available to the pharmacy department in advance of consideration by an ethics committee, so that the practical details, such as doses and method of administration, packaging, labelling, and study documentation appropriate for each individual trial, can be checked. The protocol must specify the duration of and responsibility for the storage of all pharmacy records relating to the trial.

- Failure to comply with UK law transposed from the EU Clinical Trials Directive is a criminal offence.
- On completion of a clinical trial, the sponsor must notify the competent authority within 90 days of the conclusion of the trial:
  - If the trial terminates early, the sponsor must notify the competent authority within 15 days.
- The competent authority can suspend or terminate any trial if there are doubts about the safety or scientific validity.

In summary, the Clinical Trials Directive sets standards to ensure the following:
- Safety of clinical trial participants
- Quality assurance of clinical trials and IMPs
- An appropriate regulatory approval system for clinical trials in the EU
- Ethics committees were established on a statutory basis
- Appropriate requirements for the manufacture, import, and labelling of IMPs
- Manufacture and labelling of clinical trial drugs are compliant with GMP
- Adequate safety monitoring of patients participating in trials
- Procedures for reporting and recording ADRs.

A new Clinical Trials Regulation has been approved by the EU (No 536/2014) which is planned to come into effect in 2017. The main changes that will result from this regulation are:
- direct transposition into UK law, therefore no scope for interpretation which should result in more consistency across trials run in all European countries
- formalization of the risk adaptive approach already introduced in the UK by the MHRA
- ↑ requirement for retention of documentation relating to clinical trials to 25 years.

There do not appear at the time of publication to be any major pharmacy relevant changes; however, clarification of certain clauses is still being developed.

Clinical trials: hospital pharmacy guidance

All IMPs used in a clinical trial should be received from an approved EU supplier and must be verified by a qualified person (QP) from within the EU. Any supplies manufactured outside the EU must be imported into and released from within the EU with an import licence.

Receipt of supplies

The pharmacy department is responsible for maintaining the traceability of all IMPs used in the trial:

- All clinical trial supplies should be checked on receipt to ensure that they have been received in good condition and are in accordance with the shipping paperwork.
- Receipt of supplies may need to be acknowledged. This can be done using an electronic system or by faxing the paperwork back to the company who shipped the drug. This is to ensure that the supplies reached their intended destination.

Storage and handling

- IMPs must be kept in a separate secure storage area, with sufficient segregation to ensure that there is no confusion between trial materials. These activities are usually completed by the pharmacy department unless there are significant immediate access requirements that pharmacy operating hours are not able to adhere to.
- The designated pharmacist should ensure that the formulation, presentation, and storage of clinical trial medications are appropriate.
- Records of storage conditions must be kept, unless clearly stated as exempt from this requirement in the protocol or associated documentation.
- Clinical trial medication must be dispensed against appropriate prescription forms, which have been agreed by the trial investigators and pharmacy department and which help to clearly identify that the subject is participating in a clinical trial.
- Each clinical trial drug prescription must contain the agreed title of the study and a protocol number unique to the study to enable the study to be easily identified and avoid confusion.
- The pharmacy department should be involved in the reconciliation and disposal of unused medication. Guidance is available from the regional quality assurance pharmacists' document on waste disposal.

Labelling, packaging, and stability issues

- All IMP labels must comply with labelling requirements for IMPs, as outlined in Annex 13 of the GMP guide, unless written exemption has been provided by the competent authority.
- Pharmacists, and those working under their supervision, do not need to hold a manufacturing authorization to repackage or change the packaging of clinical trial materials if this is done in a hospital or health centre for patients of that clinical trial only.

Documentation and records

- The pharmacy department must keep appropriate records of the dispensing of clinical trial drugs and detailed drug accountability.
- Clinical trial documentation should be retained in the pharmacy for the life of the trial, and must be retained for a minimum of 15 years and in the case of a paediatric trial until the subject is 21 years of age.
- All training must be documented and available for inspection. Only people who are suitably trained in the trial procedures should be involved in the running of the trial.
- Clinical trial randomization codes should be held in the pharmacy department. Arrangements for the codes to be broken outside normal pharmacy working hours must be made. Criteria for code breaking should be available and records made in the relevant trial documentation.
- Departmental standard operating procedures must be in place, which are suitably version-controlled and reviewed at regular intervals.

Charging for clinical trials

- The pharmacy department should have a standard method of charging for clinical trials, which has been agreed with the R&D department.
- The National Institute for Health Research (NIHR) has issued a costing template to help ensure trials are costed appropriately and consistently within the NHS.
- Arrangements should be made for the levy of prescription charges in accordance with current guidance:
  - Prescription charges do not apply in trials where patients could receive a placebo substance.
  - A prescription charge should be levied (subject to the usual prescription charge exemption criteria) for trials comparing active substances or different doses of an active substance.

Ethical committees

The EU directive (2001/20/EC) ensures that there are national ethics committees operating within a legal framework, with firm deadlines for approval. The UK ethics review system is the National Research Ethics Service (NRES). Different NRES committees may be flagged for specific types of trials (e.g. paediatric, mental health).

The composition of a national research ethics committee is as follows:
- 12–18 members (lay and medical and usually including a pharmacist)
- Balanced age and gender distribution
- Subcommittees encouraged
- Lead reviewers suggested
- Quorum of seven members stipulated and defined
- Co-opted members allowed, as defined, to ensure the balance of the committee is maintained.

Ethics committees consider the following:
- The relevance of the clinical trial and trial design
- Whether the evaluation of the anticipated benefits and risks are satisfactory and conclusions justified
- The protocol
- The suitability of the investigator and supporting staff
- The Investigators' Brochure (a document that details results of previous trials and the chemical composition of the IMP)
- The consent form and patient information sheet
- The procedure to be followed for obtaining informed consent
- Justification for research on persons incapable of giving informed consent or for individual in prison
- The arrangements for the recruitment of subjects
- Provision for indemnity or compensation in the event of injury or death
- Insurance or indemnity to cover the liability of the investigator and sponsor
- The arrangements for rewarding or compensating investigators and trial subjects, including the amount, and the relevant aspects of any agreement between the sponsor and the site.

Timelines for ethics committees
- Ethics committees meet monthly.
- The ethics committee has a maximum of 60 days from the date of receipt of the valid application to give its 'reasoned opinion'.
- Ethics committees must give a favourable or unfavourable opinion within 35 days.
- There might be a single request for supplementary information.
- There is no extension to the 60-day period except for trials involving gene therapy, somatic cell therapy, or xenogenic cell therapy.

Pharmacists advising ethics committees

Pharmacists advising ethics committees should be able to use their pharmaceutical expertise to advise on issues including the following:
- Quality assurance
- GCP issues
- GMP issues
- Storage
- Issues surrounding drug administration (e.g. blinding)
- Monitoring ADRs
- Clinical trial design and randomization
- Licensing arrangements for the trial
- Indemnity arrangements for the trial
- Safety and efficacy of any drugs involved
- Appropriateness of the proposed dosage regimens
- Appropriateness of the formulation
- The method of monitoring compliance with drug regimens
- Patient education
- Continuing supply of medications for 2 years following the trial
- Availability of a QP (if required).

Further reading

Day S (2007). *Dictionary for Clinical Trials* (2nd ed). Chichester: John Wiley.

Clinical Trials Toolkit: ℘ www.ct-toolkit.ac.uk

European Clinical Trials Directive (2001/20/EC).

Medicines and Healthcare products Regulatory Agency website: ℘ https://www.gov.uk/government/organisations/medicines-and-healthcare-products-regulatory-agency.

Medicines and Healthcare products Regulatory Agency (2012). *Good Clinical Practice Guide* (The Grey Guide). London: The Stationery Office.

Medicines and Healthcare products Regulatory Agency (2015). *Rules and Guidance for Pharmaceutical Manufacturers and Distributors 2015* (The Orange Guide). London: MHRA.

National Research Ethics Service (NRES) website: ℘ http://www.hra.nhs.uk/

Hackshaw A (2009). *A Concise Guide to Clinical Trials*. Chichester: Wiley-Blackwell/BMJ Books.

Regulation No 536/2014 of the European Parliament and of the Council on clinical trials on medicinal products for human use, and repealing Directive 2001/20/EC. ℘ http://ec.europa.eu/health/human-use/clinical-trials/regulation/index_en.htm

The Medicines for Human Use (Clinical Trials) Regulations 2004 (SI 2004/1031). ℘ http://www.legislation.gov.uk/uksi/2004/1031/contents/made

The Medicines for Human Use (Clinical Trials) Amendment Regulations 2006 (SI 2006/1928). ℘ http://www.legislation.gov.uk/uksi/2004/1031/pdfs/uksi_20041031_en.pdf

The Medicines for Human Use (Clinical Trials) Amendment (No. 2) Regulations 2006 (SI 2006/2984). ℘ http://www.legislation.gov.uk/uksi/2006/2984/pdfs/uksi_20062984_en.pdf

The Medicines for Human Use (Clinical Trials) and Blood Safety and Quality (Amendment) Regulations 2008 (SI 2008/941). ℘ http://www.legislation.gov.uk/uksi/2008/941/contents/made

Controlled drugs

Suspected loss of controlled drugs within hospitals

Ward or clinic level

On discovering a discrepancy in a stock balance, two nurses, midwives, or operating department practitioners (ODPs) must immediately check the following:

- All requisitions received have been entered on the correct page of the record book(s)
- Administered controlled drugs prescribed for in-patients have been entered into the controlled drug record book (or the patients' own controlled drug record book)
- No item has been accidentally put in the wrong place or cupboard
- All calculations of previous balance checks are correct.

If the error or omission is traced, the two nurses, midwives, or ODPs must make an entry in the controlled drug record book (or the patients' own controlled drug record book), clearly stating the reasons for the entry and the correct balance, and sign the entry.

If no reason for the error or omission is found it must be reported to the ward pharmacist (if available—resident pharmacist out of hours) without delay, and an incident form and suspected loss of controlled drug form completed.

If the pharmacist confirms the discrepancy, the accountable officer must be informed immediately by the pharmacist.

The Health Act 2006 created a new role of accountable officer for controlled drugs who is charged with the responsibility for the safe, appropriate, and effective management and use of controlled drugs within their organization.

It is the responsibility of the accountable officer or chief pharmacist to inform the police if criminal activity is reasonably suspected. The police should *not* be contacted by ward staff unless instructed to do so.

If theft by a member of staff involving controlled drugs is witnessed or there is strong suspicion that a member of staff has diverted a controlled drug for their own purposes, the senior nurse, midwife, or ODP in charge of the shift should deal with the issue as for any other witnessed or suspicion of theft situation as this falls under a performance and conduct issue. They must also inform the pharmacist (if available—resident pharmacist out of hours) without delay who will immediately inform the senior pharmacist on call who will in turn inform security, the accountable officer, and the chief pharmacist. The police should not be involved without prior permission from the accountable officer and the chief pharmacist.

The record of suspected losses should be reported to the clinical governance committee, or a similar body, that has responsibility for the administration of medicines.

Notes for the investigating pharmacist

On investigating identified discrepancies, it is good practice to check the following initially:
- Arithmetic details in the register
- Identify the time interval since the drug balance was correct
- Enquire about the probable number of staff (and if possible, identify them) who could have had access to the keys for controlled drug storage during the investigated period
- Check whether the senior nurse has organized all administrations for the drug to be checked against the patient's drug chart during the time period being investigated
- Ensure that regular checks of controlled drug stocks have been performed
- Check when nurse and pharmacist stock accountability was last undertaken.

Note that small discrepancies involving liquid preparations are not uncommon, but could need to be monitored in case a pattern emerges.

If an arithmetical error explains the loss, it is not usually considered necessary to complete an incident form or report the incident to senior managers.

Hospital pharmacy department

Suspicion of loss must be reported immediately to the appropriate manager, e.g. the dispensary manager or stores manager. The manager must undertake an inventory check and decide if staff are following the department's standing operating procedures for receipt and supply of controlled drugs. It is GCP to check the following:
- Arithmetic details in the register
- Identify the time interval since the drug balance was correct
- Department's standard operating procedures have been complied with—e.g. only designated staff have access to operate in controlled drug preparation area, including out-of-hours staff, and that all such staff have received appropriate training
- Receipt and invoice procedures are in place
- Access to the department by visitors is enforced and visitors have no access to controlled drug preparation areas
- All supply requisitions are checked.

If a discrepancy exists, the loss should be submitted in writing to the chief pharmacist and accountable officer, who should review the standard operating procedures. The incident should be reported to the clinical governance committee, or a similar body, that has responsibility for medicine management.

The decision to involve an external investigator must be undertaken with the involvement of the chief pharmacist and the accountable officer.

Patients' own controlled drugs in a hospital setting

Patients admitted into hospital

- Patients' own controlled drugs refer to those drugs brought in by patients when admitted to hospital and those that may be supplied as part of discharge medication (TTO).
- Whenever a patient is admitted with his/her own controlled drug(s) they should be encouraged to return these to their home via an identified adult. Responsibility for security is given to the adult, and therefore it is essential that this is recorded in the patient notes/care plan. They do not need to be entered in the patients' own controlled drug record book unless considered as an added documented precaution.
- If a patient is admitted with his/her own controlled drugs and it has been decided to retain the patient on the ward, two registered nurses should check these into the ward's patients' own controlled drugs register.
- The drug and its form, strength, and quantity should be checked, and the drug(s) should then be placed in a controlled drugs cupboard, with the details entered in a separate patients' own controlled drugs record book.
- The patient's name must be written on the label. If unlabelled strips of medicine are brought in, these should not be administered to the patient and the supplies should be highlighted to a pharmacist, who should organize their destruction or return to the patient, or their relative, on discharge.

Use of patients' own controlled drugs

Ideally, the use of the patient's own supplies for in-patients should be restricted to the following:

- Non-formulary drugs or drugs which are otherwise unavailable
- While awaiting supplies from the pharmacy
- Administration records should be completed on the relevant page of the patients' own controlled drugs record book.

Nurses should be encouraged to order supplies from their pharmacy as soon as feasible.

Return of patients' own controlled drugs

When the patient goes home, their medicines must be signed out of the patients' own controlled drug record book by the patient's nurse/midwife, which should be checked by a second nurse/midwife and handed directly to the patient, assuming that the nurse has previously checked that the patient's drug and labelled dose schedule hasn't changed during the in-patient stay.

A patient's own controlled drug should never be used to treat other patients but must be returned to the patient before their discharge if there is no change to the prescription. If they have been issued with a new and revised prescription for controlled drugs, those brought in with them must be returned to the pharmacy and destroyed after gaining the patient's permission as soon as is practical after the patient has been discharged.

Disposal and destruction of controlled drugs including patients' own medicines

- A controlled drug ceases to be classified as a controlled drug once it has been rendered irretrievable, i.e. all controlled drugs, once disposed of, should be unrecognizable as controlled drugs and non-usable as a controlled drug.
- Only small amounts of controlled drugs can be destroyed on wards, e.g. the surplus when a dose smaller than the total ampoule or vial is drawn up, when a dose is drawn up but not used, broken ampoules of controlled drugs, or left-over syringe/opiate infusion residue.
- For all other controlled drugs (e.g. expired stocks, patients' own drugs, and excess stock) the pharmacist responsible for the ward or department *must* be notified. These controlled drugs *must not* be destroyed on the ward.
- Wards and departments who do not receive a routine pharmacy visit must either arrange for a pharmacist to come to the ward or agree a mutually convenient time for the nurse, midwife, or ODP to take their controlled drugs and the controlled drug record book to the pharmacy, where a pharmacist will sign for their return.
- The process for destruction of controlled drugs in pharmacy should be found in your local standard operating procedure.

Records of destruction

All destruction must be documented in the appropriate section of the controlled drug record book or the patients' own controlled drug record book. It must be witnessed by a second person who may be another nurse, midwife, ODP, doctor, or pharmacist.

Evidence-based medicine

Evidence-based medicine and clinical pharmacy

Evidence-based medicine (EBM) has become standard practice during recent years, although it is probably more widely practised in primary care in the UK. The following definition of EBM can be adapted for clinical pharmacy.

Definition of EBM

EBM is 'the conscientious, explicit and judicious use of current best evidence in making decisions about the care of individual patients'.[1]

The authors of the definition go on to state that the practice of EBM requires the integration of individual clinical expertise with the best available external clinical evidence from systematic research.

The second definition comes from McMaster University:

EBM is 'an approach to healthcare that promotes the collection, interpretation and integration of valid, important and applicable patient-reported, clinician-observed and research-derived evidence. The best available evidence, moderated by patient circumstances and preferences, is applied to improve the quality of clinical judgements'.[2]

Evidence-based clinical pharmacy

Borrowing the Sackett definition,[1] a definition might be as follows: evidence-based clinical pharmacy is the conscientious, explicit, and judicious use of current best evidence in making decisions about the care of individual patients.

This entirely fits with the concept of pharmaceutical care (see ➲ pp. 34–6) and challenges clinical pharmacists not only to keep abreast of developments in their chosen specialty, but also to apply clinical developments to patient circumstances and preferences.

One of Bandolier's maxims is that EBM is essentially 'tools not rules'.[3] Pharmacists need to remember this when applying current best evidence to patient care.

Strengths of evidence

A hierarchy of evidence (Table 7.1) is helpful in avoiding types of studies that are inherently biased. A number of grading systems are currently available which are useful in terms of identifying the level of evidence available and as a tool for categorizing recommendations made in clinical guidelines, for example. For updated information on this topic, see the Grading of Recommendations Assessment, Development and Evaluation (GRADE) website.[4]

Some evidence tables regard large randomized trials as level I evidence. Evidence from levels IV and V should not be overlooked if it is all that is available. Conversely, recommendations should not be made on level V evidence if level I or II evidence is available.

Table 7.1 Type and strength of efficacy evidence

I	Strong evidence from at least one systematic review of multiple well-designed randomized controlled trials
II	Strong evidence from at least one properly designed randomized controlled trial of appropriate size
III	Evidence from well-designed trials without randomization, single group, cohort, time series, or matched case-controlled studies
IV	Evidence from well-designed non-experimental studies from more than one centre or research group
V	Opinions of respected authorities, based on clinical evidence, descriptive studies, or reports of expert committees

Further reading

For a useful resource for pharmacy see Moore A, McQuay H (2006). *Bandolier's Little Book of Making Sense of the Medical Evidence*. Oxford: Oxford University Press.

References

1. Sackett DL, Rosenberg WM, Gray JA, *et al.* (1996). Evidence based medicine: what it is and what it isn't. *BMJ* 312: 71–2.
2. McKibbon KA, Lokker C, Wilczynski NL, et al. (1995). The medical literature as a resource for health care practice. *J Am Soc Inf Sci* 46: 737–42.
3. Moore A, McQuay H (2006). *Bandolier's Little Book of Making Sense of the Medical Evidence*. Oxford: Oxford University Press.
4. 'GRADE' website, ℘ www.gradeworkinggroup.org

Statistical versus clinical significance

Simply because a study finding is statistically significant does not mean that the finding is important. Large trials or large meta-analyses have the potential to find very small statistically significant differences between groups. An important consideration when interpreting significant findings is assessment of how clinically significant the finding is.

'*Clinical significance*' refers to a value judgement people must make when determining the meaningfulness of the magnitude of an intervention effect.

For example, if an expensive medication was found to significantly ↓ systolic blood pressure (SBP) by an average of 2mmHg, it would be important to consider the clinical merit of the intervention. Would there be any important health benefits to a patient of a ↓ in SBP of just 2mmHg? Would it be worth investing in an expensive intervention if it delivered such a meagre ↓ in SBP?

Well-conducted rigorous RCTs should recruit enough participants to detect a difference between groups which is determined as clinically significant before the study.

Odds ratios and relative risk

What is an odds ratio?

The number needed to treat (NNT) is a very useful way of describing the benefits (or harms) of treatments, both in individual trials and in systematic reviews. Few papers report results using this easily interpretable measure. However, NNT calculations come second to working out whether an effect of treatment in one group of patients is different from that found in the control groups. Many studies, particularly systematic reviews, report their results as odds ratios or as a ↓ in odds ratios and some trials do the same. Odds ratios are also commonly used in epidemiological studies to describe the probable harm an exposure might cause.

Calculating the odds

The odds of an event occurring are calculated as the number of events divided by the number of non-events. For example, 24 pharmacists are on call in a major city. Six pharmacists are called. The odds of being called are 6 divided by 18 (the number who were not called) or 0.33. An odds ratio is calculated by dividing the odds in the treated or exposed group by the odds in the control group. In general, epidemiological studies try to identify factors that cause harm—those with odds ratios >1; for example, if we look at case–control studies investigating the potential harm of giving high doses of calcium-channel blockers to treat hypertension. Clinical trials typically look for treatments that ↓ event rates, and that have odds ratios <1. In these cases, a percentage ↓ in the odds ratio is often quoted instead of the odds ratio. For example, the Fourth International Study of Infarct Survival (ISIS-4) trial reported a 7% ↓ in the odds of mortality with captopril treatment, rather than reporting an odds ratio of 0.93.

Relative risks

Few people have a natural ability to interpret event rates that are reported in terms of odds ratios. Understanding risks and relative risks seems to be easier to grasp.

The risk (or probability) of being called in the example already described in 'Calculating the odds' is 6 divided by 24 (the total number on call) or 0.25 (25%). The relative risk is also known as the 'risk ratio', and if reporting positive outcomes, such as improvement, it can be called 'relative benefit'.

Risks and odds

In many situations in medicine, we can get a long way in interpreting odds ratios by pretending that they are relative risks. When events are rare, risks and odds are very similar. For example, in the ISIS-4 study, 2231 out of 29 022 patients in the control group died within 35 days: a risk of 0.077 (2231/29 022) or an odds of 0.083 (2231/(29 022−2231)). This is an absolute difference of 6 in 1000 or a relative error of ~7%. This close approximation holds true when we talk about odds ratios and relative risks, provided that the events are rare.

Why use an odds ratio rather than relative risk?

If odds ratios are difficult to interpret, why don't we always use relative risks instead? There are several reasons for continuing with odds ratios, most of which relate to the superior mathematical properties of odds ratios. Odds ratios can always take values between zero and infinity, which is not the case for relative risks.

The range that relative risk can take depends on the baseline event rate. This could obviously cause problems if we were performing a meta-analysis of relative risks in trials with greatly different event rates. Odds ratios also possess a symmetrical property: if you reverse the outcomes in the analysis and look at good outcomes rather than bad outcomes, the relationships have reciprocal odds ratios. Again, this is not true for relative risks.

Odds ratios are always used in case–control studies where disease prevalence is not known: the apparent prevalence depends solely on the ratio of sampling cases to controls, which is totally artificial. To use an effect measure that is altered by prevalence in these circumstances would obviously be wrong, so odds ratios are the ideal choice. This, in fact, provides the historical link with their use in meta-analyses: the statistical methods that are routinely used are based on methods first published in the 1950s for the analysis of stratified case–control studies. Meta-analytical methods that combine relative risks and absolute risk reductions are now available, but more caution is required in their application, especially when there are large variations in baseline event rates.

A fourth point of convenience occurs if it is necessary to make adjustments for confounding factors using multiple regression. When measuring event rates, the correct approach is to use logistic regression models that work in terms of odds and report effects as odds ratios. All of which makes odds ratios likely to be in use for some time—so it is important to understand how to use them. Of course, it is also important to consider the statistical significance of an effect in addition to its size: as with relative risks, it is easy to spot statistically significant odds ratios by noting whether their 95% confidence intervals do not include 1, which is analogous to a <1 in 20 chance (or a probability of <0.05 or gambling odds of better than 19:1) that the reported effect is solely due to chance.

Formula to calculate an odds ratio

$$\text{Odds ratio} = \frac{\text{odds on treatment}}{\text{odds on control}}$$

where odds ratio = 1, this implies no difference in effect.

Formula to calculate a relative risk

$$\text{Risk ratio} = \frac{\text{risk on treatment}}{\text{risk on control}}$$

where risk ratio = 1, this implies no difference in effect.

Binary and continuous data

Broadly, statistical tests can be grouped into those used to compare *binary* (also called 'dichotomous') outcome data and those used to compare *continuous* outcome data. Binary outcomes are those that can only take two possible values, such as dead or alive, pain or no pain, and smoker or non-smoker. Statistical tests on binary data, such as relative risks, compare the rate of an event between the groups; it also makes the calculation of NNT possible. Continuous outcomes are derived from data that can take any value on a scale. Some examples of continuous data include height, BP, time, or the score in a test. Statistical tests on continuous data (e.g. compare the difference between means of each group; see ➜ 'Mean difference and standardized mean difference', p. 131).

L'Abbé plots

L'Abbé plots are named after a paper by Kristen L'Abbé and colleagues and are an extremely valuable contribution to understanding systematic reviews. The authors suggest a simple graphical representation of the information from trials. Each point on a L'Abbé scatter plot represents one trial in the review. They are a simple and effective way to present a series of results, without complex statistics. The proportion of patients achieving the outcome with the experimental intervention is plotted against the event rate in the control group. Even if a review does not show the data in this way, it is relatively simple to determine this if the information is available.

For treatment, trials in which the experimental intervention was better than the control are in the upper-left section of the plot, between the y-axis and the line of equality. If the experimental intervention was no better than the control, the point falls on the line of equality, and if the control was better than the experimental intervention, the point is in the lower-right section of the plot, between the x-axis and the line of equality (Fig. 7.1).

For prophylaxis, this pattern is reversed. Because prophylaxis ↓ the number of bad events (e.g. death after myocardial infarction following the use of aspirin), we expect a smaller proportion of patients harmed by treatment than in the control group. So if the experimental intervention is better than the control, the trial results should be between the x-axis and the line of equality.

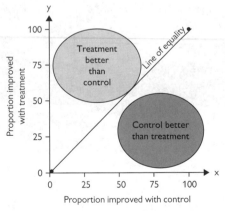

Fig. 7.1 L'Abbé plot for treatment.

Mean difference and standardized mean difference

Analyses of continuous data often show the difference between the means of the groups being compared. In a meta-analysis, this can involve either comparing the mean difference of trials in two groups directly if the unit of measurement of the outcome is the same (e.g. if height is the outcome of interest and all trials measure height in centimetres) or standardizing the outcome measure and comparing the difference between the standardized means if different assessment scales are used to measure subjective conditions, such as mood, depression, or pain.

In a meta-analysis of continuous data, if an experimental intervention has an identical effect as a control (or comparison), the mean difference or standardized mean difference is zero. Therefore if the lower limit of a confidence interval around a mean difference or standardized mean difference is >0, the mean of the experimental intervention group is significantly greater than that of the control group. Similarly, if the upper limit of the confidence interval is <0, the mean of the experimental intervention is significantly lower than that of the control. However, if the confidence interval incorporates the value 0, there is no significant difference between the means of the groups being compared.

Consider the output from a Cochrane review which compared the effect of very low-calorie diets (VLCDs) with other interventions for weight loss in patients with type 2 diabetes mellitus (Fig. 7.2). In this case, weight loss is measured in kilograms so there is no need for standardization. As can be seen, the meta-analysis of the two trials indicated that the mean difference in weight between the management with a VLCD and other interventions is −2.95kg. This suggests that patients with type 2 diabetes mellitus on a VLCD are, on average, 2.95kg lighter than patients with type 2 diabetes mellitus on the comparison interventions. However, the range of the 95% confidence intervals includes 0, which indicates that the difference in weight loss between the two groups is not statistically significant.

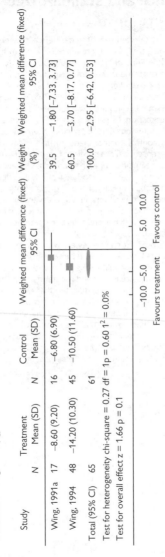

Review: Long-term non-pharmacological weight loss interventions for adults with type 2 diabetes mellitus
Comparison: 01 VLCD vs different intervention (1–10: fixed models. 11–20: random models, rho = 0.75)
Outcome: 01 weight loss (kg)

Study	Treatment		Control		Weighted mean difference (fixed)	Weight	Weighted mean difference (fixed)
	N	Mean (SD)	N	Mean (SD)	95% CI	(%)	95% CI
Wing, 1991a	17	−8.60 (9.20)	16	−6.80 (6.90)		39.5	−1.80 [−7.33, 3.73]
Wing, 1994	48	−14.20 (10.30)	45	−10.50 (11.60)		60.5	−3.70 [−8.17, 0.77]
Total (95% CI)	65		61			100.0	−2.95 [−6.42, 0.53]

Test for heterogeneity chi-square = 0.27 df = 1p = 0.60 I^2 = 0.0%
Test for overall effect z = 1.66 p = 0.1

-10.0   -5.0   0   5.0   10.0

Favours treatment   Favours control

Fig. 7.2 Meta-analysis of a VLCD versus other interventions for weight loss in patients with type 2 diabetes mellitus.

Number needed to treat

The number needed to treat (NNT) is a measure of clinical significance and changes view from 'Does a treatment work?' to 'How well does a treatment work?'. This concept is widely used and useful not only in its own right, but also to enable direct comparisons of treatments. The league table of treatments from the Oxford Pain Research Unit (Fig. 7.3) illustrates the value of such an approach. Ideally, we would want an NNT of 1. Although there are treatments that meet this criterion (e.g. anaesthetic agents), in practice NNTs are >1 for the reasons discussed here.

The NNT is defined as follows: the number of people who must be treated for one patient to benefit. The NNT is expressed in terms of a specific clinical outcome and should be shown with confidence intervals.

Calculating the NNT for active treatments

- The NNT calculation is based on the understanding of risk ratios (Fig. 7.4). Although the NNT is the reciprocal of the absolute risk reduction, it is not necessary to understand this concept to calculate the NNT. A worked example is included so that the process is transparent. The equation is quite simple, and it is easy to calculate the NNT in published trials using a pocket calculator.
- The NNT was initially used to describe prophylactic interventions. The NNT for prophylaxis is given by the following equation:
  - 1/(proportion of patients benefiting from the control intervention minus the proportion of patients benefiting from the experimental intervention).
- The NNT for active treatment is given by the following equation:
  - 1/(proportion of patients benefiting from the experimental intervention minus the proportion of patients benefiting from the control intervention).

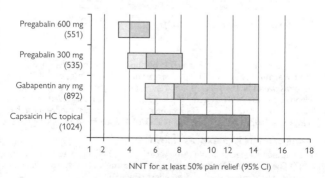

Fig. 7.3 Table of NNTs showing benefit of treatments in painful diabetic neuropathy. Participant numbers in brackets. CI, confidence interval; HC, high concentration.

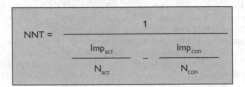

	Controls	Active treatment
Number of patients	N_{con}	N_{act}
Improved = clinical end point	Imp_{con}	Imp_{act}

$$NNT = \frac{1}{\dfrac{Imp_{act}}{N_{act}} - \dfrac{Imp_{con}}{N_{con}}}$$

Fig. 7.4 Number needed to harm (NNH).

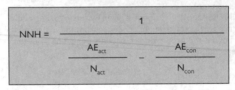

	Controls	Active treatment
Number of patients	N_{con}	N_{act}
Number of patients with the adverse event (AE)	AE_{con}	AE_{act}

$$NNH = \frac{1}{\dfrac{AE_{act}}{N_{act}} - \dfrac{AE_{con}}{N_{con}}}$$

Fig. 7.5 Number needed to treat (NNT).

From the equation in Fig. 7.5 it should be apparent that any response in the control arm leads to a NNT >1. People often ask what a good NNT is: it depends whether the NNT is for treatment (ideally in the range 2–4) or prophylaxis (the NNT is generally larger). Issues such as toxicity have an influence, including the cost. For example, a cheap and safe intervention that prevents a serious disease but has a NNT of 100 might well be acceptable.

Using the NNT to express harm

The number needed to harm (NNH) can also be helpful, in addition to the NNT. The NNH is calculated using a similar formula derived from data for adverse events rather than desired effect (Fig. 7.4).

Confidence intervals

Most pharmacists are aware of *p*-values in terms of an answer being significant (in a statistical sense) or not. However, the use of *p* is increasingly redundant, and new methods of reporting significance have emerged.

The most common method is the confidence interval, which enables us to estimate the margin of error. For example, if we measured BP in 100 adults, we could derive a mean result. If we then took a further 100 adults and repeated the experiment, we would arrive at a similar, but not identical, figure. The confidence interval, expressed as a percentage, enables calculation of the margin of error and tells us how good our mean is. Generally, the figure is set at 95%, so we can be confident that the true mean lies somewhere between the upper and lower estimates (Fig. 7.6). Expressed a different way, there is only a 5% chance of the result being outside the calculated limits.

The statistics involved are derived from a range of 1.96 standard deviations above and below the point estimated. For a 99% confidence interval, a figure of 2.58 standard deviations is used.

Calculating confidence intervals

Although the formulae are available in standard statistics publications, there are a number of confidence interval calculators on the Internet that require the use of the calculated point estimate and the number of samples to derive the confidence interval at a given percentage.

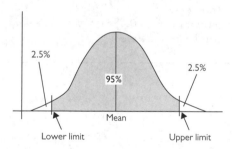

Fig. 7.6 Illustration of the data incorporated within a 95% confidence interval.

Assessing the quality of randomized studies

Assessment tools for randomized studies are widely available and all have problems because they do not cover all the issues that could be considered to be important. This simple method picks up on the main issues of randomization, blinding, and patient withdrawal from studies (Table 7.2).[5] The maximum quality score is 5 if all the criteria are fulfilled.

In addition, a more general appraisal tool is presented (Box 7.1). It picks up details from the scoring system described in Table 7.2.

Table 7.2 Simple assessment tool for a randomized trial

	Score
Is the study randomized?	
• Yes	1
Is the randomization appropriate?	
• Yes—e.g. random number tables	1
• No—e.g. alternate patients, date of birth, or hospital number	−1
Was the study double blind?	
• Yes	1
Was blinding correctly carried out?	
• Yes—e.g. double dummy	1
• No—e.g. treatments did not look identical	−1
Were withdrawals and drop-outs described?	
• Yes	1

Box 7.1 General appraisal tool for a randomized trial

- Was the method of randomization appropriate (e.g. computer generated)?
- Was the study described as 'double blind'? And was the method of blinding adequate (e.g. double dummy, or identical tablets)?
- Was the trial sensitive, i.e. able to detect a difference between treatment groups (e.g. use of a placebo, or additional active groups)?
- Were baseline values for each treatment group adequate for trialists to measure a change following treatment?
- Were the groups similar at the start of the trial?
- Similar patients?
- Diagnostic criteria clearly stated?
- Similar baseline measures?
- Was the size of the trial adequate?
- How many patients were there in each group?
- Were outcomes clearly defined and measured appropriately?
- Were they clinically meaningful?
- Were they primary/surrogate outcomes?
- Were the outcome data presented clearly?
- If multiple tests were conducted, were single positive results inappropriately presented?
- Quality score:
  - Randomization
  - Double-blinding
  - Withdrawals/drop-outs
  - Total score.

Reference

5. Jadad A, Moore RA, Carroll D, et al. (1996). Assessing the quality of reports of randomized clinical trials: is blinding necessary? Control Clin Trials 17: 1–12.

Critical appraisal of systematic reviews

Systematic reviews are considered to be the best level of evidence if they are well conducted and evaluate a number of randomized trials. They can be particularly useful when seeking to answer clinical questions. However, they are only reliable if the process of the review has followed rigorous scientific principles. Authors should explicitly state the topic being reviewed and have made a reasonable attempt to identify all the relevant studies. The 10 questions listed in Box 7.2 help in that assessment. If the study fails either of the first two questions, it is not worth proceeding further.

Box 7.2 Ten questions to make sense of a review
For each question answer: 'Yes', 'No', or 'Don't know'.

Are the results of the review valid?
1. Did the review address a clearly focused issue (e.g. the population, intervention, and/or outcomes)?
2. Did the authors look for the appropriate sort of papers?
   • Check that the authors looked for randomized controlled trials or had clear reasons for including other types of studies.

Is it worth continuing?
3. Do you think the relevant important studies were included?
   • Look for search methods, use reference list, unpublished studies, and non-English-language articles.
4. Did the authors do enough to assess the quality of the studies included?
   • This would routinely be in the form of an assessment tool for randomized controlled trials.
5. If the results of studies were combined, was it reasonable to do so?

What are the results?
6. What is the overall result of the review?
   • Is there a clear numerical expression?
7. How precise are the results?
   • What were the confidence intervals?

Will the results help my local situation?
8. Can the results be applied locally?
9. Were all important outcomes considered?
10. Are the benefits worth the harms and costs?

Based on information from Oxman AD et al. (1994). Users guide to the medical literature. VI: How to use an overview. *Journal of the American Medical Association* 272: 1367–71.

Critical assessment of papers

When reading a clinical trial paper, it is too easy to read the abstract quickly and skim through the main text. Taking the time to critically evaluate the paper might seem daunting and too time-consuming. In many situations a quick read through is all that is needed. However, if the information gleaned from the paper is going to be used to decide on treatment options or might be used to support a formulary application, a more thoughtful approach is required. The information in this section specifically relates to critically evaluating a clinical trial paper, but the same process, adapted to the content, can be used for other types of clinical paper.

It is not necessary to be a statistician or an expert in trial design to critically evaluate a paper. Much of the evaluation is common sense. A full critical evaluation should take all the following points into account, but even simply bearing them in mind will help you get more out of any paper you read.

- Title—does this accurately reflect the content of the paper? Ideally, the title should state the question under investigation, rather than potentially biasing readers by declaring the results. Cryptic titles are a popular way of attracting readers' attention, but if it is too obscure, could it be because that the authors don't really know what they are writing about? Before progressing, consider how useful this trial is in the clinical setting. If it is too esoteric, it might not be worth reading any further!
- Authors—should be from professions/institutions appropriate to the subject studied. Be cautious with papers authored by pharmaceutical industry employees, but don't dismiss these out of hand. Too many authors might mean that the work is scrappy. Multicentre studies should list the key authors and acknowledge other participants at the end of the paper. Is a statistician listed as an author or acknowledged? This should provide reassurance that the statistics are correct.
- Journal—don't assume that because a paper is published in a main-stream journal it is a good paper. However, be more cautious about papers from obscure journals.
- Introduction—should give relevant background information, building logically to the study topic. If the introduction is waffly or irrelevant, ask yourself if the authors really know what they are writing about.
- Method—a well-written method should give sufficient information for another person to reproduce the study. The information given should include the following:
  - Type of study (e.g. randomized controlled trial, cohort, or case study).
  - Numbers involved, ideally including details of powering.
  - Patient selection and randomization—details of patient demographics should be given and the baseline characteristics of each group should be roughly the same (and should be acknowledged if not).
  - Inclusion/exclusion criteria—consider whether these are appropriate. If there are too many exclusion criteria, the study might not be relevant to the clinical setting.

- Outcome measurements—by now, the question that the authors are trying to answer should be clear. The factors used to measure the outcome should be appropriate and, if possible, directly related to the question. Be cautious of surrogate markers. In many clinical settings, it might be unethical, too invasive, or take too long to use the target outcome. However, check that the surrogate marker closely reflects the target outcome as a whole and not just one aspect of it.
- An appropriate comparator drug should be used at its standard dose. Any new drug should be tested against standard therapy. If a drug is compared with placebo or an outdated or rarely used drug, ask yourself why. With the exception of the study treatment, all other interventions should be the same.
- A randomized controlled trial should ideally be double-blinded (i.e. neither the study participants nor the investigators know which subjects are receiving the study drug and which subjects are receiving the comparator). Sometimes this is not feasible or ethical, but there might be bias if the trial is open-label (both subjects and investigator know who is receiving which treatment) or single blind (the investigator but not the participants know who is receiving each treatment).
- Be cautious with crossover trials—if the disease studied could improve with time without treatment (especially if it is self-limiting or seasonal), a crossover trial is inappropriate. An adequate 'washout' period between treatments is essential.
- The details of statistical tests should be given—the tests should be appropriate to the type of data presented. Beware of trials that use numerous statistical tests. Why are so many tests needed? Is it that there is nothing to prove? Further discussion of statistical tests is beyond the scope of this topic. Consult relevant textbooks for further information.
- Results—should answer the question originally asked and be easy to comprehend:
  - Graphs and tables should be relevant and clear. Too many graphs and tables suggest that the authors are having difficulty proving their point! Watch labelling of axes on graphs. Sometimes labelling is skewed (e.g. does not start at zero) to give more impressive results.
  - If means are quoted, the variance and/or median should also be quoted. This helps determine whether the mean is a true 'average' or whether extreme values have skewed the results.
  - The results might be statistically significant, but are they clinically significant? Results presented as odds ratios, relative risks, or NNT are generally easier to apply to a clinical setting.
- Discussion—should logically build from the results to answer the original question, one way or another. If the authors make statements such as 'further study is required …', ask yourself why. Is this because the original study design was unsuitable? Any doubts or inconsistencies should be dealt with satisfactorily, not just explained away.
- Conclusion—should be appropriate to the data presented and give a definite final answer. If the conclusion is woolly, was there any point in the study in the first place or were the authors just 'paper chasing'?

- Bibliography—should be up to date and relevant. Beware of too many references from obscure journals. You should be able to satisfactorily follow up statements made in the rest of the paper by reference to the original papers quoted.
- Acknowledgements—look for any specialists not in the author list, which might provide reassurance if you had any doubts about the authors' expertise in any angle of the study. Watch out for funding or sponsorship from parties with a vested interest in the outcome of the study (notably the pharmaceutical industry!). However, don't dismiss studies sponsored by the pharmaceutical industry out of hand. Much good work is supported by the pharmaceutical industry.

Further reading

Jones C (2009). Evidence-based medicine. 1: Research methods. *Pharm J* 268: 839. ℛ www. pharmaceutical-journal.com/learning/learning-article/evidence-based-medicine-1-research-methods/10979165.article

Straus SE, Glasziou P, Richardson WS, *et al.* (2010). *Evidence-Based Medicine: How to Practice and Teach It* (4th ed). London: Churchill Livingstone.

Guidelines

Guideline development is a common way of either seeking to introduce new practices or attempting to stop some current practices. Guidelines can be time-consuming and costly to develop. There is evidence that they can be effective if carefully prepared and peer reviewed. Shekelle et al.[6] proposed the following key steps that need to be followed:

- Identify and refine the subject area
- Create a guideline development group
- Based on systematic reviews:
  - Assess the evidence about the clinical question or condition
  - Translate the evidence into a recommendation within the guideline
- Ensure that the guideline is externally reviewed.

A useful checklist for guidelines is provided by Shaneyfelt et al.[7] This review of some 270 guidelines lists some 25 points to consider when preparing a guideline. These include stating the purpose of the guideline, using an expiry date, and grading the recommendations according to the strength of the evidence.

References

6. Shekelle PG, Woolf SH, Eccles M, *et al*. (1999). Developing clinical guidelines. *WJM* 170: 348–51.
7. Shaneyfelt TM, Mayo-Smith MF, Rothwangl J (1999). Are guidelines following guidelines? *JAMA* 281: 1900–5.

Herbal medicines

Herbal drugs

The efficacy and safety of herbal drugs present a number of issues to pharmacists. Herbal drugs are more often complex mixtures of active constituents that vary in quality for a number of reasons, such as environmental and genetic factors. Furthermore, the constituents responsible for the claimed therapeutic effects are frequently unknown or only partly explained.

The position is further complicated by the traditional practice of using combinations of herbal drugs, and it is not uncommon to have as many as five or more herbal drugs in one product. There is potential risk from impurities/adulterations of herbal medicine mixed with toxic plant extracts because of misidentification or intentional addition of allopathic drugs.

The European pharmacopoeia includes 120 monographs on herbal drugs. Control of the starting materials is essential to ensure the reproducible quality of herbal medicinal products. Herbal drugs must be accurately identified by macroscopic and microscopic comparison with authentic material. Herbal drugs are referred to by their binomial Latin names of genus and species; only permitted synonyms should be used. Different batches of the same herbal ingredient can differ in quality because of a number of factors:

- Inter- or intra-species variation
- Environmental factors
- Time of harvesting
- Plant part used—active constituents usually vary between plant parts, and it is not uncommon for a herbal drug to be adulterated with parts of the plant that are not normally used
- Storage conditions and processing treatments can greatly affect the quality of a herbal ingredient
- Instances of herbal remedies adulterated with other plant material and conventional medicines
- Extraction/drying methods.

Identity tests establish the botanical identity of a herbal drug:

- Chemical (e.g. colour or precipitation) and chromatographic tests are used for identification of the ingredients.
- Assay—a herbal drug with known active principles should have an assay established to set the criterion for the minimum acceptable percentage of active substance(s).

Legislation of herbal drugs

Although herbal drugs have been used as traditional remedies for centuries and are perceived by many to be without major safety problems, the UK has a series of controls to limit general availability.

Hazardous plants, such as digitalis, rauwolfia, and nux vomica, are specifically controlled under the Medicines Act as prescription-only medicines (POMs).

Certain herbal ingredients are controlled under the Medicines (Retail Sale and Supply of Herbal Remedies) Order, 1977, SI 2130. This Order (part I) specifies 25 plants that cannot be supplied except by a pharmacy, and includes well-known toxic species such as areca, crotalaria, dryopteris, and strophanthus.

Herbal remedies exempt from licensing fall under two main categories:
- Subject to the provisions of section 12 of the Medicines Act 1968, products can be compounded and supplied by a herbalist on their own recommendation.
- If no medical claims are made that are attributable to the herbal product, it can be sold as a food supplement.

Efficacy

Herbs used medicinally normally have a traditional reputation for their uses, but generally there is little scientific documentation of their active constituents, pharmacological actions, and clinical efficacy.

The current emphasis on EBM requires evidence of efficacy from rigorous randomized controlled trials. Several systematic reviews have been prepared by the Cochrane Collaboration. These reviews highlight that, in some cases, the evidence base is weak and studies are often flawed. Evidence from randomized controlled trials has confirmed the efficacy of St John's wort products versus placebo in the treatment of mild to moderate depression.

If the active constituents of a herbal drug are known, it is possible and, in most cases, desirable to standardize the extract. The aim of standardization is to obtain an optimum and consistent quality of a herbal drug preparation by adjusting it to give a defined content of a constituent or group of constituents with known therapeutic activity. Examples include senna, frangula, digitalis, belladonna, and horse chestnut.

In the case of St John's wort, early studies concentrated on the hypericin constituents, but more recent work suggests that hyperforin and, possibly, flavonoids also contribute to the antidepressant properties.

Safety and adverse effects

Information on herbal medicines is lacking in many areas including active constituents, metabolites, pharmacokinetics, pharmacology, toxicology, adverse effects, long-term effects, use by specific patient groups, and contraindications.
- Herbal drugs could present a potential risk to health from exposure to contaminants present in the herbal product and result in ADRs (Table 8.1).
- Reliance on self-administration of herbal drugs or products could delay a patient seeking qualified advice or cause a patient to abandon conventional treatment without appropriate advice.
- In some cases, herbal medicines could compromise the efficacy of conventional medicines through herb–drug interactions.

Table 8.1 Adverse reactions associated with herbal medications

Adverse reaction	Herbal medication
Cardiotoxicity	Aconite root tuber, ephedra (ma huang), ginger, liquorice root
Cross-sensitivity with ragweed	Arnica, calendula, dandelion, echinacea, feverfew, German chamomile, golden rod, march blazing star, milk thistle, mugwort, pyrethrum, stevia, tansy, wormwood oil, yarrow
Gastrointestinal (nausea, emesis, dyspepsia, etc.)	Echinacea, ephedra, evening primrose oil, garlic, ginger, milk thistle, soy
Hepatotoxicity	Borage, calamus, chaparral, Chinese herbs, coltsfoot, echinacea, ephedra, germander, kava rhizome, kombucha, life root, pennyroyal, sassafras, skullcap, soy, valerian
Neurotoxicity	Aconite root tuber, ephedra, ginkgo seed or leaf, kava rhizome, penny royal
Renal toxicity	Chinese yew, hawthorn, impila root, penny royal, star fruit
Sedation	Chamomile, ginger, St John's wort, valerian

General information about commonly used herbal medications

See Table 8.2.

Table 8.2 General information about commonly used herbal medications

Herbal drug	Use(s)	Proposed mechanism of action	Other considerations
Black cohosh	• Treat PMS and dysmenorrhea • Reduce menopausal symptoms such as hot flushes	• Possibly has oestrogen-like activity • Suppresses luteinizing hormone secretion	• Not recommended for >6 months • May relieve vasomotor symptoms • Effect on breast cancer, osteoporosis, and cardiovascular risk is not known
Chamomile	• Reduce anxiety and insomnia • Relieve GI spasms	• Contains flavonoids which are the active component • Benzodiazepine receptor binding ligand	• Allergic reactions reported esp. if patient has ragweed allergy • Sedation is additive with other therapies
Echinacea	• Treat and prevent colds • Stimulate the immune system	• ↑ phagocytosis and lymphocyte activity • Anti-inflammatory	• Not recommended for >8wks • Can worsen asthma
Evening primrose oil	• Treat symptoms of PMS and menopause	• Active component probably linoleic acid	• Evidence is controversial • Side effects include headache, nausea, and diarrhoea
Feverfew	• Prevent migraines • Relieve dysmenorrhea • Improve inflammatory processes	• Inhibits prostaglandin synthesis • Analgesic properties	• Rapid with 'post feverfew syndrome' which includes anxiety, headaches, and insomnia • Must be taken daily for migraine prevention • Not used for migraine treatment • Contraindicated in pregnancy

(Continued)

Table 8.2 (Contd.)

Herbal drug	Use(s)	Proposed mechanism of action	Other considerations
Garlic	• Lower cholesterol • Treat hypertension • Prevent stomach and colon cancer	• Antioxidant and antiplatelet activity • Smooth muscle relaxant and vasodilator • HMG-CoA reductase inhibitor	• Odourless preparations have less of the active component • Enteric coating ensures proper absorption
Ginger	• ↓ GI upset and nausea • Reduce post-surgical nausea	• Serotonin antagonist at 5-HT$_3$ receptor in ileum • Anti-inflammatory	• Toxicity includes sedation and arrhythmias • Adverse effects include gas, heartburn, and bloating
Ginkgo biloba	• Enhance memory • Treat or prevent dementia	• Antioxidant • ↑ blood circulation by ↓ viscosity • Regulates vascular smooth muscle	• Uncooked seeds contain ginkgo toxin which can cause seizures
Ginseng	• Stimulate the immune system • Improve blood glucose and BP control	• ↑ cortisol concentrations • Stimulates natural killer cells	• Limit use to 3 months • May cause sleep disturbances • Avoid large amounts of caffeine
Hawthorn	• Treat heart failure • Improve hypertension • Treat coronary heart disease	• Anti-inflammatory properties • Lipid-lowering properties	• May ↓ dyspnoea and fatigue • No mortality or morbidity data
Horse chestnut	• Improve symptoms of chronic venous insufficiency • ↓ leg oedema	• Seeds contain aescin which reduces venous capillary permeability • Anti-inflammatory • Weak diuretic activity	• May ↑ bleeding when in combination with warfarin • Can turn urine red • Can cause kidney or liver damage
Liquorice	• Treat stomach ulcers • Relieve constipation	• Glycyrrhizin and glycyrrhetinic acid prevent the degradation of prostaglandins in the gastric mucosa • Antioxidant activity	• Can cause sodium and water retention and hypokalaemia • Avoid in patients with cardiovascular or renal disorders

Table 8.2 (Contd.)

Herbal drug	Use(s)	Proposed mechanism of action	Other considerations
Milk thistle	• Protect the liver	• Seeds contain silymarin • Antioxidant, anti-inflammatory activity • Inhibits mitochondrial damage	• GI side effects are common including nausea, diarrhoea, and fullness • Cross-sensitivity to ragweed allergy
Pepper mint	• Reduce nausea and indigestion • Treat headaches • Improve irritable bowel syndrome	• Direct relaxing on GI smooth muscle • Inhibits potassium depolarization in intestine	• Avoid in patients with pre-existing GI disorders • May ↓ absorption of iron
Saw palmetto	• Treat benign prostatic hyperplasia	• May inhibit 5α-reductase • Local anti-androgenic and anti-inflammatory effects on prostate	• Symptom improvement similar to that seen with finasteride • No long-term data
Soy	• ↓ cholesterol • Relieve menopausal symptoms • Improve bone mineral density	• Isoflavones bind to A and B oestrogen receptors	• Causes nausea, bloating, and constipation
St John's wort	• Treat depression and anxiety	• Active components, hypericin and hyperforin, inhibit serotonin, dopamine, and norepinephrine (noradrenaline) re-uptake	• May cause photo-sensitivity • Avoid in patients with psychiatric illness including bipolar disorder and schizophrenia • May have withdrawal effect after chronic use
Valerian	• Treat anxiety and insomnia	• Binds with GABA receptor in CNS	• Can cause excitability with high doses • Takes weeks for effect

Chinese herbal medicine

Most of the substances used in Chinese herbal medicine originate from China. The Chinese pharmacopeia lists >6000 different medicinal substances; there are currently >600 different herbs in common use. Herbs are used for their abilities to treat specific Chinese diagnoses and alleviate specific complaints. For example, there are assortments of herbs that can alleviate coughing, but each one is appropriate for a cough with a different Chinese diagnosis. The variety and degree of different combinations of herbal medicines makes Chinese herbal medicine very complex.

Combination of herbal products

The one characteristic of Chinese herbal medicine that most differentiates it from other types of herbal medicine is the degree of combination undertaken. Chinese herbalists very rarely prescribe a single herb to treat a condition; instead, a mixture could contain >20 herbs. Pre-prepared formulas are available; however, these products are not usually as potent as the traditional preparation of 'decoction'.

Decoction is the traditional method of preparing herbal medicine. A decoction is a concentrated form of tea. The practitioner weighs out a day's dosage of each herb and combines them in a bag. A patient is given a bag for each day the herbal formula must be taken. The herbs are then boiled in water by the patient at home; the boiling process takes 30–60min and the resulting decoction is consumed several times during the day.

Quality issues

The quality and safety of Chinese herbs has repeatedly come into question after media coverage of concerns over heavy-metal contamination, adulteration, and use of endangered animal species. Heavy-metal contamination has been detected in several Chinese herbal products, usually as a result of poor manufacturing. Adulteration of herbal medicines with prescription drugs has been found in a few herbal products. The use of endangered animals in Chinese herbal medicine is very rare.

Herbal interactions

Information on herb–drug interactions (Table 8.3) is generally limited to case reports, although recognition is improving, with the result that clinically important interactions are increasingly being identified and prevented by HCPs.

Variability of constituent ingredients and the pharmaceutical quality of unlicensed herbal products can often be the main reason for the low incidence of reported interactions.

Types of interaction

Pharmacokinetic interactions with drugs
- Absorption
- Distribution
- Metabolism
- Excretion.

Pharmacodynamic interactions with drugs
- One substance affecting the response of another at its site of action.

Herb–disease interaction
Certain underlying diseases could be exacerbated by ingestion of herbal ingredients with the following properties:
- Hypertensive properties
- Hyperglycaemic/hypoglycaemic activity.

Table 8.3 Some important herb–drug interactions

Herb	Drug interaction	Considerations
Black cohosh (*Actaea racemosa*)	Antihypertensives	May ↓ BP
Chamomile (*Chamaemelum nobile*)	Anticoagulants	Consider discontinuing 2wks before surgery
Echinacea purpurea	Immunosuppressants (e.g. corticosteroids)	Immune suppression can result from prolonged use for >14 days Loss or ↓ in therapeutic effect of some drug therapies; probably induction of CYP enzymes
Ephedra (ma huang)—active constituent is ephedrine	Will have the same interactions as ephedrine	Misuse has resulted in death
Evening primrose oil	Could interact with anti-coagulants or antiplatelet drugs Can ↓ seizure threshold	
Feverfew (*Tanacetum parthenium*)	Could interact with anti-coagulants or antiplatelet drugs	Consider discontinuing 2wks before surgery

(Continued)

Table 8.3 (Contd.)

Herb	Drug interaction	Considerations
Fish oil supplements (omega-3 fatty acids)	Reports of ↓ platelet aggregation	Unlikely to have clinical significance
Garlic (*Allium sativum*)	Could interact with anti-coagulants or antiplatelet drugs	Consider discontinuing 2wks before surgery Loss or ↓ in therapeutic effect of the drug therapies; probably induction of CYP enzymes
Ginger (*Zingiber officinale*)	Could interact with anti-coagulants or antiplatelet drugs	Consider discontinuing 2wks before surgery
Ginkgo biloba	Could interact with anti-coagulants or antiplatelet drugs	Consider discontinuing 2wks before surgery
Ginseng (*Panax ginseng*)	Could interact with anti-coagulants or antiplatelet drugs Interacts with hypoglycaemic drugs Avoid concurrent monoamine oxidase inhibitors (MAOIs)	Varying effects on BP Hypoglycaemia Could potentiate action of MAOIs Limit use to 3 months
Hops (*Humulus lupulus*)	Could have additive effect with CNS depressants	Avoid in depressive states
Horse chestnut (*Aesculus hippocastanum*)	Could interact with anti-coagulants or antiplatelet drugs	↑ risk of bleeding
Passion flower (*Passiflora incarnate*)	Additive effects with CNS depressants Avoid concurrent MAOIs	Reports of hepatic and pancreatic toxicity
Saw palmetto (*Serenoa serulata*)	Caution with finasteride	Potential of additive effect
St John's wort (*Hypericum perforatum*)	Anticonvulsants Ciclosporin Digoxin Protease inhibitors and non-nucleoside reverse transcriptase inhibitors (NNRTIs) Oral contraceptives Theophylline Warfarin Irinotecan	Loss or ↓ in therapeutic effect of the drug therapies; probably induction of CYP enzymes by St John's wort constituents
Valerian (*Valeriana officinalis*)	Additive effects with CNS depressants	
Milk thistle (*Silybum marianus*)	CYP3A4 enzyme inducer Protease inhibitors and NNRTIs Phenytoin	↓ blood levels and hence chance of treatment failure

Please note that this is not an exhaustive list but a point of general reference. New information about herbal interactions can be obtained from ℘ www.mhra.gov.uk

Perioperative considerations for herbal drugs

- Herbal medicines have the potential to pose problems in the peri-operative setting because patients often fail to communicate concurrent herbal remedies during DHx taking by HCPs.
- Few data exist in the medical literature regarding the use of herbal products and the development of ADRs or interactions associated with anaesthesia.
- The most important risks associated with herbal products during the perioperative and immediate postoperative periods are cardiovascular, coagulation, and sedative effects.
  - Cardiovascular effects—ephedra, ginseng, garlic, guarana, aconite, and liquorice:
    —Ephedra can cause a dose-dependent ↑ in heart rate and BP.
    —Ginseng ↑ BP and its use is not recommended during the surgical period in patients with cardiovascular disease.
    —Garlic could ↓ BP, but its effects are normally brief and usually require high dosages.
    —Guarana can ↑ BP and cause heart palpitations.
    —Use of aconite has been documented to cause ventricular arrhythmias as well as complete cardiovascular collapse.
    —Liquorice can cause ↑ BP, heart failure, and cardiac arrest, usually if used in high dosages for long periods.
  - Bleeding effects—garlic, ginseng, gingko, evening primrose oil, saw palmetto, danshen, dong quai, feverfew, fish oils, ginger, horse chestnut, and kava kava.
  - Sedative effects—chamomile, kava kava, valerian, hops, passion flower, and St John's wort.
- Although there continues to be debate on the incidence of reactions to herbal products during the perioperative period, it might be prudent to recommend discontinuation of these agents for at least 2wks before surgery.

Advising on herbal remedies

Background

Herbal medicine is the use of plant remedies in the treatment or prophylaxis of disease, and many currently used conventional medicines have their origins in herbal products and plant materials. Herbal products exhibit a dose–response pharmacology where the biological response varies in direct proportion to the dose or concentration of the product. Herbal products are known to cause adverse effects and to interact with conventional medicines.

Pitfall for pharmacists and technicians

When it comes to herbal products, pharmacists must ensure the approach to evidence isn't forgotten, and not adopt a 'what the public wants, the public gets' attitude. Of course, patient choice is important. A multitude of factors contribute to customer decisions on herbal products, including culture and health beliefs.

Consumer watchdog investigations often evaluate the quality of advice on herbal medicines given in pharmacies at the point of sale and their published findings have judged the advice and support by pharmacy staff to be below par for products such as dubious herbal slimming tablets, topical oils that reduce scarring, and other alternative remedies.

Patient and public perceptions

The phrases natural, herbal, and sourced from plants do not necessarily mean safe. Among the public there is the perception that natural equates to safe and, therefore, many herbal medicine users would not realize that a herbal remedy may be responsible for unpleasant symptoms they have experienced or be aware of drug interactions.

Evidence shows that most people do not tell their doctor or pharmacist that they are taking a herbal remedy and most healthcare workers do not ask and so would have no reason to suspect that symptoms or changes in efficacy or side effects were linked to consumption of a herbal remedy.

Often, pharmacists working in large chain and independent pharmacies have no influence over the range of herbal products on sale, and the historical good reputation of such organizations helps fuel the patient's perception that herbal remedies are safe and effective.

Evidence

Few herbal products have been subjected to randomized clinical trials (RCTs) under the International Conference on Harmonization (ICH) Good Clinical Practice Guidelines to determine their efficacy and/or safety. Proof of efficacy or safety for the vast majority of herbal medicine is now only starting to be established through an evidence-based approach.

Quality

Fundamental to assuring the efficacy and reproducibility of any medicinal agent, be it a single chemical or a complex herbal mixture, is the assured quality of the product.

Compared to single chemical drugs whose specifications are listed in a pharmacopeia, herbal medicines, be they single herbs or polyherbal products, suffer from a lack of uniformity in their chemical and physical qualities due to various factors such as plant growth variation as a result of seasonal influences and time of harvesting, storage conditions, etc.

Sources of evidence

Cochrane database
℘ www.thecochranelibrary.com

In helping the public decide on choosing a herbal product for a condition, one of the best sources is the Cochrane library, which is probably the best database of systematic reviews.

During December 2014, searching under herbal medicines resulted in 8630 records, from which there were 113 systematic reviews.

Of these systematic reviews, most involved traditional Chinese remedies in a variety of clinical indications that ranged from neonatal jaundice, perimenopausal symptoms, and treatment of influenza through to advanced cancer.

Generally, the authors' conclusions tend to advise in most reviews that evidence cannot be assured concerning the effectiveness of the intervention over placebo.

Cochrane database evidence concerning herbal medicines relates to registered clinical trials involving Asian herbal remedies in Asian populations.

Trip database
℘ www.tripdatabase.com

This is a valuable tool to recommend to patients and the general public, and the presentation and search tools will probably be easier to use for patients. In fact, there are a range of media including videos and images that will enable understanding of topics involving herbal medicines.

HerbMed database
℘ www.herbmed.org

Again, this is a useful depository of relevant information, presented as an interactive, electronic herbal database providing hyperlinked access to the scientific data underlying the use of herbs for health. This public site provides free access to information about 20 of the most popular herbs.

The 'HerbMedPro' option contains a more comprehensive range of herbal product reviews, but a subscription is required.

Medical gases

Clinical uses

Air

Clinical indications

- In ventilators and incubators—to provide uncontaminated and controlled airflows
- Replacement for contaminated atmospheric air
- Carrier for volatile anaesthetic agents
- Power source for pneumatic equipment.

Carbon dioxide

Clinical indications

- To rapidly ↑ depth of anaesthesia when volatile anaesthetic agents are administered
- To facilitate blind intubation in anaesthetic practice
- To facilitate vasodilatation, lessening the degree of metabolic acidosis during the induction of hypothermia
- To ↑ cerebral blood flow in arteriosclerotic patients undergoing surgery
- To stimulate respiration after a period of apnoea
- To prevent hypocapnia during hyperventilation
- For clinical and physiological investigations—e.g. insufflation into Fallopian tubes
- For tissue-freezing techniques.

Entonox® (50:50 mixture of nitrous oxide and oxygen)

Clinical indications

Used exclusively for the relief of pain:

- Trauma
- Dental work
- Wound and burn analgesia
- Childbirth analgesia.

Administration of Entonox®

The gas is administered using a facemask or mouthpiece; gas flow is controlled by a sensitive demand valve which is activated by the patient's inspired breath. This enables pressurized gas from the cylinder to flow through a pressure regulator into the lungs at a steady rate. Longer and deeper breaths enable greater volumes of gas to be taken into the lungs, if necessary.

The gas is rapidly absorbed on inhalation, providing analgesia within minutes. The patient safely controls the dosage and, under normal conditions, there is no risk of overdose because the patient's level of consciousness governs their ability to maintain the flow of gas.

Helium

Clinical indications

Helium is used with at least 21% O_2 to:

- assist O_2 flow into the alveoli of patients with severe respiratory obstruction
- prevent atelectasis
- gas-transfer lung function tests.

Oxygen

Clinical indications
- To provide life support by restoring tissue O_2 levels—e.g. asthma, myocardial infarction (MI), and sickle cell crisis
- Management of sudden cardiac or respiratory arrest
- Resuscitation of the critically ill
- Anaesthesia.

O_2 delivery systems are listed in Table 9.1.

Typical dosing for O_2 in acute conditions
- Cardiac or respiratory conditions: 100%
- Hypoxaemia with $Paco_2$ <5.3kPa: 40–60%
- Hypoxaemia with $Paco_2$ >5.3kPa: 24% initially.

Long-term O_2
Used to improve mortality and morbidity in patients with chronic hypoxia caused by chronic obstructive pulmonary disease (COPD), pulmonary malignancy, heart failure, and other lung diseases such as cystic fibrosis and interstitial lung disease. Should be considered if arterial Pao_2 <7.3kPa or 7.3–8kPa if the patient has polycythaemia or evidence of pulmonary hypertension.

Nitrous oxide

Clinical indications
- Nitrous oxide is used as an inhalation anaesthetic in combination with either a volatile or an IV anaesthetic agent.
- Used in combination with 50% O_2 as an analgesic agent.

Table 9.1 Oxygen delivery systems

Type	Flow rate	Inspired O_2 concentration
Low flow (Ventimask®-controlled)		24%/28%/31%
Nasal prongs	1–2L	24–28%
High-flow mask	1–15L	24–60%
Non-rebreathing mask		≤90%
Anaesthetic mask or endotracheal tube		100%

Cylinder identification coding

Cylinders are made either from steel or, more recently, aluminium wrapped with Kevlar®. Each cylinder is marked with a specific colour for each gas type, according to standards BS1319C and ISO 32, and fitted with outlet valves of various types. The top of the cylinder has a tapered thread into which is permanently fitted a valve. The valve can be opened by a hand-wheel, thumbwheel, or special key. The gas outlet from this valve is connected to a pressure-reducing regulator, pressure gauge, and other devices, depending on the application.

Four main types of cylinder outlet valves are in use: bullnose, pin index, handwheel, and valve and side spindle pin-index valves. More recently, cylinders have been introduced that carry an integrated valve/regulator. These are also known as 'star valves' or 'combi-valves'.

The most important valve in use is the pin-index valve, which has a system of non-interchangeable valves designed to ensure that the correct gas is filled into the cylinder and that the cylinder can only be connected to the correct equipment.

Medical gas flowmeters

Medical O_2 and air flowmeters normally have differently calibrated flow tubes, but the fitting of the cylinder onto the regulator is the same. The Entonox® cylinder is fitted with a demand valve, because administration depends on patient demand.

The cylinder labelling includes details of the following (Fig. 9.1):

- Product name, chemical symbol, and pharmaceutical form
- Safety phrases
- Cylinder size code
- Nominal cylinder contents in litres
- Maximum cylinder pressure in bars
- Product shelf-life and expiry date
- Reference to the medical gas data sheet (which details clinical indications, dosage schedules, and contraindications—ensure that you are aware of location of this information in the pharmacy)
- Storage and handling precautions.

At the pressures used, some gases liquefy within the cylinder and therefore behave differently during storage and delivery.

O_2 and Entonox® remain gases, whereas nitrous oxide and CO_2 liquefy. The liquids will cool considerably during expansion and this can cause problems, although this drawback is put to good use in cryosurgery where nitrous oxide evaporation and expansion are used as the energy source. Entonox® should not be stored below freezing point (0°C) because the mixture (50% nitrous oxide and 50% O_2) can separate.

◉ Oxygen — Integral valve

Cylinder order code	CD	ZD	HX	ZX	ZH[1]	DF[1]
Cylinder order code	101-CD	101-ZD	101-HX	101-ZX	101-ZH	101-DF
Nominal contents (litres)	460	600	2300	3040	2400	1360
Nominal cylinder pressure (bar)	230	300	230	300	300	137
Nominal outlet pressure (bar)	4	4	4	4	4	4
Valve outlet flow connection	6mm firtree	6mm firtree	6mm firtree	6mm firtree	6mm firtree	6mm firtree
Valve outlet pressure connection	Oxygen Schrader (BS 5682)	Oxygen Schrader (BS 5682)	Oxygen Schrader (BS 5682)	Oxygen Schrader (BS 5682)	Oxygen Schrader (BS 5682)	Oxygen Schrader (BS 5682)
Valve operation	handwheel	handwheel	handwheel	handwheel	handwheel	handwheel
Flow-rate (litres/min)	Firtree: 1-15/Schrader: 40	Firtree: 1-15/Schrader: 40	Firtree: 1-15/Schrader: 40	Firtree: 1-15/Schrader: 40	Firtree: 2-4/Schrader: 40	Firtree: 2-4
Dimensions* L × D (mm)	520 × 100	525 × 101	930 × 140	930 × 143	595 × 175	690 × 175
Water capacity (litres)	2.0	2.0	10.0	10.0	8.0	9.4
Nominal weight full (kg)	3.5	4.06	19.0	14.0	14.0	12.0

Cylinder code	ZA	ZB	ZC[1]	AD[1]	DD[1]
Cylinder order code	101-ZA	101-ZB	101-ZC	139-AD	109-DD
Nominal contents (litres)	300	300	300	460	460
Nominal cylinder pressure (bar)	300	300	300	230	230
Nominal outlet pressure (bar)	4	4	4	4	4
Valve outlet flow connection	6mm firtree	6mm firtree	6mm firtree	6mm firtree	6mm firtree
Valve operation	handwheel	handwheel	handwheel	handwheel	handwheel
Flow-rate (litres/min)	0.1-15	1-15	0.1-5	8	
Dimensions* L × D (mm)	390 × 85	390 × 85	390 × 85	480 × 100	520 × 100
Water capacity (litres)	1.0	1.0	1.0	2.0	2.0
Nominal weight full (kg)	1.75	2.7	2.7	4.0	3.5

◉ Oxygen — Standard valve

Cylinder code	AZ	C	D	E	J
Cylinder order code	298121-AZ	101-C	101-D	101-E	101-J
Nominal contents (litres)	170	170	340	680	6800
Nominal cylinder pressure (bar)	137	137	137	137	137
Valve outlet connection	Pin-index	Pin-index	Pin-index	Pin-index	Pin-index (side spindle)
Valve outlet specification	ISO 407	ISO 407	ISO 407	ISO 407	ISO 407
Valve operation	key	key	key	key	key
Dimensions* L × D (mm)	290 × 106	430 × 89	535 × 102	865 × 102	1320 × 229
Water capacity (litres)	1.2	1.2	2.3	4.7	47.2
Nominal weight full (kg)	2.5	2.5	3.9	6.5	78.0

Cylinder code	AF[1]	F	G
Cylinder order code	101-AF	101-F	101-G
Nominal contents (litres)	1360	1360	3400
Nominal cylinder pressure (bar)	137	137	137
Valve outlet connection	5/8" BSP (F)	5/8" BSP (F)	5/8" BSP (F)
Valve outlet specification	BS 341 No.3 (Bullnose)	BS 341 No.3 (Bullnose)	BS 341 No.3 (Bullnose)
Valve operation	key	key	key
Dimensions* L × D (mm)	670 × 175	930 × 140	1320 × 178
Water capacity (litres)	9.4	9.4	23.6
Nominal weight full (kg)	12.0	17.0	39.0

Key notes: (1) The indicated cylinders are for specialised applications and availability is restricted. (2) For domiciliary use only. * (inc valve)

Fig. 9.1 Medical cylinder data. Information is current and is UK specific. Reproduced with permission from BOC Medical, part of the BOC Group PLC. ℞ www.bochealthcare.co.uk/en/index.html

Nitrous oxide — Standard valve

Cylinder code	AZ	C	D	E	F	G	J
Cylinder order code	298122-AZ	141-C	141-D	141-E	141-F	141-G	141-J
Nominal contents (litres)	450	450	900	1800	3600	9000	18000
Nominal cylinder pressure (bar)	44	44	44	44	44	44	44
Valve outlet connection	Pin-index	Pin-index	Pin-index	Pin-index	11/16" × 20 TPI (M)	11/16" × 20 TPI (M)	11/16" × 20 TPI (M)
Valve outlet specification	ISO 407	ISO 407	ISO 407	ISO 407	BS 341 No 13	BS 341 No 13	BS 341 No 13
Valve operation	key	key	key	key	handwheel	handwheel	handwheel
Dimensions* L × D (mm)	290 × 106	430 × 89	535 × 102	865 × 102	930 × 140	1320 × 178	1520 × 229
Water capacity (litres)	1.20	1.20	2.32	4.68	9.43	23.60	47.20
Nominal weight full (kg)	3.0	2.0	5.0	9.0	22.0	52.0	105.0

ENTONOX® (50% O_2/50% N_2O) — Integral valve

Cylinder code	EA	ED	HX	EX
Cylinder order code	211-EA	211-ED	211-HX	211-EX
Nominal contents (litres)	350	700	2200	3500
Nominal cylinder pressure (bar)	217	217	137	217
Nominal outlet pressure (bar)	4	4	4	4
Valve outlet connection	Entonox Schrader (BS 5682)	Entonox Schrader (BS 5682)	Entonox Schrader (BS 5682)	Entonox Schrader (BS 5682)
Valve operation	handwheel	handwheel	handwheel	handwheel
Valve outlet specification	Schrader-40	Schrader-40	Schrader-40	Schrader-40
Dimensions* L × D (mm)	366 × 85	520 × 100	940 × 140	940 × 140
Water capacity (litres)	1.0	2.0	10.0	10.0
Nominal weight full (kg)	2.4	4.0	19.0	19.8

ENTONOX® (50% O_2/50% N_2O) — Standard valve

Cylinder order code	211-D	211-F	211-G
Nominal contents (litres)	500	2000	5000
Nominal cylinder pressure (bar)	137	137	137
Nominal outlet pressure (bar)	4	4	4
Valve outlet connection	Pin-index	Pin-index	Pin-index
Valve outlet specification	ISO 407	ISO 407 (side spindle)	ISO 407
Valve operation	key	key	key
Dimensions* L × D (mm)	535 × 102	930 × 140	1320 × 178
Water capacity (litres)	2.32	9.43	23.60
Nominal weight full (kg)	4.0	18.0	43.0

Helium — Standard valve

Cylinder code	F
Cylinder order code	163-F
Nominal contents (litres)	1200
Nominal cylinder pressure (bar)	137
Valve outlet connection	5/8" BSP (F)
Valve outlet specification	BS 341 No.3 (Bullnose)
Valve operation	key
Dimensions* L × D (mm)	930 × 140
Water capacity (litres)	9.43
Nominal weight full (kg)	17.0

HELIOX21 (79% He/21% O_2) — Integral valve

Cylinder code	HX	HL
Cylinder order code	173-HX	173-HL
Nominal contents (litres)	1780	8200
Nominal cylinder pressure (bar)	200	200
Nominal outlet pressure (bar)	4	
Valve outlet flow connection	6mm firtree	Side outlet
Valve outlet pressure connection	Heliox Schrader (BS 5682)	ISO 5145 No.26
Valve operation	handwheel	handwheel
Flow-rate (litres/min)	Firtree 1-15 / Schrader-40	
Dimensions* L × D (mm)	940 × 140	1540 × 230
Water capacity (litres)	10.0	50.0
Nominal weight full (kg)	15.5	85.0

Fig. 9.1 (Contd.)

Carbon dioxide — Standard valve

Cylinder code	C	E	LF	VF
Cylinder order code	201-C	201-E	201-LF	201-VF
Nominal contents (litres)	450	1800	3600	3600
Nominal cylinder pressure (bar)	50	50	50	50
Valve outlet connection	Pin-index	Pin-index	0.860" × 14 TPI (M)	0.860" × 14 TPI (M)
Valve outlet specification	ISO 407	ISO 407	BS 341 No.8	BS 341 No.8
Valve operation	key	key	handwheel	handwheel
Dimensions* L × D (mm)	430 × 89	865 × 102	930 × 140	930 × 140
Water capacity (litres)	1.20	4.68	9.43	9.43
Nominal weight full (kg)	3.0	8.5	22.0	22.0

Air — Standard valve

Cylinder code	AZ	E	F	G	J
Cylinder order code	29813-AZ	191-E	191-F	191-G	191-J
Nominal contents (litres)	160	640	1280	3200	6400
Nominal cylinder pressure (bar)	137	137	137	137	137
Valve outlet connection	Pin-index	Pin-index	5/8" BSP (F)	5/8" BSP (F)	Pin-index
Valve outlet specification	ISO 407	ISO 407	BS 341 No.3	BS 341 No.3	ISO 407
Valve operation	key	key	(Bullnose) key	(Bullnose) key	(side spindle)
Dimensions* L × D (mm)	299 × 106	865 × 102	930 × 140	1320 × 178	1520 × 229
Water capacity (litres)	1.2	4.7	9.4	23.6	47.2
Nominal weight full (kg)	2.5	6.5	17.0	39.0	78.0

Carbon dioxide/oxygen mixtures

	(5% CO₂/95% O₂)		(10% CO₂/90% O₂)		(20% CO₂/80% O₂)	
Cylinder code	AV	L	AV	L	AV	L
Cylinder order code	299031-AV-PC	299031-L-PC	299032-AV-PC	299032-L-PC	299954-AV-PC	299033-L-PC
Nominal contents (litres)	1460	7300	1460	7300	1530	7650
Nominal cylinder pressure (bar)	137	137	137	137	137	137
Valve outlet connection	5/8" BSP (F) (Side Outlet)	5/8" BSP (F) (Side Outlet)	5/8" BSP (F) (Side Outlet)	5/8" BSP (F) (Side Outlet)	5/8" BSP (F) (Side Outlet)	5/8" BSP (F) (Side Outlet)
Valve outlet specification	BS 341 No.3	BS 341 No.3	BS 341 No.3	BS 341 No.3	BS 341 No.3	BS 341 No.3
Valve operation	(Bullnose) handwheel	(Bullnose) handwheel	(Bullnose) handwheel	(Bullnose) handwheel	(Bullnose) handwheel	(Bullnose) handwheel
L × D (mm)	680 × 180	1540 × 230	680 × 180	1540 × 230	680 × 180	1540 × 230
Water capacity (litres)	10.0	50.0	10.0	50.0	10.0	50.0
Nominal weight full (kg)	19.0	85.0	19.0	86.0	19.0	87.0

Oxygen/Carbon dioxide mixture (95% O₂/5% CO₂)

Cylinder order code	F	G	J
Cylinder order code	131-F	131-G	131-J
Nominal contents (litres)	1360	3400	6800
Nominal cylinder pressure (bar)	137	137	137
Valve outlet connection	5/8" BSP (F)	5/8" BSP (F)	5/8" BSP (F)
Valve outlet specification	BS 341 No.3	BS 341 No.3	BS 341 No.3
Valve operation	(Bullnose) key	(Bullnose) key	(Bullnose) key
Dimensions* L × D (mm)	930 × 140	1320 × 178	1520 × 229
Water capacity (litres)	9.43	23.6	47.2
Nominal weight full (kg)	17.0	39.0	78.0

Lung Function mixtures Types 1-4

Cylinder order code	AV	AK
Cylinder order code	Various	Various
Nominal contents (litres)	1500	6000
Nominal cylinder pressure (bar)	150	150
Valve outlet connection	5/8" BSP (F) (LH) (Side Outlet)	5/8" BSP (F)
Valve outlet specification	BS 341 No.3	BS 341 No.3
Valve operation	(Bullnose) handwheel	(Bullnose) handwheel
Dimensions* L × D (mm)	680 × 180	1540 × 230
Water capacity (litres)	10.0	40.0
Nominal weight full (kg)	18.0	59.0

Fig. 9.1 (Contd.)

Carbon dioxide/air mixture (5% CO_2/95% Air)

Cylinder code	AV	L
Cylinder order code	299034-AV-PC	299034-L-PC
Nominal contents (litres)	1350	6750
Nominal cylinder pressure (bar)	137	137
Valve outlet connection	5/8" BSP (F)	5/8" BSP (F)
	(Side Outlet)	(Side Outlet)
Valve outlet specification	BS 341 No.3	BS 341 No.3
Valve operation	(Bullnose)	(Bullnose)
	handwheel	handwheel
Dimensions* L × D (mm)	680 × 180	1540 × 230
Water capacity (litres)	10.0	50.0
Nominal weight full (kg)	18.0	82.0

Helium/oxygen/nitrogen mixture (56% N_2/35% O_2/9% He)

Cylinder code	AV	L
Cylinder order code	299035-AV-PC	299035-L-PC
Nominal contents (litres)	1310	6580
Nominal cylinder pressure (bar)	137	137
Valve outlet connection	5/8" BSP (F)	5/8" BSP (F)
	(Side Outlet)	(Side Outlet)
Valve outlet specification	BS 341 No.3	BS 341 No.3
Valve operation	(Bullnose)	(Bullnose)
	handwheel	handwheel
Dimensions* L × D (mm)	680 × 180	1540 × 230
Water capacity (litres)	10.0	50.0
Nominal weight full (kg)	18.0	81.0

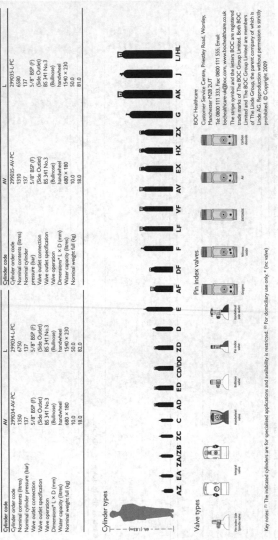

Cylinder types

AZ EA ZA/ZB ZC C AD ED CD/DD ZD D E AF DF F LF VF AV EX HX ZX G AK J L/HL

649 (1.83m)

Valve types

Pin-index side Spindle valve

Integral valve

Handwheel valve

Bullnose valve

Pin-index valve

Handwheel side outlet

Pin index valves

Oxygen   Nitrous oxide   Air   Carbon dioxide

Key notes: [1] The indicated cylinders are for specialised applications and availability is restricted. [2] For domiciliary use only. * (inc valve)

BOC Healthcare

Customer Service Centre, Priestley Road, Worsley, Manchester M28 2UT
Tel: 0800 111 333, Fax: 0800 111 555, Email: bochealthcare-uk@boc.com, www.bochealthcare.co.uk

The stripe symbol and the letters BOC are registered trade marks of The BOC Group Limited. Both BOC Limited and The BOC Group Limited are members of The Linde Group, the parent company of which is Linde AG. Reproduction without permission is strictly prohibited. © Copyright 2009

Fig. 9.1 (Contd.)

Guideline for oxygen use in adult patients

O_2 has traditionally been used in hospitals in an uncontrolled manner, sometimes with inadequate monitoring. It is a treatment that should be used with discrimination and responsibility, as with any form of treatment.

Clinical indication, policy, and potential errors

Additional inspired O_2 is used to improve O_2 delivery to the tissues, i.e. it is a treatment for hypoxaemia not breathlessness.

Each hospital should develop guidelines to ensure a requirement for O_2 to be prescribed according to a target saturation range and for those who administer O_2 therapy to monitor the patient and keep within the saturation target range.

O_2 prescription

O_2 should be prescribed to achieve a target saturation of 94–98% for the most acutely ill patients or 88–92% for those at risk of hypercapnic respiratory failure.

O_2 administration

O_2 should be administered by staff who are trained in O_2 administration. These staff should use appropriate devices and flow rates in order to achieve the target saturation range.

Monitoring and maintenance of target saturation

O_2 saturation and delivery system should be recorded on the patient's monitoring chart alongside the oximetry result. O_2 delivery devices and flow rates should be adjusted to keep the O_2 saturation in the target range.

O_2 should be signed for on the drug chart on each drug round.

Weaning and discontinuation

O_2 should be reduced in stable patients with satisfactory O_2 saturation, assuming that corrective action has been undertaken to resolve the cause of hypoxaemia. O_2 should be crossed off the drug chart once the decision has been taken to stop O_2 therapy.

Errors

- Patients with chronic ventilatory failure are sometimes given inappropriately high concentrations of O_2, which results in worsening CO_2 retention and respiratory acidosis.
- Patients who are otherwise hypoxic, including those with acute ventilatory failure, are given unnecessarily low inspired O_2 concentrations.

Management of respiratory failure

Type 1 respiratory failure (hypoxia with normal $Paco_2$)

- Occurs in a wide variety of patients with acute or chronic cardiac or respiratory disease.
- Hypoxia can be confirmed by measurements of O_2 saturation but arterial blood gas analysis is required to exclude CO_2 retention.
- The objective of treatment is to achieve normal levels of oxygenation.

Type 2 respiratory failure (hypoxia with elevated Paco₂)

Acute ventilatory failure

- This occurs in most conditions resulting in acute respiratory distress—e.g. asthma, pulmonary oedema, pneumonia, etc.
- Hypoxia can be confirmed by measurements of O_2 saturation. Blood gas analysis is required to confirm acute ventilatory failure with an elevated $Paco_2$, low pH, and normal bicarbonate (acute respiratory acidosis).
- The objective of treatment is to restore normal oxygenation. High concentrations of inspired O_2 are *not* contraindicated.
- There should be urgent assessment of the need for assisted ventilation.

Chronic ventilatory failure (± acute component)

- This should be suspected in a variety of situations including patients with chronic lung disease (COPD), neuromuscular disease, and skeletal disorders.
- It is confirmed on the basis of blood gas analysis, which shows an elevated $Paco_2$, normal or reduced pH, and elevated bicarbonate.
- The objective is to achieve safe but not normal levels of O_2. A Pao_2 of 6–8 or saturations of 80–90% are acceptable.
- Low concentrations of O_2 should be administered using a system working on the Venturi principle, which delivers precise concentrations of 24%, 28%, 31%, etc.
- If, in the chronic situation, nasal cannulae are used, O_2 saturation should be monitored to achieve saturation levels of ~85%.

Further reading

O'Driscoll BR, Howard LS, Davison AG, *et al.* (2008). BTS guideline for emergency oxygen use in adult patients. *Thorax* 63 (Suppl vi): vi1–68.

Domiciliary oxygen therapy

Domiciliary O_2 therapy, of which there are three forms, is the administration of O_2 at concentrations greater than that available in room air (which is 21%). It is prescribed for the following reasons:

- To correct hypoxaemia—a deficiency of O_2 in arterial blood, leading to an arterial O_2 tension (PaO_2) ≤7.3kPa (normal values are 11.5–13.5kPa). Complications, if left untreated, include cor pulmonale, secondary polycythaemia, and pulmonary hypertension.
- To prevent hypoxia—a lack of O_2 in the tissues resulting in cell death.

Long-term oxygen therapy

There are several conditions which may lead to long-term O_2 therapy (LTOT) being prescribed to correct the chronic hypoxaemia which can result. Screening patients with the use of pulse oximetry is advisable for those with an underlying condition, with a referral for an LTOT assessment made if O_2 saturations fall below 92%. The LTOT assessment must include arterial blood gas analysis so that O_2 and CO_2 levels can be reviewed.

The assessment should take place during a period of clinical stability and therefore requires consideration in terms of timing as the treatment for the underlying condition needs to be reviewed and optimized. If an assessment is undertaken during an exacerbation of a condition, LTOT may be inappropriately indicated and subsequently prescribed.

Conditions that could result in chronic hypoxaemia include:

- COPD (the disease for which LTOT is most commonly prescribed)
- cystic fibrosis
- bronchiectasis
- interstitial lung disease
- pulmonary lung disease
- primary pulmonary hypertension
- pulmonary malignancy
- chronic heart failure.

Studies have shown improved exercise endurance in COPD patients breathing supplemental O_2, with improved walking distance and ability to perform daily activities. Additional benefits of LTOT in COPD patients include reduction of secondary polycythaemia, improved sleep quality, and reduced sympathetic outflow, with ↑ sodium and water excretion, leading to improvement in renal function.[1–3]

The term LTOT refers to the number of hours per day therapy is used rather than the number of years it is used for, although it is likely to be lifelong treatment once commenced. This form of therapy is based on two landmark trials conducted in the 1980s, in which the main outcome was improved survival in those patients receiving O_2 for at least 15h per day and an ↑ in 5-year survival and an overall improvement in quality of life.[4,5] For this to be achieved, the following is necessary:

- The daytime O_2 tension should be kept at or above 8kPa (the equivalent to an O_2 saturation (SpO_2) ≥92%).
- The equipment used to deliver LTOT is suitable to administer O_2 therapy for at least 15h per day.

When therapy is indicated, an O_2 concentrator is a more convenient and reliable way to supply LTOT than O_2 cylinders. This runs off the normal household electricity supply and does not require replenishing like an O_2 cylinder does. However, it requires yearly maintenance. This device draws in atmospheric/room air (consisting of ~78% nitrogen and 21% O_2) and separates these gases through the use of zeolite, which captures nitrogen molecules, resulting in a continuous supply of O_2 in the home of up to a flow rate of ~5L/min. A back-up O_2 cylinder should be supplied to patients using an O_2 concentrator in case of emergencies such as mechanical break-downs or an electricity supply failure.

Nasal cannulae, designed to deliver a typical low flow of O_2 at 1–4L/min, are more frequently used than facemasks to deliver O_2 to the patient because:

• they are less obvious and obtrusive
• communication is not hindered
• the patient is able to eat and drink while using O_2.

NB: higher flows of O_2 (>4L/min) may cause the nasal passages to become dried out, resulting in inflammation, nosebleeds, and pain, which could affect adherence to treatment.

Facemasks are seldom used in LTOT as they are often considered to act as a barrier to communication and need to be removed in order for the patient to eat and drink. However, there are circumstances which would warrant provision of a facemask. Such instances include the presence of a nasal defect or high flow rates not being tolerated via nasal cannulae. When a mask is used, the most appropriate is a fixed-concentration mask in the form of a Venturi® mask which will deliver a more accurate concentration of O_2. It is also advisable to provide the patient with nasal cannulae so that O_2 can continue to be delivered during periods of eating and drinking.

Ambulatory oxygen therapy

Ambulatory O_2 therapy provides O_2 during exercise and activities of daily living for patients who have chronic hypoxaemia or exercise O_2 desaturation. It enables patients to leave home for a longer period of time to fulfil activities of daily living and improve their quality of life. Several factors need to be taken into account when deciding if a prescription of ambulatory O_2 is indicated. This may involve patients having to undertake a timed walking test or a shuttle walking test during assessment.

Patients suitable for this type of therapy can be divided into two main categories:

• Those with PaO_2 ≤7.3 kPa (i.e. those patients already on LTOT) who are also mobile
• Patients with PaO_2 of 7.3–8.0kPa who desaturate on exercise or show an improvement in exercise capacity or dyspnoea with O_2.

Different types of equipment can be used to deliver ambulatory O_2 (see Fig. 9.1):

• Portable O_2 cylinders, of which there are four types available:
  • DD—a lightweight cylinder containing 460L of O_2 that lasts for 3h 50min at 2L/min
  • F size—contains 1360L of O_2 and lasts ~11.5h at 2L/min

- PD—a smaller but heavier cylinder than the DD type which contains 300L of O_2 and lasts for 2.5h at 2L/min
- E size—a lightweight portable cylinder containing 600L of O_2 which lasts for 5h at 2L/min.
- NB: the duration of use of the chosen cylinder may be ↑ by adding an O_2-conserving device into the circuit, which ensures that O_2 is only delivered on inspiration
- Liquid O_2
- Portable concentrator.

Apart from E size portable O_2 cylinders and portable concentrators, ambulatory O_2 equipment is available on the NHS.

Short-burst oxygen therapy

Short-burst O_2 therapy (SBOT) lasts for 10–15min at a time and is frequently given to patients with normal O_2 levels to alleviate breathlessness due to hypoxia after exercise. Some patients are noted to use a burst of O_2 prior to exertion, such as climbing the stairs.

SBOT is an expensive treatment, best provided by using one or more O_2 cylinders (usually F size) placed strategically round the house, with little published evidence to support its use. It is considered for patients with episodes of severe breathlessness due to hypoxia which is not relieved by other means, such as the use of oral morphine or benzodiazepines. This mode of therapy may also be used for palliation—e.g. terminal stages of lung cancer, which causes distressing shortness of breath, where some patients describe a subjective benefit in their breathlessness from using short bursts of O_2 during this time.

The practicalities of domiciliary oxygen therapy

- Patients needing domiciliary O_2 therapy should have stopped smoking before commencing therapy. Studies indicate that the benefit of such therapy, LTOT in particular, is limited in continued smokers, with an ↑ risk of fire.[1,3]
- The specialist home O_2 assessment services should be contacted when domiciliary O_2 is indicated for a patient. This service assesses, prescribes, reviews, and follows up patients requiring domiciliary O_2 in the UK. (Previously, O_2 was prescribed by a GP following recommendation from a respiratory physician.)
- These services are funded by clinical commissioning groups, which can give details of who should be contacted if an assessment is needed.
- Once a patient has been assessed for domiciliary O_2, a home O_2 order form (HOOF) is completed by the specialist O_2 assessment service for the provision of the correct form of domiciliary O_2.
- The completed HOOF is faxed to the O_2 supplier, who then contacts the patient to arrange a date for installation. (Details of O_2 suppliers can be found on the primary care commissioning website[6].)
- Follow-up reviews of patients are carried out by the specialist home O_2 assessment service to ensure compliance and ongoing requirement for domiciliary O_2.
- Patient education in the use and maintenance of long-term, ambulatory, or short-burst oxygen therapy and maintenance of equipment is important and requires the involvement of specialist respiratory nurses.

References

1. Chapman S, Robinson G, Stradling J, et al. (eds) (2014). Long-term oxygen therapy. In: *Oxford Handbook of Respiratory Therapy* (3rd ed), pp. 708–10. Oxford: Oxford University Press.
2. National Institute of Health and Care Excellence (2010). *Chronic Obstructive Pulmonary Disease in over 16s: Diagnosis and Management*. London: NICE. ℘ www.nice.org.uk/guidance/cg101
3. Esmond G, Mikelsons C (2009). Oxygen therapy. In: *Non-Invasive Respiratory Support Techniques: Oxygen Therapy, Non-invasive Ventilation and CPAP*, pp. 47–88. Chichester: Wiley–Blackwell.
4. Nocturnal Oxygen Therapy Trial Group (1980). Continuous or nocturnal oxygen therapy in hypoxemic chronic obstructive pulmonary disease: a clinical trial. *Ann Internal Med* 93: 391–8.
5. Medical Research Council (1981). Long term domiciliary oxygen therapy in hypoxemic cor pulmonale complicating chronic bronchitis and emphysema. Report of the Medical Research Council Working Party. *Lancet* i: 681–6.
6. 'Primary Care Commissioning' website, ℘ www.pcc.nhs.uk

Patient management issues

Drug use in liver disease

Terminology used in liver disease is summarized in Table 10.1. Liver function tests are used to identify and assess liver inflammation and damage but are not direct indicators of the liver's drug handling ability. The severity and pattern of the derangement of these tests can indicate the type of liver damage (Table 10.2). There may be an overlap between liver conditions and the effects on drug handling and subsequent dose adjustments should be considered and individualized for the patient. The liver is the main site of drug metabolism and the principal location for CYP450 metabolism (see ➔ p. 24). In most cases, metabolism leads to inactivation of the drug, although some drugs have active metabolites (e.g. morphine) or require metabolism to be activated (e.g. cyclophosphamide). Despite this, it is frequently unnecessary to modify the dose (or choice) of drug in patients with liver disease, as they are at no greater risk of drug-induced liver damage than the general population (except methotrexate and sodium valproate or dose-related damage) because the liver has a large reserve of function, even if disease seems severe. However, special consideration of drugs and doses are required in the following situations:

- *Hepatotoxic drugs*—whether the hepatotoxicity is dose related or idiosyncratic, these drugs are more likely to cause toxicity in patients with liver disease and so should be avoided if possible. Consider the clinical urgency for treatment, whether a safer alternative is available, length of treatment and incidence, severity, reversibility, and type of drug-induced liver disease with the nature of the patient's pre-existing liver disease.
- *Protein binding*—the liver is the main source of synthesis of plasma proteins (e.g. albumin). As liver disease progresses and becomes chronic, plasma protein levels fall. Thus, with less protein available for binding, there is more free drug available, which can lead to ↑ effects

Table 10.1 Terminology in liver disease

Hepatocellular injury	Damage to the main cells of the liver (hepatocytes)
Hepatitis	Inflammation of the liver, a type of hepatocellular injury. Could be caused by viruses, drugs, or other agents, or could be idiosyncratic
Cirrhosis	Chronic, irreversible damage to liver cells, usually caused by alcohol or hepatitis C. If the remaining cells cannot maintain normal liver function (compensated disease), ascites, jaundice, and encephalopathy can develop (decompensated disease)
Cholestasis	Reduction in bile production or bile flow through the bile ducts
Liver failure	Severe hepatic dysfunction where compensatory mechanisms are no longer sufficient to maintain homeostasis. Could be acute and reversible, or irreversible (e.g. end-stage cirrhosis).

Table 10.2 Interpretation of liver function tests

	Reference range (adults)*	Cholestasis	Acute necrosis / injury	Chronic liver disease (compensated)	Chronic liver disease (decompensated)	Comment
Aminotransferases (alanine aminotransferase (ALT)/aspartate transferase (AST))	5–35IU/L	↔ or ↑	↑↑↑	↑	↑	↑ in circulation failure with hypoxia, AST in cardiac and skeletal muscle so↑ after MI, muscle trauma, AST:ALT ratio 2:1 indicates alcoholic liver disease
Alkaline phosphatise (ALP)	30–150IU/L	↑↑↑	↑	↕	↑	↑ in bone disease (e.g. cancer, Paget's disease, vitamin D deficiency) and in 3rd trimester of pregnancy
Bilirubin	3–17μmol/L	↑↑↑	↑↑	↑↑↑	↑↑↑	↑ in haemolytic states
Albumin	35–50g/L	↕	↕	→	→	
Gamma-glutamyl transferase (GGT)	♀: 7–33IU/L ♂: 11–51IU/L	↑↑↑	↑	↕	↕	↑ GGT with ↑ ALP confirms cholestasis, ↑ by some enzymes, drugs (e.g. phenytoin), ↑ by substantial alcohol intake
International normalized ratio (INR)/ prothrombin time (PT)	1 10–14s	↔ or ↑	↑	↕	↑	↑ in cholestasis when vitamin K absorption impaired

* Reference ranges vary with method, check laboratory for local ranges.

and toxicity, especially if the therapeutic index is narrow or the drug is normally highly protein bound (e.g. phenytoin, prednisolone). If albumin levels are significantly ↓, serum levels measured for TDM might have to be adjusted to give a corrected level.

- *Anticoagulants/drugs that cause bleeding or thrombocytopenia*—the liver is the main source of synthesis of clotting factors and there is an ↑ risk of bleeding and thrombocytopenia as liver function deteriorates. Anticoagulants should be avoided (and are rarely indicated because of the ↓ in clotting factors) and drugs that ↑ the risk of bleeding (e.g. NSAIDs, selective serotonin re-uptake inhibitors (SSRIs)) or thrombocytopenia should be used with caution. Avoid IM injections because there is a risk of haematoma.
- *Liver failure*—patients with clinical signs of liver failure (e.g. significantly deranged liver enzymes, ascites, or profound jaundice) usually have altered drug handling (Table 10.2). In addition, drugs that could worsen the condition should be avoided:
  - Hepatic encephalopathy could be precipitated by certain drugs. Avoid all sedative drugs (including opioid analgesics), drugs causing hypokalaemia (including loop and thiazide diuretics), and drugs causing constipation.
  - Oedema and ascites could be exacerbated by drugs that cause fluid and salt retention (e.g. NSAIDs and corticosteroids). Drugs with high sodium content (e.g. soluble/effervescent formulations, some antacids, and IV injections) should also be avoided.
  - Pruritus caused by cholestatic conditions can be further aggravated by drugs that can cause urticaria and pruritus. Try to avoid drugs with a high incidence of these side effects.
  - Patients with gastric and oesophageal varices associated with portal hypertension, should avoid drugs that irritate the GI tract (e.g. NSAIDs, bisphosphonates) and affect clotting, as these may ↑ the risk of bleeding.
  - In liver patients with alcohol dependence, avoid drugs that lower seizure threshold or ↑ the risk of seizures (e.g. tramadol, antidepressants).
  - Renal excretion of drugs may be affected in liver disease; therefore nephrotoxic drugs (e.g. aminoglycosides, NSAIDs) should be used with caution or avoided in patients with hepatorenal syndrome (see ➜ 'Hepatorenal syndrome', pp. 179–80).

Drug dosing in liver disease

The effects of liver disease, and consequent impairment of drug handling, are diverse and often unpredictable. Unlike renal disease, drug clearance does not ↓ in a linear fashion as liver function worsens. In addition, whereas in renal disease measuring creatinine clearance gives a good predictor of drug clearance, in liver disease there is no good clinical factor that predicts the extent to which drug clearance is affected and thus the dose adjustment required.

Impaired elimination is usually only seen in advanced liver disease. Liver dysfunction assessment should be made according to the whole clinical picture, as there is no one specific test that gives a good measure of liver dysfunction and every drug is handled differently in patients with different liver conditions. The following markers indicate significant impairment:

- ↓ albumin (↑ or ↓ in acute liver disease)
- ↑ prothrombin time
- ↑↑ liver function tests (LFTs).

The following four main factors affect drug clearance:

Hepatic blood flow

Hepatic blood flow might be altered in liver disease because of cirrhosis (fibrosis inhibits blood flow), hepatic venous outflow obstruction (Budd–Chiari syndrome), or portal vein thrombosis. Even in the absence of liver disease, hepatic blood flow might be ↓ in cardiac failure or if BP is massively ↓ (e.g. in shock).

The clearance of drugs that are highly metabolized by the liver (high-extraction/high-first-pass metabolized drugs) is directly related to blood flow. When these drugs are administered orally, their first-pass metabolism is significantly ↓ (if hepatic blood flow is ↓) and so bioavailability is ↑ leading to ↑ therapeutic and adverse effects. Administration by non-enteral routes, especially IV administration, avoids the effect of first-pass metabolism and therefore bioavailability is unaffected. Thus the effect of liver impairment on the clearance of these drugs is fairly predictable, being directly related to hepatic blood flow.

Drugs that are poorly metabolized (low-extraction/low-clearance drugs) are unaffected by changes in hepatic blood flow. Clearance of these drugs is affected by a variety of other factors.

In both situations, doses should be titrated according to clinical response and side effects (Box 10.1).

Decreased hepatic cell mass

Extensive liver cell damage can occur in both acute and chronic liver disease (especially decompensated cirrhosis), potentially resulting in less hepatic reserve to cope should hepatotoxicity occur. High-extraction drugs are metabolized less efficiently and therefore doses should be ↓ because peak plasma levels are ↑. Low-extraction drugs will have ↓ systemic clearance, leading to delayed elimination. Thus the dose should remain the same but generally the dose interval should be ↑ (Box 10.1). However, protein binding can also affect the drug pharmacokinetics and clearance.

Box 10.1 **High- and low-hepatic-extraction drugs**

High-extraction drugs

↑ dose interval in portal systemic shunting.
- Antidepressants (tricyclic antidepressants, SSRIs)
- Antipsychotics
- β-blockers (most including metoprolol and propranolol)
- Calcium channel blockers (nifedipine and verapamil)
- Glyceryl trinitrate
- Levodopa
- Lidocaine
- Opioids (including fentanyl, morphine, and pethidine (meperidine)).

Low-extraction drugs

Dose at 25% normal (all routes).
↑ dose interval.
- Amiodarone
- Anticonvulsants (most, including carbamazepine and phenytoin)
- Antimalarials
- Anti-Parkinsons medicines (except amantadine)
- Benzodiazepines (including chlordiazepoxide, diazepam, lorazepam)
- Chloramphenicol
- Digoxin
- Lansoprazole
- NSAIDs (including ibuprofen, naproxen)
- Paracetamol
- Prednisolone
- Proton pump inhibitors
- Rifampicin
- Spironolactone
- Sulfonylureas
- Theophylline
- Valproic acid
- Warfarin.

Portal systemic shunting

If cirrhosis or portal hypertension is present, a collateral venous circulation (varices), which bypasses the liver, could develop. This means that drugs absorbed by the GI tract might enter the systemic circulation directly. Thus there is minimal first-pass metabolism of high-extraction drugs and peak concentrations are ↑. The half-life of both high- and low-extraction drugs is prolonged, and so the dose interval should be ↑.

Cholestasis

In cholestasis, substances that are normally eliminated by the biliary system instead accumulate. This includes some drugs that are eliminated unchanged by bile salts (e.g. rifampicin and sodium fusidate). Because lipid absorption depends on bile salt production, it is theoretically possible that there is a

Box 10.2 General guidelines for prescribing in liver disease

- Avoid hepatotoxic drugs (note that many herbal medicines/adulterants are potentially hepatotoxic)
- Use renally cleared drugs preferentially (if renal function is normal) and monitor renal function
- Monitor closely for side effects of hepatically cleared/metabolized drugs
- Avoid drugs that ↑ the risk of bleeding
- Avoid sedating drugs if there is a risk of encephalopathy
- Avoid constipating drugs if there is a risk of encephalopathy
- In moderate or severe liver impairment, consider the following options:
  - ↓ dose of highly metabolized drugs
  - ↑ dose interval for all hepatically cleared drugs
- If albumin levels are low, consider ↓ the dose of highly protein-bound drugs
- Drugs that affect electrolyte balance should be used cautiously and monitored carefully
- In preference, use older well established drugs if there is experience of use in liver impairment
- Start with the lowest possible dose at the greatest dosing interval and ↑ cautiously, according to response or side effects
- Use drugs with shorter half-lives preferentially, avoid prolonged-release preparations
- Use drugs with narrow therapeutic index with caution
- If available, use drugs with the potential to reverse toxic effects of the drug should accumulation occur.

↓ in absorption of lipid-soluble drugs (e.g. fat-soluble vitamins), leading to reduced plasma concentrations and reduced efficacy. In cholestasis, bile salts and bilirubin accumulate in the blood. This could ↑ bioavailability of protein-bound drugs because of competition for/displacement from their binding sites. Drugs which undergo enterohepatic recirculation may be excreted more slowly than usual in cholestasis and it is difficult to predict the outcome.

Other factors to consider

- Absorption of some drugs (e.g. furosemide) is delayed in cirrhosis and ascites.
- Water-soluble drugs may distribute into ascitic fluid, reducing the concentration of the drug distributed into other areas of the body, including its site of action. Larger loading doses may be required.
- Is the drug metabolized to an active metabolite? If so, the clearance may be affected. If the drug is a pro-drug requiring activation in the liver, poor liver metabolism will reduce the rate/extent of activation leading to ↓ therapeutic effect.

- In cirrhosis, the glomerular filtration rate may be overestimated by CrCl and dose reduction may be required. For some drugs (e.g. torasemide), renal excretion may ↑ to compensate for impaired hepatic metabolism.
- LFTs should be continually monitored whilst liver dysfunction persists. Note abnormal LFTs do not always indicate liver impairment and for some drugs larger ↑ may be considered acceptable.
- See also Box 10.2.

Analgesia in liver failure

The choice of analgesic drug in liver failure is problematic because both NSAIDs and opioids are contraindicated. The analgesic of choice is paracetamol because hepatotoxicity only occurs in overdose, when glutathione is saturated. In liver failure, glutathione production is maintained. It is advisable to avoid maximum daily doses of paracetamol because this can ↑ prothrombin time.

Further reading

Das J (2011). Liver disease—pathophysiology. *Clin Pharm* 3: 140–4.
North-Lewis P (ed) (2008). *Drugs and the Liver*. London: Pharmaceutical Press.

Hepatorenal syndrome

Hepatorenal syndrome (HRS) is defined as the development of unexplained renal impairment in patients with severe liver disease. There are two types of HRS based on how quickly renal function declines and the degree of impairment:

- Acute—rapid and progressive renal failure (more serious)
- Chronic—moderate and stable reduction in the glomerular filtration rate (GFR).

The kidneys are morphologically normal and recover if liver function recovers (e.g. following liver transplantation). However, the condition has a poor prognosis, with a mortality of >50% and mean survival of <2wks. A suggested treatment regimen is shown in Table 10.3.

HRS seems to be caused by ↓ renal blood flow and perfusion consequent to the circulatory changes associated with severe liver impairment. It is characterized by oliguria, hyponatraemia, and uraemia.

Management

- Maintain renal perfusion:
  - Correct hypovolaemia—human albumin solution 4.5% is preferred (avoid glucose 5% solution because it exacerbates hyponatraemia). However, avoid excessive IV fluids to prevent fluid overload.
  - Maintain BP—if necessary using vasoconstrictor drugs. Terlipressin has been used to ↑ BP, but this is an unlicensed indication. Midodrine and octreotide (always in combination) have also been used.
- Investigate and correct other causes of renal failure:
  - Stop diuretics and all potentially nephrotoxic drugs.
  - Start empirical broad-spectrum antibacterials, investigate possible septic focus, and perform blood cultures.
  - Avoid paracentesis without colloid cover.
- Institute renal replacement therapy:
  - Because of the poor prognosis, the decision to institute dialysis should not be taken lightly and only instituted if other organs are functioning well and improvement in liver function/liver transplantation is likely.
  - Continuous haemodialysis/filtration is required because intermittent therapy can lead to significant disturbance of haemodynamics and intracranial pressure.

Table 10.3 Suggested treatment regimen for HRS

Day 1	Terlipressin 0.5mg IV twice daily
	Albumin 1g/kg body weight
Days 2–5	Albumin 20–40g/daily
	If no fall in serum creatinine by at least 25% after 72h, ↑ terlipressin dose to 1mg, 4–6-hourly up to a maximum of 2mg, 4–6-hourly*

Treatment may be continued for up to 15 days if the patient is responding to therapy.

* Note for some brands the maximum dose of terlipressin is 8mg/24h.

- • Renal replacement therapy is usually necessary until liver function improves.
- • Transjugular intrahepatic portosystemic shunt (TIPS) insertion may be performed in highly selected patients not responding to medical therapy and are well enough to undergo the procedure. Some studies suggest an improvement in renal function and survival in some patients. However the evidence for its use is not well established and the risks versus benefits of TIPS should be carefully considered.[1]
- • Molecular adsorbent recirculating system (MARS), also known as extracorporeal albumin dialysis, is a form of dialysis that removes albumin-bound toxins. Efficacy has not been established and there is limited availability in the UK.
- Liver transplantation is the only treatment shown to significantly improve survival, but it is usually inappropriate by the time HRS is established.

Reference

1. Malinchoc M, Kamath PS, Gordon FD, *et al.* (2000). A model to predict poor survival in patients undergoing transjugular intrahepatic portosystemic shunts. *Hepatology* 31:864–71.

Drugs in renal impairment

Patients with renal impairment (who frequently include elderly patients) can experience various problems with drug use and dosing. In addition to the obvious problem of ↓ excretion and thus ↑ toxicity, considerations are as follows:

- Pharmacokinetics of some drugs can be altered, including altered distribution and protein binding
- Sensitivity to some drugs is ↑, although excretion may not be impaired
- Side effects may be tolerated less well by renally impaired patients
- Some drugs (notably those that rely on urinary excretion for effect) can be ineffective if renal function is impaired.

This section mainly concentrates on the problem of ↓ excretion because this is what most pharmacists come across in their daily work. For additional information, consult the texts in the ➲ 'Further reading' section, p. 187.

Distribution

Oedema/ascites could ↑ the volume of distribution of highly water-soluble drugs, so an ↑ dose might be required. Conversely, dehydration or muscle wasting can lead to a ↓ volume of distribution, thereby requiring a ↓ dose.

In uraemic patients, plasma protein binding might be ↓, leading to ↑ levels of free drug but a shorter half-life. This might be significant for drugs with a narrow therapeutic index. In some instances, it is necessary to make compensatory adjustments when assessing plasma levels of certain drugs (e.g. phenytoin).

Metabolism

There are only two clinically significant examples of drug metabolism being affected by renal impairment:

- Insulin is metabolized in the kidney and thus ↓ doses might be required.
- Conversion of 25-hydroxycholecalciferol to 1,25-dihydroxychole-calciferol (i.e. active vitamin D; calcitriol) takes place in the kidney. This process might be inhibited in renal impairment. Thus patients with renal failure might require supplementation with α-calcidol or calcitriol.

Excretion

This is the most significant effect because ↑ renal impairment leads to ↓ clearance and the potential for drug toxicity. This includes not only the original drug, but also toxic or active metabolites (e.g. morphine).

Assessing renal function

Renal function is assessed by measuring the GFR, reflecting the number of functioning glomeruli. An estimate of the GFR can be gained by measuring or calculating the creatinine clearance (CrCl) rate. Creatinine is a byproduct of muscle metabolism and is excreted by glomerular filtration. Provided that muscle mass is stable, any change in plasma creatinine levels is directly related to GFR. Thus, measuring the rate of CrCl gives an estimate of GFR.

Measuring CrCl requires 24h urine collection (i.e. all of the patient's urine during a 24h period must be collected). The concentration of creatinine in the urine and total volume of urine is measured to establish the CrCl.

This process is inconvenient, involving a delay of ≥24h in obtaining results. Historically the most well-established estimate of CrCl can be achieved using the Cockcroft and Gault (CG) equation (Box 10.3). This equation takes into account the fact that muscle mass (and therefore serum creatinine levels) vary according to gender and weight.

Calculating the rate of CrCl in this way gives a better estimate than simply using serum creatinine, but it is not exact and tends to under- or overestimate the rate by up to 20%. Ideal body weight should be used in obese or fluid-overloaded patients. The equation is particularly inaccurate in pregnant women, children, those with very low or high muscle mass, and patients with marked catabolism or rapidly changing renal function (i.e. acute kidney injury). For children, a more accurate CrCl can be calculated (Box 10.3).[2-6]

Remember that elderly patients nearly always have some degree of renal impairment, because of the normal ageing process, but this may not be indicated by a raised serum creatinine due to reduced muscle mass.

Box 10.3 Calculating creatinine clearance

Adults

Cockcroft and Gault equation:[2]

$$\text{Creatinine clearance (CrCl)} = \frac{(140 - \text{age [years]}) \times \text{weight [kg]} \times F}{\text{Serum creatinine [micromol/L]}}$$

where $F = 1.04$ in females and 1.23 in males.

Use ideal body weight in obese or fluid-overloaded patients.

Modification of Diet in Renal Disease[3] (= eGFR):

$$\text{eGFR (mL/min/1.73m}^2) = 32788 \times \text{serum creatinine (micromol/L)}^{-1.154} \times \text{age}^{-0.203} \times X \times Y$$

where $X = 1.212$ (if African American) and $Y = 0.742$ (if female).

Absolute glomerular filtration rate:[4]

$$\text{GFR}_{\text{Absolute}} = \text{eGFR} \times (\text{individual's body surface area}/1.73)$$

Children[5]

$$\text{GFR (mL/min/1.73m}^2) = \frac{40 \times \text{height (cm)}}{\text{Serum creatinine (micromol/L)}}$$

Neonates[6]

$$\text{GFR (mL/min/1.73 m}^2) = \frac{0.55 \times \text{length (cm)}}{\text{Plasma creatinine (mg/100mL)}}$$

Despite its limitations, the CG equation is extremely useful for assessing renal impairment in this setting and is preferable to using serum creatinine alone. For example, a serum creatinine of 120micromol/L might be normal in a fit young man but could represent significant renal impairment in a frail elderly woman.

Normal CrCl in adults is ~80–120mL/min (for infants and children, see Table 10.4).

An alternative method of estimating GFR is to use the Modification of Diet in Renal Disease (MDRD) equation (see Table 10.3), which is often quoted as estimated GFR (eGFR). This equation is more reliable than the CG equation for patients with unstable renal function or acute kidney injury. However, it quotes the GFR for a standard body surface area (i.e. mL/min/1.73m²) and so it is unsuitable for patients at extremes of body weight or amputees, pregnant women, and children. It has also not been validated in certain ethnic groups.

Laboratories are now quoting eGFR in addition to serum creatinine when reporting renal function. This is appropriate in terms of giving a better indication than serum creatinine of whether the patient has any degree of renal impairment. However, most drug dosing recommendations (except the *British National Formulary*) are still based on GFR not eGFR and the two measures of renal function are not interchangeable. In practice, for most drugs and for most patients (>18 years) of average build and height, eGFR can be used to determine dosage adjustments in place of CrCl calculated by the CG equation. The exceptions to this is for toxic drugs and extremes of body weight, in which CrCl should be used to adjust drug dosages, as well as clinical response and plasma-drug concentration for toxic drugs. Alternatively, an eGFR value can be easily converted to an actual GFR value (see Table 10.3).[7,8]

Dose adjustment in renal failure

The kidney is involved in the elimination of most drugs, either in their active/unchanged form or as their metabolites, although for some drugs this might be only a very small proportion of the dose. Drugs and active metabolites for which the kidney is a major site of elimination usually require dosage adjustment, according to severity of renal impairment, to avoid accumulation and thus toxicity. Remember that some of these drugs might also be nephrotoxic and drug accumulation can make renal impairment worse.

Table 10.4 Normal creatinine clearances in infants and children

Age	Creatinine clearance (mL/min/1.73m²)
Premature	10–15
Neonate (term)	15–20
2wks	30–40
2 months	50–60
1–2 years to adult	100–120

Table 10.5 Stages of chronic kidney disease

Stage	eGFR (ml/min/1.73 m²)	Degree of impairment
1	≥90 and other evidence of renal failure	Normal or high
2	60–89 and other evidence of renal failure	Mildly ↓
3A	45–59	Mildly to moderately ↓
3B	30–44	Moderately to severely ↓
4	15–29	Severely ↓
5	<15	Kidney failure or on dialysis

In patients with mild renal impairment it might only be necessary to monitor closely for side effects, with or without further deterioration in kidney function. However, in moderate or severe renal impairment an alternative drug should be used if possible. The ideal drug in renal failure would have the following attributes:
- <25% excreted unchanged in the urine
- No active/toxic renally cleared metabolites
- Levels/activity minimally affected by fluid balance or protein-binding or tissue sensitivity changes
- Wide therapeutic margin
- Low adverse effect profile
- Not nephrotoxic
- Is able to reach the site of action in a high enough concentration even in renal impairment.

Unfortunately, it is frequently not possible to find a suitable drug that fits these criteria, in which case dose adjustment is usually necessary. Two methods of dose reduction are used, either alone or in combination:
- Give a smaller dose at the same dose interval
- Give the same dose at a longer dose interval.

It is possible to calculate a corrected dose/dose interval, but a more practical option is to use drug-dosing guidelines. The reader is referred to the sources on ➔ p. 187.

Renal impairment prolongs the half-life of any drug excreted by the kidney. The time to steady-state concentration is ~5 times the half-life. Thus, just as in patients with normal renal function, a loading dose might be needed if an immediate effect is required. This is especially true if the dose interval has been ↑. The loading dose in patients with renal impairment is the same as in patients with normal renal function.

Certain drugs should always be checked if there is any suspicion of renal impairment (Table 10.6). In many instances, not only are these drugs primarily excreted by the kidneys, but some are also potentially nephrotoxic, such that accumulation could lead to further renal impairment. In addition, side effects caused by accumulation might be mistaken for disease

Table 10.6 Checklist of drugs requiring dose adjustment in renal impairment

Commonly used drugs for which dose reduction is always necessary in moderate or severe renal impairment*

• Aciclovir	• Imipenem	• Penicillin
• Aminoglycosides	• Meropenem	• Thiazide diuretics
• Capecitabine	• Methotrexate	• Vancomycin
• Cisplatin		

Commonly used drugs for which dose reduction should be considered in moderate or severe renal impairment*

• Allopurinol	• Ethambutol	• Melphalan
• Amoxicillin	• Flucloxacillin	• Opioids
• Cephalosporins	• Furosemide	• Quinolones
• Cyclophosphamide	• Lomustine	• Sulfonamides (including
• Digoxin	• Low-molecular-weight heparins	co-trimoxazole)

* These lists are not comprehensive—check specialist references (➲ p. 187) for further information.

deterioration, and the pharmacist should be alert to this and advise medical staff accordingly. Wherever possible, avoid using potentially nephrotoxic drugs in patients with renal impairment.

Remember that renal function might improve or further deteriorate according to the patient's condition and, consequently, doses may need to be readjusted accordingly.

Drug dosing in renal replacement therapies

Renal replacement therapies (RRTs) are used in patients with chronic renal failure whose renal function is so poor that the kidneys are barely functioning. They can also be used temporarily in patients with acute kidney injury. RRT aims to remove toxins, excess fluid, and correct biochemical disturbances. Drugs which are cleared by the kidneys are usually dialysed although there are some exceptions. There are four types of renal replacement therapy in common use:

• Intermittent haemodialysis (HD)
• Continuous ambulatory peritoneal dialysis (CAPD)
• Continuous arteriovenous haemofiltration (CAV HF)/venovenous haemofiltration (CVV HF)
• Continuous arteriovenous haemodiafiltration (CAV HDF)/venovenous haemodiafiltration (CVV HDF).

Each method works on the principle of removing toxins from the blood by diffusion or osmosis across a semipermeable membrane into a dialysis solution. Therefore the factors that affect drug removal are much the same for HD, CAPD, and CAV HD. CAV HDF is a slightly different technique, removing drugs more efficiently than HD and is influenced by slightly different factors.

Dialysis-related factors

The following factors influence drug removal by dialysis or filtration:
- Duration of dialysis
- Blood flow rate in dialyser
- Type of dialyser membrane (synthetic or natural)
- Flow rate and composition of dialysate.

However, these characteristics are difficult to quantify and therefore it is hard to predict exactly what effect they will have on drug removal. In CAPD, frequent exchanges (e.g. every 1–4h) ↑ drug clearance.

Drug-related factors

It is possible to judge whether or not a drug will be significantly cleared by dialysis according to the pharmacokinetic parameters. Factors that favour drug removal are as follows:
- Low molecular weight—removal ↑ as molecular weight ↓ below 500Da
- Low protein binding (<20%)
- Low volume of distribution (<1L/kg)
- High water solubility
- High degree of renal clearance in normal renal function.

The exception is CAVH, where molecules with a higher molecular weight (up to that of insulin) are preferentially removed, but there is less removal of smaller molecules (e.g. K^+ and urea).

Drug dosing in renal replacement therapies

Accurately quantifying drug clearance during RRTs is of limited value. The equations tend to assume constant conditions, but in practice both patient and dialysis conditions can vary. For example, the patient's clinical status (e.g. BP or renal function) could change, which has an effect on drug clearance. In CAPD, peritonitis affects peritoneal permeability and thus clearance. No RRT is as effective as the kidney functioning normally, so doses used will never be larger than those recommended in normal renal function.

The most practical approach is to use empirical dosing according to theoretical GFR achieved by the dialysis technique used (Table 10.7). This

Table 10.7 Theoretical GFR in renal replacement therapy

Renal replacement therapy		Typical theoretical GFR achieved (mL/min)
HD	During dialysis	150–200
	Between dialysis periods	0–10
CAVHF		0–15
CVVHF		15–25
CAVHDF		20
CVVHDF		30–40
CAPD (4 exchanges daily)		5–10

should be backed up by close monitoring for drug response and toxicity, including TDM.

In patients receiving HD, drugs should be given after the dialysis session to avoid the possibility that the drug might be removed before it has time to act. Because CAVH and CAVD are continuous processes, doses do not need to be scheduled around dialysis sessions. The same is true for CAPD, but the dose might need to be titrated up or down if the frequency of exchanges is ↑ or ↓. Additional doses may be required depending on the dialysability of the drug and type of RRT in order to avoid subtherapeutic levels.

Further reading

Ashley C, Currie A (eds) (2008). *The Renal Drug Handbook* (3rd edn). Abingdon: Radcliffe Medical Press.

electronic Medicines Compendium (eMC). 'Summaries of Product Characteristics' ℘ www.emc. medicines.org.uk

Jogia P, O'Brien (2009). How to approach prescriptions for patients with renal impairment. *Clin Pharm* 1: 179–83.

Sexton J. (2003). Drug use and dosing in the renally impaired adult. *Pharm J* 271: 744–6.

References

2. Cockcroft DW, Gault MH (1976). Prediction of creatinine clearance from serum creatinine. *Nephron* 16(1): 31–41.
3. Levey AS, Bosch JP, Lewis JB, et al. (1999). A more accurate method to estimate glomerular filtration rate from serum creatinine: a new prediction equation. *Ann Internal Med* 130: 461–70.
4. Joint Formulary Committee. *British National Formulary* (online). London: BMJ Group and Pharmaceutical Press. ℘ www.medicinescomplete.com
5. Morris MC, Allanby CW, Toseland P, et al. (1982). Evaluation of a height/plasma creatinine formula in the measurement of glomerular filtration rate. *Arch Dis Child* 57: 611–15.
6. Schwartz GJ, Feld LG, Langford DJ (1984). A simple estimate of glomerular filtration rate in full term infants during the first year of life. *J Paediatr* 104: 849–54.
7. National Institute for Health and Care Excellence (2013). 'Acute kidney injury: prevention, detection and management', ℘ www.nice.org.uk/guidance/cg169
8. National Institute for Health and Care Excellence (2014). 'Chronic kidney disease in adults: assessment and management', ℘ www.nice.org.uk/guidance/cg182

Drugs in pregnancy

Drugs can have harmful effects on the embryo or fetus at any time during pregnancy. Therefore drugs should only be used in pregnancy if the expected benefit to the mother is thought to be greater than the risk to the fetus.

The UK Teratology Information Service (UKTIS) provides information to health professionals via a telephone information service and online through the TOXBASE® database (password required). UKTIS also produces patient information leaflets on use of medicines during pregnancy on their website for patients (see ➲ 'Further reading', p. 191).

A drug is defined as teratogenic if it crosses the placenta, causing congenital malformations. Teratogenic effects usually only occur when the fetus is exposed during a critical period of development. Even then, not all fetuses exposed will be affected, e.g. <50% of fetuses exposed to thalidomide developed congenital abnormalities. Aside from congenital malformations drugs can cause a variety of embryo/fetotoxic effects, such as spontaneous abortions, intrauterine growth retardation, prematurity, obstetric complications, neonatal postnatal effects, and withdrawal effects.

Various textbooks and reference sources (see ➲ 'Further reading', p. 191) give information on using and exposure to drugs/chemicals in pregnancy (Table 10.8[9] and Box 10.4), but these sources do not always take into account all the relevant factors when assessing risk. Absence of information for a drug does not imply safety in pregnancy. To fully evaluate the risk/benefit of a drug in pregnancy, the following factors should be taken into account.

Other possible causes

- Miscarriage occurs in ~10–20% of pregnancies. The incidence of major congenital malformations in the general population is estimated to be between 2% and 3%. Over 75% of these malformations are of unknown aetiology; only 1–2% are thought to be caused by drugs.
- Maternal morbidity or an acute exacerbation/relapse of the disease could present a higher risk to the fetus than the drug.
- The underlying maternal disease might be associated with congenital abnormalities (e.g. epilepsy).
- Smoking and alcohol use during pregnancy can lead to congenital abnormalities, growth retardation, and spontaneous abortion.

Drug characteristics

- Most drugs (an estimated 99%), cross the placenta by simple diffusion although the extent to which the drug crosses will depend on certain drug characteristics (see below), including protein binding.
  - High-molecular-weight drugs do not cross the placenta (e.g. heparin and insulin).
  - Non-ionized lipophilic drugs (e.g. labetalol) cross the placenta to a greater extent than ionized hydrophilic drugs (e.g. atenolol).
- A drug can cause fetal toxicity without crossing the placenta (e.g. any drug that causes vasoconstriction of the placental vasculature).

Table 10.8 Some drugs that should be avoided* in pregnancy

Drugs known to cause congenital malformations	
• Anticonvulsants	• Lithium
• Cytotoxics	• Retinoids (systemic)
• Danazol	• Warfarin

Drugs that can affect fetal growth and development

- ACE inhibitors (after 12wks)—fetal or neonatal renal failure
- Barbiturates, benzodiazepines, and opioids (near term)—drug dependence in fetus
- NSAIDs (after 12wks)—premature closure of ductus arteriosus
- Tetracyclines (after 12wks)—abnormalities of teeth and bone
- Warfarin—fetal or neonatal haemorrhage

* Note that if the benefit clearly outweighs the risk (e.g. life-threatening or pregnancy-threatening disease), these drugs can be used in pregnancy.

Box 10.4 Some drugs that have a good safety record in pregnancy

- Analgesics—codeine (caution near term) and paracetamol
- Antacids containing aluminium, calcium, or magnesium
- Antibacterials—penicillins, cephalosporins, erythromycin, clindamycin, and nitrofurantoin (avoid near term)
- Antiemetics—cyclizine and promethazine
- Antifungal agents (topical and vaginal): clotrimazole and nystatin
- Antihistamines—chlorphenamine and hydroxyzine
- Asthma—bronchodilator and steroid inhalers (avoid high doses in the long term), and short-course oral steroids
- Corticosteroids (topical, including nasal and eye drops)
- Insulin
- Laxatives—bulk-forming and lactulose
- Levothyroxine
- Methyldopa
- Ranitidine.

Timing

- If the drug is taken during the first 17 days after conception, there is an 'all-or-nothing' effect—i.e. if most cells are affected, this leads to spontaneous miscarriage, and if a few cells are affected, this leads to cell repair/replacement and a normal fetus.
- Exposure during the first trimester (especially weeks 3–11) carries the greatest risk of permanent congenital abnormalities, as during this embryonic phase the cells differentiate and major organs are formed.
- During the second or third trimester, the main risks are growth defects, functional loss (e.g. deafness), or fetal tissue toxicity, rather than gross structural abnormalities. However, organs such as the cerebral cortex and renal glomeruli continue to develop and are still susceptible to damage.

- Shortly before or during labour there is a risk of maternal complications (e.g. NSAIDs and maternal bleeding) or neonate complications (e.g. opioids and sedation).

Other considerations

- Consider the effect of drugs when used in ♀ of childbearing age or for ♂ trying to father a child, as drugs can have a harmful effect at any stage of pregnancy. It is unusual for an ↑ risk in congenital malformations to be associated with drugs/chemicals exposure in the father alone, unless they cause chromosomal abnormalities. It can take up to 3 months before drug-induced effects on ♂ reproduction become apparent.
- Not all the damaging effects of exposure during pregnancy are obvious at birth, some may only manifest later on in life (e.g. malignancy, intellectual, social and functional development).
- The presence or absence of teratogenic effects in animals does not necessarily translate to the same effects in humans, as their physiology, metabolism, and development are very different to humans. Think logically—if the agent causes tail shortening in rats, is this relevant in humans? Some studies use higher doses in animals than would be used in humans.
- Drugs associated with abnormalities at high doses/during the first trimester might be lower risk at low doses/during the second or third trimester (e.g. fluconazole).
- If possible, avoid all drugs in the first trimester. If treatment cannot be avoided during pregnancy, in preference use established drugs that have good evidence of safety at the lowest effective dose. (NB: sometimes a lack of reports of teratogenicity for a well-established/frequently used drug may have to be taken as evidence of safety.)
- Teratogenic effects are usually dose related (e.g. neural tube defects with anticonvulsants); thus the drug may not exert a teratogenic effects below a threshold dose. Higher doses or combining more than one drug with the same effect (e.g. antiepileptics) will ↑ the risk.
- Consider non-drug treatments (e.g. acupressure wrist bands for morning sickness) or whether treatment can be delayed until after pregnancy, or at least after the first trimester.

Maternal considerations

- Maternal drug-handling changes during pregnancy but some may revert back to pre-pregnancy levels rapidly soon after delivery. The volume of distribution ↑, protein binding ↓, and renal function ↑ gradually. Take special care with drugs that have a narrow therapeutic index.
- Remind the mother that some over-the-counter, herbal, and vitamin products should be avoided in pregnancy.
- The disease itself may be a greater fetotoxic risk than the drug therapy and this should be factored into the benefit/risk assessment and any chronic condition monitored intensively during pregnancy. Many ♀ do not comply with drug treatment during pregnancy because of safety concerns, so discuss this with the mother and reassure her.

- All ♀ should take folate supplements from the time pregnancy is planned and for the first 12 weeks of pregnancy to reduce the risks of neural tube defects in the fetus.
- Remember to consider maternal contraindications and precautions when advising on a drug in pregnancy.

Handling potentially teratogenic drugs

There is little published evidence on whether occupational exposure to potentially teratogenic drugs can ↑ the risk of congenital abnormalities. Available data investigating the risks of occupational exposure amongst pregnant ♀ provide conflicting findings. Therefore in the absence of evidence or specific guidelines, sensible precautions should be taken to reduce the risk of exposure, especially by pregnant ♀ and ♀ planning a pregnancy. A risk assessment should be performed (using COSHH (Control of Substances Hazardous to Health) data as appropriate), and pregnant ♀ should be excluded from any task that poses even a low risk.

Handling blister-packed versions of a teratogenic tablet presents (virtually) no risk and film-coated or sugar-coated versions present a low risk. A high-risk procedure might involve preparation of cytotoxic infusions or handling crushed tablets of a known teratogenic drug. This type of procedure should not be carried out by pregnant ♀. ♀ (and ♂) of child-bearing potential (especially if planning a pregnancy) should take appropriate precautions (e.g. apron, mask, and gloves). Ideally, potentially teratogenic infusions should be prepared by centralized pharmacy reconstitution service, where the use of cytotoxic cabinets further ↓ the risk of exposure.

Further reading

Briggs GG, Freeman RK, Yaffe SJ (eds) (2014). *Drugs in Pregnancy and Lactation: A Reference Guide to Fetal and Neonatal Risk* (10th ed). Philadelphia, PA: Lippincott–Williams and Wilkins.

BUMPS (Best use of medicines in pregnancy). Information factsheets for members of public produced by UKTIS. ℘ www.medicinesinpregnancy.org/

'Motherisk' website, ℘ www.motherisk.org

Schaefer C, Peters PWJ, Miller RK (2014). *Drugs during Pregnancy and Lactation* (3rd ed). London: Academic Press Inc.

TOXBASE®. Drug monographs, including pregnancy risk (password required). ℘ www.toxbase.org

Reference

9. Welsh Medicines Resources Centre (2000). Prescribing in pregnancy. *Welsh Medicines Resources Bulletin* 7: 1–5. ℘ www.wemerec.org/Documents/bulletins/03pppg.PDF

Drugs in breastfeeding

Breastfeeding has many advantages over bottle feeding. Even if the mother is taking a drug that is excreted in breast milk it can be preferable to continue breastfeeding, as the excreted amount is rarely sufficient to produce a noticeable effect on the infant. General principles to ↓ risk to babies are listed in Box 10.5. Various textbooks and reference sources give information on using drugs in breastfeeding. There is insufficient evidence for many drugs to provide guidance on use in breastfeeding and several reference sources should be used to fully evaluate the risk/benefit of a drug in breastfeeding. Absence of information does not imply safety of a drug in breastfeeding.

The main questions to consider are as follows.

- Is the drug, or an active metabolite, excreted into breast milk in quantities that are clinically significant?
- Do these drug levels pose any threat to the infant's health?
- How efficiently is the drug absorbed and metabolized by the infant?
- What clinical effect does the drug have on the infant?

To answer these questions, the following factors must be considered.

Factors that affect drug transfer into breast milk

- *Maternal drug plasma level*—usually the most important determinant of breast milk drug levels. Some drugs are not absorbed from the gut at all (e.g. nystatin, ispaghula husk, sucralfate) or absorbed very poorly (e.g. orlistat, oral vancomycin, mesalazine). Drugs enter the breast milk primarily by passive diffusion. For most drugs, the level in the maternal drug compartment is directly proportional to the maternal plasma level.

Box 10.5 General principles to decrease risk to breastfed babies

- Consider whether non-drug therapy is possible; assess the benefit/risk ratio for both mother and infant
- Can treatment be delayed until the mother is no longer breastfeeding or the infant is older and can tolerate the drug better?
- Use drugs where safety in breastfeeding has been established; avoid new drugs where possible
- Keep the maternal dose as low as possible
- In preference, use drugs with a local effect limiting systemic exposure (e.g. inhalers, creams, or drugs not absorbed orally, such as nystatin)
- Use drugs with a short half-life, high protein binding, low oral bioavailability, or high molecular weight and avoid sustained-release preparations
- Avoid polypharmacy—additive side effects and drug interactions potentially ↑ the risk
- Advise the mother to breastfeed when the level of the drug in breast milk will be lowest (this is usually just before the next dose is due) or at least wait until the peak maternal levels will have subsided.

Thus, the higher the maternal dose, the higher is the drug level in the breast milk. Diffusion of drug between plasma and milk is a two-way process and is concentration dependent. At peak maternal plasma levels (T_{max}), drug levels in breast milk are also at their highest. As the level of the drug in the plasma falls, the level of the drug in breast milk also falls as drug diffuses from the milk back into the plasma. Thus drugs that only have a short half-life only appear in breast milk for a correspondingly short time.

- During the first 4 days after delivery, drugs diffuse more readily into the breast milk because there are gaps between the alveolar cell walls in mammary capillaries. These gaps permit enhanced access for most drugs, in addition to immunoglobulins and maternal proteins. This results in ↑ drug levels in breast milk during the neonatal stage. After the first 4–7 days, these gaps close.
- Some drugs pass into breast milk by an active process, such that the drug is concentrated in the milk. This occurs with iodides, especially radioactive iodides, making it necessary to interrupt breastfeeding.

- *Lipid solubility of the drug*—lipophilic fat-soluble drugs (e.g. benzodiazepines, chlorpromazine, and many other CNS-active drugs) preferentially dissolve in the lipid globules of breast milk. As a general rule, ↑ lipid solubility leads to ↑ penetration into milk. However, lipid solubility is not a good predictor of milk levels overall because fat represents a relatively small proportion of total milk volume.
- *Milk pH levels*—breast milk has a lower pH than blood. Thus drugs that are weak bases (e.g. isoniazid, barbiturates, and atropine-like drugs) are ionized in the milk, which makes them more water-soluble and thus less likely to diffuse back into the maternal plasma circulation. This can lead to accumulation of these drugs in breast milk. Conversely, weakly acidic drugs (e.g. penicillins, aspirin, and diuretics) tend not to accumulate in breast milk.
- *Molecular size/molecular weight of the drug*—as a general rule, 'bulky' drugs do not diffuse across capillary walls because the molecules are simply too large to pass through the gaps. Drugs with a molecular weight <200 are considered to have a small molecular weight. Generally, the smaller the molecular weight, the higher the relative transfer of the drug into milk.
- *Drug protein binding*—highly protein-bound (typically greater than 90%) drugs (e.g. phenytoin, warfarin and many NSAIDs) do not normally pass into breast milk in significant quantities because only free unbound drug diffuses across the capillary walls into breast milk. Bear in mind that if a new drug is added that displaces the first drug from protein-binding sites, this could (at least temporarily) ↑ milk levels of the first drug.

Infant factors

- *Bioavailability*—drugs that are broken down in the gut (omeprazole) or are not absorbed orally (e.g. insulin and aminoglycosides) should not cause any adverse effect because the infant's absorption of the drug is negligible, if any. Similarly, infant serum levels of any drug that has high first-pass metabolism are likely to be low. However, these drugs can sometimes have a local effect on the infant's gut, causing GI symptoms such as diarrhoea and constipation, which can be profound

- *Infant status, age, and maturity* must be taken into account, as it affects their ability to handle medication. If the baby is premature, sick, or unstable, they might be less able to tolerate even small quantities of the drug. Consider whether drug side effects could exacerbate the infant's underlying disease, e.g. opioids in breast milk may be a higher risk for a baby with respiratory problems than for a healthy baby.
- *Metabolism and excretion* of some drugs are altered in infancy. Neonates, especially premature infants, are at greatest risk from drug exposure due to immature or impaired renal and hepatic function. Thus the drug effects can be greater than expected because the clearance of the drug is ↓. This can be especially marked for drugs (or their active metabolites) with a long half-life.
- *Drugs that are often administered to infants* (e.g. paracetamol, penicillin, and aciclovir) are generally safe if absorbed in breast milk. As a general rule, <1% of the maternal dose reaches the infant. Thus, if the normal infant dose is >1% of the maternal dose, it is usually safe, but side effects can still occur (e.g. antibiotic-induced diarrhoea).

Other factors to consider

- Some mothers and healthcare workers assume that because the infant was exposed to the drug during pregnancy, it will be safe in breastfeeding. However, in pregnancy it is the maternal organs that clear the drug from the infant's circulation, but during breastfeeding the infant is clearing the drug. In addition, some adverse effects, such as respiratory depression, are not relevant during pregnancy but become relevant after delivery.
- Consider avoiding the use of drugs known to cause serious toxicity in adults and children. Some drugs are toxic to infants even in small amounts and should be avoided.
- Some mothers are resistant to using conventional medicines during breastfeeding because of perceived risks and decide to use alternative therapies. Drugs which are natural to the body (e.g. iron, potassium, and ascorbic acid) are unlikely to be harmful unless large doses are used. Mothers should also be reminded that herbal or homeopathic medicines might be excreted in breast milk and cause adverse effects on the infant.
- Remember also to advise mothers that over-the-counter medicines, alcohol, and other recreational drugs may be excreted in breast milk.
- Some drugs can inhibit or even stop breast milk production. These include bromocriptine and other dopamine agonists, diuretics, and moderate to heavy alcohol intake. Drugs that ↑ breast milk production (e.g. chlorpromazine, haloperidol, and other dopamine antagonists) may lead to concern from the mother that the baby is not taking the full amount. Drugs can also inhibit an infant's sucking reflex (e.g. phenobarbital) or alter sensory qualities (e.g. affect the taste) of the milk resulting in feeding problems.
- If medication is taken over a long period, even drugs that are excreted into breast milk in relatively low levels can accumulate and cause adverse effects, as a result of prolonged half-life in infancy.

- Sometimes breastfeeding might have to be interrupted or stopped completely if there is no alternative to administering a potentially risky drug. For short courses (<48h), it might be possible to stop breastfeeding temporarily. Using a breast pump and discarding the expressed milk until such time as it is safe to resume breastfeeding should encourage continued breast milk production. Some mothers might find bottle feeding difficult because of the more complex processes involved, cost, or cultural issues and might need extra support.

Further reading

Briggs GG, Freeman RK, Yaffe SJ (eds) (2014). *Drugs in Pregnancy and Lactation* (10th ed). Philadelphia, PA: Lippincott Williams & Wilkins.

Hale TW (ed) (2014). *Medications and Mother's Milk* (16th ed). Amarillo, TX: Pharmasoft Medical Publishing.

Specialist Pharmacy Service (SPS). 'Safety in lactation' website, ℘ www.sps.nhs.uk

Toxnet. 'Drugs and Lactation Database (LactMed)' website, ℘ http://toxnet.nlm.nih.gov/new-toxnet/lactmed.htm

Drugs and dietary considerations

Dietary considerations may impact on drug therapy in various ways. In addition to drug–food interactions (see ➲ 'Drug interactions', pp. 23–5), food allergies or intolerances and cultural or religious dietary restrictions may have an impact on choice of drug therapy. Certain metabolic disorders also require restrictions on certain foodstuffs which may also be found as excipients in medicines.

Food allergy or intolerance

Food and drink allergy is reported to affect 5% of children and 3–4% of adults in Westernized countries, with the prevalence of food intolerances thought to be ↑. It is important to distinguish between a true food allergy (i.e. symptoms of hypersensitivity occur after ingestion of the food) or intolerance (e.g. proven gluten intolerance) and a perceived food intolerance and consequent food exclusion on the part of the patient.

The most common food allergens in adults and children are:

- peanuts and other nuts
- wheat
- eggs
- milk
- soy
- fish and shellfish
- food additives (colouring and flavouring agents).

In these instances, a true hypersensitivity reaction, ranging from rash to anaphylaxis, could occur as a result of exposure to the allergen even in the extremely small quantities that might be present as excipients to the drug. Nut allergy is often potentially serious, with anaphylaxis being a risk. Some people will be so sensitive to nuts (especially peanuts) that topical exposure can lead to anaphylaxis. Pharmacists need to be aware that topical agents may contain nut oils, notably arachis (i.e. peanut) oil and sesame seed oil (to which there is often cross-sensitivity).

Food and drink intolerance can vary in severity, but exposure to the offending agent in a drug may lead to GI symptoms (e.g. bloating, cramps, and diarrhoea) in some patients. Typical examples are:

- gluten (wheat, rye, barley, oats)
- lactose.

The small amounts of lactose in most pharmaceutical products are unlikely to be harmful, unless the patient has a severe intolerance.

Pharmacists need to be aware of the possibility of food allergy or intolerance in their patients and should include questioning regarding this when taking a drug history. Listing drugs which may contain food allergens is beyond the scope of this section. If a patient reports significant symptoms as a result of exposure to a food or drink substance, pharmacists should check whether any new drugs contain the offending agent. This information can frequently be found in the summary of product characteristics (SPC); however, SPCs do not always list all excipients therefore contact the manufacturer for full details.

Egg allergy is often a cause for concern with vaccinations as some vaccines are derived from egg culture. The UK Department of Health advises that a history of anaphylaxis to eggs contraindicates the yellow fever vaccine.

Individuals who have an egg allergy may be at ↑ risk of reaction to some influenza vaccines. However, there are egg-free, or very low ovalbumin content, influenza vaccines available and studies show they may be used safely in individuals with egg allergies. All other vaccines, including MMR (but check SPC as brand specific) are considered safe.

The amount of sugar (glucose and sucrose) in some medicines can occasionally be significant enough to affect blood sugar levels in diabetic patients. Also consider the sodium content of drugs if patients are on a restricted salt diet.

Cultural or religious considerations

Some drugs and formulation components (e.g. capsule shells) are derived from animal sources or may contain animal derivatives as excipients. This may affect drug choice for strict vegetarians or vegans or for those who avoid certain animal products for religious reasons. However, ingestion of the animal product may be permitted if it is for medical purposes or because it is not taken orally—e.g. Jewish law permits the use of heparins, even though they are of porcine origin, as they are not taken by mouth. It is important to remember that gelatin capsules are usually derived from animal sources and that other excipients (e.g. magnesium stearate) may be derived from plant or animal sources. The manufacturing company should be able to advise the source of the ingredient or if it is kosher or halal.

Lactose is a common excipient, but as it is milk derived it will be avoided by Jews who keep dietary laws strictly which prohibit consumption of milk and meat together. Where alcohol is avoided for religious or cultural reasons, this may also affect the choice of drug or formulation as some liquid medicines and injections contain alcohol. Some individuals will also have concerns about the use of topical agents which contain alcohol as they could inadvertently ingest it by getting the alcohol-containing product on their hands.

Fasting for religious reasons (e.g. during Ramadan) may mean that patients miss both oral and parenteral medicines. Most religions exempt people who are sick from fasting, but patients who are well and on long-term therapy may wish to observe the fasts. Pharmacists may be able to assist these patients by adjusting timings and frequency of medicines to comply with the fast. Diabetics should be advised to be cautious about fasting, as it is difficult to maintain glycaemic control. It is advised that patients with type 1 diabetes, especially if poorly controlled, or pregnant should not fast.

Metabolic disorders

A range of metabolic disorders exist whereby a genetic mutation leads to a defect in the metabolic pathway. Restriction of certain foodstuffs is often a key component of management of these disorders and certain excipients may be present in medicines which have an impact on the disease. Examples include:
- galactosaemia—avoid lactose
- phenylketonuria—avoid aspartame which is a source of phenylalanine. Aspartame is widely used as a sweetener in liquid and dispersible medicines.

Further reading
Food Additives and Ingredients Association. 'E-Numbers' website (contains detailed list of E numbers). ℘ www.faia.org.uk/e-numbers/
Gilani A (2011). Medicines management during Ramadan. *Pharm J* 286: 1–4.
Public Health England (2014). 'Immunisation Against Infectious Disease (the Green Book)', ℘ www.gov.uk/government/collections/immunisation-against-infectious-disease-the-green-book

Glucose-6-phosphate dehydrogenase deficiency

Glucose-6-phosphate dehydrogenase (G6PD) is an enzyme that produces reduced glutathione, which protects red blood cells against oxidant stress. Exposure to an oxidant in G6PD-deficient individuals can lead to acute haemolysis of RBCs. G6PD deficiency is an X-linked genetic disorder. Thus ♂ are either normal or deficient, whereas ♀ are normal, deficient, or intermediate.

G6PD deficiency is distributed worldwide, with the highest prevalence in Africa, Southern Europe, the Middle East, Southeast Asia, and Oceania. Thus patients originating from any of these areas should be tested for G6PD deficiency before being administered an at-risk drug.

There are varying degrees of G6PD deficiency, (and depending on the magnitude of G6PD deficiency and the consequent severity of haemolysis) with people of African origin generally having a lower level of deficiency (and therefore being more able to tolerate oxidizing drugs) and those of Southeast Asian and Mediterranean origin generally having a high level of deficiency. Mild deficiency is defined as 10–60% of normal activity. Note that young red cells are not deficient in G6PD. Thus false-normal levels can occur during or immediately after an acute haemolytic attack, when new red cells are being produced or when assessing neonates, who have a young red-blood cell population.

Although many people remain clinically asymptomatic throughout their lives, they are all at risk of acute haemolytic anaemia in response to one of the following trigger events:
- Infection
- Acute illness
- Some foods, typically fava (broad) beans
- Oxidizing drugs.

A haemolytic attack usually starts with malaise, sometimes associated with weakness, lumbar pain, and abdominal pain. This is followed several hours or days later by jaundice and dark urine. In most cases, the attack is self-limiting, although adults (but rarely children) can develop renal failure.

Drug treatment in G6PD deficiency

Patients in at-risk groups should be tested for G6PD deficiency. There are a number of screening tests for G6PD deficiency, which should then be confirmed by quantitative test of G6PD activity.
- Patients with severe deficiency should not be prescribed highly oxidizing drugs (Box 10.6), and drugs with a lower risk should be prescribed with caution.
- Patients with a lesser degree of deficiency may be able to tolerate even the drugs listed in Box 10.6, but exercise caution.
- Susceptibility to the haemolytic risk from drugs varies; a drug found to be safe in some G6PD-deficient patients may not be equally safe in others.
- The risk and severity of haemolytic anaemia is almost always dose related. Thus, even severely deficient patients can tolerate low doses of these drugs if there is no alternative. For example, for treatment of *Plasmodium vivax* or *Plasmodium ovale*, a dose of primaquine 45mg once

Box 10.6 Drugs to be used with caution in G6PD deficiency

Drugs with definite risk of haemolytic anaemia in most G6PD-deficient patients (avoid)

- Dapsone and other sulphones
- Methylthioninium chloride (methylene blue)
- Nitrofurantoin
- Primaquine
- Quinolones
- Rasburicase
- Sulfonamides (including co-trimoxazole).

Drugs with possible risk of haemolytic anaemia in some G6PD-deficient patients (caution)*

- Aminosalicylic acid
- Ascorbic acid
- Aspirin (doses >1g/day)
- Chloramphenicol
- Chloroquine[†]
- Hydroxychloroquine
- Isoniazid
- Levodopa
- Menadione (water-soluble vitamin K derivatives)
- Probenecid
- Pyrimethamine
- Quinidine[†]
- Quinine[†]
- Streptomycin
- Sulfonylureas.

*Use with caution; low doses probably safe.

[†]Acceptable to treat acute malaria at usual doses.

weekly for 8wks can be used instead of the usual dose of primaquine 15–30mg once daily for 14 days.
- Drug manufacturers do not routinely carry out testing to identify the potential risk of their drug to G6PD-deficient patients. Do not assume with new drugs that if there is no warning in the SPC, the drug is safe.

Treatment of a haemolytic attack
- Withdraw drug
- Maintain high urine output
- Blood transfusion, if indicated.

Further reading

Cappellini MD, Fiorelli G (2008). Glucose-6-phosphate dehydrogenase deficiency. *Lancet* 371:64–74.
'G6PD Deficiency Association' website, ✆ www.g6pd.org
Thompson A (2011). Questions from practice: G6PD deficiency. *Pharm J* 286: 205.

Drugs in porphyria

The porphyrias are a group of rare hereditary metabolic disorders in which there are defects in the haem biosynthesis pathway. In the acute porphyrias (alanine (ALA) dehydratase deficiency, acute intermittent and variegate porphyrias, and hereditary coproporphyria) there is overproduction of porphyrin precursors as well as porphyrins which can lead to systemic symptoms including:

- acute (often severe) abdominal pain, sometimes pain in back, thighs, or extremities
- constipation
- nausea and vomiting
- hypertension
- tachycardia and cardiac arrhythmias
- muscle weakness and loss of sensation that can lead to paralysis
- convulsions
- confusion, disorientation, hallucinations, paranoia
- hyponatraemia and hypokalaemia.

Several factors may work together to induce an acute porphyria attack, which may include alcohol, endogenous hormone changes, infection, weight loss, calorie restriction, smoking stress, major surgery, and drugs.

Numerous drugs have been linked to precipitating an acute porphyria attack, but these are mostly based on animal or *in vitro* studies. Pharmacists need to be aware of which drugs should be avoided and which are considered safe in porphyria, as an acute attack is serious and potentially life-threatening. The National Acute Porphyria Service (NAPS) provides specialist clinical support and treatment on porphyria. One of the NAPS centres, the Welsh Medicines Information Centre (WMIC) publishes a list of drugs considered safe in acute porphyria.[10] The European Porphyria Network also publishes a drugs list based on the WMIC list and includes an unsafe drugs list too.[11] Absence of a drug from the lists does not necessarily imply that the drug is safe, as there is no information on safety in porphyria for many drugs. Check general statements for groups of drugs first where possible.

In serious or life-threatening conditions a drug should not be withheld just because it is not on the 'safe' list. If there is no alternative 'safe' drug, treatment should be commenced and urinary porphobilinogen measured before treatment and regularly during treatment. If levels ↑ or symptoms of an acute attack occur, the drugs should be stopped and the acute attack treated.

Patients with acute porphyrias need to be aware that drugs can precipitate an attack and to inform healthcare professionals that they have porphyria. Relatives of affected patients should be screened and advised on the potential risks with certain drugs. The British Porphyria Association publishes a series of fact sheets for patients including advice on drugs.[12] The European Porphyria Network also publishes similar information in various languages.[11]

Treatment of an acute attack is symptomatic and supportive, ensuring that the drugs used are those considered safe in porphyria (Table 10.9). Specific treatment is with haem arginate, which replenishes the body's haem stores and so through negative feedback reduces the production of porphyrins and porphyrin precursors.

Table 10.9 Drug treatments in acute porphyria: symptomatic treatment

Condition	Drug category	Drug*
Abdominal pain	Analgesics	Aspirin
		Diamorphine
		Dihydrocodeine
		Ibuprofen
		Morphine
		Paracetamol
		Pethidine (meperidine)
Vomiting	Antiemetics	Chlorpromazine
		Ondansetron
		Prochlorperazine
		Promazine
Hypertension and tachycardia	Antihypertensives	β-blockers, e.g. atenolol, labetalol, propranolol
Neurosis, psychosis, and seizures	Sedatives, tranquillizers, and anticonvulsants	Chlorpromazine
		Clonazepam
		Lorazepam
		Promazine
Constipation	Laxatives	Bulk-forming (ispaghula)
		Lactulose
		Senna

* Drugs are listed alphabetically rather than preferred order of treatment. Management of symptoms should be individualized to meet the needs of the patient.

The non-acute or cutaneous porphyrias are associated with skin photosensitivity but do not show the serious systemic symptoms associated with the acute porphyrias. Thus it is not necessary to avoid exposure to 'unsafe' drugs in these conditions (with the exception of chloroquine and related drugs in antimalarial treatment and prophylactic doses in patients with porphyria cutanea tarda). Patients should avoid exposure to the sun by sun avoidance and wearing appropriate clothing, as the majority of sun screens do not filter out the long UVA wavelengths and visible light which activate porphyrins. In mild cases, some high-factor UVA sunblocks may provide adequate protection.

Further reading

'European Network Project' website, ℘ www.porphyria-europe.org
NHS Wales. 'Porphyria Service Cardiff' website (diagnostic and clinical advisory service), ℘ http://www.cardiffandvaleuhb.wales.nhs.uk/national-acute-porphyria-service-naps
Welsh Medicines Information Centre. 'Porphyria Information Service' website, ℘ http://www.ukmi.nhs.uk/activities/specialistServices/default.asp?pageRef=6

References

10. Welsh Medicines Information Centre. 'Drugs considered "safe" in the acute porphyrias' website, ℘ http://wmic.wales.nhs.uk/wp-content/uploads/2016/07/2016-porphyria-safe-list-FINAL.pdf
11. 'European Network Project' website, ℘ www.porphyria-europe.org
12. British Porphyria Association. 'Leaflets' website, ℘ www.porphyria-europe.org.uk/?page_id=508

Patient-specific issues

Medicines for children: introduction

Children represent a significant proportion of patients in both primary and secondary care. It is important to remember that children are not small adults, and neither are they a homogenous group. Drug handling in children can be quite different to that in adults and can also be different at different ages. For medical and pharmaceutical purposes, children are usually grouped according to the following ages:

- Premature—born before 37wks of gestation
- Neonate—≤4wks old (if premature, add the number of weeks premature, e.g. if born 2wks premature, the baby would be considered a neonate until it was 6wks old)
- Infant—4wks to 2yrs
- Child—2yrs to (usually) 12yrs
- Adolescent—(usually) 12–18yrs.

From 12yrs old onwards, drug handling and dosing is usually the same as for adults, but adolescents require special consideration in terms of social and emotional needs.

Medicines for children: pharmacokinetics and pharmacodynamics

Virtually all pharmacokinetic parameters change with age. An understanding of how drug handling changes with age is essential to avoid toxicity or underdosing.

Absorption

GI absorption may be slower in newborns and infants than in adults. Newborns have a prolonged gastric emptying time. Lower levels of gastric acid in newborns might ↓ absorption of some drugs (e.g. itraconazole). Whereas drugs which are broken down by acid may have an ↑ bioavailability (e.g. ampicillin). Drugs that bind to calcium or magnesium should not be given at the same time as milk feeds.

IM absorption requires muscle movement to stimulate blood flow and so could be erratic in newborns who are relatively immobile. In addition, blood supply to the muscles is very variable. Low muscle mass and pain associated with IM injections may make administration of drugs undesirable.

Topical absorption of agents is enhanced in neonates and infants because the skin is thinner and better hydrated. This age group also has a proportionally larger body surface area for weight than older children (see ➔ Table 11.1, p. 209). Thus, topical agents applied over a large area can provide a significant systemic dose.

Rectal absorption of agents may differ from that of adults as infants have ↑ rectal contractions, which may reduce the duration of retention.

Distribution

Total body water changes with age:
- Premature—80% of body weight
- Newborn—75% of body weight
- Children—60–65% of body weight
- Adults—60% of body weight.

This affects the volume of distribution of water-soluble drugs, and higher doses per kilogram might be required for premature or newborn infants.

Protein binding

In neonates, protein binding of drugs is less than in adults, but within a few months after birth it is similar to adult levels. ↓ protein binding might account for the ↑ sensitivity of neonates to some drugs due to the ↑ free drug in the body (e.g. theophylline).

Metabolism

Premature and newborn infants metabolize drugs more slowly than adults, due to immature metabolism at birth. This can mean higher loading doses are required, due to a larger volume of distribution but with reduced frequency. However, young children have a faster metabolic rate, which ↓ to adult levels with ↑ age. Thus doses of highly metabolized drugs are proportionally lower per kilogram for neonates and infants and higher for young children. As the child grows, doses should be frequently recalculated not only to allow for differing rates of drug metabolism, but also to allow for ↑ height and weight.

Premature infants and neonates have immature renal function, with the neonatal GFR being 0.6–0.8mL/min/1.73m^2, whereas term neonates have a GFR of 2–4mL/min/1.73m^2. Thus doses should be ↓ accordingly. After infancy, plasma clearance of some drugs is significantly ↑ because of both ↑ hepatic elimination and ↑ renal excretion.

Pharmacodynamics

Children's response to medication is not fully researched. However, it is known that children do not respond to medication in the same way as adults. Density and sensitivity of receptors may differ leading to unexpected sensitivities to drugs. An example of this is ciclosporin, where lower levels can produce a greater immunosuppressive response. Drugs may also lead to unexpected or more severe adverse effects when compared to adult dosing, such as selective serotonin receptor inhibitors and suicide risk in teenagers.

Medicines for children: licensing

It is believed that across Europe 40% of prescribing in children is unlicensed or 'off label'—i.e. the drug is not licensed for use in that age range, route, dose, or indication.

Extemporaneous preparations and imported and specials products are effectively 'named patient' and thus unlicensed. Until such time as a wider range of formulations is available or drug manufacturers perform the relevant trials to obtain licences for paediatric use or indications, this is an unavoidable practice.

To address this inequality, the European Union created regulation to encourage medicines information and high-quality research for paediatric medication. This is leading to more licensed drugs and a greater quality of information for medicines use in children. The use of unlicensed and off-label medication, may give rise to an ↑ risk of adverse effects. Therefore, it is important that appropriate medicines information is available to inform healthcare professionals involved in prescribing and supplying of unlicensed and off-label medication.

The Royal College of Paediatrics and Child Health and the Neonatal and Paediatric Pharmacists Group (NPPG) have issued a joint declaration stating the following:

'The informed use of unlicensed medicines, or of licensed medicines for unlicensed applications, is necessary in paediatric practice.'

Pharmacists should ensure that licensed preparations are used wherever possible. If there is no alternative, they should ensure that both prescribers and parents (and the child, as appropriate) are informed of unlicensed or off-label use. It is especially important to ensure that parents or carers do not feel that the medicine is 'sub-standard' or 'second best' because it is unlicensed. In general, it is not considered necessary to obtain formal consent for the use of unlicensed medicines in this context. The NPPG has produced leaflets suitable for parents and older children to explain the need to use unlicensed and off-label medicines. These are available on the NPPG website (see also ➔ p. 211). Local guidelines on documentation and consent for use of unlicensed medicines should be complied with.

It is important that pharmacists ensure a continued supply of unlicensed, extemporaneous, and special medicines by liaising with and providing product information to GPs and community pharmacists.

Medicines for children: calculating children's doses

A reputable reference source should be used for children's doses. Doses may be calculated in different ways and it is important to be clear how the dose is calculated to avoid the risk of overdose. Doses are usually quoted as follows:

- The total dose in mg/kg body weight per day, and the number of doses it should be divided into (e.g. xmg/kg daily, in four divided doses)
- The individual dose in mg/kg body weight per dose, and the number of doses that should be given each day (e.g. xmg/kg four times a day).

Most doses are based on weight, although doses based on body surface area are more accurate because this takes into account the child's overall size (Table 11.1). Body surface area dosing is more frequent for drugs if accurate dosing is critical (e.g. cytotoxic drugs). Nomograms for calculating body surface area can be found in paediatric drugs handbooks, or the following equation can be used:

$$\text{body surface area}\,(m^2) = \sqrt{\frac{\text{body weight}\,(kg) \times \text{height}\,(cm)}{3600}}$$

Very rarely it is impossible to find a published and validated children's dose for a drug, in which case it can be estimated from the adult dose based on physiological or pharmacokinetic factors[1] or using approximate proportions (Table 11.2). This should only be used as a last resort. This method tends to give an underdose. Calculated doses should usually be rounded up, rather than down, and the dose titrated according to clinical response, as necessary. However, caution should be taken due to the unknown pharmacodynamics that may occur.

Always take into account the usual and maximum doses in adults. Many sources that quote children's doses will give a maximum dose. If the calculated dose for a child exceeds the usual adult dose and no maximum is quoted, consider whether this dose is appropriate (e.g. if it is known that children of that age metabolize the drug faster than adults). For obese children it may be more appropriate to use ideal body weight. If in any doubt seek expert advice.

Table 11.1 Approximate surface area and weight*

	Weight (kg)	Surface area (m²)
Newborn	3	0.20
1yr	10	0.50
3yrs	15	0.65
5yrs	20	0.80
9yrs	30	1.0
14yrs	50	1.5
Adult	70	1.9

. * Note that many children in developing countries might only weigh 60–80% of the average weight.

Table 11.2 Estimating children's doses as a proportion of the adult doses*

Weight	Age	Proportion of adult dose
3–5kg	0–5 months	1/8
6–10kg	6 months–1 yr	1/4
11–20kg	1–6yrs	1/3
21–30kg	7–10yrs	1/2
>30kg	11–15yrs	3/4

* Note that this method tends to result in an underdose. This method should only be used where no other validated paediatric dose is available.

Reference

1. Bartelink IH, Rademaker CM, Schobben AF, et al. (2006). Guidelines on paediatric dosing on the basis of development physiology and pharmacokinetic considerations. *Clin Pharmacokinet* 45: 1077–97.

Medicines for children: adherence

Counselling on medicine use and adherence issues is important for children. Parents might be familiar with taking medicines themselves but this doesn't necessarily mean that they will cope with giving medicines to their child, especially if they are distressed by the child's diagnosis or the child is uncooperative. The toddler age group is often the most difficult because at this age they can be uncooperative but lack the language ability and insight needed for parents to reason with them.

- Wherever possible and within the child's level of understanding, pharmacists should aim to involve the child in discussions about their medicines.
- Ideally, counselling about medicine use and adherence should involve both parents (or two carers), especially if the therapy is complex and/or long term. As appropriate, also involve other people, such as school nurses, although it is best to avoid giving doses during school time if at all possible.
- Always aim to involve the child/parents/carers in discussions about medicines and never assume what a child's preference is. Some children/adolescents may prefer some drugs as liquids and other medicines in tablet/capsule form depending upon taste, size/volume, and consistency.
- The most appropriate delivery form should be selected. Most parents find an oral syringe easy to use but some children can object to this, and once measured the medicine might have to be transferred to a spoon. Ensure advice on how to use syringes, bungs, and spoons is provided.
- Parents and carers might find it easier to give the medicine mixed with a small amount of food or drink. They should be taught how to do this correctly so that the child takes the full dose. Medicines should not be added to baby's bottle feeds because the full quantity might not be taken.
- If a child is spitting out doses or vomiting after a dose due to an unpleasant taste, consider if there is an alternative liquid, 'melt formulation', or if a tablet can be crushed/dissolved in water, or if the contents of a capsule can be mixed with a small amount of food such as apple sauce or mixed with a sweet liquid such or cordial to mask the medication/taste. Always check for interactions/compatibility before advising. 'Specials' or 'named-patient' unlicensed formulations may also be an option, if available. However, continuity of supply should be considered and planned before commencing. Tips on making medicines more palatable for children are given in Box 11.1.
- Be aware that some patient information leaflets might be for indications other than the one for which the medicine is being used.
- Explain to the child, parent, or carer why the child needs to take their medicine in simple terms, allowing for any limitations on disclosure of the diagnosis—e.g. a child may not be aware of their diagnosis, but might have been told that they need medicine to help them get better.
- For complex medication regimens, additional written information such as a medication administration record (MAR) chart may be useful to aid administration. Discuss with families if this would be helpful.

Box 11.1 Tips on making medicines more palatable

- Chill the medicine (but do not freeze it).*
- Take the medicine through a straw.
- Use an oral syringe to direct the medicine towards the back of the mouth and away from the tongue (and therefore away from the highest concentration of taste buds).
- Chocolate disguises many flavours—try mixing the medicine with a small amount of chocolate milk, spread, or syrup.*
- Coat the tongue and roof of the mouth with a spoonful of peanut butter or chocolate spread before taking the medicine.
- Suck an ice cube or ice lolly immediately before taking the medicine.
- Brush teeth after taking the dose.
- Eat strongly flavoured food after the dose—e.g. crisps, Marmite®, or citrus fruit (small amounts of these foods should not adversely affect drug absorption).

* Check drug compatibility and storage temperature requirements.

- Encourage parents/carers to involve the child in the administration process. From quite a young age (and with appropriate supervision and support), children can be taught to measure doses of liquid medicines, make up a Monitored Dosage Systems (MDS) such as a Dosette® box, or even self-administer insulin.
- Help parents/carers to think ahead to how medicines will be administered during the school day or on a school or youth organization residential event. Tailoring the regimen to once-daily or twice-daily dosing means that drug administration during school hours can usually be avoided.
- Consider the family situation; some children may require additional supplies of medication such as inhalers or insulin pens or duplicate copies of information leaflets if they live at more than one address.
- Adolescents might wish to discuss their medicines without their parents present. Non-adherence in adolescents is not uncommon as a way of expressing independence and requires sensitive handling.

Further reading

'Neonatal and Paediatric Pharmacists Group' website ℘ www.nppg.org.uk

Pharminfotech. Advice on administering medicines to children, formulae for extemporaneous preparation, ℘ www.pharminfotech.co.nz

Paediatric Formulary Committee (2016). *BNF for Children*. London: BMJ Group, Pharmaceutical Press, and RCPCH Publications. ℘ www.bnfc.org

Royal College of Paediatrics and Child Health and the Neonatal Paediatric Pharmacists Group (2014). 'Medicines for Children – information for parents and carers', ℘ http://www.rcpch.ac.uk/child-health/childrens-medicines/information-parents-and-carers

Royal Pharmaceutical Society (2013). 'Medicines Optimisation: Helping patients to make the most of medicines. Good practice guidance for healthcare professionals in England', ℘ www.rpharms.com/promoting-pharmacy-pdfs/helping-patients-make-the-most-of-their-medicines.pdf

'Pill school': teaching children how to take tablets and capsules

Background

Children, especially small children, will usually take their medicines as liquids. This may be because the dose can only be accurately measured as a liquid, because the child is too small or unwell to swallow tablets or capsules, or because they have a fear of choking. However, a solid-dose formulation may be preferable if the liquid has a bad taste or a suitable liquid formulation is not available. To aid swallowing some tablets can be halved or quartered using a tablet cutter, or crushed and dispersed in liquid or food, and some capsules can be opened. A pharmacist should advise on whether a medicine is suitable for crushing or dividing, e.g. controlled-release tablets should not be crushed as this would affect their release mechanism.

Where it is desirable for the child to take their medicine as a tablet or capsule, the following technique (sometimes known as 'pill school') can be used.

Preparation

- Discuss the child's ability to swallow food, especially hard or chewy food, with the parents. Ask the parents, and the child if possible, whether they think the child would be able to swallow tablets or capsules.
- Ask whether the child has had any previous experience of taking tablets and capsules and whether this was successful.
- Check any dietary issues with respect to the placebo capsules to be used, e.g. allergies to food colouring or consumption of gelatin products.
- Ask parents to ensure that the child has not eaten or drunk anything immediately before the session so that they are not too full to swallow the capsules or water.
- Arrange the appointment for a time when the child will be alert and cooperative—e.g. not straight after school or nursery when they may be tired.
- Advise parents and other healthcare workers not to tell the child in advance what the session is about because this might create anxiety and resistance.
- To avoid possible disruption, ensure that the child has been to the toilet before starting the session.

Equipment

- Prepare a series of capsule shells of different sizes containing sugar strands and place in bottles labelled with the sizes. Place some loose sugar strands in a bottle. Keep bottles and labels hidden from the child's view.
- Two cups (one for the child and one for you) and a bottle of water.
- Two small trays or containers (e.g. weighing boats), one on which to place capsules and one to use if the child spits out a capsule.
- Tissues for mopping-up purposes.

Environment

- The room should be quiet, without distractions such as books or toys.
- Have only one other person present (as a chaperone) and ask them to sit behind the child out of view. Advise them not to intervene at any stage It may be preferable for this to be a 'neutral' person rather than a parent.
- Sit across the table from the child.

Process

- Explain the purpose of the session to the child in simple terms. Talk enthusiastically and mention good things about taking tablets or capsules—e.g. avoiding bad-tasting medicine.
- Show the bottle of sugar strands and place a few on the tray. Ask the child to show you that they can swallow these.
- Place two of the smallest capsules on the tray. Explain to the child that now you want them to try swallowing the sugar strands inside a capsule. Explain how to swallow a capsule without chewing and demonstrate this:
  - Sit or stand upright
  - Take a breath
  - Put the pill in the middle of your tongue
  - Take a mouthful of water and swallow
  - Keep your head straight.
- Show the child that you have swallowed the capsule by opening your mouth and sticking out your tongue. Make the process fun, but be firm if necessary.
- Ask the child to show you that they can do the same with the other capsule.
- Get them to show you that their mouth is empty by opening their mouth and sticking out their tongue. Praise the child for their success.
- If the child has been successful, repeat the process with the next size of capsule, again demonstrating how to swallow it if necessary. State that it is the next capsule, not that it is larger. Give praise and encouragement at each stage.
- If the child has difficulties swallowing a capsule at any stage, get them to spit it out. Encourage them to try again with the same size of capsule.
- If the child is unsuccessful at the second attempt or if they refuse to try again, stop the session. Do not pressure the child because this could create an association between capsule taking and distress. Praise the child for trying hard.
- At the end of the session, if the parents have not been present, bring them into the room so that the child can demonstrate successful capsule swallowing.
- Give the parents a supply of the largest size swallowed and written instructions on how to take capsules for further practice at home.
- Explain to the child that the medicines they will take could look different to the sample capsules but they should be able to swallow them in the same way.

After the session

- Discuss the child's achievement with medical staff.
- Review current or planned medication to establish whether it can be dispensed as tablets or capsules of a suitable size and shape.
- Bear in mind that uncoated and/or round tablets are harder to swallow than capsules, coated tablets, or oval/capsule-shaped tablets.

Medicines for older people: introduction

Older people are high consumers of medicines, both prescribed and non-prescribed. In the UK, 50% of NHS drug expenditure is consumed by medicines for older people. Prescribing for older people is often provided as 'repeats', without regular review. This can lead to prescribing for 'conditions' that are actually ADRs. Minimizing the risk of inappropriate polypharmacy[2] is a challenge in the care of older people, balancing the benefit of the use of evidence-based medicines with the risks from high pill burdens, poor adherence, ADRs, and drug interaction.

In the UK, the NSF for Older People[3] has a specific section on medicines management, with the following primary aims:

- Ensuring that older people gain maximum benefit from their medication to maintain or ↑ their quality and duration of life
- Ensuring that older people do not suffer unnecessarily from illness caused by excessive, inappropriate, or inadequate consumption of medicines.

Older people are at ↑ risk of medication-related problems:

- ↑ risk of ADRs (many preventable) caused by polypharmacy, drug interactions, and changes in pharmacokinetics and pharmacodynamics
- Underprescribing of some medicines—e.g. thrombolysis in MI
- Non-adherence
- Repeat medicines not being reviewed, leading to unnecessary long-term therapy and stockpiling
- Difficulty in accessing the GP practice and/or pharmacy.

References

2. The King's Fund (2013). 'Polypharmacy and medicines optimisation: Making it safe and sound'. ℘ www.kingsfund.org.uk/publications/polypharmacy-and-medicines-optimisation

3. Department of Health (2001). *National Service Framework: Older People*. London: Department of Health. ℘ www.gov.uk/government/publications/quality-standards-for-care-services-for-older-people

Medicines for older people: pharmacokinetics and pharmacodynamics

Physiological changes that occur with age affect drug handling and sensitivity. Predicting at what age these changes become significant is almost impossible because people 'age' at different rates, depending on environmental, social, and other factors. However, the pharmacist should be alert to possible changes in drug handling and sensitivity in any patient >75yrs of age.

Absorption

- Ageing rarely has a significant effect on absorption. Delayed gastric emptying ↑ time to peak concentrations (C_{max}) but is rarely clinically significant.
- ↓ production of gastric acid can lead to ↓ absorption of drugs that require an acid environment for absorption (e.g. itraconazole), but can slightly ↑ the amount absorbed of drugs that are broken down by gastric acid (e.g. penicillins).
- Bioavailability of levodopa is ↑ in older people, possibly because of ↓ levels of dopa decarboxylase in the gastric mucosa.
- ↓ regional blood flow might ↓ the rate of absorption of drugs administered by the IM or SC route, but the total amount absorbed is the same.

Distribution

- Lean body mass ↓ with age, leading to ↑ levels of drugs distributed in the muscle (e.g. digoxin).
- Adipose tissue ↑ up to the age of 85yrs, leading to ↑ tissue levels and thus prolonged duration of effect of lipid-soluble drugs (e.g. diazepam). Patients >85yrs tend to lose adipose tissue.
- ↓ in total body water leads to ↑ in the serum concentration of water-soluble drugs (e.g. gentamicin and digoxin).
- ↓ serum albumin (common in underweight older people) leads to ↑ levels of free drug for highly protein-bound drugs (e.g. NSAIDs, sulfonylureas, and warfarin). In the acute phase, homeostatic mechanisms usually counteract the ↑ drug effects. ↑ level of free drug also means ↑ amounts for clearance, so the effect is rarely significant in the long term.

Metabolism

Older people can have up to a 40% ↓ in hepatic blood flow. Drugs with high first-pass metabolism can be significantly affected (see ➡ 'Hepatic blood flow', p. 175). There might be up to 60% ↓ in metabolism of some drugs, such as NSAIDs and anticonvulsants, leading to ↑ concentration, duration of action, and possibly accumulation.

Excretion

The natural ageing process between the ages of 20 and 80yrs leads to a 30–35% loss of functioning of glomeruli, with a consequent up to 50% loss of normal renal function. Serum creatinine levels might be normal or near normal because of ↓ muscle mass, but creatinine clearance will be ↓. Acute illness and dehydration can cause a rapid decline in renal function, which can be exacerbated by the use of potentially nephrotoxic drugs, including high-dose antibacterials. Even a fairly well older patient may tolerate a combination of potentially nephrotoxic drugs (e.g. diuretic plus NSAID), but the addition of one more nephrotoxic drug (e.g. an antibacterial) can tip the balance towards renal impairment.

It is advisable to calculate the creatinine clearance (using the Cockcroft and Gault equation (see ➔ Box 10.3, p. 182)) for any patient >70yrs who is prescribed renally cleared or potentially nephrotoxic drugs. Remember that drugs such as morphine have active metabolites that are renally cleared. Drugs that rely on excretion into the urine for their effect—notably nitrofurantoin—can be ineffective in older people. Beware of low serum creatinine in older people with low muscle mass as the result may underestimate the degree of renal impairment.

Pharmacodynamic changes

As the body ages, there is a natural loss of function at a cellular level. This can lead to ↑ or ↓ drug sensitivity. Changes in receptor–drug interactions can occur—e.g. there is a ↓ response to both β-adrenoceptor agonists and β-adrenoceptor antagonists.

Homeostatic responses can be blunted in old age—e.g. postural hypotension is more likely to be caused by blunting of reflex tachycardia, and cardiac failure might result from fluid overload caused by over-enthusiastic rehydration or NSAIDs combined with ↓ cardiac output and renal function.

There is ↑ susceptibility to CNS effects of drugs. Even drugs that are not normally associated with CNS effects can cause such symptoms in older people (e.g. histamine H_2 receptor antagonists and diuretics). These effects can occur without changes in kinetics, probably because of ↑ CNS penetration or altered drug response. For example, confusion and disorientation are more common in older people receiving benzodiazepines, antidepressants, and NSAIDs, even at standard doses. In addition, changes in kinetics can lead to CNS effects not usually seen in younger people—e.g. ↓ renal function can lead to confusion associated with ↑ levels of drugs such as ciprofloxacin and aciclovir.

Medicines for older people: medication review

See also ➲ 'Medication review', pp. 60–1.

Regular medication review is an essential aspect of good quality care for older people. While medical professionals may undertake reviews, pharmacists in all sectors can contribute to effective review with patients. In a hospital setting, opportunities for medication review include medicines reconciliation at admission, during the hospital stay, and at discharge prior to writing the discharge prescription. Communication with the next sector of care about changes is essential for safe practice and good continuity of care. In primary care all patients >75yrs should have their drugs reviewed at least annually at their GP practice. Community pharmacists have funded opportunities to review medicines use through the New Medicines Service (NMS) and the Medicines Use Review Service (MUR) including post-hospital discharge. Patients who will most benefit from review can be prioritized according to their risk of medication-related problems. Risk factors include:

- patients taking four or more drugs
- patients recently discharged from hospital
- patients taking 'high-risk' medicines:
  - hypnotics—drowsiness and falls
  - diuretics—dehydration, renal failure, and confusion caused by hypokalaemia
  - NSAIDs—fluid retention and GI bleeds
  - antihypertensives—falls resulting from postural hypotension
  - digoxin—nausea, vomiting, and confusion could be missed as signs of toxicity
  - warfarin—bruising and bleeding.

Other factors that can ↑ the risk of medication-related problems are as follows:

- Social—lack of home support
- Physical—poor vision, hearing, and dexterity
- Mental—confusion, depression, and difficulty in understanding instructions.

Older people are often high users of over-the-counter medicines and the pharmacist should be alert to this. Many over-the-counter drugs can:

- be unnecessary
- ↑ the risk of drug interactions
- ↑ the risk of additive side effects
- be an indicator for ADRs to other medicines (e.g. high antacid consumption could point to NSAID-induced gastric irritation).

Be aware that patients may also take medication from other sources including relatives or friends or may be given treatments by other health practitioners.

Patients and/or carers (formal and informal) should be involved in every medication review in order to provide patient-centred care and not least because they are the ones who will be implementing changes in drug regimens. If reviews are conducted by the pharmacist alone, results/recommendations must be communicated in a timely way to all relevant health and social care professionals involved in the patient's care, e.g. GP practice, documentation in patient's hospital notes, with a copy to the patient. If patients are attending the clinic for a review, they should be asked to bring all medications with them ('brown-bag review') as an aid. A useful opening question for medication review is 'Tell me how medicine taking fits into your day'.

Effective medication review needs to address both clinical and behavioural issues in medicine-taking to support good adherence. Exploration of patient's beliefs, attitudes, and concerns about medication is important as poor adherence is often something which appears to be a practical issue, e.g. forgetting, but is actually psychological, e.g. the medicine isn't a priority, it doesn't help me.

Discussion in a medication review can also include addressing:

- stockpiling
- out-of-date medicines
- problems with reading or interpretation of medicine labels
- strategies for self-administration—e.g. marking containers or transferring medicines to other containers
- problems with manipulation—e.g. opening bottle caps or using technologically difficult products, such as inhalers or eye drops
- use of over-the-counter or herbal medicines.

The NO TEARS tool is a useful model both for medication review and when considering initiating a new drug:[4]

- **N**eed and indication.
  - Is the drug really necessary?
  - Is it being used to treat an adverse effect?
  - Can it be stopped?
- **O**pen questions.
  - Ask non-directive questions about the medication, such as:
    —Any problems?
    —Tell me how/when you take these medicines?
- **T**ests and monitoring.
  - Ensure that appropriate monitoring is being done for both desired effect and checking for ADRs.
  - Where possible ensure that tests, such as TDM and INR, are done beforehand so that the results can be used to inform the review.
  - Check adherence (see ➔ Chapter 1).
- **E**vidence and guidelines.
  - Ensure that treatment is evidence-based and complies with up-to-date local and national guidelines. If it doesn't comply, the reason should be rational and documented.
- **A**DRs.
  - Ask about ADRs.
  - Check whether a medicine is being used to treat side effects and, if possible, stop or change the causative drug.
- **R**isk reduction and prevention.
  - Pay special attention to 'high-risk' drugs. Are they really necessary?
  - Could the dose be reduced?
  - If initiating a drug, start at the lowest dose and cautiously titrate according to the response.
- **S**implification and switches.
  - Could a change of drug or formulation simplify the regimen or make self-administration easier?

Reference
4. Lewis T (2004). Using the NO TEARS tool for medication review. *BMJ* 329: 434.

Dealing with injecting drug users in hospital

Injecting drug users and people who misuse other drugs, including alcohol, can present behavioural, in addition to medical, challenges on admission to hospital. An awareness of the issues involved is important, but equally healthcare staff should not assume that all drug misusers are 'difficult' patients. Drugs of misuse include the following:

- Opioids
- Benzodiazepines
- Other prescription or over-the-counter drugs (e.g. anticholinergics)
- Cocaine
- Cannabis
- Alcohol.

Managing behaviour

- Don't assume that all drug misusers will misbehave. Treat the patient with respect, as you would any other patient. A suspicious or negative manner from the healthcare professional is more likely to generate negative behaviour from the patient.
- Remove temptation—ensure that all drug cupboards and trolleys are locked and drug deliveries are put away immediately.
- Use a firm no-nonsense approach. Guidelines or a contract for acceptable behaviour might be helpful (see ➔ 'Dealing with aggressive or violent patients', pp. 66–7).
- Liaise with local addiction teams for advice and support.

Patients who misuse drugs on the ward

Healthcare professionals should be aware that patients (or their visitors) might misuse drugs on the ward. Indicators for this are as follows:

- Large numbers of visitors and/or visitors at odd times.
- Signs of intoxication or a behaviour change, often after receiving visitors or temporarily leaving the ward.
- Actual evidence (e.g. empty syringe).

Management depends on local policy, but this type of behaviour should not be tolerated. A senior doctor or nurse will normally be the member of staff who addresses this issue with the patient. Other healthcare staff should ensure that their dealings with the patient are consistent with agreed management policies. A suggested approach is as follows:

- Do not condone or tolerate the behaviour; make it clear that it is unacceptable.
- Give a warning that the behaviour will not be tolerated and the patient will be discharged if it is repeated.
- Consider limiting the number of visitors and the time during which they can visit.
- Involve hospital security or the police, especially if the safety of other patients or healthcare staff is compromised.
- Liaise with senior managers/hospital legal advisers to ensure that action taken is within the law.

Handling illegal drugs

Pharmacists could be asked to take possession of illegal drugs that ward staff have taken from a patient. This might include schedule 1 drugs, which normally require a licence for possession. However, UK law allows pharmacists to take possession of illegal (including schedule 1) drugs for the following purposes:

• Destruction of the drug.
• Handing the drug over to the police.

In this situation, it can be difficult to maintain the patient's rights and confidentiality while remaining within the law.

If a sufficiently large quantity is involved, such that it is clear that the drug is not just for personal use, it might be deemed that the public interest outweighs patient confidentiality and the police should be called. The decision to involve the police should only be taken after consultation with senior management and legal advisers.

If the quantity involved is small and clearly for personal use, the drugs should be destroyed. The patient's authority is required to remove and destroy the drug, and if they refuse to hand it over, consideration should be given to discharging the patient or involving the police. Returning the drug to the patient is not an option, because this would make the pharmacist guilty of unlawful supply of a controlled drug.

Managing patients who are opioid dependent

Patients who are maintained on opioid-replacement therapy (e.g. methadone or buprenorphine) in the community should have this continued in hospital.

• Verify the dose independently—e.g. by contacting the GP, addictions service, or community pharmacist.
• Notify the community pharmacist of the patient's admission (to ensure the patient doesn't 'double up' by obtaining supplies from the community, in addition to the hospital supply) and discharge (to ensure that community supply is restarted).
• Liaise with the GP and addictions service to ensure a consistent approach.
• As a rule, it is best to avoid providing more than one or two doses of replacement therapy on discharge. Liaise with the GP/community pharmacist to ensure that valid prescription is available for therapy to be continued in the community after discharge.
• Avoid prescribing other opioids if at all possible, especially short-acting opioids (e.g. pethidine).
• Benzodiazepines should only be prescribed if medically indicated (e.g. for alcohol withdrawal). If night sedation is required, prescribe in accordance with local addictions service guidance.
• If a dose adjustment of the replacement therapy is required (e.g. because of drug interactions), liaise with the local addictions service.

Patients dependent on opioids who are not on replacement therapy require careful management.

• Methadone or buprenorphine should only be prescribed if there are objective signs of withdrawal.[5,6]
• The dose should be titrated according to objective withdrawal symptoms, not according to the patient's reported use of street opioids. A suggested regimen is as follows:

Day 1
- Objective signs of withdrawal—methadone 20mg single dose (stat).
- Further signs of withdrawal—methadone 10mg single dose can be repeated after 4h.
- Maximum dose of methadone in the first 24h is usually 40–50mg.

Day 2 onwards
- Total dose given in the first 24h should be prescribed as a single daily dose.
- Up to two additional doses of methadone (10mg) can be given every 24h if further objective signs of withdrawal occur. Rewrite the maintenance dose each day to include additional doses until dose titration is achieved.
- A dose of methadone 80mg daily is usually considered the maximum maintenance dose, but some centres use higher doses.
- At all times, doses should only be ↑ if there are objective signs of withdrawal. Bear in mind that methadone has a long half-life, and so it takes several days to reach steady-state concentrations.
- Additional doses should not be prescribed 'as required' (*pro re nata*, PRN)—the patient should be assessed each time by a doctor and any extra doses (if needed) prescribed as a single dose.
- If the patient wishes to continue replacement therapy after discharge, they should be referred to the local addictions service as soon as possible.
- Patients who do not wish to continue replacement therapy might require a rapid reduction of the therapy before discharge. Note that these patients will usually return to using street opioids on discharge; thus the risk of withdrawal is minimal.

It is advisable for hospitals to produce written guidelines on opioid replacement therapy in consultation with the local addictions service. This ensures continuity of care and can also be a great help to junior doctors, who may be pressurized by patients to prescribe replacement therapy inappropriately.

Managing alcohol withdrawal
See ➲ 'Treatment of alcohol withdrawal', pp. 658–60.

Management of concurrent illness
In general, concurrent illnesses in patients who misuse drugs should be managed in the same way as for any other patient. However, the following points should be considered:
- Avoid opioids, benzodiazepines, and other drugs that could be misused.
- Be aware that enzyme inducers and inhibitors can affect methadone levels.
- If the patient has a chaotic lifestyle, avoid drugs with a narrow therapeutic index—e.g. direct oral anticoagulants (such as apixaban) may be preferable to warfarin for deep vein thrombosis (DVT).

Pain control
Pain should be managed in the same way as for any other patient. Many HCPs assume that patients on opioid replacement therapy require less analgesia, and the patient might insist that they require extra analgesia because

of tolerance. If the patient is experiencing pain, it is clear that the replacement therapy is not blocking all opioid receptors and analgesia is required. Ideally, opioids—both weak and strong—should be avoided. If an opioid is required, a long-acting opioid is preferred. Tramadol has no advantage over codeine in this setting.

Because buprenorphine is a partial antagonist, it can present a specific problem in patients who require opioid analgesia (e.g. postoperatively). It might be appropriate to convert the patient to an equivalent dose of morphine before surgery. The local addiction service should be contacted for advice.

References

5. Wesson DR, Ling W (2003). The Clinical Opiate Withdrawal Scale (COWS). *J Psychoactive Drugs* 35(2): 253–9.
6. Sullivan JT, Sykora K, Schneiderman J, *et al.* (1989). Assessment of alcohol withdrawal: The revised Clinical Institute Withdrawal Assessment for Alcohol scale (CIWA-Ar). *Br J Addiction* 84: 1353–7.

Discharge prescriptions for opioid-replacement therapy

Injecting drug users who are stabilized with methadone (IV or oral) or buprenorphine might require a supply on discharge from hospital. It is usually not advisable to give more than a 24–48h discharge supply, especially if opioid-replacement therapy is new or the patient usually gets their supply on a daily basis from the community pharmacist. Sometimes there can be a delay before a prescription for a community pharmacy supply can be arranged (e.g. at weekends or on bank holidays). On these occasions, it might be appropriate to use a prescription issued by the hospital, which can be dispensed in the community (FP10 in the UK).

Things to consider

• Could an alternative arrangement be made—e.g. could the patient attend the ward/out-patient clinic for a supply?
• In the UK, only Home Office-registered doctors can prescribe diamorphine, cocaine, or dipipanone to injecting drug users, but any doctor can prescribe any other replacement therapy.
• Close liaison with the local addiction service/GP/community pharmacist is important to ensure continuity of care.

Writing the prescription (guidelines refer to UK law)

Normal writing rules for controlled drug prescriptions apply:
• FP10 prescriptions cannot be used for instalment prescribing. If a daily pick-up is required, a separate prescription must be written for each day.
• FP10(MDA) prescriptions (HBP(A), in Scotland, WP10(MDA) in Wales) can be used by any doctor to write instalment prescriptions. The prescription must specify the total quantity required, the amount of the instalments to be dispensed, and the intervals to be observed between instalments.
• A maximum of 14 days' supply of schedule 2 controlled drugs can be prescribed by instalments for the treatment of substance misuse.
• FP10 prescriptions have a potential street value and may be sold to other injecting drug users. Consider posting or delivering the prescription to the community pharmacy, rather than handing it to the patient. Check normal practice with the local addiction service/GP.

Perioperative medicine management

Patients are often not given essential regular medicines before operations that can potentially cause an exacerbation of their chronic condition or adverse effects from abrupt drug withdrawal. It is not justified to simply omit an oral medication without first clarifying the instruction from an anaesthetist/pharmacist. It may be appropriate to give the oral medicine or to change to an alternative product using an alternative route.

However there are a number of medicines that should be discontinued in advance to reduce the risk of thromboembolism or haemorrhage.

Patients may be labelled 'nil by mouth' (NBM) for several reasons including unconsciousness, to rest the gut, impending surgery or postoperatively as a result of the surgery itself. This review is aimed at the latter two situations; however, some of the commentary may be appropriate when patients develop an intolerance of oral medicines at any time during a stay in hospital, e.g. because of nausea or vomiting.

It is imperative that a comprehensive DHx is undertaken for all patients admitted to hospital for surgery. The DHx should include regular, if needed, and recently stopped or withheld medications. Over-the-counter and herbal products need to be documented.

- Medicines used to control life-threatening conditions should be continued.
- Optimize the treatment of chronic diseases before admission for surgery—e.g. for asthma and COPD.
- For surgical emergencies, e.g. abdominal aortic aneurysm (AAA), it might not be possible to optimize drug therapy preoperatively and the pharmacist needs to highlight any possible complications relating to a recently administered drug that otherwise should have been stopped or dose-modified.

In general, with the exception of those drugs noted in this section, few drugs need to be stopped before surgery.

NBM period

- Patients are at risk of aspirating their stomach contents during general anaesthesia. They are usually prevented from eating within 6h of surgery. However, clear fluids leave the stomach within 2h of ingestion, and thus free clear fluids that enable a patient to take routine medication are allowed up to 1h presurgery and with up to 150mL water pre-procedure (for children 30min and 75mL).
- After surgery, oral medicines can be restarted at their previous preoperative dose as soon as the patient can swallow small amounts of fluid.
- If a patient is likely to be NBM for a long time (e.g. surgeon's plan and postoperative nausea and vomiting (PONV)), the drug can be given by an alternative route—e.g. rectal, transdermal, parenteral, or feeding tube delivery.
- Drugs with a long half-life (e.g. levothyroxine) or long duration of action (e.g. antidepressants) shouldn't cause a problem if they have to be omitted for several days.

Reviewing a patient's medication during the NBM period

The risks and benefits must be considered when deciding to continue or suspend medication. For example, the consequences of stopping long-term therapy for conditions such as osteoporosis or osteoarthritis in the NBM period might be considered non-problematic in the majority of patients.

To avoid interrupting appropriate long-term therapies, oral medicines can be administered with sips of clear oral fluid in the NBM period.

The anaesthetist should be contacted if there is any doubt about a patient's specific medication plan—e.g. if a drug is known to have potential interaction with anaesthetic agents.

There are a few significant interactions between drugs used during surgery and routine medications that require the drugs not to be administered concurrently. This is usually managed by the anaesthetist, by their choice of anaesthetic technique. Significant interactions are as follows:

- Enflurane can precipitate seizure activity in patients taking tricyclic antidepressants.
- Pethidine can precipitate fatal 'excitatory' reactions in patients taking monoamine oxidase inhibitors and can cause serotonin syndrome in patients taking SSRIs.
- The effects of suxamethonium (succinylcholine) can be prolonged by neostigmine.
- The metabolism of midazolam is significantly ↓ by protease inhibitors and efavirenz.

Advice for adjustment of specific medication during the pre-, peri-, and postoperative periods

Hormone-replacement therapy (HRT)

Women on HRT have an ↑ risk of developing venous thromboembolism (VTE) after major surgery compared with controls. The MHRA advise that there is no need to stop HRT unless patients have other predisposing risk factors for VTE; such patients require suitable thromboprophylaxis.

For patients with predisposing risk factors, HRT should be stopped 4wks before major surgery.

Combined oral contraceptives

Again, there is an ↑ risk of VTE in patients having therapy with COCs. Therapy should be discontinued 4wks before major elective surgery and all leg surgery. However, the risks and consequences of pregnancy versus VTE must be discussed with patients.

COCs should be restarted at the first menses that occurs at least 2wks after full mobilization.

Tamoxifen

Patients on tamoxifen therapy have a higher risk of VTE after surgery. However, tamoxifen treatment for breast cancer should be continued during surgery unless directed by the patient's oncologist, and close monitoring of VTE symptoms for 3 months post surgery should be planned.

Patients having tamoxifen treatment for fertility should have treatment suspended 6wks before major surgery.

Methotrexate

Fluid restriction, hypovolaemia, and renal hypoperfusion can result in ↓ clearance; it is advisable to suspend methotrexate for 2 days before surgery and check renal function before recommencing therapy.

Monoamine oxidase inhibitors

MAOIs can result in hypertensive crisis if used concurrently with interacting drugs (e.g. pethidine, dextromethorphan, and pentazocine). They are usually withdrawn 2wks before surgery. However, the risk of psychiatric relapse must be considered. If necessary, MAOIs can be substituted with a short-acting form, such as moclobemide (which can be withheld on the morning of surgery). If withdrawal is not possible, avoid pethidine and indirectly acting sympathomimetics—use isoprenaline instead. Phentolamine can be used to ↓ BP in the event of a hypertensive crisis.

Corticosteroids

Stress caused by surgery is associated with ↑ cortisol production. Prolonged corticosteroid therapy, especially at high doses, can cause adrenal atrophy, an impaired stress response, and risk of hypoadrenal crisis, manifesting in circulatory collapse and shock.

The risk of hypothalamic–pituitary–adrenal (HPA) axis suppression should be considered if patients have been on steroids for 1–2wks before surgery or within the last 6 months. The dose and duration of steroids determine the risk, in addition to the type of surgery. Therefore these patients will require IV hydrocortisone cover. The usual dose is 50–100mg of hydrocortisone given preoperatively, intraoperatively (if necessary), and every 6–8h for 2–3 days after surgery. Normal preoperative steroid doses should be restarted 2 days after surgery (no gradual dose reduction is needed from postoperative cover).

Lithium

Lithium prolongs the action of depolarizing and non-depolarizing muscle relaxants. Ideally, stop therapy 24–72h before major surgery, but therapy can continue during minor surgery. If it is not possible to stop therapy, ensure adequate fluid intake during and after surgery. Monitor U&Es regularly; measure lithium blood levels if necessary.

Diuretics

Omit K^+-sparing diuretics on the morning of surgery because ↓ kidney perfusion in the immediate postoperative period can predispose to hyperkalaemia. Thiazide and loop diuretics need not be omitted. Any electrolyte imbalance should be corrected before surgery.

Beta-blockers

Anaesthesia and surgery can provoke tachycardia and ↑ BP in patients with hypertension. β-blockers can help to suppress these effects and therefore are usually continued perioperatively.

Antiplatelet drugs

Aspirin/clopidogrel should be stopped when the risks of postoperative bleeding are high or if the consequences of, even minor, bleeding are significant (e.g. retinal and intracranial bleeding). This must be balanced against the risk of precipitating thromboembolic complications if these drugs are stopped, particularly in patients with unstable angina. If low-dose aspirin or clopidogrel are stopped, this is generally 7–10 days before surgery to enable recovery of adequate platelet function. It is not usually necessary to stop dipyridamole before surgery, but if complete absence of antiplatelet effect is desired, it should be stopped 24h before surgery.

Vitamin K antagonists (e.g. warfarin)

Vitamin K antagonists ↑ the risk of bleeding complications and should, ideally, be stopped 3–4 days before surgery to allow the INR to fall below 1.5. Prophylaxis for thromboembolism with LMWH or heparin can be given in the interim as appropriate. If not possible to stop, the effects can be reversed with oral vitamin K within 12h, 6–8h with IV vitamin K, or immediately with Beriplex®.

Novel oral anticoagulants (NOACs)

Rivaroxaban and apixaban should be discontinued for 48h prior to elective surgery or invasive procedures with a moderate or high risk of bleeding and for 24h prior to elective surgery or invasive procedures with a low risk of bleeding. Dabigatran should be discontinued in accordance with Table 11.3. Patients on NOACs should have their PT and APTT measured prior to surgery.

Anti-Parkinson's drugs

There is a small risk of arrhythmias or hypertension during anaesthesia in patients with Parkinson's disease. However, anaesthesia can worsen symptoms of Parkinson's disease after surgery and uncontrolled symptoms ↓ mobility and impede recovery. These drugs should be continued wherever possible. Procyclidine can be given by injection to relieve rigidity and tremor if the patient is unable to take oral medication after surgery.

Antipsychotics, anxiolytics, and clozapine

Generally these agents are continued to avoid relapse of the condition. Antipsychotics can ↓ anaesthetic requirements and potentiate arrhythmias. However, clozapine should be stopped 24h before surgery. Therefore if the patient is on the morning list, do not give medication on the day before surgery, in addition to the day of surgery itself. There are no withdrawal problems associated with doing this. If the patient is unable to take clozapine for >2 days because of being NBM, the drug must be gradually re-titrated up from the starting dose (12.5mg once or twice daily).

Table 11.3 Discontinuation of dabigatran

Renal function CrCL (mL/min)	Standard risk	High risk of bleeding or major surgery
>80	1 day	2 days
>50–<80	2 day	3 days
>30–<50	3 days	4 days

Oral hypoglycaemics

It is important to gain optimal glycaemic control perioperatively for patients with diabetes. To ensure this is done, patients with diabetes should ideally be admitted to hospital the day before surgery. This will give the medical and nursing teams time to assess each patient's control.

For major surgery, most patients with type 2 diabetes benefit from IV insulin therapy, especially if a prolonged NBM period is expected or if the stress from surgery has led to unacceptable hyperglycaemia.

However, the following guidance can aid your patient management:

- Glibenclamide—switch to a sulfonylurea with a shorter half-life 3 days before surgery or switch to soluble insulin.
- Gliclazide/glipizide/tolbutamide—omit therapy on the day of surgery.
- Metformin—to ↓ the risk of lactic acidosis, withdraw the drug 48–72h before surgery and restabilize 48h after surgery.

Further reading

UpToDate®. 'Perioperative medication management', ℛ www.uptodate.com/contents/peri-operative-medication-management

Pharmaceutical calculations

Concept of ratio and proportion

Ratio

- Used in numerous applications in everyday life and is very common concept in pharmacy practice.
- Used when two expressions are directly related to one another, e.g. if 100g of sweets costs us £1, how much will 500g cost? Answer: £5.
- Both expressions contain cost per weight; if set up as ratios, once the problem is solved, both ratios must be equal.
- A ratio is the relation between like numbers or values or a way to express a fractional part of a whole, and can be displayed in three differing ways—our two examples can be expressed in the following ways:
  - As a fraction: £1/100g and £5/500g
  - With a ratio sign(:) £1:100g and £5:500g
  - Using 'per': £1 per 100g and £5 per 500g
  - Strength or concentration of various drugs can be expressed as a ratio
  - E.g. gentamicin 40mg/1ml or 40mg per ml or 40mg:1mL.

Proportion

A proportion consists of two equal ratios and is essentially a statement of equality between two ratios, e.g.:

$$2/5 = 4/10$$

You have a 10-ml vial of aminophylline labelled '25mg per mL'. How many millilitres must be injected to administer a dose of 125 mg?

$$25mg/1mL = 125mg/XmL$$

$$(25mg) \times (XmL) = (1mL) \times (125mg)$$

$$(XmL) = (1mL) \times (125mg)/(25mg)$$

$$XmL = 5mL$$

Concentrations

Pharmaceutical preparations usually consist of a number of different ingredients in a vehicle. The ingredients can be solid, liquid, or gas.

'Concentration' is an expression of the ratio of the amount of an ingredient to the amount of product. Units of concentrations can therefore also be defined in several ways depending on the physical composition:

- Solutions of solids in liquids, denoted by w/v
- Solutions of liquids in liquids, denoted by v/v
- Admixtures of liquids in solids (v/w) or solids combined with solids (w/w).

Concentrations are expressions of ratios and are written in different formats that can cause confusion. Formats traditionally used are as follows:

- Amount strengths
- Ratio strengths
- Parts per million (ppm)
- Percentage strength.

Amount strengths

A preparation contains 900mg of sodium chloride dissolved in water to make a final volume of 100mL. The concentration of this solution can be written as an amount strength in units of 900mg/100mL, 9mg/mL, 0.9g/100mL, or 9g/L.

Ratio strengths

Convention states that when ratio strength represents a solid in a liquid, involving units of weight and volume, the weight is expressed in grams and the volume in millilitres.

A 1 in 50 sodium chloride in water preparation is a solid in a liquid (w/v) ratio strength. This means that the solution contains 1g of sodium chloride made up to 50mL with water.

A 14 in 100 sulphuric acid in water preparation is a liquid in liquid (v/v) ratio strength, i.e. 14mL of sulphuric acid in 86mL of water.

Parts per million (ppm)

This expression is used when the ratio of ingredient to product is very small, by convention 1ppm weight in volume is 1g in 1 000 000mL. 1ppm weight in weight is 1mg per 1 000 000mg or 1g per 1 000 000g. In volume, it is 1mL in 1 000 000mL or 1L in 1 000 000L.

Percentage strength

'Percentage' in pharmaceutical calculations is quantified as the amount of ingredient in 100 parts of the product.

By convention, % w/v indicates the number of grams of ingredient in 100mL of product. Therefore 900mg of sodium chloride made up to 100mL with water can be expressed as 0.9g in 100mL and the percentage strength is 0.9% w/v.

A 1 in 1000 adrenaline injection is equivalent to 0.1% w/v or, by convention, 1g of adrenaline made up to 1000mL with water.

A 1 in 10 000 adrenaline injection is equivalent to 0.01% w/v or, by convention, 1g of adrenaline made up to 10000mL with water.

Calculations

For example, how many millilitres of a 1 in 50 w/v solution are required to make 500mL of a 0.02% solution?

By convention, 1 in 50 means 1g in 50mL and 0.02% w/v means 0.02g in 100mL. Let the number of millilitres of the 1 in 50 solution be y and let the amount of ingredient in grams in 500mL of 0.02% solution be x. The amount of ingredient in grams in ymL of a 1 in 50 solution will also be x.

Setting up proportional sets

For 1 in 50:

Ingredient (g)	1	x	1g
Product (mL)	50	y	to 50mL

For 500mL of 0.02%:

Ingredient (g)	0.02	x	0.02g
Product (mL)	100	500	to 100mL

By 'spotting' $x = 0.1$; substitute into the first pair of proportional sets.

For 1 in 50:

Ingredient (g)	1	0.1	1g
Product (mL)	50	y	to 50mL

By 'spotting' $y = 5$. Therefore 5mL of a 1 in 50 w/v solution is required to make 500mL of a 0.02% w/v solution.

Alternatively, how many grams in 500mL of 0.02% solution?

0.02% $= 0.02$g in 100mL

in 500mL $= 0.02 \times 5 = 0.1$g

1 in 50 solution, by convention 1g in 50mL

Then, to calculate the volume containing 0.1g, 1/10 of 1g or 1/10 of 50mL = 5mL.

Moles and millimoles

The atomic and molecular weights of a drug can be used as methods of defining the amount of drug. The substance can be atoms, molecules, or ions; a mole is the weight expressed in grams. The mole is the SI base unit for the amount of a substance—e.g. the atomic weight of iron is 56 and 1 mole of iron weighs 56g.

The molecular weight of a drug (e.g. sodium chloride) is the sum of all the atomic weights of the individual atoms in the molecule. A molecule of sodium chloride consists of one sodium ion and one chloride ion:

- 1 mole sodium ions weighs 23g
- 1 mole chloride ions weighs 35.5g
- Hence the molecular weight of sodium chloride is 58.5g.

In the same way that the systems of weights and volumes have multiples and subdivisions (e.g. milli-, micro-, and nano-), so the mole has similar subdivisions and multiples:

- 1 mole contains 1000 millimoles (mmol)
- 1mmol contains 1000 micromoles (μmol)
- 1micromol contains 1000 nanomoles (nmol)
- 1nanomol contains 1000 picomoles (pmol).

Amount of substance concentration

In clinical chemistry, laboratory results are usually written in terms of mol/L (or mmol/L or micromol/L).

Example

How many millimoles of sodium chloride are there in a litre of sodium chloride 0.9% w/v?

First calculate the weight of sodium chloride in a litre:

0.9g in 100mL

=0.9g × 10 in 1000mL

=9g in 1000mL.

For the molecule sodium chloride: 1mole = 58.5g

$$58.5g = 1000mmol$$
$$9/58.5 = x/1000$$
$$x = 9000/58.5$$
$$x = 153mmol.$$

Alternatively, to calculate the number of millimoles contained in 1g of substance, use the following formula:

$$mmol = \frac{1000 \times \text{number of specified units in one unit (atom, molecule or ion)}}{\text{atomic, molecular, or ionic weight}}$$

Number of mmol of sodium in 1g of sodium chloride (molecular weight = 58.5):

$$\text{mmol} = \frac{1000 \times 1}{58.5}$$

$$= 17 \text{mmol in 1g or 153 mmol in 9g}$$

For $CaCl_2, 2H_2O$ (molecular weight = 147):

$$\text{mmol of calcium in 1g } CaCl_2, 2H_2O = \frac{1000 \times 1}{147} = 6.8 \text{mmol}$$

$$\text{mmol of chloride in 1g } CaCl_2, 2H_2O = \frac{1000 \times 2}{147} = 13.6 \text{mmol}$$

$$\text{mmol of water in 1g } CaCl_2, 2H_2O = \frac{1000 \times 2}{147} = 13.6 \text{mmol}$$

i.e. each gram of $CaCl_2, 2H_2O$ represents 6.8 mmol of calcium, 13.6 mmol of chloride, and 13.6 mmol of water of crystallization.

Practical issues involving pharmaceutical calculations

- Compound glucose, sodium chloride, and sodium citrate oral solution BP 2015. Make 200mL (see Table 12.1).
- Use double checks: 4g is 1/5 of 20g and 0.7g is 1/5 of 3.5g.
- Don't forget your units: 1g = 1000mg = 1 000 000 micrograms.

Preparing dilutions

- Ensure correct choice of diluent
- Calculate dilution factor
- Correctly express the concentration of the diluted product on the label.

Example 1

Calculate the amount of benzalkonium chloride solution BP 2004 needed to prepare a 150mL of a solution of benzalkonium chloride 10% w/v. Benzalkonium chloride solution BP 2004 is a 50% w/v concentration.

Calculation of dilution factor
Method 1:

$$\frac{\text{Strength of concentrate}}{\text{Strength of dilute solution}} = \text{dilution factor}$$

$$\frac{\text{Strength of concentrate}}{\text{Strength of dilute solution}} = \frac{50\% \, \text{w/v}}{10\% \, \text{w/V}} = 5 \, \text{times}$$

$$\text{To prepare dilute solution} = \frac{\text{final volume}}{\text{dilution factor}}$$

$$150/5 = 30\text{mL of concentrate solution}$$

The diluted solution is obtained by using 30mL of BP solution and diluting with 120mL of water.

Table 12.1 Pharmaceutical calculations

Ingredients	Master formula	Scaled quantities
Anhydrous glucose	20g	4g
Sodium chloride	3.5g	0.7g (700mg)
Sodium citrate	2.5g	0.5g (500mg)
Water	To 1000mL	To 200mL

Method 2:
Product of volume and concentration:

$$V_c \times C_c = V_d \times C_d \text{ where}$$
$$V_c \times 50 = 150 \times 10$$
$$V_c = 150/5$$
$$V_c = 30\text{mL}$$

V_c = volume of concentrated solution
C_c = concentration of concentrate
V_d = volume of diluted solution
C_d = concentration of diluted solution

Example 2

Calculate the quantity of potassium permanganate 0.25% w/v solution that is required to produce 100mL of a 0.0125% w/v solution of potassium permanganate.

Calculation of dilution factor

$$V_c \times C_c = V_d \times C_d$$

V_c = volume of concentrated solution	= unknown
C_c = concentration of concentrate	= 0.25%
V_d = volume of diluted solution	= 100mL
C_d = concentration of diluted solution	= 0.0125%

$$V_c \times 0.25\% = 100\text{mL} \times 0.0125\%$$
$$V_c = 1.25/0.25$$
$$= 5\text{mL}.$$

Dilution instructions

5mL of potassium permanganate solution 0.25% w/v must be diluted to 100mL with water to produce a 0.0125% w/v solution.

Pharmaceutical calculations involving drug administration

Calculations

- Calculations usually involve fairly straightforward theory, but difficulties can arise as a result of interruptions, tiredness, or lack of experience or not respecting the importance of the correct units.
- In preparing infusions, the mathematics normally involves translating units such as micrograms/kg body weight/min into a practical number of millilitres of diluted infusion solution per hour.

Examples

A patient requires a parenteral loading dose of 0.5mg of digoxin. Digoxin is available as an injection containing 250 micrograms/mL. How many millilitres of injection will supply the required dose?

First convert mg to micrograms:

   0.5mg=500 micrograms

Setting up a proportional set

Weight of digoxin (mg)	250	500
Volume of injection (mL)	1	y

250 multiplied by 2 gives 500, so 1 is multiplied by 2 to give $y = 2$.

Because the injection contains 250 micrograms in 1mL, a 500-microgram dose will be provided in 2mL.

ITUs prepare dobutamine as a standard concentration of 250mg in 50mL 5% dextrose solution. You need to confirm that the prescribed 5 micrograms/kg/body weight/min dose for a 70kg patient is correctly delivered by the volumetric hourly rate set by the nurse.

Standard concentration = 250mg in 50mL (patient 70kg)

To calculate the hourly rate: = 5 micrograms × kg body weight × min

   = 5 × 70 × 60 (min)

   = 21 000 micrograms/h

Concentration of dobutamine = 250mg in 50mL

(convert to micrograms)   = 250 × 1000 (micrograms) in 50mL

   = 250 000 micrograms in 50mL

   = 5000 micrograms in 1mL

Volume per hour requires 21 000 micrograms to be administered:

   = (21 000 micrograms/h)/(5000 micrograms/mL)

   = 4.2mL/h

Interfacing your calculation skills with nursing and medical staff

Flow rate calculations

Flow rate is the speed at which an IV solution is delivered.

Function of volume per time—usually reported in millilitres per hour.

The magical formula:

volume ÷ time = flow rate

Always be sure which time and volume units you are being asked to solve for, is it mL/min ? Or L/h? Something else?

A patient receives 1L of IV solution over a 3h period.

Calculate the flow rate in mL/h.

Note: the volume given is in litres, but the answer asks for millilitres. If the conversion wasn't so obvious, we would first need to do a conversion of L per ml.

volume ÷ time = flow rate

1000mL ÷ 3h = 333mL/h

Solve for time

By manipulating the rate formula, we can solve for time.

The equation becomes:

volume ÷ rate = time

If an IV is run at 125mL/h, how long will 1L last?

volume ÷ rate = time

1000mL ÷ 125mL/h = 8h

Solving for volume

Rearrange the formula and we can solve for volume.

The equation becomes:

rate × time = volume

How many mL of IV solution would be required to run an IV for 8h at a rate of 60mL/h?

rate × time = volume

60mL/1h × 8h = 480mL

Medicines management

Introduction to medicines management

Medicines management can be described as using the right medicine for the right patient at the right time. The goal of medicines management is to ensure that medicines use is safe and effective, optimizing the benefits of treatment to ensure the best outcome for patients. Medicines management encompasses both:
- the clinical and cost-effective use of medicines
- the safe and secure handling of medicines.

Safe and effective medicines management ensures that processes are in place at all stages of the medicines journey, including manufacturing and marketing, procurement, selection, prescribing, dispensing, sale or supply, patient use, and disposal.

Each hospital should have a strategic plan for medicines management, which reflects the following:
- The strategic direction for the local health economy.
- Priorities of the local population.
- Targets relating to Commissioning Guidance and implementation of NICE guidance.
- Communication strategy for the dissemination of information.
- Clinical governance arrangements for medicine management including controls and assurance arrangements.

Hospitals should ensure that the following systems are in place to ensure effective medicines management:
- Drug and therapeutics committee (or equivalent).
- Targeting clinical pharmacy activity to patients requiring early assessment following hospital admission.
- A medicines reconciliation should be completed within 24h of hospital admission.
- Acute medical admissions should be prioritized and, if possible, seen by a pharmacist.
- Patient's own drugs (PODs) should be used if they have been reviewed and considered suitable for continued use.
- As appropriate, all patients should be given the option of self-administering their own medicines while in hospital.
- Dispensing for discharge (or one-stop dispensing) systems should be in place to ensure that patients receive their discharge medication in sufficient quantity and in a timely manner, with the appropriate patient information leaflet.

The multidisciplinary team should be trained on medicines management:
- All doctors, nurses, pharmacists, and other relevant healthcare professionals should receive training on medicines management as part of their induction programme, including the legislative and good clinical practice (GCP) aspects of controls assurance (in particular, the safe and secure handling of medicines) and clinical and cost-effective use of medicines.
- Medicines management systems and policies should be incorporated into ongoing clinical training programmes.

- Information technology system support should be available to provide healthcare staff with accurate information on the use of medicines.
- The risk of medication errors occurring should be minimized.

Medicines management policies and procedures should be in place to mini-mize the risk of medication errors occurring during the medication process, i.e. for prescribing, dispensing, and administration.

Further reading

Audit Commission (2001). *A Spoonful of Sugar. Medicines Management in NHS Hospitals*. London: Audit Commission.

Department of Health (2003). *A Vision for Pharmacy in the New NHS*. London: Department of Health. http://webarchive.nationalarchives.gov.uk/20130107105354/http://www.dh.gov.uk/prod_consum_dh/groups/dh_digitalassets/@dh/@en/documents/digitalasset/dh_4070099.pdf

Nursing & Midwifery Council (2010). *Standards for Medicines Management*. London: NMC. https://www.nmc.org.uk/globalassets/sitedocuments/standards/nmc-standards-for-medi-cines-management.pdf

NICE. 'Medicines management'. https://www.nice.org.uk/guidance/service-delivery--organisation-and-staffing/medicines-management/medicines-management--general-and-other

Smith J (2004). *Building a Safer NHS for Patients: Improving Medication Safety*. London: Department of Health.

The King's Fund. *Effective Medicines Management*. https://www.kingsfund.org.uk/projects/gp-commissioning/ten-priorities-for-commissioners/medicines-management

Medicines optimization

Medicines optimization is defined as 'a person-centred approach to safe and effective medicines use, to ensure people obtain the best possible outcomes from their medicines'[1]. It ensures that the correct patients receive the correct medicine at the correct time to improve outcomes. Medicines optimization requires patient engagement and the collaboration of healthcare professionals across all health and social care settings to individualize patient treatment with the best outcomes.[1-3] Pharmacists should use the principles of medicines optimization in their routine practice.[2]

Medicines optimization ensures that:
- there is a patient-centred approach
- there is an evidence-based use of medicines
- patients take ownership of their medicines
- patients avoid taking unnecessary medicines
- adherence is improved
- the incidence of medicine-related adverse effects is reduced
- medicines safety is improved
- medicines wastage is reduced
- there is a reduction in medicines related admissions

There are four principles to medicines optimization:[2]

Aim to understand the patient's experience

It is important that patients are engaged and understand about their medicines, so that they can take their medicines as agreed in the shared decision-making process between the patient and the healthcare professionals. Patients must have the opportunity to share their experience of medicine taking, which may change with time. This includes reasons why they may not be taking certain medicines, and why they are taking some of their medicines routinely.

Evidence-based choice of medicines

The most clinically and cost-effective medicines should be prescribed using an evidence base, e.g. NICE, systematic reviews, or local formularies, that best meet the needs of the patient.

Ensure medicines use is as safe as possible

Safety encompasses adverse effects, interactions, safe processes and systems, and effective inter-professional communication. It is essential to ensure that avoidable harm from medicines is minimized so that medicines can be used as safely as possible.

Make medicines optimization part of routine practice

Ensure that patients and healthcare professionals from all sectors review medicines to ensure the best outcomes with consistent communication between providers.

The priorities for implementing medicines optimization include:[1]

- systems for identifying, reporting, and learning from medicines-related patient safety incidents
- communications systems about medicines when patients move between care settings
- medicines reconciliation
- self-management plans
- patient decision aids used in consultations involving medicines
- clinical decision support
- medicines-related models of organizational and cross-sector working.

References

1. NICE (March 2015). 'Medicines optimisation: the safe and effective use of medicines to enable the best possible outcomes (NG9)', ℘ www.nice.org.uk/guidance/ng5
2. Royal Pharmaceutical Society (2013). 'Medicines Optimisation: Helping patients to make the most of medicines. Good practice guidance for healthcare professionals in England', ℘ www.rpharms.com/promoting-pharmacy-pdfs/helping-patients-make-the-most-of-their-medicines.pdf
3. NHS England (2014). Medicines Optimisation Dashboard', ℘ https://www.england.nhs.uk/ourwork/pe/mo-dash/

Evaluating new medicines and formulary applications

New medicines appear on the market regularly and healthcare professionals are constantly bombarded with promotional material from the pharmaceutical industry either directly or via ads in the medical press. The pharmaceutical industry's business is to sell medicines in order to survive. All promotional material should be reviewed with a critical eye.

A medicine may receive regulatory approval, but that does not necessarily mean that it is a clinically significant advance. Most regulatory authorities evaluate quality, safety, and efficacy, not therapeutic value. Assessments of the value of new medicines from Canada, France, and the United States have shown that, at best, only one-third offer some additional clinical benefit and as few as 3% are a major therapeutic advance.[4]

Premarketing trials are often placebo controlled, so they give an indication of effectiveness but do not give comparative data. Ideally, a trial should compare the new medicine with an established reference treatment. Even if the trial compares the new medicine with a reference treatment, it might be too small in terms of participants or too short in time to provide meaningful data—in particular, uncommon ADRs or differences in response in subgroups of patients are unlikely to be identified.

Much of the data presented by the pharmaceutical industry is disease orientated rather than patient orientated, and this can make a difference to the patient outcome. For example, disease-orientated evidence (DOE) demonstrates that cyclooxygenase 2 (COX2) NSAIDs cause fewer endoscopically detected ulcers than standard NSAIDs. However, many of these ulcers would not be clinically significant. A more relevant evaluation is to determine the difference between COX2 NSAIDs and standard NSAIDs in causing symptomatic or bleeding ulcers. The STEPS acronym is a useful tool for evaluating new drugs:[5]

Safety

Evaluate the safety of the new drug versus a standard reference preparation, ideally using comparison studies that reflect the real-life situation. Pharmaceutical companies often highlight differences in ADRs that are relatively trivial or rare. Check especially for ADRs that would place the patient at particular risk, notably the following:

- Liver, kidney, or bone marrow toxicity
- Cardiovascular events
- CNS events (e.g. fits)
- Significant skin or hypersensitivity reactions (e.g. Stevens–Johnson syndrome)
- GI bleeding
- Congenital abnormalities.

Look at the frequency of these events versus the significance of the disease. A 5% risk of hepatotoxicity in a life-threatening disease is a more acceptable level of risk than if the disease is self-limiting.

Tolerability

Are side effects likely to affect adherence? Look at drop-out rates in clinical trials. If there is a high drop-out rate because of ADRs versus the reference drug, this makes the new drug of less therapeutic value. If patients don't take the drug, it won't work!

Effectiveness

Look at head-to-head trials of the new drug versus the reference drug, rather than comparing different trials. Ask: 'Does this new drug work as well or better than the reference drug?' The numbers needed to treat (NNT) is the best way of assessing therapeutic value. If the NNT of the new drug is the same or lower than the reference drug, it is worth considering.

Price

Consider all the costs associated with the new drug versus the reference, not just the purchase price. This might include the following:

- Administration cost (e.g. IV giving sets)
- Monitoring costs
- Additional time/travel if patient has to attend more frequently at the start of therapy.

Simplicity of use

Is it relatively easy for the patient to use the drug? This includes considering the following:

- Dosage schedule
- Number of tablets
- Liquid versus tablets
- Parenteral versus enteral administration
- Special storage requirements (e.g. refrigeration).

WHO criteria for drug selection are listed in Box 13.1.[6]

Box 13.1 WHO criteria for drug selection

- On the WHO essential drug list
- Relevance to pattern of prevalent disease
- Proven efficacy and safety
- Evidence of performance in different settings
- Adequate quality, bioavailability, and safety
- Favourable cost–benefit ratio, in terms of total treatment cost
- Preference for drugs that are well known or familiar to use and locally manufactured
- Single compounds.

Formulary applications

The evaluation of new medicines is an important aspect of a formulary application. The hospitals' Drug and Therapeutics Committee or Medicines committee (see ➔ pp. 253–4) is usually responsible for the maintenance of the hospital formulary. A formulary is a continually updated list of medicines that is preferred for use by the hospital, which identifies medicines that are most medically appropriate and cost-effective for the patient population. Any new medicine to be used in an organization should be approved for inclusion on the formulary.

The benefits of a local formulary include:
- improving patient outcomes by optimizing the use of medicines
- supporting the inclusion of patient factors in decision-making about medicines
- improving local care pathways
- improving collaboration between clinicians and commissioners
- improving quality through access to cost-effective medicines
- supporting the supply arrangements of medicines across a local health economy
- supporting financial management and expenditure on medicines across health communities
- supporting prescribers to follow guidance published by professional regulatory bodies in relation to medicines and prescribing.

Formulary applications should be evidence based and need to be submitted to the appropriate committee, who decides whether a medicine is suitable for inclusion on the formulary. Specific formulary application forms may be used that require sign off by, for example, the requesting consultant, senior pharmacist, senior manager, and senior finance manager.

The formulary application includes information that enables the committee to assess the suitability of the medicine for inclusion in the formulary, including clinical safety, efficacy and cost-effectiveness. The financial impact plan and implications in primary care are also assessed. Procurement, safe storage, and administration of the medicine are also reviewed.

A formulary application requires the following information:
- Medicines information:
  - Medicine name, strength, and form
  - Pharmacological action
  - Intended indication
  - Dose
  - Duration of treatment
  - Details whether the medicine should be available for general or restricted use
  - Whether the medicine should be restricted to a specific indication or patient group
  - Whether the medicine would replace a medicine or therapy currently on the formulary.
- Clinical information:
  - Has the medicine been recommended by a national medicines review, e.g. NICE?
  - What is the place of the medicine in therapy, e.g. first line, second line?
  - How patients should be selected
  - Implications if patients do not receive this medicine
  - Whether the prescribing of the medicine is supported by primary care.

- Pharmaceutical information:
  - Manufacturer
  - Country of origin
  - Whether the medicine is unlicensed or will be used for an unlicensed indication
  - Route of administration
  - Storage
  - Whether aseptic dispensing is required
  - Control of Substances Hazardous to Health (COSHH) assessment
  - Shelf life
  - Packaging
  - Details of how the dose will be measured
  - Whether reconstitution is required
  - Whether there are any special handling precautions
  - Whether any specialist training is needed
  - Whether the medicine would be kept as ward stock.
- Financial information:
  - Average duration of treatment (days)
  - Average number of dosage units per day
  - Cost per dosage unit
  - Cost per standard course
  - Additional costs per patient per course, e.g. monitoring, administration, training
  - Total annual cost per patient
  - Expected number of patients per year
  - Annual cost
  - Difference (new cost—current cost)
  - Proposed source of funding
  - Whether the medicine will bring about a change in current practice
  - Whether the service is commissioned
  - Whether the medicine is available on contract.
- Information about continuing treatment in the community or primary care:
  - Whether the medicine is likely to be prescribed by GPs
  - Whether there is a shared care protocol in place
  - Cost in primary care.
- Declaration of interest:
  - Whether the requesting consultant has been involved in clinical trials of the medicine.
  - Whether the requesting consultant has been approached by the pharmaceutical manufacturer to include this medicine in the formulary.
  - Whether the requesting consultant has any direct interest with the manufacturer, e.g. being a shareholder or a director of the company, acting as a lecturer or consultant to a company, or any relationship where they have personally received money or payment in kind in the last 12 months.
  - Whether the requesting consultant has any indirect interests with the manufacturer, e.g. them or their co-workers receiving money, equipment or salaries over the last 12 months that has been used to contribute to the running of research or clinical activities.

- Additional information.
- Signatures of requesting consultant, senior pharmacist, senior finance manager, senior manager.

The possible outcomes of a formulary application are:
- formulary—the medicine can be used throughout the hospital for its licensed indications
- restricted formulary—the medicine can be used following certain restrictions
- non-formulary—the medicine remains non-formulary.

There is usually an appeal process in place to appeal a decision made by the drug and therapeutics committee, e.g. if the published formulary process has not been followed, if there is significant new information that has become available and requires a reconsideration of the evidence, or if the decision was based on inaccurate or incomplete information.

Formularies are tried and tested and while logical, there is little evidence to support their effectiveness for patient benefit or managing costs. In addition, formularies should not be so restrictive that a patient who does not benefit from one medicine in a class cannot be prescribed another within that class.

References

4. Lexchin J (2004). Are new drugs as good as they claim to be? *Aust Prescr* 27: 2–3.
5. Preskorn SH (1994). Antidepressant drug selection: criteria and options. *J Clin Psychiatry* 55(suppl A): 6–22, 23–4, 98–100.
6. World Health Organization (1988). *How to Develop and Implement a National Drug Policy* (2nd ed). Geneva: WHO. ℘ http://apps.who.int/iris/bitstream/10665/42423/1/924154547X.pdf

How to write a drug protocol

Drug protocols are evidence-based documents that specify the indications for which a drug treatment can be prescribed within defined clinical settings. They help to ensure that drugs are used cost-effectively and safely within the clinical setting.

The need for a drug protocol is usually highlighted for an area by the multidisciplinary team. Initially, the evidence base must be established. Literature searches, protocols from other hospitals or institutions, and information on local practice are used as the basis for the protocol.

Ensure that local practice is followed to implement new drug protocols. This might include approval by a hospital or primary care committee, such as a drugs and therapeutics or formulary committee.

A drug protocol should include the following:
- Drug name—international approved name and trade name
- Formulation
- Dose
- Frequency of administration
- Administration details
- Side effects and their treatment
- Dose reductions required for changes in organ function—e.g. impaired renal or liver function
- Drug interactions
- Indications for use
- Place in therapy—e.g. if another option should be tried first (especially if use is restricted)
- Restrictions of use
- Cost
- References.

Stages of protocol development

Identification of need

A new or existing practice is recognized as being cumbersome, unsafe, or otherwise in need of revision. For example, a new use for a drug is developed that requires compounding in a specific way, additional monitoring, and adjunctive medication therapy. It has begun use with these orders written in longhand, but the inconsistency of this practice and ↑ likelihood of error make clear the need for a pre-written protocol.

Assignment of responsibility

A leader should be identified for the project. Although a group may be responsible for the final form, projects such as this typically require a leader who is responsible for moving the work along.

Gathering evidence and best practice

The leader and group obtain other similar protocols and enquire about their strengths and weaknesses. Other departments that will be affected by the protocol or whose work contributes to the project should be contacted with questions, although they may not need to sit on the committee. Literature searches are made to collect current evidence and best practices. These data should be reviewed and vetted, and the most useful results distributed to those working on the project, if applicable.

Draft compilation

After reviewing the available evidence, the leader or committee drafts a protocol. The protocol should be reviewed and revised by the committee or its writer until no major flaws remain. At times, substantive decisions must be delayed until the protocol can be reviewed by the next committee, or committee members from the next committee may be asked their opinion so that the protocol-drafting group can deliver a better result. After the draft has been rewritten and edited, the protocol is submitted to the appropriate hospital committee. After review by this committee, the protocol should assume a final or near-final form.

Education and roll-out

The completed protocol is often submitted to an education department to gain their expertise in training staff members. The date to begin using the protocol may also be set according to the time it will take for staff to be educated. It is important to remember that implementation of a protocol may need to be delayed after its approval if staff education is required. Staff members should be allowed to have the opportunity to familiarize themselves with a protocol before being expected to act on it.

It is imperative that pharmacists are able to review a protocol during its development. The protocol should be reviewed with great scrutiny because it will be used many times. A protocol containing drugs or focused on drug therapy should be reviewed for the following details:
- Generic and trade names for each drug, with emphasis on the generic name.
- Correct route, dose, and frequency for each medication.
- Frequency of administration.
- Dilution instructions for each drug present.
- All ambiguous statements clarified.
- Contraindications or reasons not to use drugs prominently placed.

Limitations

A protocol may not be made to deal with every eventuality. Rather, a well-designed protocol will succinctly provide a framework for dealing with a particular set of circumstances. Patients will inevitably fall outside these circumstances; thus a protocol should be developed with these limitations in mind so that it does not become inappropriately complex.[7]

Reference

7. American Society of Health-System Pharmacists (2014). *ASHP Best Practices 2014–2015*. Bethesda, MD: ASHP.

Unlicensed use of medicines

- The product licence of a medication defines the therapeutic purpose for which the product can be used.
- Unlicensed medicines have not been formally assessed through the licensing process for safety, quality, and efficacy. The risks associated with their use might not have been evaluated. Some unlicensed medicines may have been fully evaluated and licensed in another country, but not in the country of use.
- If a prescriber uses a licensed medicine for an unlicensed indication, this is outside its product licence and is sometimes referred to as 'off licence' or 'off label'.
- The same principles apply to unlicensed medicines as to licensed medicines used for unlicensed indications, e.g. in paediatrics (see ➌ 'Medicines for children', p. 207).
- Medicines that are not covered by a product licence include the following:
  - Medicines prepared by a manufacturer but not on sale in this country. A specialist importer with the appropriate importing licences can obtain these.
  - Medicines prepared for a specified patient in accordance with a prescriber's instructions. This includes any form of extemporaneous dispensing.
  - Unlicensed medicines obtained from a hospital or a commercial supplier with a special manufacturing licence. These medicines are often known as 'specials'.
  - Manipulated products—medicines in which the formulation has been altered, e.g. by crushing tablets or opening capsules, and may be undertaken by a pharmacist as extemporaneous dispensing or by the medicines administrator/carer.
  - Repacked medicines—the product licence regulates the container in which a medicine is sold. If a medicine is removed from its original container and repacked, it technically becomes an unlicensed product.
- Implications for the prescriber, pharmacist, and nurses of prescribing, dispensing, and administering unlicensed medicines are as follows:
  - Prescribers need to be aware of the licence status of medicines they prescribe. The responsibility of prescribing unlicensed medicines lies with the prescriber. The manufacturer takes no responsibility for any safety or efficacy of unlicensed medicines.
  - A pharmacist shares the responsibility with the prescriber, as the product purchaser, or if the pharmacist's actions or omissions have contributed to any harm.
  - Pharmacists should ensure that before the product is ordered and administered, the prescriber is aware that they are prescribing an unlicensed medicine, or a medicine outside its licence.
  - Nurses are responsible for administering medication that is administered outside of its licence and must ensure that the relevant hospital or institution policies have been adhered to.

- A hospital or institution should have a clear written policy for the 'use of unlicensed medicines', outlining the responsibilities of all those involved in the prescribing, purchase, supply, and administration of this category of medicines. It should be a summary document, supported by standard operating procedures and making reference to existing documents and sources of information. The drugs and therapeutics committee, or equivalent, should approve this.
- The use of unlicensed medicines in a hospital or institution needs to be controlled and monitored. A risk assessment should be undertaken before an unlicensed medicine, or medicine prescribed outside of its license, is prescribed. This is often done through the drugs and therapeutics committee, or equivalent.
- Written notification, signed by the prescriber and returned to the pharmacy department, is usually used. This usually includes the patient details, the name of the product and its specification, the reason for using an unlicensed medicine, and the prescriber's name and signature. The manufacturer, date ordered, quantity ordered, and batch number received are usually recorded in the pharmacy department. Check what documentation is used in your local hospital or institution.
- Some hospitals or institutions require that informed consent is obtained from patients for some unlicensed medicines to be supplied.
- Prescribing a medicine by a route for which it is not licensed is unlicensed but is often 'accepted practice' (e.g. SC cyclizine).

Further reading

Department of Health (2003). *A Vision for Pharmacy in the New NHS*. London: Department of Health.

General Pharmaceutical Council (2014). 'Guidance for registered pharmacies preparing unlicensed medicines', ℘ www.pharmacyregulation.org/sites/default/files/guidance_for_registered_pharmacies_preparing_unlicensed_medicines_23_05_14.pdf

Medicines and Healthcare products Regulatory Agency (MHRA) (2009). 'Off-label or unlicensed use of medicines: prescribers' responsibilities', ℘ https://www.gov.uk/drug-safety-update/off-label-or-unlicensed-use-of-medicines-prescribers-responsibilities

Medicines and Healthcare products Regulatory Agency (MHRA) (2014). 'The supply of unlicensed medicinal products 'specials (MHRA guidance note 14)', ℘ https://www.gov.uk/government/uploads/system/uploads/attachment_data/file/373505/The_supply_of_unlicensed_medicinal_products__specials_.pdf

NHS Choices (2016). 'Medicines information—Licensing', ℘ http://www.nhs.uk/Conditions/Medicinesinfo/Pages/Safetyissues.aspx

Royal Pharmaceutical Society (2015). 'Professional Guidance for the Procurement and Supply of Specials', ℘ http://www.rpharms.com/support-pdfs/rps---specials-professional-guidance.pdf

Medicines committees

Each hospital has a drug and therapeutics committee, or an equivalent medicines committee. This committee is responsible for ensuring that the introduction of new medicines to the hospital formulary is cost-effective, safe, and has an acceptable (or reliable) evidence base. Before new medicines are bought by the pharmacy department and used in the hospital, they need to be approved by the drug and therapeutics committee using the principles of evidence-based medicine (EBM). The cost of new medicines being licensed causes financial pressures on hospitals, which leads to some prioritization of medicines available for use.

Generally, the membership of a drug and therapeutics committee comprises representatives from the following disciplines:
- Medical staff—including medical director, surgeon, anaesthetist, clinical pharmacologist, and paediatrician
- Nurse (chief nurse or nominee)
- Pharmacist—chief pharmacist and medicines management/formulary pharmacist
- Finance (director or nominee)
- Commissioner
- Primary care prescribing lead
- Specialists—e.g. paediatrics, oncology, or clinical pharmacology
- Public health
- Medical microbiologist
- Patient representative/lay member
- Management
- Administration
- Executive board member (if not one of the disciplines already listed)
- Other members are co-opted, as needed.

The drug and therapeutics committee should have terms of reference and a membership list. There may be subcommittees, to whom decision-making may be devolved for some specialist areas (e.g. antimicrobials), which are responsible to the drug and therapeutics committee. In addition to making decisions on the introduction of new medicines into a hospital according to assessment of the clinical evidence, a drug and therapeutics committee can also have a role in the following areas:
- Maintenance and updating of a hospital formulary.
- Review of medicines expenditure.
- Horizon scanning of medicines to be licensed or those with national approval.
- Prioritization of new drugs.
- Overseeing safe medication practice systems, including maintaining policies and procedures for medicines, overseeing education and training for safe medication practice, and analysing medication error incident reports.

Evidence that is used by drug and therapeutics committees includes the following based on a thorough search of the medical databases:
- Results of clinical trials
- Scientific evidence
- Cost-effectiveness
- Safety
- Effect of adopting a new drug
- Pre-existing prescribing
- Decisions of drug and therapeutics committees in other hospitals
- Restrictions of use of a new drug
- NICE appraisals.

Drug and therapeutics committees should meet regularly (monthly or bimonthly). Decisions made at the committee meetings are made available through minutes, newsletters, e-mail, or intranets.

Further reading

Department of Health. *A Vision for Pharmacy in the New NHS* (2003). London: Department of Health. இ www.dh.gov.uk).

Fullerton DS, Atherly DS (2004). Formularies, therapeutics, and outcomes: new opportunities. *Med Care* **42**(4 Suppl): III39–44.

Holloway K, Green T (2003). *Drug and Therapeutics Committees: A Practical Guide*. Geneva: World Health Organization. இ http://apps.who.int/medicinedocs/pdf/s4882e/s4882e.pdf

Jenkings KN, Barber N (2004). What constitutes evidence in hospital new drug decision making? *Soc Sci Med* **58**: 1757–66.

Martin DK, Hollenberg D, MacRae S, *et al.* (2003). Priority setting in a hospital drug formulary: a qualitative case study and evaluation. *Health Policy* **66**: 295–303.

Schumock GT, Walton SM, Park HY, *et al.* (2004). Factors that influence prescribing decisions. *Ann Pharmacother* **38**: 557–62.

Patient group directions

Definition

- Patient group directions (PGDs) are written instructions for the sale, supply, and/or administration of medicines to groups of patients who may not be individually identified before presentation for treatment.
- PGDs allow a range of authorized healthcare professionals to supply and/or administer medicines directly to a patient with an identified clinical condition, without them necessarily seeing a prescriber. The healthcare professional working within the PGD is responsible for assessing that the patient fits the criteria set out in the PGD.
- Implementing PGDs might be appropriate both in circumstances where groups of patients might not have been previously identified (e.g. minor injuries and first-contact services) and in services where assessment and treatment follow a clearly predictable pattern (e.g. immunization and family planning).
- In general, a PGD is not meant to be a long-term means of managing a patient's clinical condition. This is best achieved by a healthcare professional prescribing for an individual patient on a one-to-one basis.
- Legal requirements and guidance on PGDs are set out in the circular HSC 2000/026.

Health professionals allowed to use PGDs (only as named individuals)

- Nurses
- Midwives
- Health visitors
- Optometrists
- Pharmacists
- Dental hygienists
- Dietitians
- Occupational therapists
- Chiropodists and podiatrists
- Radiographers
- Orthoptists
- Physiotherapists
- Ambulance paramedics
- Dental therapists
- Orthotists and prosthetists
- Speech and language therapists.

The pharmacist's role in PGDs

Apart from developing practice using a PGD, pharmacists are expected to be involved in various aspects of PGDs:

- Development of a PGD for other healthcare professionals.
- Making sure the PGD is signed by a doctor (or dentist), a pharmacist and authorized by the relevant appropriate body as set out in the legislation.
- Responsibility to ensure that only fully competent, qualified, and trained professionals operate within PGDs.

- Organization of arrangements for the security, storage, and labelling of PGD medicines. Such medicines would normally be expected to be supplied pre-packaged and a robust reconciliation system for stock use is established.
- Checking that the use of the medicine outlined in a specific PGD is consistent with the SPCs, although off-licence use could be considered in exceptional circumstances, provided that it is justified by current best clinical practice.
- Ensuring that a patient information leaflet is provided to patients who have a medicine supplied under a PGD.

Medicines and healthcare products excluded from PGDs

- Unlicensed medicines
- Dressings, appliances, and devices
- Radiopharmaceuticals
- Abortifacients, such as mifepristone
- Nebulizer solutions.

Controlled drugs that can be included in PGDs are shown in Table 13.1.

Antimicrobials

- Should only be included if clinically essential and will not jeopardize strategies to combat ↑ resistance.
- A local microbiologist should be involved in drawing up the PGD.

Table 13.1 Controlled drugs that can be included in PGDs

Schedule	Controlled drug	Additional comments/exceptions
2	Morphine Diamorphine	Only to be used by registered nurses and pharmacists, for the immediate necessary treatment of a sick or injured person (except for treating addiction)
3	Midazolam	
4	All drugs	Except anabolic steroids and injectables used for treating addiction
5	All drugs	

Further reading

'Department of Health' website (UK) has PGDs for drugs and chemical and biological counter-measures, ℘ http://www.dh.gov.uk

Medicines & Healthcare products Regulatory Agency (2014). 'Patient Group Directions (PGDs)'. ℘ https://www.gov.uk/government/publications/patient-group-directions-pgds

NHS (2015). 'What is a Patient Group Direction (PGD)?', ℘ www.sps.nhs.uk/articles/what-is-a-patient-group-direction-pgd

NICE (2013). 'Patient Group Directions (MPG2)', ℘ www.nice.org.uk/guidance/mpg2

Non-medical prescribing

Pharmacists in the UK can train to become non-medical prescribers when they are registered pharmacists, and have completed a non-medical prescribing education and training programme at a designated university, which includes a period of supervised practice. Pharmacists can practise as both independent and supplementary prescribers. It is usually advisable to have at least 2yrs of experience practising as a clinical pharmacist, prior to training as a non-medical prescriber.

Pharmacists are able to prescribe any licensed or unlicensed medicine for any medical condition for which they are competent and experienced to prescribe. Pharmacists are able to prescribe licensed medicines for unlicensed indications, i.e. 'off label', if it is accepted clinical practice and supported by a local policy. Pharmacist prescribing must be in accordance with the General Pharmaceutical Council's (GPhC's) *Standards of Conduct, Ethics and Performance*.[8] Pharmacists are required to demonstrate continuing professional development in their area of prescribing practice. Organizations should have a 'non-medical prescribing policy' in place to support pharmacist prescribing. Some specialist organizations also have guidance on pharmacist prescribing in a specialist area—e.g. the British Oncology Pharmacy Association (BOPA) *Guidance for the Development of Pharmacist Non-Medical Prescribing and Review of Patients Receiving Anticancer Medicines*.[9] The pharmacist prescriber must ensure that their prescriptions are checked and dispensed by another pharmacist, in accordance with local clinical governance procedures that are in place for all prescribers.

Definitions

The Department of Health defines independent prescribing as 'prescribing by a practitioner (e.g. doctor, dentist, nurse, pharmacist) responsible and accountable for the assessment of patients with undiagnosed or diagnosed conditions and for decisions about the clinical management required, including prescribing'.[10]

Supplementary prescribing is a 'voluntary partnership between an independent prescriber (doctor or dentist) and a supplementary prescriber to implement an agreed patient-specific clinical management plan with the patient's agreement'.[11]

Independent prescribing

The practitioner is required to assess the patient, interpret the assessment, and make a decision on the appropriate therapy including safety and a process for monitoring. Independent prescribing usually takes place as part of a multidisciplinary team using a single healthcare record, and the practitioner is accountable for their prescribing. Patients need to be informed that a non-medical practitioner is prescribing their medicine and give their consent.

Supplementary prescribing

There are some key principles that underpin supplementary prescribing:
- The independent prescriber is a doctor or dentist, and is responsible for the assessment and diagnosis of patients, and deciding on the clinical management required, which includes prescribing.
- The supplementary prescribing pharmacist is responsible for prescribing for patients who have been clinically assessed by the independent prescriber according to an agreed patient-specific clinical management plan (Fig. 13.1).

Hospital name and department
Clinical management plan

Name of patient:
Patient medication sensitivities/allergies:
Patient identification (e.g. ID number or, date of birth):
Independent prescriber(s): Name and profession
Supplementary prescriber(s): Name and profession

Condition(s) to be treated:
Might be specific indications or broader terms and might also include treating side effects of specified drugs/classes of drug (e.g. treatment of HIV and related opportunistic infections/complications or treatment of side effects of antiretrovirals and other drugs used in treatment of HIV).

Aim of treatment:
Medicines that could be prescribed by supplementary prescriber:
  Preparation
  Drug names and preparations
  Can also be drug classes (e.g. antiretrovirals)
  Indication—does not have to be very specific
  Dose schedule—does not have to be very specific (e.g. could say 'as *BNF*')

Specific indications for referral back to the independent prescriber:

Guidelines or protocols supporting the clinical management plan:

Frequency of review and monitoring by:

  Supplementary prescriber

  Supplementary prescriber and independent prescriber

Process for reporting ADRs:

Shared record to be used by independent prescriber and supplementary prescriber:

Agreed by independent prescriber(s): (signature and name)

Agreed by supplementary prescriber(s): (signature and name)

Date agreed with patient/carer:

Fig 13.1 Example of a clinical management plan for supplementary prescribers.

- The patient must be treated as a partner in their care and be involved at all stages of decision-making, including consenting for part of their care to be delivered by supplementary prescribing.
- There must be a written clinical management plan relating to a named patient and to that patient's specific conditions. Both the independent and supplementary prescribers must record agreement to the plan before supplementary prescribing begins.

- The independent and supplementary prescribers must share access to, consult, and use the same common patient record.

Benefits

The benefits of pharmacist prescribing are to improve patient care without compromising patient safety, make it easier for patients to get the medicines they require, ↑ patient choice, make better use of healthcare professional skills, and contribute to more flexible team-working in the NHS.

References

8. General Pharmaceutical Council (2010). 'Standards of Conduct, Ethics and Performance', http://www.pharmacyregulation.org/standards/conduct-ethics-and-performance
9. British Oncology Pharmacy Association (2015). 'Guidance for the Development of Pharmacist Non Medical Prescribing and Review of Patients Receiving Anti-cancer Medicines', http://www.bopawebsite.org/
10. Department of Health (2006). *Improving Patients' Access to Medicines: A Guide to Implementing Nurse and Pharmacist Independent Prescribing within the NHS in England*. London: Department of Health. http://webarchive.nationalarchives.gov.uk/20130107105354/http://www.dh.gov.uk/en/Publicationsandstatistics/Publications/PublicationsPolicyAndGuidance/DH_4133743
11. Department of Health. 'Prescribing by non-medical healthcare professionals'. https://www.health-ni.gov.uk/articles/pharmaceutical-non-medical-prescribing

Incident reporting

- Each hospital or institution should have a policy in place for reporting incidents. An incident reporting policy often covers all incidents, including adverse events, hazards, and near misses of an adverse event or hazard. Such a policy applies to all hospital staff. An induction programme to a hospital usually covers details of any local policy.
- An incident reporting programme identifies, assesses, and manages risks that could compromise or threaten the quality of patient services or staff working in a safe environment, as part of the overall management of risk. It is a confidential process, and all staff should complete the appropriate documentation if they are involved in, or aware of, an incident.
- An 'incident' is usually defined as an event or circumstance that could have, or did, lead to unintended or unexpected harm, loss, or damage. Incidents might involve actual or potential injury, damage, loss, fire, theft, violence, abuse, accidents, ill health, and infection.
- It is necessary for incidents to be reported to ensure that the hospital can analyse the data for trends, causes, and costs. Action plans can then be developed to minimize future similar incidents. Reporting of incidents is also a mechanism for staff to have input into change of practice and procedures. Incident reporting follows a 'no-blame' culture.
- Medication incidents must be reported through this mechanism to ensure that there can be a review of trends, a root cause analysis, arrangements for improvement, and a follow-up audit. This is a requirement of medicines management in hospitals.
- The types of incident that a pharmacist can report include medication errors and failure of systems or processes that affect patient care.
- In addition to reporting an incident, a pharmacist must also deal with an incident by communicating with the relevant members of staff involved (see ➔ 'Dealing with mistakes', pp. 64–5).

Further reading

NHS England. 'Reporting Patient Safety Incidents', ℜ https://www.england.nhs.uk/patientsafety/report-patient-safety/

Medical representatives

- Medical representatives provide information to healthcare practitioners, but their prime function is to promote and sell their products and services.
- Medical representatives should provide their services according to the Association of the British Pharmaceutical Industry (ABPI) code of practice (or similar). If the code of practice is breached, medical representatives can be reported to the director of the Prescription Medicines Code of Practice Authority (PMCPA).
- Most hospitals have a policy for dealing with medical representatives—check the local policy.
- Some hospitals do not allow medical representatives to leave samples. Check the policy for the local hospital before accepting trial samples from medical representatives.
- It is GCP for medical representatives to make an appointment before meeting with a member of staff. Some hospital policies restrict the grades of staff that are allowed to meet with medical representatives.
- Medical representatives are not allowed to promote unlicensed indications for their products or products that have not yet been licensed.
- Hospital drug prices are confidential to the hospital and under no circumstance must they be revealed to a medical representative.
- Most hospitals limit the level of hospitality provided by representatives. For example, it is reasonable for representatives to provide food for a working lunch, but not expensive meals at a restaurant.

Further reading

Association of the British Pharmaceutical Industry. 'Guidance Notes for Health Professionals, Understanding the ABPI Code of Practice for the Pharmaceutical Industry and Controls on the Promotion of Prescription Medicines in the UK', ℘ http://www.abpi.org.uk

Overseas visitors

- The term 'overseas visitor' is used for patients who have fallen ill unexpectedly while visiting the UK and who, consequently, require standard NHS emergency care.
- People who do not normally live in the UK are not automatically entitled to use the NHS free of charge.
- Patients who are eligible for full NHS treatment include the following:
  - Anyone legally living in the UK for ≥12 months.
  - Permanent residents.
  - Students in the UK for >6 months.
  - Refugees or asylum seekers who have made an application to remain in the UK and are waiting for a decision on their immigration status.
  - People detained by the immigration authorities.
  - People from countries with a reciprocal agreement—e.g. European Union residents.
- Patients who are not eligible for full NHS treatment include the following:
  - Students on courses in the UK for <6 months.
  - Refugees or asylum seekers who have not yet submitted applications to the Home Office.
  - Those who have had an asylum application turned down and exhausted the appeals process.
  - Illegal immigrants.
- The NHS hospital is legally responsible for establishing whether patients are not normally resident in the UK.
- If patients are not eligible for free NHS care, the hospital must charge the patient for the costs of the NHS care.
- When the patient is charged depends on the urgency of the treatment needed:
  - For immediately necessary treatment, treatment must not be delayed or withheld while the patient's chargeable status is being established.
  - For urgent and non-urgent treatment, patients should pay a deposit equivalent to the estimated full cost of treatment in advance.
  - Any surplus can be returned to the patient on completion of the treatment.
- Treatment that is available to overseas patients free of charge is as follows:
  - A&E visits. However, treatment in other departments following an A&E visit (e.g. X-ray) is charged.
  - Emergency or immediately necessary treatment.
  - Treatment of sexually transmitted diseases (except HIV).
  - Treatment of diseases that are a threat to public health (e.g. tuberculosis (TB)) and acute treatment of all infectious diseases.
  - Family planning.
  - Compulsory psychiatric treatment.
- If an overseas visitor chooses to be treated privately, they are classed as an 'international private patient'. These patients are treated as private patients (see → 'Private patients', p. 263).

Further reading

Department of Health (2015). 'Guidance on implementing the overseas visitors hospital charging regulations'. ℘ www.gov.uk/government/uploads/system/uploads/attachment_data/file/496951/Overseas_visitor_hospital_charging_accs.pdf

Private patients

In the UK, patients can choose to have treatment either from the NHS or privately. Private patients usually have private health insurance, which covers some, or all, of the costs of private treatment. Patients can be treated privately either in a private hospital or in NHS hospitals. Private patients treated in NHS hospitals are discussed in this section.

- NHS hospitals either have specific wards for private patients or private patients are treated on the same ward as NHS patients, often in a side room.
- Patients who are treated privately either have private health insurance or are paying themselves.
- Before the patient receives treatment, the private health insurance company must confirm what they will cover, according to the patient's insurance policy.
- Patients' medicines must be charged accurately to the private health insurance companies to ensure that the NHS generates income from using NHS facilities to treat these patients.
- If a patient is having private treatment, this should be annotated in some way on the patient notes or identification labels.
- Any prescription for a private patient must be annotated as 'private patient' to ensure that the pharmacy department can charge appropriately for the drugs.
- Private patients do not have to pay NHS prescriptions charges.
- Charging and systems can vary for in-patients and out-patients.
- An on-cost is usually added to the medicine price when charging for private patients' medicines.
- Clinical pharmacists' input into patient care for medicines review and counselling might be appropriate.
- Check what systems are in place for private patients' medicines in your hospital.
- Patients can choose to change from being a private patient to an NHS patient between consultations.

In 2009, the Department of Health issued guidance for patients to enable them to remain NHS patients, but to pay for additional private care, such as medicines, not available in or funded by the NHS.[12] The NHS continues to provide the care the patient is entitled to in the NHS, and the private care has to be delivered separately from the NHS care. Hospitals should have specific policies in place for patients requesting additional private care in accordance with this guidance.

Reference

12. Department of Health (2009). 'Guidance on NHS patients who wish to pay for additional private care', ℘ https://www.gov.uk/government/uploads/system/uploads/attachment_data/file/404423/patients-add-priv-care.pdf

Responsible pharmacist

The responsible pharmacist

The responsible pharmacist regulations came into effect in the UK on 1 October 2009. Prior to this date, in order to conduct a retail pharmacy business lawfully, the Medicines Act 1968 specified that there had to be a pharmacist in 'personal control'. 'Personal control' meant that the pharmacist needed to be physically present in the pharmacy. Furthermore, sales of pharmacy and prescription-only medicines had to be under the supervision of a pharmacist. However, the Medicines Act did not define 'supervision', although it was interpreted as needing a pharmacist to be able to 'intervene and advise'.

It was recognized that, to improve the range of services available in pharmacies, pharmacists must be able to work more flexibly and be allowed to undertake their role out of the pharmacy for a limited period to make better use of their clinical training and the skills of pharmacy staff, and hence the concept of the responsible pharmacist was developed.

The Health Act 2006 amends relevant sections of the Medicines Act 1968. Instead of requiring a pharmacist in 'personal control', there must be a 'responsible pharmacist' in charge of each registered pharmacy.

Responsible pharmacists—community pharmacists

The responsible pharmacist has to:
- secure the safe and effective running of the pharmacy, including during periods of absence
- display a notice with their name, registration number, and the fact that they are in charge of the pharmacy at that time
- complete the pharmacy record to identify who the responsible pharmacist was for a pharmacy at any one time
- establish (if not already established), maintain, and keep under review procedures for safe working.

Responsible pharmacists—hospital pharmacists

The responsible pharmacist changes to the Medicines Act only affect those hospitals that have registered all or part of their pharmacy premises with the General Pharmaceutical Council.

Hospitals may choose to have registered pharmacy premises for a number of reasons including the following:
- Operation of a retail pharmacy, which allows dispensing of prescriptions that have not originated within their hospital and selling prescription medicines to visitors and staff.
- To allow the dispensing of private prescriptions when consultation is not covered as part of the business of the hospital.
- To allow for self-prescribing by medical staff.

If you have a registered pharmacy within the hospital, the law and standards for responsible pharmacists will apply. This means that the registered pharmacy is required to have a responsible pharmacist when it is operating as a pharmacy business. As a hospital pharmacist you are advised to ensure you are clear what the responsible pharmacist requirements are within your pharmacy.

Requirements of responsible pharmacist legislation

The law covers four key areas:

- Have a responsible pharmacist to secure the *safe and effective* running of the pharmacy.
- Conspicuously display to the public the name and registration number of the current responsible pharmacist.
- Maintain a pharmacy record detailing who has been the responsible pharmacist at any particular time.
- Maintain and operate pharmacy procedures on a range of specified matters.

The responsible pharmacist is the pharmacist appointed by the employer, who is responsible for securing the safe and effective running of the pharmacy at that time. The responsible pharmacist continues to be responsible for securing the safe and effective running of the pharmacy during any periods of absence.

If there is more than one pharmacist working in the pharmacy at any one time, only one can be the responsible pharmacist. A pharmacist cannot be the responsible pharmacist for more than one pharmacy at any one time.

A hospital department has to be registered with the Council for 3yrs before EU-trained pharmacists can assume responsible pharmacist responsibility.

Pharmacy record

This is an important legal document, it should show who the responsible pharmacist is on any particular given day and time.

The record must be kept for at least 5yrs and must be available at the premises for inspection.

Notice display

The notice is important to ensure that the public can identify the pharmacist who is responsible for the safe and effective running of the registered pharmacy.

Absence of the responsible pharmacist

A responsible pharmacist can be absent from the pharmacy for a maximum of 2h during the business hours of the pharmacy when the pharmacy is operational. The responsible pharmacist continues to be responsible for the safe and effective running of the pharmacy throughout this absence. A responsible pharmacist must comply with the conditions for absence, which are as follows:

- They remain contactable throughout their absence.
- They return with reasonable promptness.
- In the event that they cannot remain contactable, they must arrange for another pharmacist to provide advice during their absence.

Examples of pharmacy procedures that need to be established

- Medicine management standard operating procedures that describe procedures for ordering, storage, preparation, sale and supply, delivery, and disposal.
- Advice about medicinal products that includes:
  - staff training to be undertaken to provide advice
  - those products for which staff may/may not provide advice
  - when staff should refer to a pharmacist and what to do if a pharmacist is not physically present.
- Pharmacy staff listing based on competency.
- Management of records including controlled drugs, invoices, and training details.
- Arrangements during absence.
- Change of responsible pharmacist.
- Complaints and incidents procedures.
- Changes to the pharmacy procedures and how staff are notified.

Further reading

Royal Pharmaceutical Society (2016). *Medicines, Ethics and Practice: The Professional Guide for Pharmacists* (40th ed). London: Royal Pharmaceutical Society.

Gene therapy

The development of genetically modified viruses and advances in cloning and sequencing the human genome have offered the opportunity to treat a wide variety of diseases using 'gene therapy'. The term 'gene therapy' applies to any clinical therapeutic procedure in which genes are intentionally introduced into human cells. Gene therapy clinical trials have been undertaken in cystic fibrosis, cancer, cardiac disease, HIV, and inherited genetic disorders.

Gene therapy can be divided into two main categories: gene replacement and gene addition. Gene replacement tends to be used for monogenic diseases, in which a single 'faulty' gene can be replaced with a normal gene. For example, an abnormal cystic fibrosis transmembrane conductance regulator (CFTR) gene can be replaced in cystic fibrosis. Currently, the majority of gene therapy clinical trials use a gene-addition strategy for cancer, whereby a gene or genes can be 'added' to a cell to provide a new function, e.g. addition of tumour suppressor genes to cancer cells.

For gene therapy to be successful, a therapeutic gene must be delivered to the nucleus of a target cell, where it can be expressed as a therapeutic protein. Genes are delivered to target cells by vectors in a process called 'gene transfer'. The greatest challenge to gene therapy is finding a vector that can transfer therapeutic genes to target cells specifically and efficiently. Gene transfer vectors can be broadly divided into non-viral and viral systems. Non-viral vectors, such as liposomes, have limited efficiency. Genetically modified viruses have proved to be the most efficient way of delivering DNA. Viruses are merely genetic information protected by a protein coat. They have a unique ability to enter (infect) a cell, delivering viral genes to the nucleus using the host cell machinery to express those viral genes. A variety of viruses have been used as vectors, including retroviruses, herpes viruses, and adenoviruses. Many viral vectors have been genetically modified so that they cannot form new viral particles and so are termed 'replication-deficient' or 'replication-defective'. Replication-deficient viruses have had the viral genes required for replication and the pathogenic host response removed. This prevents the virus replicating and the potential for the therapeutic virus to reverse back to a pathogenic virus. The deleted genes are replaced by a therapeutic gene, thus allowing the delivery and expression of the therapeutic gene without subsequent spread of the virus to surrounding cells. Some gene therapy vectors are able to replicate under genetically specified conditions.

There is the potential for infectious hazards with gene therapy, including possible transmission of the vector to hospital personnel. Therefore, consideration has to be given to protecting both the environment and the staff handling these agents, because of the uncertain effects of specific genes on normal human cells, potential for operator sensitization on repeated exposure, and the potentially infective nature of some products. Some gene therapy agents might require handling in negative-pressure isolators in separate specific aseptic facilities.

Trusts undertaking clinical trials with gene therapy products should have a local Genetic Modification Safety Committee, a Trust biological safety officer, and local biological safety officers for the units handling these trials.

Gene therapy trials fall under the Health and Safety Executive Genetically Modified Organisms (Contained Use) Regulations 2014. Any area handling gene therapy must have standard operating procedures in place.

Genetically modified organisms are classified as one of four classes (1, 2, 3, and 4) and their classification determines the level of containment required to control the risk. There are four corresponding levels of containment (1, 2, 3, and 4). Class 1 activities involve the least and class 4 the highest risk. Class 1 activities are unlikely to result in harm to humans or the environment and require containment level 1. Agents that are able to cause human disease are categorized as class 2 or higher. This is the same classification as used for microbiological organisms, e.g. HIV is classified as class 3.

A risk assessment should be made for each gene therapy product, with input from the lead investigator or Trust biological safety officer, because they should have a good understanding of molecular biology and virology. The assessment should include details of the class of the gene therapy (class I or II, class I being of minimal risk), the containment level required (containment level 1 or 2 respectively), the control measures that need to be in place to handle the product, an assessment on the risk to human health and safety to the environment, identification of the harmful effects including details of the severity and risk, the characteristics of the proposed activity, the properties of the genetically modified organism, and the disposal methods required.

Further reading

Brooks G (ed) (2002). *Gene Therapy: The Use of DNA as a Drug*. London: Pharmaceutical Press.

Searle PF, Spiers I, Simpson J, *et al.* (2002). Cancer gene therapy: from science to clinical trials. *Drug Deliv Systems Sci* 2: 5–13.

Simpson J, Stoner NS (2003). Implications of gene therapy to pharmacists. *Pharm J* 271: 127–30.

Stoner N (2009). Gene therapy applications. *Clin Pharm* 1: 270–4.

Stoner NS, Gibson RN, Edwards J (2003). Development of procedures to address health and safety considerations for the administration of gene therapy within the clinical setting. *J Oncol Pharm Pract* 9: 29–35.

Stoner NS *et al.* (2006). Appendix 6—Gene therapy. In Beaney AM *Quality Assurance of Aseptic Preparation Services* (4th edn), pp. 123–33. London: Pharmaceutical Press.

UK Health and Safety Executive (2014). 'Genetically Modified Organisms (Contained Use)', ℘ www.hse.gov.uk/biosafety/GMO/index.htm

Vulto AG, Stoner N, Balasova H, *et al.* (2007). European Association of Hospital Pharmacists (EAHP) guidance on the pharmacy handling of gene medicines. *Eur J Hosp Pharm Pract* 13: 29–39.

Watson M, Stoner N (2007). Safe handling of gene medicines. *Eur J Hosp Pharm Pract* 13: 24–6.

Pharmacogenetics

Pharmacogenetics is defined as the study of human genetic variation, which causes different responses to drugs. The differences in response can be both in the therapeutic effect and in ADRs.

For example, genetic make-up may determine variations in liver enzymes that are produced, which in turn affect drug metabolism. One of the cytochrome P450 liver enzymes, CYP2D6, metabolizes drugs (e.g. β-blockers, antidepressants, and opioids) in the liver so that they can be eliminated. The level of this enzyme in the liver is genetically determined. Patients are classified as 'slow metabolizers' if they have low levels of CYP2D6 in the liver, which means that the drug is eliminated from the body more slowly, resulting in additional toxicity. 'Fast metabolizers' have a high level of CYP2D6 in the liver and therefore metabolize the drug more quickly, resulting in a possible reduced therapeutic effect. In practice, 'slow metabolizers' may require a lower dose of drug than 'fast metabolizers' for the same effect. An example of a drug metabolized through this mechanism is warfarin: 40% of the variability in warfarin levels is accounted for by the CYP2C9 enzyme.

Another example of genetic influence on drug response is via receptors. If drugs bind to specific receptors to generate a response and the number of receptors present is genetically determined, the response to the drug will vary according to the patient's genetics. This has enabled drug development to be much more targeted, so that only patients with specific characteristics receive the appropriate drugs. For example, breast cancer patients who have the HER2 receptor present on their breast cancer cells will be the only group of breast cancer patients who respond to trastuzumab. In cancer patients, the presence or absence of some genes will determine the patient's response to some anticancer drugs.

Genetic testing of individuals is usually done from a saliva or blood sample. There will be issues regarding the quality of the tests, their initiation, communication to the patient, and the implication of the test to treatment. The general public would need to be more widely educated about pharmacogenetics and its implications. Tests would need to be rigorously evaluated. Currently there are some home test kits available, but the sale of these is not regulated. This means that some of the test kits available have no guarantee of being validated or of producing accurate results.

There are ethical issues that need to be considered in genotyping individuals. (The genotype is the genetic make-up of a cell or individual. Genotyping is the process of determining an individual's genotype using biological assays to find out the genetic make-up of an individual.) This could lead to discrimination of individuals who carry specific genes and affect the allocation of resources. For example, there is concern that some individuals may not be able to obtain insurance policies if their genetic test results are considered negatively. There is also concern about the privacy and confidentiality of genetic information, where it should be stored, and who would have access to it. Drug companies may only research drugs for diseases that are straightforward to treat, rather than those that could be used for rarer diseases. In addition, pharmacogenetic testing may predict for future risks of disease or raise implications for other family members, which adds to the ethical issues of informing patients and their families.

Pharmacogenetics will enable more cost-effective and targeted prescribing that will optimize the use of drugs, avoiding the prescribing of drugs that will be ineffective, and reduce the medical and financial impact of adverse drug reactions. This means that in the future, patients will be prescribed drugs specific to their conditions, taking into account genetic factors when deciding on dosage regimens. However, targeted drugs may be more expensive. In addition, there may be a loss of any benefit of, for example, racemic mixtures.

Standards of business conduct for clinical pharmacists

Declaration of interests has become an integral part of professional life, and pharmacists are not exempt from showing that they are independent and unbiased. In addition, clinical pharmacists have access to valuable confidential data and can influence purchasing decisions that can have a major effect on a particular company's products. Therefore it is important that pharmacists are aware of relevant guidelines. In the UK, Department of Health guidelines have been produced on these issues and it is prudent to have a local policy designed using this or similar guidance.

The Department of Health guidelines cover the standards of conduct expected of all NHS staff, where their private interests could conflict with their public duties, and the steps that NHS employers should take to safeguard themselves and the NHS against conflict of interest.

Details can be found in the Code of Conduct for NHS Managers 2002; which is available on the Department of Health website.[13] Some key relevant issues are as follows:

- Avoid conflicts of interest between private and NHS interests. It is a well-established principle that public sector bodies, which include the NHS, must be impartial and honest in the conduct of their business, and that their employees should remain above suspicion.
- NHS staff are expected to ensure that the interest of patients is paramount at all times, to be impartial and honest in the conduct of their official business, and to use the public funds entrusted to them to the best advantage of the service, always ensuring value for money.
- It is also the responsibility of staff to ensure that they do not abuse their official position for personal gain or to benefit their family or friends.
- Modest hospitality, provided that it is normal and reasonable in the circumstances (e.g. lunches in the course of working visits), are acceptable, although it should be similar to the scale of hospitality that the NHS, as an employer, would probably offer. Anything else should be declined.
- Casual gifts can be offered by contractors or others (e.g. at Christmas time). Such gifts should nevertheless be politely, but firmly, declined. Articles of low intrinsic value, such as diaries or calendars, or small tokens of gratitude from patients or their relatives, need not necessarily be refused.
- NHS employers need to be aware of all cases in which an employee or their close relative or associate has a significant financial interest in a business.
- Individual staff must not seek or accept preferential rates or benefits in kind for private transactions carried out with companies with which they have had, or might have had, official dealings on behalf of their NHS employer.
- All staff who are in contact with suppliers and contractors, in particular those who are authorized to sign purchase orders or place contracts for goods, are expected to adhere to professional standards of the kind set out in the ethical code of the Chartered Institute of Purchasing & Supply.[14]

- Fair and open competition between prospective contractors or suppliers for NHS contracts is a requirement of NHS standing orders and of EC directives on public purchasing for works and supplies.
- NHS employers should ensure that no special favour is shown to current or former employees in awarding contracts to private or other businesses run by them.
- NHS employees are advised not to engage in outside employment that could conflict with their NHS work or be detrimental to it.
- Acceptance by staff of commercial sponsorship for attendance at relevant conferences and courses is acceptable, but only if the employee seeks permission in advance and the employer is satisfied that acceptance will not compromise purchasing decisions in any way.
- Pharmaceutical companies, for example, might offer to sponsor, wholly or partially, a post for an employing authority. NHS employers should not enter into such arrangements, unless it has been made abundantly clear to the company concerned that the sponsorship will have no effect on purchasing decisions within the authority.
- Staff should be particularly careful of using, or making public, internal information of a 'commercial in confidence' nature, if its use would prejudice the principle of a purchasing system based on fair competition.
- Finally, many employers maintain a record of interests and pharmacists should cooperate with such practices.

References

13. Department of Health (2002). *Code of Conduct for NHS Managers*. London: Department of Health. 🔗 www.nhsemployers.org/~/media/Employers/Documents/Recruit/Code_of_conduct_for_NHS_managers_2002.pdf
14. 'Chartered Institute of Purchasing & Supply' website, 🔗 www.cips.org

Waste management of medicines

Pharmaceutical waste refers to the disposal of unwanted medicines, out-of-date or obsolete stock, sharps, and waste arising from diagnostic testing. The current regulations are detailed in the Hazardous Waste Regulations 2009, and further guidance specifically for community pharmacies are detailed in the Department of Health document *Health Technical Memorandum 07-01: Environment and Sustainability—Safe management of healthcare waste.*[15]

The legislation relevant to pharmaceutical waste derives mainly from European directives. The storage, carriage, processing, and supply of waste are all subject to stringent controls designed to minimize the negative effects of waste on the environment.

The Environment Agency or the relevant local authority is the enforcement authority for the legislation. Depending on the circumstances, and in cases of doubt, either can be contacted for advice. The Environment Agency general enquiries number is 03708 506 506.

Policies

Hospital or community pharmacies must have a waste management policy that details general themes, including dealing with pharmaceutical waste such as cytotoxics. Key requirements that need specification in the policy are as follows:
- Detail how returned controlled drugs should be denatured and recorded—see the Royal Pharmaceutical Society publication on the denaturing of controlled drugs.[16]
- Include a list of hazardous medicines that may be encountered in the pharmacy.
- Include instructions to staff on dealing with products other than medicines that are handed in to the pharmacy.
- Include instructions on identifying incompatible products such as flammable products and oxidizing agents.
- Include the protective measures to be adopted by staff when segregating controlled drugs and incompatible products.
- Include reference to monitored dosage system trays and the disposal of blister packs.
- Set out the retention and audit requirements for transfer notes, consignment notes, and quarterly returns.

The guidance also details the types of containers that need to be used for segregation and transportation of the different types of waste. For example:
- A purple-lidded sharps bin should be used for medicines or sharps contaminated with cytotoxic or cytostatic medicines.
- A yellow-lidded sharps bin should be used for all other medicines or sharps contaminated with non-hazardous medicines.
- A blue-lidded sharps bin or container should be used for disposing of medicinal or pharmaceutical waste including contaminated items such as glassware containing residual medicines, syringes, IV lines and giving sets.
- Patient-identifiable data must be disposed of as confidential waste or made unreadable.

When completing any documentation needed for the transfer and transportation of waste from the pharmacy, pharmacies are advised to ensure that all waste coding and descriptions are robust and accurate, particularly with regard to the presence of medicinal waste and medicinally contaminated sharps.

Waste generated

The waste generated is likely to consist of the following:

Community pharmacy

- Pharmaceutical products returned from individuals and households as part of the essential services (i.e. the disposal of unwanted medicines—a service provided by all pharmacies).
- Out-of-date or obsolete stock.
- Needles and syringes.
- Waste arising from diagnostic testing such as blood glucose and cholesterol monitoring.

Hospital pharmacy

- Unwanted items from ward/department, including controlled drugs, PODs, fridge items, and hazardous, harmful, or toxic pharmaceuticals, require processing as many items can be recycled if storage conditions have been complied with.
- Otherwise waste will contain out-of-date dispensary stock, items that are not economically viable to recycle, and PODs that may have been returned to pharmacy for a variety of reasons.

Medicines brought into hospital by patients

Medicines brought into hospital by the patient are the property of the patient and should only be sent to pharmacy for destruction with the prior agreement from the patient or their agent. It is GCP to record the details of PODs sent to the pharmacy for destruction.

Carriage of waste and community pharmacy

Ensure that a carrier's licence is held if the pharmacy carries waste medicines from a patient's home or residential home to the pharmacy.

Handling waste within the pharmacy

The Hazardous Waste Regulations 2005 introduced significant changes for pharmacies. They required pharmacies to separate hazardous waste medicines from non-hazardous waste.

Staff safety is paramount. Handling of waste should be minimal and carried out with great care. Acceptance of waste other than medicines returned from households should not be undertaken.

Hazardous waste medicines and non-hazardous waste medicines must be separated before they are sent to a suitably authorized waste contractor for incineration. Whenever waste that may contain some hazardous waste medicine is sent for incineration, it is required to be consigned as though it were hazardous and needs to be accompanied by a hazardous waste consignment note.

▶ Under the Hazardous Waste Directives, only cytotoxic or cytostatic medicines are classified as hazardous waste.

As an aid to pharmacists, a suitable starting point for identifying hazardous medicines is to adopt the list of hazardous drugs provide by the National Institute for Occupational Safety and Health (NIOSH).

Liquid medicines

Liquids should generally not be decanted and mixed. Where liquid medicines are being discarded, they should be retained within their individual containers and placed in the waste bins provided for the purpose.

If the waste contractor has provided a waste bin specially designed for liquids and suggests that the liquid medicines can be emptied from containers and mixed in the waste bin, the pharmacist has a duty of care to ensure that only compatible products are mixed.

Empty medicine containers that have held liquids must be disposed of as waste medicines for incineration as it is not possible to ensure that the contents have been completely removed (containers cannot be rinsed into the sewerage system). If residues of liquid controlled drugs are present, these should be emptied, as far as possible, and denatured before the container is placed in the waste container.

If segregation is not being undertaken, purple-lidded burn bins should be used for all pharmaceutical waste, including cytotoxic agents and antibiotic products.

Transfer of waste to a waste carrier

A consignment note is required to list the hazardous medicines that are being consigned so that they can be handled safely and disposed of appropriately. A waste transfer note is required for non-hazardous waste. Refer to *Health Technical Memorandum 07-01*[15] for details of completing required documentation.

Radioactive waste

Radioactive waste is governed by the Environmental Agency, which issues organizations with certificates of authorization that regulate the routes of disposal, limits of disposal, and type of radioactive material disposed of.

Disposal and destruction of controlled drugs

A controlled drug ceases to be classified as a controlled drug after it has been rendered irretrievable, i.e. all controlled drugs that are disposed of should be unrecognizable as controlled drugs (Misuse of Drugs Act 1971).

Hospital only—controlled drugs must be returned to pharmacy

All controlled drugs (e.g. expired stocks, PODs, and excess stock) must be notified to the pharmacist responsible for the ward/unit/department. These controlled drugs must not be destroyed on the ward.[16]

The pharmacist must return the controlled drugs to the pharmacy to either the pharmacy controlled drug record book for destruction (in the case of expired stock or PODs) or the pharmacy controlled drug record book (in the case of excess stock of controlled drugs, which can be entered back into pharmacy stock).

Departments who do not receive a pharmacy visiting service must either arrange for a pharmacist to come to the ward or agree a mutually convenient time for the nurse to take their controlled drugs and the controlled drug record book to the pharmacy, where a pharmacist will sign for their return.

Records of controlled drug destruction

In both cases outlined, an entry must be made in the ward controlled drug record book or the patient's own controlled drugs record book on the appropriate page for the drug in question, specifying 'destruction' or 'return to pharmacy', the quantity involved, the new stock balance, and the signatures of the two persons involved.

Prefilled PCA/PCEA/epidural syringes and opiate infusions

Part contents of opiate infusions/PCA/PCEA/epidural syringes that were initially set up and issued in theatres but are no longer needed must be destroyed on the ward where the patient resides.

Opiate infusions/PCA/PCEA/epidural syringes containing residual unused injections must be emptied into an in-use sharps bin, in addition to the empty syringe. Empty bags can be disposed of in a clinical waste bag according to procedure for disposing of empty infusion bags. This must be witnessed by a second person. One of the two witnesses should be the nurse looking after the patient.

References

15. Department of Health (2013). 'Health Technical Memorandum 07-01: Environment and Sustainability – Safe management of healthcare waste', ℘ www.gov.uk/government/uploads/system/uploads/attachment_data/file/167976/HTM_07-01_Final.pdf
16. Royal Pharmaceutical Society of Great Britain (2005). 'The Safe and Secure Handling of Medicines: A Team Approach', ℘ http://www.rpharms.com/support-pdfs/safsechandmeds.pdf

Interface issues between primary and secondary care

Interface medicines management is a component of the overall medicines management agenda. Primary and secondary care should be working in collaboration to promote seamless care for patients.

The following examples illustrate some of the interface considerations:

Seamless care

Patients should experience a smooth transition as they move between the primary and secondary care sectors during admission to, or discharge from, hospital. The efficient and accurate transfer of information is an essential part of this process, if unintended changes in medication are to be avoided. An accurate up-to-date list of medication should be available to the admitting clinicians and a comprehensive discharge summary outlining current medication and changes should be available to the patient's GP. NHS Summary Care records are available throughout England, which is an electronic system used by GPs to summarize patients' medication history. This allows appropriate healthcare professionals, such as pharmacists and clinicians, to access a patient's medication history on admission. This information would support medicines reconciliation on admission. Similarly, at discharge, medication changes at point of discharge should be communicated to patients' GPs. This can be done via discharge summaries including electronic prescriptions. There is a huge risk to patient safety when this information is completed inaccurately. Some primary care organizations and hospitals are reporting such issues via their incident reporting systems to understand the magnitude and address concerns in a joined-up approach.

Formulary

Due to the vast number of medicines available, it is imperative to rationalize medicines across the interface to promote evidence-based, cost-effective prescribing. Primary care and hospitals work together to consider the impact of new guidance such as that issued by national groups (e.g. NICE in England) at appropriate drug and therapeutics committees. Issues can arise if the prescribing formulary in primary care differs to that in the local hospital setting. For example, patients may be switched to a similar drug within the same class (e.g. statins or angiotensin-converting enzyme (ACE) inhibitors) when admitted to hospital or vice versa. This can cause various issues including confusion for patients and GPs and result in an ↑ in the cost of medicines when transferring from one care setting to another. Some primary care organizations and hospitals have worked together to develop a 'joint prescribing formulary' (primary/secondary care) with a view to minimizing this. In some instances, these formularies have various categories such as 'Specialist only drugs', 'Shared care' and 'Blacklisted'. Primary care organizations usually have an Area Prescribing Committee (APC) where new medicines and prescribing protocols are considered. They have representation from both primary care and the local hospitals.

Hospital discounting

The NHS and pharma have come to expect this in the past, though the changing NHS landscape has altered the way discounts are used for leverage. So 'loss leaders' (where drugs are provided to hospitals for pennies when they cost significant money in the community) have slowly become politically incorrect as joint formularies have become the norm within health economies.

Antimicrobial steering/stewardship group

Antimicrobial stewardship is an important element of the both the UK Five-Year Antimicrobial Resistance Strategy and the 2011 Chief Medical Officer report. The aims of such stewardship initiatives are to improve the safety and quality of patient care and to contribute significantly to reductions in the emergence and spread of antimicrobial-resistance. These aims are ultimately achieved by improving antimicrobial prescribing through an organized antimicrobial management programme. This usually involves a microbiologist in the Trust, whilst infection control nurses and various pharmacists are typically within primary care and hospitals. Any prescribing guidelines or recommendations affecting primary and secondary care should be considered via due process—such as the APC.

Shared care

A shared care agreement outlines ways in which the responsibilities for managing the prescribing of a medicine can be shared between the specialist and a primary care prescriber. Primary care prescribers are invited to participate. If they are unable to undertake these roles, then he or she is under no obligation to do so. In such an event, the total clinical responsibility for the patient for that diagnosed condition remains with the specialist.

Issues may arise when patients requiring Specialist medicines are discharged back to the community (i.e. GP). An example being disease modifying anti-rheumatic drugs (DMARDs) for rheumatoid arthritis. Primary care organizations and hospitals work together to produce shared care protocols outlining any special monitoring requirements that need to be undertaken, the dosing regimen of medicine, and roles and responsibilities of the individuals involved.

Acute commissioning

Primary care organizations commission services from hospitals. Since they commission the majority of the services for their local population, this is associated with a drugs budget and with the quality of the medicines management services delivered. It is therefore imperative that senior pharmacists in Clinical Commissioning Groups (CCGs) and hospital Trusts work together across the interface on a number of issues including acute commissioning. This involves managing the payment by results (PbR) excluded drugs, which includes identifying the responsible commissioner and monitoring use of these high-cost drugs.

Service redesign

With the trend towards an ageing population, the focus is on long-term conditions, empowering patients and bringing care closer to home. There are some exciting projects and examples whereby primary and secondary care can work together to facilitate this. For example, in an area with a high rate of COPD admissions—the primary care organization and local hospitals may want to work together to reduce admissions and empower patients to manage their condition in the community where possible. An example of this service would be to have a shared point of access whereby GPs can refer complex patients to a specialist clinician across a certain geographical area.

Reducing medicines waste

A report by the Department of Health estimates that unused medicines cost the NHS around £300 million per annum, with an estimated £110 million worth of medicine returned to pharmacies, £90 million worth of unused prescriptions being stored in homes, and £50 million worth of medicines disposed of by care homes.

Joint working across primary and secondary care (including community pharmacies), has been shown to help tackle this via initiatives such as social marketing campaigns, zero tolerance on pharmacy returns in secondary care, and improving inhaler technique. The 'Green Bag Scheme' is a national initiative that encourages patients to bring in their medicines from home when attending and/or being transferred between care settings. This means that their own medicines can be used if they are admitted to hospital.

There are many solutions to dealing with interface issues such as the following:

- Discharge information (including an explanation of the discharge prescription), is faxed/electronically transferred from the hospital to the GP, community pharmacist, and primary care pharmacist.
- Patients at risk of medication problems after discharge are identified in hospital and then referred to a named pharmacist or technician to follow-up at the patient's home.
- Patients are helped to self-administer medicines in hospital so they become accustomed to their new medicines before they are discharged.
- Discharge planning starts as early as possible in the hospital stay, even before admission for planned procedures, and should involve a multidisciplinary approach.
- Joint formularies between primary and secondary care are used to help prevent medicines being changed purely because they are not on the formulary.
- Tackling medicines waste across primary and secondary care.

Interface pharmacy encompasses a range of opportunities for collaborative working across primary and secondary care to improve the safety of patients, promote cost-effective and evidence-based prescribing, tackle medicines waste, and bring care closer to home.

Further reading

Bellingham C (2004). How to improve medicines management at the primary/secondary care interface. *Pharm J* 272: 10–11.

British Medical Association (2016). 'The structure of the new NHS', ℘ www.bma.org.uk/collective-voice/policy-and-research/nhs-structure-and-delivery/nhs-structure-new

Department of Health (2010). *Equity and Excellence: Liberating the NHS*. London: Department of Health. ℘ www.gov.uk/government/uploads/system/uploads/attachment_data/file/213823/dh_117794.pdf

Department of Health (2012). *Improving the Use of Medicines for Better Outcomes and Reduced Waste*. London: Department of Health. ℘ www.gov.uk/government/uploads/system/uploads/attachment_data/file/212837/Improving-the-use-of-medicines-for-better-outcomes-and-reduced-waste-An-action-plan.pdf

Public Health England (2015). 'Start Smart – then focus. Antimicrobial Stewardship Toolkit for English Hospitals', ℘ www.gov.uk/government/uploads/system/uploads/attachment_data/file/417032/Start_Smart_Then_Focus_FINAL.PDF

The Kings Fund (2015). 'An alternative guide to the new NHS in England', ℘ www.kingsfund.org.uk/projects/nhs-65/alternative-guide-new-nhs-england

Technician role in clinical pharmacy

Pharmacy technicians play a vital role in supporting clinical pharmacists. Pharmacy technicians work with pharmacists in clinical areas to improve patient care and deliver cost savings. The diverse role of a pharmacy technician continues to expand and develop, creating more responsibilities and opportunities for technicians.

Technicians are able to complete many tasks traditionally undertaken by pharmacists. Once accredited, an experienced technician is able to independently carry out drug histories and medicine reconciliation, as well as in-patient and one-stop ordering. In addition to these clinical duties, technicians carry out drug returns, expenditure reporting, auditing, ward-based dispensing, controlled drug returns and destruction, stock management, and assisting with timely discharges.

Pharmacy technicians are invaluable when there is a need for fast discharges, either due to a bed crisis or a patient at risk of leaving without their medication. A ward technician is usually able to fast-track the discharge prescription (TTO) through pharmacy, thus avoiding the usual waiting time. In addition, ward-based dispensing of discharge medication has been adopted successfully in various Trusts. Although only a basic list of drugs is available to be dispensed on the ward, a significant number of simple prescriptions are being turned around more promptly, thus allowing for more timely discharges. This task requires two members of pharmacy staff, so the presence of a ward technician avoids the necessity for two pharmacists per prescription. The technician or pharmacist can also counsel the patient on their medication, thus saving nursing time during discharges.

Technicians help to reduce the occurrence of delayed or missed doses by checking drug charts alongside the pharmacist. A technician may identify newly prescribed items, which need to be ordered from pharmacy, before the pharmacist has seen the chart. In doing so, the request can be brought to the pharmacist's attention and sent to pharmacy earlier, which also helps avoid work being sent to pharmacy late in the day. With the experience gained during time spent on the ward, technicians will become more aware of certain clinical issues and be able to highlight these to the pharmacist. Common examples are ensuring the correct dose or formulary choices of medicines are prescribed, avoiding accidental omission of regular medication or prolonged courses of antibiotics, for example. Although technicians are not authorized to request or suggest a change to patients' medication, they can hand-over to the pharmacist who then brings it to the attention of the doctor and/or nurse. It is vital that a technician works within their professional responsibilities.

With technicians developing their roles and supporting the pharmacists with the clinical pharmacy workload, pharmacists can focus on developing their roles further. This provides an essential skill mix for successful pharmacy teams.

Electronic prescribing

Electronic prescribing is defined as follows by NHS Connecting for Health:
  'The utilization of electronic systems to facilitate and enhance the communication of a prescription or medicine order, aiding the choice, administration and supply of a medicines through knowledge and decision support and providing a robust audit trail for the entire medicines use process'.[17]

Electronic prescribing has been implemented in many hospitals in the UK to varying extents including:

- to support discharge prescribing
- in highly specialized areas—e.g. critical care, oncology, and renal
- whole process—prescribing, review, administration, and supply of medication.

The main drivers for implementing electronic prescribing are improved patient safety and improved documentation. Electronic prescribing systems can be set up to flag interactions (medicine and allergies), incorrect dosing, prescribing errors, and provide additional information for safe medicines administration. These systems require input and maintenance by pharmacy and information technology teams. It is very important to have support from all members of the multi-disciplinary teams, and identifying key champions within each team of professionals will aid in the successful implementation of a system.

Benefits

- ↓ in certain types of medication errors.
- Improved quality and safety of prescribing.
- Improved safety of prescribing medication to patients with drug allergies.
- Prescriptions are legible.
- Accessibility of information between primary and secondary care.
- Improved protocol compliance.
- Management of formulary compliance.
- Supports decision-making when prescribing.
- Implementation of policy decisions.
- Improved use of staff time due to less time spent looking for patients' notes or drug charts.
- Pharmacy can make early identification of new scripts for screening and supply, and have access to more information when screening from dispensary.
- Detailed audit trail.
- Drug-usage reports for individual patients.
- Aids clinical audit.
- Improved access to patient records.

Potential problems

- New prescribing errors, such as the selection of the wrong formulation may occur.
- ↑ time—especially initially due to lack of familiarity.
- Resistance to change.
- Healthcare professionals spending less time with the patient, as most information is on the screen.
- Ability to prescribe remotely.

Training

Providing training to all members of staff for a hospital is a huge task. The training needs to be at the most appropriate time, and the most suitable training package will vary depending on the clinical group. Classroom training, e-learning packages and one-to-one training all have their advantages and disadvantages. User guides for the system are useful, and can be developed locally to encompass departmental procedures. The most effective way to become competent at using a system is to use it regularly.

Security

It is essential that there is good security for any electronic prescribing system. Only people that need access should be granted access, with restrictions to certain functionality or areas of the system if appropriate.

Electronic systems will require maintenance, so there needs to be a plan to account for this. System downtime may be planned; alternatively, due to various reasons there may be unplanned downtime. A robust back-up system is essential to ensure all the information up to the point of downtime is accessible.

Further reading

Donyai P, O'Grady K, Jacklin A, et al. (2008). The effects of electronic prescribing on the quality of prescribing. *Br J Clin Pharmacol* 65: 230–7.
Smith J (2004). *Building a Safer NHS for Patients: Improving Medication Safety*. London: Department of Health.

Reference

17. NHS Connecting for Health (NHS CFH) (June 2009). 'Electronic prescribing in hospitals—challenges and lessons learned', ↷ http://www.lse.ac.uk/LSEHealthAndSocialCare/pdf/information%20systems/eprescribing_report.pdf

Medicines safety

Medication safety is a key aspect of the role of a pharmacist, members of the pharmacy team, as well as that of the wider healthcare team. In the UK the emphasis on medication safety ↑ as increasingly complex medicines are available for patients with increasingly complex health needs.

In the UK, the national patient safety agenda has been heightened following the Francis and Berwick reports. Moreover, NHS England has established a Patient Safety Domain which promotes patient safety within the NHS and aims to identify, understand, and manage risks to the safety of patients. National reporting of incidents from organizations across the country helps to ensure continual learning and ensure improvements in processes are shared with others. Transparency is a key part of the patient safety focus.

Initiatives which have been adopted by NHS England include the following:

- National Patient Safety Alerting System (NaPSAS) which alerts members of the healthcare team to risks which may lead to harm or death by providing timely guidance on how to prevent potential incidents (examples available on NHS England website).
- Published data around *never events** to promote transparency:
  - *Never events are 'serious, largely preventable patient safety incidents that should not occur if the available preventable measures have been implemented'. Examples of drug-related never events include wrongly prepared high-risk injectable medication; maladministration of a potassium-containing solution; wrong route administration of chemotherapy. In the 'Never Events List 2013/14', 25 never events are listed, nine of which are related to medications.
- Patient Safety Collaboratives established to support healthcare staff and patients locally to focus on safety matters and discover solutions to improve systems.

In addition, NHS England and the Medicines Healthcare products Regulatory Agency (MHRA) are working to minimize harm from medication errors through simplification of, and emphasis on, reporting in order to improve learning and guide practice in primary and secondary care. Medication Safety Officers (MSOs) have been appointed in hospital Trusts and primary care groups in order to act as a contact to improve the learning from errors, and ensure processes and systems are in place to improve safety. Prior to the establishment of NHS England, the National Patient Safety Association (NPSA) produced alerts giving advice on how to make certain medicines safer. These alerts are still accessible online.

Pharmacy staff have an essential role in helping to improve the safety of medicines for patients by:

- being a role model for safety
- ensuring safe procurement, storage, prescribing, supply, and administration of medicines
- ensuring accurate medicines reconciliation on admission and discharge from hospital or other care settings
- minimizing risk associated with medicines
- development of guidelines and protocols
- communication with patients and counselling on medicines to ensure they are taken as intended

- monitoring patients with multiple co-morbidities and those on high-risk medicines
- giving feedback and advice to other healthcare professionals relating to errors and safe use of medicines
- training of staff
- reporting medication errors.

Medication errors

A medication error occurs due to an unintentional failure in the medication process which has the potential to cause harm to a patient.

Medication errors are one of the most common treatment errors. It is thought that generally as many as one out of five prescriptions contains an error. Between 2005 and 2010, ~87 000 medication incidents were reported to cause actual patient harm, with 822 resulting in death or severe harm.

- Medication errors may occur at any stage of the medication process—prescribing, dispensing, preparation, administration, monitoring, or advice given (see Table 13.2).
- Most errors do not result in patient harm but in order to eliminate the risk of actual harm to patients, we need to be aware of all errors (including those 'near misses' which do not cause harm) to try to minimize risk of patients.
- Errors are rarely caused by one flaw in the system or one mistake by one person. Often errors result from a number of 'holes' in the process and it is important to understand all of the underlying causes to prevent errors occurring.

Pharmacists are in a key position to try to reduce the risk of medicines to patients; however, a whole team approach is required. The healthcare team must be aware and educated on medication safety issues.

High-risk medicines

A high-risk medicine is one which has the potential to cause significant harm to a patient when an error occurs. Mistakes are not necessarily more common with these medicines, but the consequences of an error are more severe.

Medicines may be higher risk due to a narrow therapeutic window, pharmacokinetic interactions with other medicines, complex dosing or monitoring schedules, as well as the medicines listed in Table 13.3. As pharmacists it is particularly important to be vigilant when these medicines are prescribed and to be aware of the potential to cause harm.

Special safeguards will often be implemented to try to reduce the risk of errors with these medicines. Some strategies include the following:

- Standardization to reduce reliance on memory.
- Simplification of the process—e.g. pre-printed prescriptions.
- Improving access to information about the medicines—e.g. guidelines, education, and training.
- Monitor and control use:
  - Limit access to high-risk medicines—e.g. only certain patients, prescribed only by particular consultants, held as stock medicines on certain wards, hospital prescribing only.
  - Monitor compliance to guidelines.
  - Monitor patient and response to medication.

Table 13.2. Potential medication safety issues and examples of strategies to reduce risk

Potential medication safety issues	Examples of strategies to reduce risk
Prescribing: unclear/illegible/ incomplete; incorrect dose, frequency, route/rate/time of administration; prescribing wrong medicine or for the wrong patient; abbreviations e.g. 'u' instead of 'Units'; trailing zeros 5.0mg which is read as 50mg; verbal orders for prescriptions misunderstood; incomplete information about patient/medicine; omissions or unintentional prescription of medicines when moving healthcare facilities; prescribing medicine patient is allergic to; poor documentation; calculation errors	• Access to electronic systems for patient records • Electronic prescribing systems • Tailor prescriptions to individual patient needs • Guidelines and resources in place to advise on prescribing • Pharmacist review of prescribing prior to administration of medicines • Including medicines reconciliation on admission to hospital • Zero tolerance for abbreviations • Use generic names for prescribing (unless brand is required, e.g. lithium) • Involvement of patients in decision-making
Administration: wrong patient, drug, strength, dose, time, route; wrong use of medical equipment; miscalculation of doses; lack of monitoring; missed doses; poor documentation of administration	• Drug standardization—use of premixed IV solutions where possible • High-risk medicines to be stored separately and only on certain ward areas • Like medicines and different concentrations stored separately • Limit stock of medicines available to be given • Limit the variety of infusion pumps available and train staff in their use • Independent double-checking of certain medicines • Use oral syringes which do not fit the IV ports on lines so oral medicines are not given by the wrong route • Only staff who have been trained can give certain medicines, e.g. cytotoxic medicines • More than one medication chart for patient resulting in medicines being overlooked • Access to medicines out of normal pharmacy working hours
Dispensing: wrong selection of medicine due to packaging or labelling; stock management/ delivery problems; unlabelled medicines or obscuring of vital information with labels;	• Reduce the risk of storing similar sounding/ packaged medicines in the same area • Warning labels to identify different doses/ strengths • Use of robotic systems • Use of tall-man letters e.g. hydrOXYzine and hydrALAZINE • Well-designed workflow in the dispensary • Purchase medicines from different manufacturers to reduce selection errors if similar packaging

Table 13.3. High-risk medicines

	Rationale for inclusion in high-risk medicines list
Insulin	Wrong dose of insulin given due to wrong prescription (including unclear prescription), supply, and administration could lead to overdose of insulin and result in hypoglycaemia, coma, or even death
Opiates including epidurals	Risks to patients include over-sedation, hypotension, delirium, and lethargy Risk of wrong selection of product, strength, wrong rate of administration Wrong route may lead to paralysis or death
Concentrated electrolytes : Potassium [conc] >40mmol/L/potassium phosphate	Maladministration of potassium may lead to patient death or serious injury or disability. It is not possible to reverse the effects when concentrated electrolytes are not given properly Wrong administration can also cause arrhythmias
Anticancer (cytotoxic) agents	Cytotoxic chemotherapy can cause adverse effects such as nausea, vomiting, bone marrow suppression, stomatitis, diarrhoea, hand–foot syndrome, peripheral and central neurotoxicity, renal and liver dysfunction Wrong route of administration, e.g. IV vincristine given by the incorrect route, could lead to paralysis and death
Concentrated unfractionated heparin	Narrow therapeutic index which means careful titration to clotting factors. Potential for clot or bleed Interactions with other medicines may alter the effects of heparin
Anticoagulants (including the new oral anticoagulants (NOAC): dabigatran, rivaroxaban, apixaban)	Narrow therapeutic range for vitamin K antagonists which requires monitoring of INR and adjustment of doses. Interaction with certain medicines or co-morbid states may also affect this measure of INR For the NOAC medicines there is a risk of haemorrhage as for all anticoagulants and lack of reversal agents for this group of medicines may potentially ↑ the risk for patients
Injectable sedatives e.g. midazolam	Could lead to over-sedation, hypotension, delirium, or lethargy

- Using alert systems or labelling to highlight risk.
- Use of forcing functions—e.g. oral syringe port cannot be added to an IV line due to the syringe design; only certain staff allowed to administer certain medicines.
- Automation for prescribing (see ➋ 'Electronic prescribing', pp. 281–2).
- Monitoring patient for effects of medicine.
- Independent double-checking of high-risk medicines.
- Record keeping.
- Involve patients in the process and provide the necessary information.

The failure, mode, and effects analysis (FMEA) is a useful to identify why a medication process or the equipment may fail and how it could be made safer.

In addition to high-risk medicines, there are some patients who would be considered high-risk patients, i.e. they are more likely to experience adverse reactions:

- Paediatric and neonatal patients:
  - Pharmacokinetics of medicines change quickly during development
  - Many medicines are unlicensed in children
  - Liquid medicines may not be available leading to inaccuracies of measuring small doses
  - Multiple calculations required to individualize doses.
- Patients on multiple medicines or with multiple co-morbidities, particularly the elderly.
- Patients who are not actively involved in their medication use.
- Patients who cannot communicate well.
- Patients who have more than one healthcare professional involved in their care.

Error reporting

- Reporting of medication errors is vital in order to establish which medicines are high-risk medicines or processes.
- Reporting systems help identify causes of errors and how they have been prevented to reduce patient harm.
- An open reporting culture is important in an organization, with a 'no-blame' culture which aims to learn from mistakes made.
- Anyone who is involved, witnessed, or discovered the problem is responsible for reporting the error.
- Reporting should occur as soon as possible after the event has happened.
- Patients and/or carers should be informed of any error and any implications.
- Pharmacy staff involved in investigations of incidents should feedback outcomes to the staff member who reported the incident as well as any patients or staff involved.
- Reporting via the organization's local incident report system is essential in order for action to be taken locally and nationally.
- Analysis of errors is vital, looking at a whole-system approach, often using root cause analysis:
  - What happened?
  - Why did it happen?
  - What will prevent it happening in the future?

Collaboration of all staff is required and an open culture of reporting and sharing of errors is needed to ensure learning.

Human factors

As more people are involved in patient safety, and in particular medication safety, quality improvement and 'human factors' are increasingly being used to identify reasons errors occur. Healthcare staff do not want to make mistakes which may harm their patients, but unfortunately this does not stop it happening. Even the most competent practitioner can make an error—we are all human!

Taking the system as a whole, the human factors approach encompasses everything which influences people and their behaviour:

* *Environmental*—factors affecting one's ability to function optimally at work, e.g. heating, poor lighting, noise, overcrowding.
* *Equipment and resources*—includes appropriately skilled staff in a team being used in the correct way, training schemes, equipment and technology required, facilities which assist in the safe and effective delivery of certain tasks, storage of medicines (look-alike medicines should not be stored together), lack of standardization, e.g. prefilled syringes of high-risk medicines to prevent preparation errors.
* *Organizational*—inherent and embedded factors in the organization, restriction of high-risk medicines; electronic prescribing systems with appropriate use of alert systems and access to patient information in a timely way.
* *Education and training*—availability of programmes which provide effective training and assessment of the necessary skills, lack of knowledge about medicine/patient/rules; patient education.
* *Individual factors*—this may include psychological, home life, work-relationships, health or lack of sleep, etc.

Being aware of the factors just listed and how they affect the way we work is vital in helping understand how errors happen and can therefore help prevent potential fatalities. In healthcare, human factors approaches aim to understand the effects of teamwork, tasks, equipment, workspace, culture, and organization on human behaviour.

Adverse drug reactions

Even when the prescription is correct, the drug has been administered correctly and the medicine was deemed appropriate for the patient, bad outcomes may follow. When a response to a medicinal product is noxious and unintended, this is known as an adverse drug reaction (ADR).

ADRs can happen within the licence of the drug or when used outside the licence (e.g. off label, overdose).

It is important to report suspected ADRs. The MHRA yellow card reporting scheme is in place to report ADRs (⌘ www.yellowcard.mhra. gov.uk). It is thought that ADRs account for 1 in 16 hospital admissions and may occur in 10–20% of hospital inpatients. ADRs are costly not just to the health service but also to the patient and may lead to reduced quality of life for some patients. It is therefore important to take a thorough drug history related to the complaint, including herbal and over-the-counter medicines.

What to report?

* If you are unsure whether an ADR should be reported, then it is best to report. Some safety alerts concerning medicines have only been issued years after the medicine first went to market.

Do you suspect an adverse drug reaction?

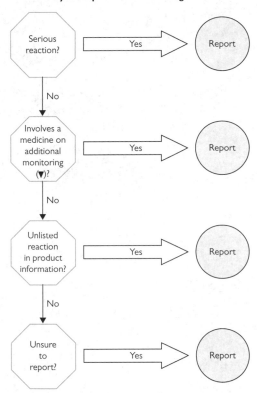

Fig 13.2 What should be reported. Reprinted from https://www.gov.uk/
government/uploads/system/uploads/attachment_data/file/403078/Specific_
areas_of_interest_for_adverse_drug_reaction_reporting.pdf with permission.

- Fig 13.2 shows a quick reference guide of what should be reported.
  Further information is detailed in the *BNF* or online at ℘ https://www.
  gov.uk/topic/medicines-medical-devices-blood/vigilance-safety-alerts.
- The MHRA also issue alerts relating to medicines following yellow card
  reports.
- An MHRA email alerting system is available which updates on recent
  changes to classification of medicines or safety concerns, as well as
  highlighting safety concerns for defective products which is important to
  relay to patients and ward areas, particularly if drug recall is required.

Research

Clinical audit and research

Sometimes there is a blurred distinction between clinical audit and research. Pharmacists need to consider projects carefully and ensure that they comply with local requirements. Research on humans should be subject to ethical committee review. Clinical audit does not usually require ethics committee review. Some of the differences between clinical audit and research are described in this section.

Clinical audit

- The principal point of clinical audit is that it measures the present level of care against a recognized standard with the aim of introducing usually a single intervention with the intention of repeating the initial measurement to assess impact
- Involves an intervention that is already in use
- Aims to improve quality of care and outcomes for patients
- Is not randomized
- Is usually initiated and conducted by those providing the clinical specialty
- Involves review of recorded data by those entitled to have access to such data, e.g. electronic medical records, clinical information systems, or other non-clinical data
- May include patient satisfaction questionnaires
- Does not normally require ethical review
- See the clinical audit cycle in Fig. 14.1.

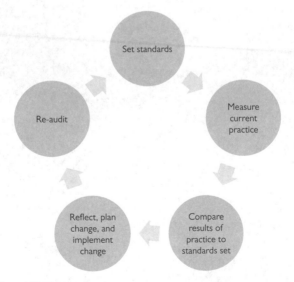

Figure 14.1 Clinical audit cycle.

Research

- Systematic investigative process to increase knowledge, establish facts, and reach new conclusions
- Addresses clearly defined questions, aims, and objectives
- Requires ethical review
- Randomized studies
- Interventions involving contact with patients by a health professional
- Questionnaires asking for personal data or sensitive sociodemographic details
- If patients or volunteers have any procedure or treatment additional to normal medical care
- If patient samples of any sort are taken additional to normal medical care
- Collection of data additional to that required for routine care
- See Chapter 5, 'Clinical trials' (pp. 105–15), for further information, including details on National Research Ethics Service (NRES).

Writing a research proposal

Follow 'SMART' principles when writing a research proposal to improve reasonable outcomes:
- Specific
- Measurable
- Attainable
- Relevant
- Time-related.

Structure of a research proposal
- Title of project
- Purpose of project (e.g. aims and objectives)
- Background of project
- Central research question(s)
- Research design
- Data analysis
- Timetable
- Research staff required
- Resources required
- Proposed budget
- Contingency measures
- Knowledge translation plans
- References.

Title of project
- Descriptive
- Clear
- Succinct
- Use recognizable keywords
- Comprehensible (to non-specialists)
- Should not imply an expected outcome.

Examples
- 'A randomized controlled trial of amitriptyline in chronic pain'
- 'A controlled evaluation of advice giving for low back pain'
- 'A descriptive study of the needs of patients on an orthopaedic surgery ward'

Purpose of project
- Why undertake the project?
- Who will benefit?
- Academic potential/contribution?
- Clinical potential/contribution?
- Patient potential/contribution?
- What gaps are likely to be filled?

Background of project
- Literature review
- Critical appraisal of literature/evidence
- Establish scientific adequacy of evidence
- Establish clinical and social adequacy of evidence

- Identify positive evidence and the potential to support, replicate, or challenge it
- Identify negative evidence and the potential to support, replicate, or challenge it
- Identify uncertain evidence and the potential to clarify, support, or reject it
- Identify lack of evidence and potential to remedy this
- Justify research questions.

Research questions
- Clear
- Specific
- Distinctive
- Comprehensible (to self and others)
- Answerable
- Feasible (human resources, scientific and financial).

Research design
- Type of research design, e.g.:
  - Randomized controlled trial
  - Case–control studies
  - Matched comparison
  - Cohort study
  - Single-case study
  - Surveys
  - Descriptive/ethnographic
  - Qualitative—involves studying how interventions are experienced
  - Quantitative—evaluates or compares interventions
- Sampling frame
- Sample selection criteria
- Consideration of power calculations and type 1 and 2 errors
- Baseline and follow-up strategy
- Measures/data to be collected (methods/outcome/satisfaction/costs)
- Access to data arrangements (Data Protection Act might apply)
- Use of Confidential Advisory Group (CAG)
- Ethical considerations—research often requires approval from an ethics committee or equivalent body (see ➲ 'Clinical audit and research', pp. 292–3):
  - Requirement for patient information leaflets and consent forms
- Consideration as to what insurance/indemnity you are required to have in place and who will be providing it
- Consideration of involvement of R&D departments.

Data analysis
- How data will be stored and who will have access to it:
  - Manually and computerized
  - Coded
  - Entered
  - Confidentiality and anonymity
- Considerations if data is to go outside of the EU
- How data will be retrieved from computer

- How data will be manipulated, e.g.:
  - Descriptive versus inductive
  - Univariate/bivariate/multivariate analysis
  - Tests of significance
  - Qualitative data handling
- Which statistical/epidemiological package (e.g. SPSS/EpiInfo/NUDIST)?
- Data presentation strategy:
  - Report writing strategy (e.g. report/journal publications/book/meeting presentation/poster)

Timetable
- Preparation time
- Start/baseline data collection
- Follow-up data collection
- End of data collection
- Data retrieval time
- Data manipulation and analysis
- Report preparation, writing, and dissemination
- Do not underestimate the time involved—be realistic and keep to the schedule.

Research staff required
- Self
- Research assistants
- Interviewers
- Secretarial/administrative support
- Data entry, retrieval, and handling staff
- Consultancies (statistician/specialist advice/support).

Resources required
- Staff
- Accommodation (office space and storage space)
- Equipment:
  - Computer hardware/software
  - Telephones/fax/email
  - Furniture/filing cabinets/storage
  - Audio/video recording machinery
  - Specialist/technical equipment
- Laboratory time/access
- Books, journals, and library services
- Printing and stationery
- Postage
- Travel (both staff and reimbursement for participants in the study)
- Overheads (staff and agency).

Dissemination of results
- Consideration of what is going to happen with the results and what impact your study will have.

References
- Provide supporting references in a standard format, such as Vancouver (see ➲ pp. 297–8).

Citations in documents and articles for publication

A variety of styles are used to cite publications in the medical literature. Editors of several medical journals have established guidelines for the format of manuscripts submitted to their journals. This group, known as the International Committee of Medical Journal Editors (ICMJE), has broadened its focus beyond manuscript and reference formatting to include ethical principles related to publication in biomedical journals. Many journals now follow the ICMJE's *Recommendations for the Conduct, Reporting, Editing and Publication of Scholarly Work in Medical Journals* (ICMJE Recommendations; formerly known as the *Uniform Requirements for Manuscripts Submitted to Biomedical Journals: Writing and Editing for Biomedical Publication*).[1] Review of the ICMJE Recommendations is beyond the scope of this book but it should be consulted by those preparing materials for publication.

The commonly used methods of citation are listed here with examples. For further details see the BMA website.[2]

Harvard style

In the Harvard style, references are cited using the author–date system. For example:
- Journal/book articles—in the text:
  - Davies and Mehan (1988) have argued …
- Journal/book articles—in the reference list:
  - Davies, P.T. and Mehan, H. (1988). Professional and family understanding of impaired communication. *British Journal of Disorders of Communication* **23**, 141–51.
- Books—in the text:
  - Davies (1983) has argued that …
- Books—in the reference list:
  - Davies, PT (1983). *Alcohol Problems and Alcohol Control in Europe*. London: Croom Helm.

List all authors (up to a maximum of six) in the reference list.

Vancouver style

In the Vancouver style, references are cited using the author–number system:
- Journal/book articles—in the text:
  - Onghena and Van Houdenhove[4] have argued …
- Journal/book articles—in the reference list:
  - 4. Onghena P, Van Houdenhove B. Antidepressant-induced analgesia in chronic pain: a meta-analysis of 39 placebo controlled studies. *Pain* 1992 May; **49**(2): 205–19.

- Books—in the text:
  - Colson and Armour[5] have argued …
- Books—in reference list:
  - 5. Colson JH, Armour WJ. *Sports Injuries and their Treatment* (2nd rev. edn). London: S Paul; 1986.
  - List all authors (up to a maximum of six) in the reference list.

References

1. International Committee of Medical Journal Editors (2015). 'ICMJE Recommendations ("The Uniform Requirements")', ℘ www.icmje.org/about-icmje/faqs/icmje-recommendations/
2. British Medical Association (2016). 'Reference styles', ℘ www.bma.org.uk/library/library-guide/reference-styles

Therapy-related issues: gastrointestinal

Diarrhoea

Description and causes

There is no universally agreed definition for diarrhoea but the British Society of Gastroenterology defines diarrhoea as the abnormal passage of loose or liquid stools more than three times daily and/or a volume of stool >200 g/day. Acute diarrhoea is usually defined as that lasting <4wks and chronic diarrhoea as that lasting >4wks.

- 'Diarrhoea' is a term generally understood to mean an ↑ frequency of bowel movement relative to normal for an individual patient.
- The normal bowel habit in Western society lies somewhere in the range between two bowel actions/week and three bowel actions/day.
- The mechanisms that result in diarrhoea are varied and include ↑ secretion or ↓ absorption of fluid and electrolytes by cells of the intestinal mucosa and exudation resulting from inflammation of the intestinal mucosa.
- Diarrhoea is a non-specific symptom that is a manifestation of a wide range of GI disorders, including inflammatory bowel disease, irritable bowel syndrome, GI malignancy, a variety of malabsorption syndromes, and acute or subacute intestinal infections and infestations.
- Diarrhoea can be an unwanted effect of almost any drug, particularly those listed on ➲ 'Medications commonly causing diarrhoea', p. 301.

Assessment

- Determine the frequency and severity of symptoms, including the quantity and character of the stools (e.g. watery, fatty, containing blood or mucus).
- Enquire about the presence of red flag symptoms:
  - Blood in the stool
  - Antibiotic treatment
  - Persistent vomiting
  - Weight loss
  - Painless, watery, high-volume diarrhoea
  - Nocturnal symptoms disturbing sleep—organic cause likely.
- Assess for complications of diarrhoea, such as dehydration.

Clinical features of dehydration

- *Mild dehydration*: commonly no specific symptoms, though lassitude, anorexia, nausea, light-headedness, or postural hypotension can be experienced.
- *Moderate dehydration*: apathy, tiredness, dizziness, muscle cramps, dry tongue or sunken eyes, reduced skin elasticity, postural hypotension, tachycardia, oliguria.
- *Severe dehydration*: profound apathy, weakness, confusion (leading to coma), shock, tachycardia, marked peripheral vasoconstriction, systolic BP <90mmHg, oliguria, or anuria.

Medications commonly causing diarrhoea

- Osmotic (drugs that create a hypertonic state in the intestine)
  - Acarbose, magnesium salts
- Secretory (↑ intestinal ion secretion or inhibit normal active ion absorption)
  - Antineoplastics, digoxin, metformin, NSAIDs, misoprostol, and olsalazine
- Disturbed motility (leading to shortened transit time)
  - Erythromycin, levothyroxine
- Exudative (drugs that cause inflammation and ulceration)
  - Antineoplastics, NSAIDs, and simvastatin
- Malabsorption or impaired digestion of fat or carbohydrates
  - Aminoglycosides, colestyramine, metformin, orlistat, and tetracyclines
- Microscopic colitis (drugs causing a submucosal band of collagen in the intestine, resulting in a watery diarrhoea)
  - Cytotoxic agents, budesonide, carbamazepine, ciclosporin, co-beneldopa, ranitidine, and simvastatin
- All patients presenting with diarrhoea should be questioned about the relationship between symptoms and changes in medications
- If an underlying cause of diarrhoea can be identified, management is directed at the cause rather than the symptom of diarrhoea.

Treatment

- Management is usually supportive with attention to fluid intake and nutrition. The priority when treating acute diarrhoea is the prevention or reversal of fluid and electrolyte depletion.
- The underlying cause may require specific treatment.
- Management of complications, especially dehydration.

Fluid and electrolyte therapy

Even in the presence of severe diarrhoea, water and salt continue to be absorbed by active glucose-enhanced sodium absorption in the small intestine. Oral replacement solutions are effective if they contain balanced quantities of sodium, potassium, glucose, and water. Glucose is necessary to promote electrolyte absorption.

Proprietary soft drinks and fruit juices may be inadequate treatment for individuals in whom dehydration poses a significant risk—e.g. the elderly and patients with renal disease.

In adults, an oral rehydration solution should be considered for patients with mild to moderate dehydration (loss of <6% of body weight). Solutions should be made up freshly according to manufacturers' recommendations, refrigerated, and replaced every 24h.

Several proprietary rehydration products are available and are made up according to brand recommendations. The recommended ranges of concentrations for rehydration solutions for use are as follows:
- sodium 50–60mmol/L
- potassium 20–35mmol/L
- glucose 80–120mmol/L.

For adults, encourage 2–3L of rehydration solution orally to be taken over 24h. This will provide 100–180mmol of sodium and 40–105mmol of potassium. Once rehydration is complete, further dehydration is prevented by encouraging the patient to drink normal volumes of an appropriate fluid and by replacing continuing losses with an oral rehydration product.

Drug therapy

Antimotility drugs may be of symptomatic benefit in adults with mild or moderate acute diarrhoea. Their most valuable role is in short-term control of symptoms during periods of maximum social inconvenience (e.g. travel and work). They are contraindicated in patients with severe diarrhoea, and in patients with severe inflammatory bowel disease or dilated or obstructed bowel. However, antimotility drugs are also sometimes useful for control of symptoms if treatment of the underlying cause is ineffective or the cause is unknown. Antimotility drugs are never indicated for management of acute diarrhoea in infants and children <12yrs.

If an antimotility drug is considered appropriate, it is reasonable to use one of the following regimens:
- Loperamide 4mg orally initially, followed by 2mg orally after each unformed stool (maximum of 16mg/daily).
- Diphenoxylate 5mg + atropine 0.05mg orally three to four times daily initially (↓ dose as soon as symptoms improve).
- Codeine phosphate 30–60mg orally up to four times daily.
- Colestyramine provides symptomatic relief of diarrhoea following ileal disease or resection.

Adsorbents, such as kaolin and activated charcoal, have not been shown to be of value in the treatment of acute diarrhoea. They could interfere with absorption of other drugs and should not be used.

Antibacterials are rarely indicated in uncomplicated infective diarrhoea, except to treat properly diagnosed enteric infections such as dysentery and antibacterial-associated colitis or for some bacterial causes of gastroenteritis such as *Campylobacter* enteritis, shigellosis and salmonellosis.

Diarrhoea can reduce the absorption of medicines. Drugs that may be affected clinically significantly include antiepileptics, modified release formulations, antidiabetic agents, anticoagulants, antimalarials, antiretrovirals, and oral contraceptives.

Constipation in adults

Description and causes of constipation in adults

- Defined as a ↓ frequency of defecation.
- The normal frequency of bowel motions in Western countries varies from three times/day to twice/wk.
- A person might complain of constipation for the following reasons.
  - Defecation occurs less frequently than usual.
  - Stools are harder than usual.
  - Defecation causes straining.
  - Sense of incomplete evacuation.

There are a large number of causes of constipation, including common dietary problems, medical conditions, mechanical obstruction, commonly used drugs and other factors such as immobility, stress, or undiagnosed conditions. Constipation can be acute or chronic and one of the most common causes is a low-residue diet.

Some medications commonly causing constipation

- $5\text{-}HT_3$ antagonists (e.g. ondansetron)
- Aluminium- and calcium-containing antacids
- Amiodarone
- Anticholinergic agents (e.g. tricyclic antidepressants, antipsychotics and antispasmodics, antiparkinsonian agents)
- Antidiarrhoeals
- Antihistamines and antipsychotics
- Calcium supplements
- Calcium-channel blockers
- Diuretics
- Iron preparations
- Lithium
- NSAIDs
- Opioids.

Changing or stopping these drugs might be all that is required to restore normal bowel function.

Most of the factors predisposing to constipation are potentially magnified or compounded in the older patient. In this group, particularly, prolonged constipation can lead to faecal impaction, causing urinary and faecal over-flow incontinence. The latter is sometimes misdiagnosed and treated as diarrhoea. It is an avoidable cause of hospital admission.

Medical conditions such as irritable bowel syndrome, intestinal bowel obstruction, cancer, pregnancy, hormonal disturbances such as hypothy-roidism and diabetes, hypercalcaemia, depression, Parkinson's disease, and stroke can all cause constipation.

Blood in stools, severe abdominal pain, unintentional weight loss, coexist-ing diarrhoea, persistent symptoms, tenesmus (feeling or urgency without production), and failure with over-the-counter laxatives can all be signs of more complex conditions (e.g. colorectal cancer).

Treatment of constipation in adults

Patients, especially if ambulant and otherwise healthy, should be encouraged to control their bowel activity by attention to diet and exercise. The diet should contain adequate amounts of fibre and fluid. Physical exercise has been shown to ↓ intestinal transit time and is believed to stimulate regular bowel movements.

If these measures are ineffective, intermittent or regular use of a laxative might be necessary (Table 15.1). The duration of treatment with laxatives should be limited to the shortest time possible. The undesirability of long-term laxative use should be explained to the patient.

Diet

The major lifestyle factor leading to constipation is inadequate dietary fibre intake. Dietary fibre consists of plant complex carbohydrates that escape digestion in the small intestine and are only partly broken down by bacterial enzymes in the large intestine. The ingestion of dietary fibre ↑ stool bulk by ↑ both solid residue and stool water content. This results in ↓ intestinal transit time and ↓ water absorption in the large bowel, resulting in stools that are softer, wetter, and easier to pass.

The recommended amount of dietary fibre is 30g/day. The fibre content of the diet should be built up gradually to avoid adverse effects, such as bloating or flatulence. Patients should be encouraged to choose a wide variety of fibre sources (e.g. wholegrain or wholemeal products such as breads, cereals, pastas and rice, fruits and vegetables, legumes, seeds, and nuts) rather than adding a few very high-fibre foods (e.g. unprocessed bran) to the diet. Ensure that adequate fluid intake is encouraged.

Drug therapy

There is little clinical evidence on which to judge the relative effectiveness and tolerability of individual laxatives. Therefore choice should be based on symptoms, patient preferences, side effects, and cost of medicines.

First-line therapy

If dietary management is not sufficient, bulk-forming agents are the laxatives of choice for mildly constipated individuals. Provided that good fluid intake is maintained, use oral bulk-forming agents, e.g. ispaghula husk.

The effect of bulk-forming laxatives is usually apparent within 24h, but 2–3 days of medication might be required to achieve the full effect.

Second-line therapy

- Osmotic laxative—a recent Cochrane review has preferred macrogols sachets (one or two sachets twice a day) over lactulose syrup (10–30mL orally twice or three times daily) for use in the treatment of chronic constipation. Lactulose syrup is contraindicated in bowel obstruction and galactosaemia. The laxative can take 48h to work, so it must be taken regularly. Laxido®/Movicol®, one to three sachets daily in divided doses; each sachet should be dissolved in 125mL of water. Macrogols are contraindicated in patients with intestinal obstruction or perforation caused by disorder of the gut wall, ileus, and patients with severe inflammatory conditions of the intestinal tract. Evidence suggests that macrogols work faster than lactulose and result in fewer side effects.

Table 15.1 Laxative choice

Constituent(s), form, and preparation	Dose (adult dose, unless otherwise specified)	Time to onset
Note: it is recommended that osmotic and bulk-forming agents be taken with adequate fluid		
Bulk-forming laxatives		
Ispaghula granules	1 sachet or 5mL spoonful, twice daily Child 6–12yrs: 50% adult dose	Usually 24h, 2–3 days for full effect
Sterculia	1–2 heaped 5mL spoonfuls twice daily Child 6–12yrs: 50% adult dose	Usually 24h, 2–3 days for full effect
Osmotic laxatives		
Macrogols	1–3 sachets in 125mL water daily	1–3 days for full effect
Lactulose syrup	15mL twice daily, adjusted according to response Child, <1yr: 2.5mL twice daily Child, 1–5yrs: 2.5–10mL twice daily Child, 5–18yrs: 5–20mL twice daily	1–3 days
Phosphate enemas	See product information	2–5min
Stool-softening laxatives		
Docusate tablets	200mg twice daily	1–3 days
Arachis oil (rectal) (contraindicated in peanut allergy)	See product information	1 day
Stimulant laxatives		
Bisacodyl 5mg tablets	1–2 tablets daily	6–12h
Bisacodyl 10mg suppositories	1 suppository daily	15–60min
Senna 7.5mg tablets	2–4 tablets daily Child >6yrs: 1–4 tablets adjusted according to response	6–12h
Lubricant laxatives		
Glycerol/glycerin suppositories	1 suppository, as required	15–30min
Liquid paraffin oral emulsion	10–30mL at night	8–12h

Note: prolonged use of liquid paraffin oral emulsion can cause deficiency of fat-soluble vitamins and is associated with lipoid pneumonia

- Stimulant laxative—senna 7.5mg or bisacodyl 5mg, one or two tablets daily (interchangeably). The agents used for second-line therapy can also be used as first-line therapy in acute illness or for hospitalized patients.
- Although stool-softening agents, such as docusate salts, are often used in the treatment of constipation, they have limited effectiveness as monotherapy.

Third-line therapy

If constipation is resistant to the first- and second-line therapies, there should be a re-evaluation of the underlying cause(s), including impaction. For further therapy, use a stimulant agent (e.g. senna 15–30mg or bisacodyl 5–10mg) orally daily at night.

If required, consider the following regimens:

- Glycerin suppository rectally (allow to remain for 15–30min)
- Phosphate enema rectally.

Fourth-line therapy

In a minority of patients all three therapies are unsuccessful and repeated enemas, macrogols (polyethylene glycol, e.g. Laxido® or Movicol®, sodium phosphate, or sodium picosulfate bowel preparations) and/or manual evacuation might be required, sometimes after admission to hospital.

Opioid-induced constipation

When an opioid is first prescribed, a macrogol and senna at night should be added as a prophylactic measure. (Sometimes the dosage must be ↑ to two capsules twice daily acutely, and then reduced to one or two at night.)

Management of nausea and vomiting

Nausea and vomiting are common and distressing symptoms, which can lead to the following clinical conditions:
- Poor hydration and nutrition
- Electrolyte imbalances (e.g. hypokalaemia, metabolic alkalosis)
- Pulmonary aspiration
- Weight loss
- Depression
- ↑ length of stay
- Poor adherence to oral medicines.

Nausea and vomiting are symptoms not a diagnosis. Always consider the underlying cause. Long-term treatment should be of the cause, rather than with antiemetic drugs.

Causes of nausea and vomiting
- Chemical:
  - Exogenous (e.g. microbial toxins and drugs)
  - Endogenous (e.g. uraemia and hypercalcaemia)
- CNS:
  - Emotional and anxiety
  - CNS lesions
  - Vestibular
  - ↑ intracranial pressure
- Obstructive:
  - Constipation
  - GI tumours.

Patient factors that can ↑ the risk or severity of nausea and vomiting include the following:
- Female
- Tendency to nausea and vomiting (e.g. motion sickness and drug intolerance)
- Non-smoker
- History of migraine
- Pain
- Anxiety
- Anticipated use of opioids postoperatively.

Management of nausea and vomiting requires accurate diagnosis of the cause and knowledge of control pathways and the ways in which antiemetics work.

Like the treatment of pain, the treatment of nausea and vomiting should be based on avoidance and prophylaxis as opposed to waiting for symptoms to occur before dealing with them.

Four steps to managing nausea and vomiting
- Identify the cause—this is not always easy because nausea and vomiting are often multifactorial, but it is important because antiemetics are not equally effective against all types of nausea and vomiting. Take an accurate and detailed history, including prescribed and over-the-counter drugs.

- Remove or correct cause if possible—e.g. stop NSAIDs or prescribe laxatives if constipated.
- Treat according to cause—start an appropriate treatment according to the diagnosis (Tables 15.2 and 15.3). About 10% of cases require more than one drug. These should preferably be from different groups (but anticholinergics and opioids antagonize the prokinetic effect of metoclopramide and domperidone, reducing their efficacy). Parenteral administration is frequently more appropriate than oral if vomiting.
- Review frequently and regularly—if nausea and vomiting persist, change from oral to parenteral administration, ↑ dose, or try drugs from a different therapeutic class. Allow a 24h trial of each intervention before trying another option.

Table 15.2 Recommended antiemetic treatments for specific indications: excludes treatment recommendations for chemotherapy or radiotherapy-induced nausea (see ➲ Box 22.3, p. 535), nausea and vomiting in palliative care, hyperemesis, or bowel obstruction

Antiemetic	Drug class	Recommended indication
Betahistine	Histamine analogue	Ménière's disease
Cinnarizine	Antihistamine	Nausea/vomiting, vertigo, Ménière's disease
Cyclizine	Antihistamine	Nausea/vomiting, vertigo, PONV, opioid-induced (unlicensed), Ménière's disease, Nausea/vomiting associated with mechanical bowel obstruction, raised intracranial pressure
Dexamethasone	Steroid	PONV, chemotherapy
Domperidone	Dopamine receptor 2 antagonist	Nausea/vomiting
Haloperidol	Antipsychotic	Nausea/vomiting in palliative care
Hyoscine	Antimuscarinic	Motion sickness
Metoclopramide	Dopamine receptor antagonist	Nausea/vomiting, GORD, opioid-induced (unlicensed), delayed gastric emptying, chemotherapy
Levomepromazine	Antipsychotic	Nausea/vomiting in palliative care
Ondansetron	5-HT$_3$ antagonist	PONV, chemotherapy
Prochlorperazine	Dopamine receptor type 2 antagonist	Nausea/vomiting, vertigo, PONV, opioid-induced (unlicensed), Meniere's disease
Promethazine	Antihistamine	Nausea/vomiting, vertigo

Table 15.3 Doses and contraindications/cautions of common antiemetics

Antiemetic	Dose	Contraindications (C/I)/cautions
Betahistine	16mg three times daily PO	C/I: Parkinson's disease; additive effects with CNS depressants
Cinnarizine	30mg three times daily PO	Cautions: Parkinson's disease, additive effects with CNS depressants Antagonizes the prokinetic effect of metoclopramide and domperidone.
Cyclizine	50mg three times daily PO/IV/IM	Caution: elderly may be more prone to side effects; risk of tachycardias, epilepsy, glaucoma, severe heart failure, GI obstruction, porphyria. Addictive effects with other CNS depressants, e.g. anaesthetics, alcohol Reports of abuse have been noted due to euphoric effects—avoid in patients with a current or past history of drug misuse Antagonizes the prokinetic effect of metoclopramide and domperidone
Dexamethasone	4mg IV at induction PONV	
Domperidone	10mg three times daily PO	Domperidone does not cross the blood–brain barrier and so is a suitable alternative to metoclopramide in young (♀) patients C/I: prolactinoma, GI obstruction, perforation or haemorrhage Not suitable for PONV MHRA warning over ventricular arrhythmias and sudden cardiac death; MHRA limits use to nausea and vomiting only and advises a low dose and short-term use
Haloperidol	1.5mg–10mg/day	Caution: elderly at risk of extrapyramidal side effects
Hyoscine		C/I: myasthenia gravis, paralytic ileus, pyloric stenosis, toxic megacolon, prostatic enlargement
Metoclopramide	10mg three times daily PO/IV/IM	C/I: phaeochromocytoma, GI obstruction, perforation or haemorrhage, epilepsy, Parkinson's disease Caution: elderly and <20yrs –↑ risk of extrapyramidal side effects MHRA warning related to neurological effects and dosage
Levomepromazine	6.25mg at night–25mg twice daily PO/SC	Administer in low doses and titrate cautiously due to sedative and hypotensive effects at higher doses

(Continued)

Table 15.3 (Contd.)

Antiemetic	Dose	Contraindications (C/I)/cautions
Ondansetron	Prophylaxis: 4mg IV Treatment 4mg IV stat Oncology—dose variable	Cautions: QT interval prolongation, correct electrolyte imbalance; constipating MHRA warning: QT prolongation with IV use
Prochlorperazine	5–10mg three times daily PO 3–6mg twice daily buccal 12.5mg three times daily IM	C/I: Parkinson's disease, epilepsy, narrow-angled glaucoma, hepatic insufficiency, phaeochromocytoma Cautions: elderly at risk of extrapyramidal side effects and hypotension, VTE Additive effects with other CNS depressants, e.g. anaesthetics, alcohol
Promethazine	Prophylaxis: 25mg PO at night Treatment: 25mg stat PO then 25mg at night 3 days	C/I: CNS depression, MAOI therapy Caution: elderly may be more prone to side effects; asthma, epilepsy, narrow-angle glaucoma, severe coronary artery disease

Specialist advice should be sought for patients with chemotherapy or radiotherapy-induced nausea (see ➔ 'Antiemetics for the prophylaxis of chemotherapy-induced nausea and vomiting', pp. 531–9), nausea and vomiting in palliative care, hyperemesis, or bowel obstruction.

Tolerance to opioid-induced nausea and vomiting usually develops after 7–10 days. A prophylactic antiemetic should be used initially and the continued need reviewed after 7–10 days.

Postoperative nausea and vomiting (PONV)

PONV is a highly undesirable complication of surgery, which affects 20–30% of patients. It is defined as any nausea, retching, or vomiting occurring within 24h after surgery. In addition to the consequences of nausea and vomiting already described, severe retching and vomiting postoperatively can delay recovery, put tension on suture lines, cause haematomas below surgical flaps, and ↑ postoperative pain.

PONV can be caused by a combination of factors including:
- use of inhaled anaesthetics (including nitrous oxide)
- duration of anaesthesia
- anaesthetic reversing agents (e.g. neostigmine doses >2.5mg)
- use of opioids
- disturbance of GI function or vestibular mechanisms by the surgical procedure
- perioperative dehydration.

Limiting the listed factors can reduce the baseline risk of PONV.

For non-emergency surgery, preoperative assessment of patient factors (described previously) that could contribute to PONV as well as consideration of the surgical procedure is essential to enable optimum prophylactic management. Several risk scoring systems are published in the literature; the higher the number of risk factors, the higher the predicted chance of PONV.

Identify risk factors and correct or minimize wherever possible.

Assess unavoidable risk factors:

- If one risk factor or fewer, no prophylaxis is required
- If two risk factors, give prophylactic antiemetic at induction (e.g. dexamethasone 4mg IV)
- If three risk factors, give antiemetic at induction (e.g. dexamethasone 4mg IV) and at end of operation (e.g. ondansetron 4mg IV)
- If four risk factors or more (i.e. high risk), give antiemetics at induction and end of operation and use total IV anaesthesia containing propofol.

If rescue therapy is required postoperatively despite prophylaxis, an alternative agent from a different class to that used intraoperatively should be used (e.g. cyclizine or prochlorperazine). Ondansetron is licensed as a single dose postoperatively. Nausea and vomiting continuing for >24h despite regular antiemetics should be reviewed to rule out other causes (e.g. postoperative ileus).

Further reading

Aptel CC, Läärä E, Koivuranta M, et al. (1999). A simplified risk score for predicting postoperative nausea and vomiting. Anesthesiology 91: 693–700.

Golembiewski J, Chemin E, Chopra T (2005). Prevention and treatment of postoperative nausea and vomiting. Am J Health Syst Pharm 62:1247–60.

Dyspepsia, peptic ulcer disease, and gastro-oesophageal reflux disease

Dyspepsia

- Broad range of symptoms related to dysfunction of the upper GI tract from oesophagus to duodenum. Also described as bad indigestion or heartburn.
- Symptoms include recurrent upper epigastric pain or discomfort, acid reflux, fullness, bloating, wind, nausea/vomiting, early satiety, flatulence. It affects 40% of the UK population a year.
- Conditions associated with dyspeptic symptoms include gastro-oesophageal reflux disease (GORD), which accounts for 25–50% of cases, peptic ulcer disease (PUD), gastritis, oesophagitis, gastric, pancreatic, or oesophageal cancer, biliary disease, liver cirrhosis, CRF, Crohn's disease.

GORD

- Acid pepsin or bile reflux into oesophagus from the stomach due to reduced sphincter tone, hiatus hernia, or abnormal oesophageal clearance.
- Symptoms include heartburn, acid regurgitation, and sometimes dysphagia.
- GORD can be complicated by strictures, ulceration, aspiration, Barrett's oesophagus, and adenocarcinoma.

PUD

- Discontinuity/breach in the entire thickness of the gastric or duodenal mucosa of >5mm in diameter with associated inflammation. Commonly involves the stomach (gastric ulcer (GU)), duodenum (duodenal ulcer (DU)), and oesophagus.
- In GUs, symptoms of upper abdominal pain are precipitated by eating and weight loss is common. 5% of GUs are malignant.
- In DUs, symptoms of pain are usually nocturnal, before meals, and are relieved by food or antacids. Weight gain is common.
- 10% of the population will suffer a peptic ulcer in their lifetime. A DU is more common than a GU.
- Despite changes in management, PUD is one of the most common causes of an upper GI bleed which is regarded as a medical emergency with a 10% hospital mortality rate.
- Other complications of PUD include perforation and subsequent peritonitis, chronic iron deficiency anaemia, gastric and oesophageal cancers.

Pathology of ulcer formation

Due to imbalance of injurious and protective factors:

- *Injurious factors*—pepsin, bile reflux, gastric acid, *Helicobacter pylori*, rapid gastric emptying, lifestyle (e.g. stress, alcohol, smoking, obesity, fatty diet, chocolate, caffeine,) co-morbidities, drugs (e.g. NSAIDs, aspirin,

clopidogrel, corticosteroids, SSRIs, calcium-channel antagonists, nitrates, bisphosphonates, theophylline, potassium chloride SR).
- *Protective factors*—mucus, bicarbonate, prostaglandins, mucosal renewal, mucosal blood flow:
  - Acid secretion is under nervous and hormonal control.
  - The most common factors contributing to ulcer formation are *H. pylori* and NSAIDs. They are independent risk factors for bleeding and ulceration.

Helicobacter pylori

- *H. pylori* found in gastric antrum predisposes to duodenal ulceration (majority of cases). Infection of proximal stomach predisposes to gastric ulceration.
- Eradication reduces recurrence of gastric and DUs and risk of re-bleeding
- There is little evidence that *H. pylori* is involved in the aetiology of GORD.
- Urea breath test—used to confirm presence of *H. pylori* prior to pre-eradication treatment or post-eradication if symptoms persist or there are complications (e.g. haemorrhage). PPIs should be stopped 2wks prior to test (false-positives) and antibacterials 4wks prior to test. Biopsy and stool antigen tests are alternative methods for detecting *H. pylori*.

NSAIDs

- NSAIDS reduce the production of mucosal gastroprotective prostaglandins by inhibiting the enzyme COX. They can also cause superficial erosions/haemorrhage and silent ulcers (asymptomatic).
- ↑ risk during first month of use, elderly, ♀, high dose/potency, PUD history, smoking, other antiplatelets or anticoagulants, co-morbidities (e.g. rheumatoid arthritis (RA) (fivefold ↑), cardiac (two- to fivefold ↑).
- Dual antiplatelet (e.g. low-dose aspirin plus clopidogrel) ↑ risk of ulcer fivefold.
- Corticosteroids alone are insignificant ulcer risk but potentiate NSAIDs.
- SSRIs potentiate NSAIDs and ↑ risk of bleed sixfold.
- Topical and enteric-coated NSAIDs can also cause ulceration.
- COX-2 inhibitors have equal efficacy to non-selective NSAIDs but are not without ulcer risk. PPI cover is still recommended in high-risk patients. They are also associated with ↑ risk of thrombotic events (e.g. MI, stroke) and are contraindicated in patients with ischaemic heart disease, peripheral arterial disease, moderate to severe heart failure or cerebrovascular disease.

Referral for endoscopy

Endoscopy is indicated in patients with the following:
- Significant upper GI bleed.
- Dyspepsia associated with alarm symptoms (urgent) defined as any age with any of the following: chronic GI bleeding, weight loss, progressive dysphagia, persistent vomiting, iron-deficiency anaemia (if not on NSAIDs and no menorrhagia), epigastric mass.

Consider if >55yrs old *and* persistent symptoms despite *H. pylori* testing and acid suppression plus one or more of the following:
- Continuing need for NSAIDs
- Previous GU or surgery
- Raised risk of anxiety of gastric cancer.

Treatment options
- Lifestyle—e.g. reduce alcohol, stop smoking, stress relief, weight loss, fatty foods, caffeine
- Rationalize use of NSAIDS and aspirin and other drugs associated with PUD/GORD
- Drugs
- Surgery
- 60–80% with successfully treated GORD will relapse within a year.

Antacids/alginates
- Symptomatic relief of PUD especially ulcer dyspepsia and GORD. Not effective in severe disease—do not affect acid secretion.
- Cheap and simple; available over the counter. Take when symptoms occur or are expected.
- Some have high sodium content (caution liver disease, hypertension, pregnancy). Aluminium-based—constipating; magnesium-based—diarrhoea. Liquids better than tablets.
- Added ingredients include alginates (Gaviscon®, Rennie®), which form a raft over stomach contents and may help in reflux oesophagitis, or simethicone (Infacol®) which is an antifoaming agent to relieve flatulence.

Proton pump inhibitors
These include lansoprazole, omeprazole, pantoprazole, rabeprazole, esomeprazole. Most effective drugs for PUD/GORD—faster healing rates than H_2 antagonists.

Act by blocking acid pump (H^+/K^+-ATPase) of gastric parietal cell and cause almost total acid suppression for >24h. Inactive pro-drugs with high affinity for acidic environments. Different PPIs bind different sites on the proton pump which may account for variation in potency.

Indications for oral PPIs
- Short-term treatment—reflux oesophagitis, benign gastric and duodenal ulcer, *H. pylori* eradication, NSAID-associated ulceration, high-output stomas (e.g. ileostomy). Therapeutic trial in cardiac patients (recommend 2wks and review).
- Long-term treatment/prophylaxis—maintenance therapy with PPIs is usually limited to patients with Barrett's oesophagus, hyper-secretory conditions (e.g. Zollinger–Ellison syndrome), complicated oesophagitis (strictures, ulceration, haemorrhage), oesophageal reflux that relapses on stopping therapy. *For these indications, full treatment doses may be needed long term.*
- High risk factors for GI bleeding that require long-term NSAID use (e.g. the elderly).

- There is no indication for PPI cover in patients prescribed corticosteroids alone:
  - PPIs are generally well tolerated. Haematological effects are rare. There is a reported association with ↑ risk of hip fracture rates and long-term PPI use. Monitor for hypomagnesaemia (usually occurs after 3–12 months of use).Caution should be taken in severe liver disease, pregnancy, and breastfeeding.
  - PPIs may mask the symptoms of gastric cancer and particular care is required in those presenting with 'alarm features'. In such cases gastric malignancy should be excluded before treatment is commenced.
  - Co-administration of PPIs and antibacterials ↑ risk of *Clostridium difficile* two- to threefold. Review all PPIs on admission, especially if high risk of *C. difficile*-associated diarrhoea (CDAD).
  - Drug interactions—PPIs reduce conversion of clopidogrel, a pro-drug, to its active form by competitively inhibiting CYP450 2C19. This leads to reduced effectiveness of clopidogrel and ↑ risk of MI, stroke, etc. The interaction is not seen with H$_2$ antagonists or pantoprazole which are not metabolized by this enzyme. In practice, the interaction is not considered clinically significant.
  - PPIs should be reviewed regularly to ensure that patients are not continued unnecessarily.
  - NICE recommends that the least expensive appropriate PPI (within its licensed indications) should be used. There is little difference in efficacy between them.

H$_2$ antagonists
E.g. ranitidine, cimetidine, nizatidine, famotidine. Act by blocking histamine receptors on gastric parietal cell, preventing acid secretion into stomach. Indications are broadly similar to PPIs, but as PPIs have generally superseded H$_2$ antagonists the latter are usually only used if PPIs are not tolerated or where drug interactions are an issue.

Sucralfate
Complex of aluminium hydroxide and sulphated sucrose which has mucosal protective properties but minimal antacid properties. Sometimes used in stress ulcer prophylaxis. Side effects are constipation, aluminium toxicity, bezoar formation—care in ITU patients.

Bismuth chelate (tripotassium dicitratobismuthate)
Ulcer healing properties comparable to H$_2$ antagonists, but not in maintaining remission. Used in *H. pylori* regimens—toxic to *H. pylori*.
   Blackens stools and tongue and may accumulate in impaired renal function.

Misoprostol
Synthetic prostaglandin E$_1$ analogue with antisecretory and protective properties (stimulates mucus and bicarbonate secretion). Use is limited by adverse effects (e.g. diarrhoea). Combination products do not provide sufficient GI cover.

Prokinetics
No longer recommended for dyspepsia/PUD or GORD.

Treatment

H. pylori eradication therapy

- Long-term healing of GU and DU can be achieved by eradicating
  H. pylori. *H. pylori* should be confirmed first.
- Several equally effective regimens available—no large randomized
  comparable trials; 85% eradication with published regimens.
- Recommended eradication regimens consist of a 7-day, twice-daily
  course of a PPI and antibacterials. E.g.:
  - Omeprazole 20mg twice daily (any PPI)
  - Clarithromycin 500mg twice daily
  - Amoxicillin 1g twice daily or metronidazole 400mg twice daily (if
    penicillin allergic)
  - Quinolones, tetracyclines, and bismuth are sometimes used if drug
    allergies or previous exposure to the earlier-listed drugs.
- 14-day triple regimens offer higher eradication rate but are offset by
  more ADRs and poor compliance. 2-week dual regimens are licensed
  but have poor efficacy and are not recommended.
- Antibacterial-associated CDAD is an uncommon risk.
- PPI should be continued for a further 3wks if ulcer is large or
  complicated by haemorrhage or perforation.
- Always give these regimens orally or via a nasogastric tube. Do not start
  the eradication therapy until the patient can take the full 7-day course
  by these routes. There is no place in therapy for IV *H. pylori* eradication
  regimens.
- 5–20% of patients will not respond because of poor compliance
  and/or bacterial resistance. Missing a dose can reduce success rates.
  Adherence (aided by good counselling) is essential, e.g. purpose, dose
  and frequency, duration (complete the course), avoidance of alcohol
  with metronidazole (sickness and headache), common side effects. Also
  advise on general lifestyle changes.

PUD

- Withdraw NSAID/COX-2 if possible and substitute with simple
  analgesia or use lowest dose possible. Review need or NSAID regularly.
- Full-dose PPI or H_2 antagonist for 2 months.
- Eradicate *H. pylori* if present.
- Offer long-term prophylaxis with PPI or H_2 antagonist if NSAID cannot
  be withdrawn.
- Exclude non-adherence, malignancy, and other co-morbidities in
  non-healing ulcers.

Functional dyspepsia and uninvestigated dyspepsia

Eradicate *H. pylori* if present. Use simple antacids and PPIs for 4 weeks.

GORD

Antacids and alginates are ineffective in severe disease. Higher doses of PPI
may be required initially. Long-term use of a PPI is usually required (often
intermittent use is sufficient).

Upper GI bleed

- *Haematemesis*—bleed proximal to duodenal–jejunal junction:
  - Large volume, bright red—*rapid, large bleed*
  - Small amount, dark red, 'coffee grounds'—*small bleed altered by gastric acid.*
- *Melaena*—proximal to and including caecum. Black tarry appearance, >60mL blood:
  - PUD is most common cause of upper GI bleed—up to 50% due to chronic PUD
  - Risk ratio: threefold ↑ if taking NSAIDs
  - Risk of mortality from upper GI bleed assessed via the Rockall score[1]
  - If large bleed or clinical signs of shock, restore blood volume and BP
  - Stop NSAIDs/aspirin, review anticoagulants, SSRIs, aspirin, corticosteroids, antihypertensives.
- *Endoscopy* will define cause of bleeding in most patients and therefore is the best treatment. Perform within 24h. Emergency scope and/or surgery candidate if continued bleeding, re-bleed. Consider antibacterial prophylaxis if heart valves etc. Test for *H. pylori.*

Endoscopic therapy

The most effective intervention for those at highest risk of re-bleed and death from PUD.

- Non-variceal: NICE recommends (1) clips with or without adrenaline, (2) thermal coagulation with adrenaline (epinephrine), or (3) fibrin or thrombin with adrenaline.
- Variceal—band ligation (oesophageal); N-butyl-2-cyanoacrylate injection (gastric). Transjugular intrahepatic portosystemic shunts (TIPS) should be considered if bleeding is not controlled by these methods.

Drug therapy

Aims to stabilize clots, and reduce the risk of further bleeding in high-risk patients and the need for surgery. Most deaths from upper GI bleeding are due to respiratory, cardiac, or renal decompensation. Mortality 10–14%.

PPIs

- Effective in prevention of re-bleeding from PUD but do not affect overall mortality.
- For major peptic ulcer bleeding (following endoscopic treatment), an IV loading dose of omeprazole 80mg, followed by a continuous infusion of 8mg/h for 72h should be given. This IV regimen is unlicensed but NICE approved. On completing the infusion, patients should receive oral omeprazole 40mg daily (high dose) for 8wks, and *H. pylori* eradicated if positive. This is essential if there are complications, e.g. haemorrhage or perforation or surgery is required:
  - Pantoprazole/omeprazole is currently unlicensed for this indication but used in practice. Esomeprazole is licensed.
  - There is debatable evidence to show that PPI prior to endoscopy has an effect on re-bleeding, need for surgery, or risk of death.
  - Ranitidine IV no longer has a place in management.
  - Tranexamic acid (antifibrinolytic) may be of value in patients with risk of high mortality (Rockall score >3) and confirmed peptic ulcer.

- Terlipressin—variceal bleed (see ➲ p. 317).
- Prokinetics—a stat dose of either metoclopramide or erythromycin at the time of endoscopy will induce gastric emptying and improve mucosal views.
- Once haemostasis has been achieved, patients on low-dose aspirin for secondary prevention of vascular events should be restarted. Low-dose PPI is recommended. The risks and benefits of continuation of antiplatelets/anticoagulants should be reviewed.

Further reading

'British Society of Gastroenterology' website, ℘ www.bsg.org.uk

NICE (2014). 'Gastro-oesophageal reflux disease and dyspepsia in adults: investigation and management [CG184]', ℘ www.nice.org.uk/guidance/cg184

NICE (2016). 'Acute upper gastrointestinal bleeding in over 16s: management [CG141]', ℘ www.nice.org.uk/guidance/cg141

SIGN (2008). 'Guideline 105: Management of acute upper and lower gastrointestinal bleeding', ℘ www.sign.ac.uk/guidelines/fulltext/105/index.html

Reference

1. Rockall TA, Logan RF, Devlin HB, et al. (1995). Incidence of and mortality from acute upper gastrointestinal haemorrhage in the United Kingdom. *BMJ* 311: 222–6.

Pharmaceutical care in gastrointestinal stoma patients

A GI stoma is a surgically created opening between the GI tract and the skin. These stomas can be temporary or permanent. A stoma may be formed during surgery for cancer, inflammatory bowel disease, or trauma. Patients with GI stomas are susceptible to certain conditions such as ↓ output and dehydration or ↓ output and obstruction, but the presence of a stoma can also influence the choice of drug therapy as it may affect the pharmacokinetics of the chosen formulation.

Dietary advice for stoma patients is provided by specialist dieticians and stoma therapists. Long-term vitamin B_{12} supplementation will be required in patients with an ileostomy because of loss of the terminal ileum.

Management of constipation

Constipation in colostomy patients is usually managed by manipulation of the diet and fluid intake. If drug therapy is considered necessary, its effect should be monitored closely to avoid high output and dehydration. Sodium docusate or balanced osmotic laxatives such as Movicol®/Laxido® are suitable. Lactulose should be avoided as flatulence makes management of the stoma bag difficult.

Laxative enemas and suppositories can be administered via the colostomy but should only be carried out by experienced practitioners. After insertion of the suppository, a dressing has to be placed over the stoma to allow the suppository to dissolve; this takes ~20min. The stoma appliance can then be applied. This is a time-consuming method of medication administration.

Constipation is highly unlikely in ileostomy patients, and a lack of output from an ileostomy is usually an indication of obstruction and should be referred for expert management. Laxatives should never be used in ileostomy patients.

Management of a high-output stoma

A normal stoma output will depend on the position of the stoma along the GI tract and the clinical condition of the patient. Colostomy output is usually formed stools. Ileostomy output is more liquid and usually ~1L/day. When output is ↑ the patient will lose different electrolytes depending on the site. Colostomy patients will lose K^+ and fluid; ileostomy patients will lose fluid, Na^+, Mg^{2+}, and possibly Ca^{2+}.

Primary therapy is aimed at removing the cause of the ↑ output such as infection or bacterial overgrowth, but drug therapy should also be reviewed as a possible cause of rapid gut transit. Once any causative factors have been removed or treated, the ongoing output is controlled using loperamide and/or codeine. The dose used depends on the site of the stoma and the output. For colostomy patients, a regular dose of loperamide 2mg one to three times daily can be effective. For patients with high-output ileostomies or those with a shortened length of gut, loperamide doses of up to 24mg four times daily have been used. This should be under expert supervision. For very high-output patients a PPI may also be added to reduce the fluid and acid production of the stomach. Not only does this reduce the volume, but it also reduces the acidity and ↑ the transit time. Occasionally a high-strength salt solution such as 'St Mark's rehydration solution'[2] or oral rehydration sachets (e.g. Dioralyte®) made to double strength can be used to encourage salt and water reabsorption in the small bowel. The sodium concentration should be >90mmol/L.

Octreotide is not considered effective in management of high-output stomas and is usually considered as a last resort. This should be used in specialist centres only.

High-output ileostomy management
- Expert dietetic advice
- High-dose loperamide—e.g. 6–24mg four times daily 30min before meals
- High-dose PPI—e.g. omeprazole 40mg twice daily
- Codeine phosphate 30–60mg four times daily 30min before meals
- High-strength salt solution.

Bowel preparation in stoma patients

Bowel preparation is rarely used prior to surgery or procedures now. However, if necessary, standard therapies can be used in colostomy patients. Bowel preparation should never be used in ileostomy patients; a clear liquid diet in the 24h prior to the procedure is sufficient in these patients.

Medication choice in patients with GI stomas

Where possible, modified and slow-release preparations should be avoided as these patients tend to have a reduced GI transit time and the formulation may not have time to release the dose. For ileostomy patients, the transit time can vary on a daily basis and variability of absorption can be a problem. Conventional-release preparations should be first choice. There is no advantage in using liquid preparations, and occasionally the high sugar or sorbitol content can ↑ the output.

Medication that affects gut transit time should be used with caution and output monitored closely—e.g. metoclopramide, domperidone, or erythromycin in patients with an ileostomy; opiates and ondansetron in patients with a colostomy.

Patients should be counselled on any medication that may colour stool output (e.g. iron preparations) as this can be distressing.

Reference

2. St Mark's Hospital. 'Information for patients', ℘ www.stmarkshospital.nhs.uk/wp-content/uploads/2014/05/High-output-stoma-2014.pdf

Therapy-related issues: cardiovascular system

Angina pectoris

Definition

Typical angina is defined and diagnosed by three clinical criteria:

- Pain in the anterior chest area, often described as a tightness or heaviness. The discomfort is diffuse and can radiate to the arms, neck, or jaw.
- Precipitated by physical exertion or emotional stress.
- Relieved by rest or use of sublingual nitrates.

Angina is the main symptom of myocardial ischaemia due to coronary artery disease (CAD) restricting oxygen delivery. Risk factors for CAD include a positive family history, smoking, hyperlipidaemia, hypertension, obesity, and diabetes mellitus.

Types of angina

- Stable angina—pain induced by exertion and relieved by rest.
- Unstable angina (crescendo)—pain occurs at minimal exertion or at rest with ↑ frequency or severity, associated with an ↑ risk of myocardial infarction (MI).
- Decubitus angina—pain precipitated by lying flat.
- Variant (Prinzmetal) angina—pain caused by coronary artery spasm.

Severe obstructive coronary atherosclerosis restricts myocardial blood flow reducing oxygen supply to the myocardium. Exercise or emotional stress ↑ myocardial oxygen demand which cannot be achieved because of the obstruction leading to myocardial ischaemia. Other causes/exacerbations of angina include anaemia (↓ oxygen delivery), tachycardia, and left ventricular hypertrophy (↑ oxygen demand).

Onset of pain is often sudden and resolves promptly with rest as oxygen demand subsides. Some patients do not experience chest pain (silent ischaemia). Others experience atypical pain, shortness of breath, or light headedness.

Aims of treatment

- To reduce symptoms.
- To improve prognosis—e.g. prevent progression of cardiovascular disease (CVD) such as MI and stroke.

Assess the occurrence of pain in relation to the patient's lifestyle. Give advice regarding avoidance of precipitating factors, e.g. heavy, sudden, and unaccustomed exertion, exertion in cold weather and acute emotional stress, where possible.

Initiate optimal drug treatment including use of one or two antianginal agents plus drugs for secondary prevention of CVD. Ensure patients understand the importance of taking medication regularly and consider potential barriers to medication adherence/concordance.

Provide lifestyle advice including smoking cessation, encouraging regular moderate exercise, healthy eating, and weight loss.

Antianginal drugs: acute attack

Nitrates act mainly by venous and coronary artery vasodilatation reducing preload and improving coronary blood flow. At the onset of an attack the patient should rest and use a short-acting nitrate preparation:

- Glyceryl trinitrate (GTN) metered dose spray 400–800 micrograms (1–2 sprays) sublingually, repeat after 5 min if pain persists. GTN spray is easy to use, has a long expiry date, and is preferred by patients.
- GTN tablets 300–600 micrograms sublingually, repeat after 5min if pain persists. GTN tablets have a limited 8wk shelf-life once opened (ensure patients are informed). Tablets can be discarded from the mouth once symptoms are relieved to reduce side effects.

If pain has not gone 5min after taking the second dose, patients should be advised to call for an ambulance.

When using GTN, especially for the first time, the patient should sit down or have something to hold on to in case of dizziness/light headedness due to hypotension. Other side effects include headache and flushing. GTN may also be used prophylactically 5min before exertion to prevent attacks.

Serious hypotension can occur when nitrates are used with selective phosphodiesterase type 5 inhibitors (PDE5 inhibitors). Nitrates should be avoided if the patient has used sildenafil in the previous 24h or tadalafil in the previous 48h.

Antianginal agents: prevention of attacks

Use a β-blocker or a calcium channel blocker (CCB) first line to prevent anginal attacks. Choice depends on co-morbidities, contraindications, and patient preference. If the initial drug is not tolerated, then consider the other option, e.g. if a β-blocker is not tolerated, switch to a CCB.

If symptoms are not controlled with a single agent then consider switching to the other option or use a combination of a β-blocker and a dihydropyridine CCB. Other antianginal agents should not be used routinely as first-line treatments for stable angina.

Beta-blockers

β-blockers reduce myocardial oxygen demand by lowering heart rate (HR), BP, and contractility. The resulting bradycardia also prolongs diastole which improves coronary blood flow and myocardial perfusion. Side effects of β-blockers include fatigue, impaired glucose tolerance, peripheral vasoconstriction, sexual dysfunction, and bronchoconstriction. Cardioselective (β_1) agents (e.g. atenolol, metoprolol, and bisoprolol) are preferred due to reduced β_2 mediated side effects (e.g. bronchospasm and peripheral vascular constriction). The dose should be titrated to achieve a resting HR of between 55 and 60 beats/min:

- Atenolol 25–100mg orally once daily.
- Bisoprolol 1.25–10mg orally once daily.
- Metoprolol 25–100mg orally twice daily.

Calcium channel blockers

CCBs inhibit L-type calcium channels in vascular smooth muscle, the myocardium, and cardiac conduction tissues.

The dihydropyridine (DHP) CCBs have greater selectivity for vascular smooth muscle, with little effect on conduction tissue, resulting in peripheral and coronary vasodilatation, reducing afterload and improving coronary perfusion. Side effects include reflex tachycardia, flushing, headache, and ankle oedema. Long-acting DHPs or once-daily modified-release formulations are preferred to avoid rapid falls in BP:

- Amlodipine 2.5–10mg orally once daily.
- Nifedipine modified-release 10–40mg orally twice daily or 30–90mg orally once daily (24h preparation e.g. Adalat® LA).
- Felodipine modified-release 2.5–10mg orally once daily.

The non-selective CCBs (e.g. diltiazem and verapamil) have a greater effect on nodal tissue and the myocardium. They reduce workload of the heart by slowing nodal conduction reducing HR, and have a depressant effect on the myocardium, reducing contractility. These CCBs are contraindicated in heart failure, bradycardia, or heart block and should not be used with β-blockers:

- Diltiazem 'standard formulation' 60–120mg orally three times a day; diltiazem modified-release 90–180mg orally twice daily or 180–500mg orally once daily (depending on preparation used).
- Verapamil 80–120mg orally three times a day; verapamil modified-release 240mg orally twice daily or 240–480mg orally once daily.
- Diltiazem and verapamil are moderate inhibitors of the hepatic cytochrome 3A4 isoenzyme (CYP3A4), and verapamil is also a potent P-glycoprotein inhibitor. Consult the BNF and manufacturer's SPCs for information on drug interactions. Also see ➔ 'Secondary prevention', pp. 325–6, for information on the use of statins.

Third-line antianginal agents

If β-blockers and CCBs are contraindicated or not tolerated consider therapy with third-line agents which may be added to existing therapy if symptoms are not controlled. Choice of agent depends on co-morbidities, contraindications, patient preference, and drug costs.

Nitrates are available in many forms, oral nitrates are commonly used but careful dosing is required to reduce tolerance (see later):

- Isosorbide mononitrate 20–120mg orally twice daily.
- Isosorbide mononitrate modified release 30–120mg orally once daily.

Nicorandil has a nitrate-like effect and is also a potassium channel activator causing arterial vasodilation. It may also have a cardioprotective effect, reducing ischaemic myocardial injury. It is licensed for use as monotherapy but is commonly used as add-on therapy to control symptoms. Side effects are similar to nitrates and also include GI ulceration:

- Nicorandil 5mg to 30mg oral twice daily.

The newer agents, ranolazine and ivabradine, are used if symptoms are not controlled with, or if side effects prevent use of established antianginal agents.

Ranolazine's mechanism of action is not fully understood. It inhibits slow sodium channels reducing intracellular sodium and calcium which reduces intracellular ionic imbalances during ischaemia. Reduction in calcium improves myocardial relaxation ↓ left ventricular stiffness. Ranolazine does not significantly affect HR or BP. Side effects include dizziness, headache, constipation, and nausea. Ranolazine also causes QT prolongation and is contraindicated in patients with long QT syndrome. Concurrent use with other drugs known to prolong the QT interval should be avoided if possible.

Ranolazine is metabolized by hepatic CYP3A4 and CYP2D6 isoenzymes and is also a substrate for P-glycoprotein. Inhibitors of these enzymes will ↑ ranolazine plasma concentrations—refer to the *BNF* and manufacturer's SPC for full details.

- Ranolazine modified-release 375mg orally twice daily slowly ↑ to a maximum of 750mg oral twice daily.

Ivabradine selectively inhibits the *I*f current in the sino-atrial node, lowering HR and reducing myocardial oxygen demand. It may be useful when β-blockers are not tolerated. Side effects include bradycardia, heart block, and visual disturbances. It is important to avoid bradycardia in angina patients as this may be associated with adverse cardiovascular outcomes. Treatment should be discontinued if HR becomes too low or symptoms of bradycardia persist (MHRA advice June 2014). Treatment should also be discontinued if there is no improvement in symptoms after 3 months.

- Ivabradine 5mg orally twice daily; reduce dose in patients >75yrs of age to 2.5mg orally twice daily.
- ↑ dose after 3–4wks to 7.5mg twice daily (in patients receiving 5mg twice daily) or 5 mg twice daily (in patients receiving 2.5mg twice daily). Maximum dose is 7.5mg twice daily.

Secondary prevention

Secondary prevention treatment aims to reduce progression of CVD and improve long-term outcomes.

Antiplatelet agents inhibit platelet aggregation and may prevent formation of coronary artery thrombus. Consider use of aspirin to reduce risk of MI and vascular events in high-risk patients. Use should be balanced against bleeding risk and co-morbidities.

- Aspirin 75mg orally once daily or clopidogrel 75mg oral once daily (if intolerant of aspirin).

ACE inhibitors are venous and arterial vasodilators, reducing preload, afterload, and improving cardiac output. Consider use of ACE inhibitors in patients with angina and diabetes. ACE inhibitors should be offered or continued in people with other coexisting conditions (e.g. hypertension and heart failure) in line with relevant NICE guidance.

- Ramipril 1.25–2.5mg orally once daily, ↑ to 10mg orally once daily as tolerated.

Angiotensin receptor II antagonists (ARBs) may be an alternative if patients are intolerant to ACE inhibitors but there are no clinical outcome studies of ARBs in angina.

Statins should be used in line with NICE guidance on lipid modification (2014). Start high-dose statin therapy in people with CVD, e.g. atorvastatin 80mg daily. Use a lower dose if there are potential drug interactions (see next paragraph), a high risk of adverse effects, or if patient preference.

Concurrent use with potent CYP3A4 inhibitors may inhibit the metabolism of certain statins, especially simvastatin, resulting in ↑ statin concentrations and an ↑ risk of myopathy and/or rhabdomyolysis. Refer to MHRA guidance (August 2012) for full advice. Of particular importance, with respect to other cardiovascular drugs, is the maximum recommended dose of 20mg of simvastatin when used in conjunction with amiodarone, amlodipine, diltiazem, or verapamil. Patients taking simvastatin should also avoid grapefruit juice. Refer to the *BNF*, and the manufacturer's SPC for full details on statin interactions.

Treat hypertension in line with NICE guidance (see ➔ 'Treatment of hypertension', pp. 335–9).

Further reading

European Society of Cardiology (2013). '2013 ESC guidelines on the management of stable coronary artery disease', ℘ www.escardio.org/Guidelines/Clinical-Practice-Guidelines/Stable-Coronary-Artery-Disease-Management-of

MHRA (2012). 'Drug Safety Update', Volume 6, Issue 1:S1, August 2012, ℘ http://webarchive.nationalarchives.gov.uk/20150122075153/http://www.mhra.gov.uk/home/groups/dsu/documents/publication/con180638.pdf

MHRA (2014). 'Drug Safety Update', Volume 7, Issue 11:S1, June 2014, ℘ http://webarchive.nationalarchives.gov.uk/20150122075153/http://www.mhra.gov.uk/home/groups/dsu/documents/publication/con428334.pdf

NICE (2011, updated 2016). 'Stable angina: management (CG126)', ℘ www.nice.org.uk/guidance/cg126

NICE (2014, updated 2016). 'Lipid modification: risk assessment and reduction, including lipid modification (CG181)', ℘ www.nice.org.uk/guidance/CG181

Tolerance to nitrate therapy

The regular use of nitrates leads to the development of tolerance with reduction in therapeutic effect. The mechanism of tolerance is not fully understood but may involve impaired nitrate activation, induction of oxidative stress, and endothelial dysfunction.

Tolerance can be prevented by allowing a 'nitrate-free' interval of a few hours every day, timed to coincide with the period of lowest risk for angina attacks (usually night-time).

Nitrate-free periods can be achieved by administering modified-release isosorbide mononitrate oral preparations once a day or using eccentric twice-daily dosing of immediate-release preparations (e.g. at 8am and 2pm).

The use of GTN patches has been largely replaced by oral nitrates due to the ↑ problem of tolerance associated with continuous transdermal GTN release. Although wearing patches for between 12 and 16h a day may reduce tolerance, this relies on patients remembering to remove the patch before bedtime. Also, rebound ischaemia can occur when the patch is not worn.

There is no advantage in using more than one type of regular nitrate preparation and combinations may limit the nitrate-free period and result in tolerance.

Heart failure

Heart failure is a complex condition ultimately resulting in failure of the heart to deliver enough oxygen to meet the metabolic demands of the body. Underlying causes and/or precipitating factors include the following:
- Hypertension
- Coronary artery disease—most commonest cause
- Valvular heart disease
- Cardiomyopathies—e.g. hypertrophic, amyloidosis
- Congenital heart disease
- Arrhythmias
- Hyperthyroidism particularly associated with rapid atrial fibrillation (AF)
- Myocarditis caused by toxins—e.g. alcohol
- Pericarditis, pericardial effusion
- Obstructive sleep apnoea.

Heart failure can affect the left or right ventricles. Left-sided heart failure is associated with fatigue and breathlessness due to pulmonary congestion and reduced cardiac output, whereas right-sided heart failure is associated with raised venous pressure, peripheral oedema, and hepatic congestion. In the majority of patients, both ventricles are affected, known as biventricular failure. Heart failure has a poor prognosis—30–40% of patients will die within 1yr of diagnosis.

Common signs and symptoms of heart failure include the following:
- Fatigue
- Dyspnoea
- Orthopnoea
- Peripheral oedema (ankle and leg swelling)
- Raised jugular venous pressure
- Third heart sound
- Tachycardia
- Displaced apex beat
- Basal crepitations.

Heart failure can be classified according to severity of symptoms using the New York Heart Association (NYHA) classification system (Table 16.1). Although the system can be subjective, it is commonly used to assess patients and progression of their condition.

Table 16.1 Management of heart failure

Class	Definition
I	No limitation of physical activity. Ordinary physical activity does not cause undue breathlessness, fatigue or palpitations
II	Slight limitation of physical activity. Comfortable at rest but ordinary activity results in undue breathlessness, fatigue or palpitations
III	Marked limitation of physical activity. Comfortable at rest but less than ordinary activity results in undue breathlessness, fatigue, or palpitations
IV	Symptomatic at rest. Unable to carry out any physical activity without discomfort.

Aims of treatment are to relieve/control symptoms, to slow disease progression, and to improve survival. Heart failure is a chronic condition and for patients their quality of life and ability to continue with normal daily activities is important.

Use of specialist heart failure teams both within hospital and community are crucial to optimize management of heart failure and improve prognosis.

Non-drug interventions

Lifestyle changes

Patients should be encouraged to make lifestyle changes to improve their health and reduce their overall cardiovascular risk:

- Stop smoking.
- ↑ physical activity—with guidance.
- Weight loss in obese patients.
- Healthy diet—reduce salt intake, aim for five portions of fruit or vegetables per day and low saturated fat intake.
- Alcohol intake within government guidelines.

Fluid restriction—to avoid fluid overload, patients are usually encouraged to limit the amount of fluid consumed per day. Typical restrictions may be <2L per day but will be tailored to the individual.

Non-surgical devices

Implantable cardiac defibrillators are used to prevent sudden cardiac death, a major cause of death in heart failure patients. Cardiac resynchronization devices can be used to improve the pumping function of the heart if the atria and ventricles are out of sync with one another due to conduction abnormalities.

Revascularization

If heart failure is due to reversible ischaemic disease, percutaneous coronary intervention or coronary artery bypass grafting revascularization procedures may improve myocardial function.

Valve replacement

Heart failure due to valve stenosis or regurgitation may be improved by replacement or repair of the affected valve.

Heart transplant

Certain patients with severe heart failure may meet the criteria to be considered for a heart transplant after all other pharmacological and non-pharmacological options have been exhausted.

Drug interventions

Optimization of therapy can take several months and requires close monitoring of symptoms, fluid status, renal function, and electrolyte levels. Most of the evidence for treatment is for patients with left ventricular systolic dysfunction, who have a reduced ejection fraction (EF), typically <40%. This is known as heart failure with reduced ejection fraction (HFREF). For other patients who have heart failure symptoms but without ventricular dysfunction and a normal or slightly reduced EF, the mainstay of treatment is symptom control only with diuretics. This is known as heart failure with preserved ejection fraction (HFPEF). Patients with HFPEF have a better prognosis than those with HFREF.

Diuretics—symptom control

Diuretics are used for the symptomatic treatment of fluid retention and overload in heart failure. However, with the exception of aldosterone antagonists, diuretics have little effect on progression of the disease.

The aim of treatment is to maintain patients at their 'dry weight' and prevent sudden ↑ in fluid retention and symptoms of fluid overload. Patients can monitor their fluid levels by weighing themselves daily and adjusting their diuretic dose to treat fluid retention.

Loop diuretics such as furosemide and bumetanide are used first line as they are the most effective, especially in pulmonary oedema due to left-sided heart failure. Thiazide diuretics produce a more sustained, gradual diuresis and are used to treat fluid retention in mild heart failure (e.g. peripheral oedema). The combination of a loop and thiazide diuretic can cause a profound diuresis and may be used in patients who develop 'resistance' to loop diuretics. Alternatively, loop diuretics may be administered IV, for an ↑ effect (see ➡ 'Diuretics', p. 333). Over-diuresis should be avoided as this may lead to renal impairment. Generally diuretic treatment in acute fluid overload should aim to remove no more than 1L of fluid per day (1kg weight loss per day).

The adverse effects of diuretics include renal failure, hypotension, hyponatraemia, hypokalaemia, fatigue, and gout. Hypokalaemia should be treated by using a potassium-sparing diuretic or potassium supplementation. Maintenance of potassium levels is important to reduce the risk of cardiac arrhythmias. Serum electrolytes, renal function, and weight should be monitored regularly during treatment especially after any ↑ in diuretic dosage.

First-line treatment

The use of β-blockers and ACE inhibitors have shown significant clinical benefits in the treatment of heart failure, reducing mortality and heart failure related hospital admissions by about one-third. Both drugs should be offered to all patients with left ventricular systolic dysfunction as soon as possible after diagnosis, unless contraindicated, starting at a low dose and titrating upwards as tolerated. Clinical judgement should be used when deciding which drug to start first, considering patient factors such as co-morbidities, renal function, BP, HR, etc. Patients should be advised that it may take a few months for their symptoms to improve after starting treatment and the importance of long-term adherence to therapy should be stressed.

Beta-blockers

β-blockers block the effect of the sympathetic nervous system, which is activated in heart failure, reducing pre-load and afterload resulting in an ↑ in cardiac output. Due to their potential benefits they should be used in patients who may normally be considered unsuitable for β- blocker therapy, e.g. patients with peripheral vascular disease, erectile dysfunction, diabetes, or COPD. Currently only bisoprolol, carvedilol, and nebivolol are licensed in the UK for treatment of heart failure.

β-blockers may temporarily worsen symptoms of heart failure due to their negative inotropic effects and should only be initiated in patients with stable heart failure. To minimize such effects treatment is started at a low dose and slowly up titrated, e.g. start bisoprolol 1.25mg daily or carvedilol 3.125mg twice daily and double dose at 2- to 4-weekly intervals depending on response, to the target dose or maximum tolerated dose. During up-titration, HR, BP, and signs and symptoms of heart failure should be monitored and if necessary a temporary ↑ in diuretic dose may be needed.

ACE inhibitors

ACE inhibitors block conversion of angiotensin I to angiotensin II. Angiotensin II causes vasoconstriction, remodelling of the heart, and stimulates aldosterone release causing sodium and water retention. Treatment should be started at a low dose and up-titrated to the target dose or maximum tolerated dose. In a community setting the dose can be doubled every 2wks; in hospital, the up-titration may be quicker. Urea, creatinine, and electrolytes should be monitored 1–2wks after initiation and up-titration. Creatinine and potassium may ↑ with ACE inhibitor therapy, if creatinine ↑ by >50% or potassium rises above 5.5mmol/L the ACE inhibitor treatment should be stopped and specialist advice sought. Other adverse effects include dizziness, low BP, cough, and rarely angio-oedema. Cough may not always be related to the ACE inhibitor and other reasons for a cough should be excluded. If the cough is proved to be related to the ACE inhibitor and it is troublesome, switch to an angiotensin II receptor antagonist (angiotensin receptor blockers, ARB).

Second-line treatments

Aldosterone receptor antagonists

Spironolactone and eplerenone are aldosterone antagonists. As well as causing salt and water retention, aldosterone has a number of non-renal effects such as stimulating myocardial fibrosis and remodelling, endothelial dysfunction, and cardiac excitability, which are important in the pathophysiology of heart failure. Both drugs have been shown to reduce mortality and hospital admissions. Based on clinical trials the drugs are licensed for slightly different indications. Spironolactone is licensed for use in severe heart failure and eplerenone is licensed for use in post-MI heart failure and moderate heart failure (class II).

Treatment should be started at 25mg once a day and up-titrated if required within 1 month. Aldosterone antagonists can cause hyperkalaemia, in particular in patients already taking an ACE inhibitor or those with impaired renal function. Urea, creatinine, and electrolytes should be checked 1wk after initiation and regularly during treatment. The dose can be reduced to as low as 12.5mg on alternate days, as necessary if hyperkalaemia occurs. Spironolactone can cause gynaecomastia, which may prove uncomfortable and embarrassing for patients, this side effect is uncommon with eplerenone.

Angiotensin II receptor antagonists

ARBs block the angiotensin II receptor binding site, blocking the effects of angiotensin II on the renin–angiotensin–aldosterone system. They can be used in patients who are intolerant of ACE inhibitors, e.g. develop cough, but both classes of drug have very similar contraindications, e.g. renal artery stenosis. There is some evidence that ARBs reduce morbidity and mortality in heart failure especially for valsartan and candesartan, but this evidence is less strong than for ACE inhibitors or aldosterone receptor antagonists. Therefore it is preferable to optimize the dose of ACE inhibitor and add an aldosterone antagonist where possible. The combination of an ACE inhibitor and ARB should only be used under specialist guidance due to the risk of renal dysfunction and hyperkalaemia. The combination of an ACE inhibitor, ARB, and aldosterone antagonist should not be used.

Ivabradine

Ivabradine selectively inhibits the I*f* current in the sino-atrial node, lowering HR and reducing myocardial oxygen demand. It has been approved by NICE for use in stable heart failure patients who have a left ventricular EF of <35%, and a HR of 75 beats/min or greater despite standard treatment or in patients who are unable to tolerate β-blockers.

Hydralazine and nitrate

The addition of a combination of hydralazine and a nitrate (e.g. isosorbide mononitrate) to standard treatment with an ACE inhibitor, β-blocker, and/or aldosterone antagonist and diuretic may provide further benefits. However, this combination may be poorly tolerated due to side effects such as dizziness and headache. This combination may also be considered in patients in whom ACE inhibitors or aldosterone antagonists are contraindicated (e.g. in renal impairment).

Digoxin

Digoxin has two indications in heart failure: the first is treatment of AF associated with heart failure, although other rate control strategies may be preferred. The second is as add-on therapy for heart failure patients in sinus rhythm who are still symptomatic despite first- and second-line therapy. Digoxin has been shown to reduce hospital admissions due to heart failure but has little effect on overall mortality. If digoxin is used for patients in sinus rhythm, a loading dose is not required and sub-therapeutic levels may still provide clinical benefit. Patients should be monitored for adverse effects or signs of toxicity (e.g. bradycardia), and have periodic monitoring of serum digoxin levels, renal function, and electrolytes, especially potassium as hypokalaemia can ↑ sensitivity to digoxin.

Further reading

European Society of Cardiology (2012). Guidelines for the diagnosis and treatment for acute and chronic heart failure. *Eur Heart J* 33: 1787–847.

NICE (2010). 'Chronic heart failure (CG108)', ℰ www.nice.org.uk/cg108

NICE (2012). 'Ivabradine for treating chronic heart failure (TA267)', ℰ www.nice.org.uk/guidance/ta267

Acute heart failure

Acute heart failure can be defined as the rapid onset of severe heart failure symptoms. It can present as new-onset heart failure or as acute decompensation of chronic heart failure with pulmonary oedema, cardiogenic shock, or acute right-sided failure. It is a medical emergency that requires urgent hospital admission and is the leading cause of hospital admission for people aged 65yrs and over in the UK.

Patients should be managed by a specialist heart failure team usually based on a cardiology ward. In patients newly presenting with suspected acute heart failure, measurement of serum natriuretic peptides (B-type natriuretic peptide, BNP or N-terminal pro-B-type natriuretic peptide, NT-proBNP) should be taken to aid diagnosis. Heart failure diagnosis can be ruled out if:

- BNP <100ng/L
- NT-pro-BNP <300ng/L.

Initial treatment—stabilize the patient (based on NICE guidelines 2014)

Oxygen

Initial oxygen therapy via a face mask at an appropriate percentage to maintain oxygen saturation may be needed if the patient is hypoxic; caution should be exercised in certain patients (e.g. COPD). Consider non-invasive ventilation such as continuous positive airways pressure (CPAP) or non-invasive positive pressure ventilation (NIPPV) in patients with deteriorating respiratory function (e.g. cardiogenic pulmonary oedema with severe dyspnoea and acidosis). Further respiratory support with invasive ventilation may be required in patients with respiratory failure and physical exhaustion.

Diuretics

Patients will usually require IV loop diuretic treatment either as bolus or infusion therapy. Acute pulmonary oedema is initially treated with IV bolus doses of furosemide 40–80mg repeated as necessary. For acute fluid overload, intermittent or continuous infusions are used, e.g. 240mg over 4–6h or given more slowly over 24h. The IV dose will usually be higher than the patient's usual oral maintenance dose and the addition of a thiazide diuretic such as metolazone may also be required, especially in patients with resistance to conventional diuretic therapy. Patient's renal function, weight, and urine output should be closely monitored.

Beta-blockers

If patients are already taking β-blockers, do not routinely stop unless HR is <50 beats/min or there is second- or third-degree atrioventricular block or cardiogenic shock.

Opiates

Are no longer routinely recommended for use in acute heart failure unless necessary for the management of pain.

Vasodilators

Vasodilators such as nitrates are no longer recommended as first-line treatment but may be considered in patients with concomitant ischaemia, hypertension, or regurgitant mitral valve disease. IV glyceryl trinitrate infusion at a rate of 1–10mg/h may be used. The infusion rate is titrated upwards slowly, aiming to maintain systolic BP above 100mmHg. The use of sodium nitroprusside, an alternative vasodilator, is no longer recommended.

Inotropes and vasopressor

Inotropes and vasopressors may be useful in patients with potentially reversible cardiogenic shock to stabilize the patient and allow reversible causes of acute heart failure to be treated. They must be administered in a high care setting via central venous access and require invasive haemodynamic monitoring.

Low-dose dopamine may improve renal blood flow (mediated by dopaminergic stimulation) and theoretically improve diuresis and renal function. Although evidence for benefit is inconclusive, low-dose dopamine is sometimes added to diuretic therapy to improve diuresis and help protect renal function.

Levosimendan, a newer inotrope, is a calcium sensitizer which does not ↑ myocardial oxygen consumption with additional vasodilatory properties. There is evidence that it may improve symptoms and reduce mortality in acute decompensated failure. It is currently unlicensed in the UK.

Other, non-pharmacological interventions that may be considered in some patients include an intra-aortic balloon pump or a ventricular assist device. These may provide a 'bridge to recovery' in patients with potentially reversible severe acute heart failure or a 'bridge to transplantation' in patients who are candidates for transplantation.

Once a patient has recovered from the episode of acute heart failure, e.g. once IV diuretics are no longer needed, it is important to initiate or restart any long-term disease-modifying treatments in patients with impaired left ventricular function to improve long-term prognosis. Prior to discharge, the patient should be stable on a diuretic regimen as well as first- and second-line therapies (e.g. β-blocker, ACE inhibitor, and aldosterone antagonist) unless contraindicated. Patients should have a follow-up assessment by a member of the heart failure specialist team within 2wks of discharge.

Further reading

NICE (2014). 'Acute heart failure (CG187)', ℔ www.nice.org.uk/cg187

Treatment of hypertension

High BP or hypertension is a major risk factor for stroke, MI, chronic kidney disease (CKD), heart failure, peripheral vascular disease, cognitive decline, and premature death. It is one of the most preventable causes of premature morbidity and mortality in the UK.

Risk factors for developing hypertension include ↑ age, ethnicity (hypertension is more common in patients of black African/Caribbean descent), obesity, lack of physical activity, excess salt intake, excess alcohol intake, stress, diabetes, sleep apnoea, and CKD.

Primary hypertension, which accounts for ~95% of cases, is defined as sustained high BP with no obvious cause. Secondary hypertension, which accounts for the remaining 5% of cases, is diagnosed when a specific cause can be identified (e.g. renovascular disease, phaeochromocytoma, primary hyperaldosteronism, Cushing's syndrome).

Certain medicines can cause hypertension:
- NSAIDs—including COX-2 inhibitors
- 5-HT$_1$ receptor agonists—e.g. sumatriptan, rizatriptan
- Corticosteroids
- Oral contraceptives
- Topical or oral decongestants
- Ciclosporin
- Recreational drugs—e.g. cocaine, amphetamines, ecstasy.

Diagnosis

Hypertension is typically asymptomatic and diagnosis is often made during opportunistic screening. For initial assessment, measure BP in both arms—if the difference in readings is >20mmHg then repeat measurements should be taken. If the difference remains, subsequent measurements should be taken from the arm with the higher reading.

If clinic BP is 140/90 mmHg or higher, offer ambulatory blood pressure monitoring (ABPM) to confirm the diagnosis. Home blood pressure monitoring (HBPM) can be considered as an alternative if the patient is unable to tolerate ABPM. Diagnosis of hypertension is confirmed if average readings from ABPM or HBPM are >135/85mmHg.

Whilst awaiting confirmation of diagnosis, further investigations for target organ damage and a formal assessment of cardiovascular risk should be carried out. When assessing cardiovascular risk it is important to consider a patient's overall risk profile. Various risk tools are available which use gender, age, smoking status, diabetic status, lipid profile, and BP to estimate an individual's 10yr risk of developing CVD.

If hypertension is not diagnosed, clinic BP should be checked at least every 5yrs, or more frequently (e.g. annually) if BP is on the higher side of normal (e.g. close to 140/90 mmHg).

Classification of hypertension

- *Stage 1 hypertension*—clinic BP 140/90 mmHg or higher and subsequent average daytime ABPM or average HBPM is 135/85mmHg or higher.
- *Stage 2 hypertension*—clinic BP 160/100mmHg or higher and subsequent average daytime ABPM or average HBPM is 150/95mmHg or higher.
- *Severe hypertension*—clinic systolic BP 180mmHg or higher, or clinic diastolic BP is 110mmHg or higher.

Non-drug treatment

Non-pharmacological measures to reduce both BP and cardiovascular risk should be offered to all patients with hypertension. Effective measures include the following:

- Smoking cessation.
- Weight reduction in obese patients.
- Reduction of excessive alcohol intake, defined as >14 units/week for men and women.
- Healthy diet and regular exercise.
- Moderate sodium restriction by reducing sodium intake e.g. no-added-salt diet or use of salt substitutes.
- Management of sleep apnoea.
- Stress reduction and relaxation therapies.
- Avoiding excessive consumption of caffeine-rich products.

Calcium, magnesium, or potassium supplements should not be offered as a method to reduce BP. Obstructive sleep apnoea is a strong independent risk factor for stroke and cardiovascular events. Effective management can help reduce the risk of CVD. Management of other cardiovascular risk factors (e.g. hyperlipidaemia and diabetes mellitus) is also important.

Recent trials using the interventional technique renal denervation to achieve renal nerve ablation and reduce BP in patients with resistant hypertension have not shown any consistent benefit. Therefore this intervention is not currently recommended for routine use.

Drug treatment

All patients with severe hypertension should be initiated on drug treatment without waiting for the results of ABPM or HBPM.

Drug treatment should be initiated in patients with stage 2 hypertension and in patients with stage 1 hypertension with one or more of the following: 10yr risk of CVD of 20% or greater or existing CVD, renal disease, diabetes, or evidence of target organ damage.

For patients under the age of 40 with stage 1 hypertension but no CVD risk factors or evidence of target organ damage, referral to a specialist should be considered for evaluation of secondary causes of hypertension.

For treatment of hypertension in specific patient groups (e.g. pregnancy, diabetes, CKD) refer to specific guidelines in the ➋ 'Further reading' section, p. 339.

Current treatment of hypertension is based on the NICE guideline (2011) which uses a four-step approach (see Table 16.2). Choice of initial treatment depends on the age and ethnicity of the patient. Drugs are prescribed alone or in combination with the aim of controlling BP (see ➋ 'Target blood pressure for treatment', p. 339) whilst minimizing side effects.

Angiotensin-converting enzyme inhibitors and angiotensin II receptor antagonists

ACE inhibitors lower BP through inhibition of ACE leading to a reduction in angiotensin II and aldosterone levels. ARBs block the angiotensin receptor. An ACE inhibitor or low-cost ARB is recommended as first-line treatment in patients under 55 years of age (step 1).

Table 16.2 Guidance on treatment of hypertension

Drug	Compelling indications	Possible indications	Compelling contraindications	Possible contraindications

STEP 1. Hypertensive patients aged 55yrs and over or black patients (African/Caribbean origin) of any age: offer a CCB. If CCB not tolerated or concurrent heart failure or peripheral oedema, offer a thiazide-like diuretic

Drug	Compelling indications	Possible indications	Compelling contraindications	Possible contraindications
Low-dose thiazides or thiazide-like drugs	Heart failure Peripheral oedema Elderly patients		Gout Diabetes	Dyslipidaemia Symptomatic orthostatic hypertension
CCBs	Angina Elderly patients	Peripheral vascular disease	Heart block	Congestive heart failure

STEP 1. Hypertensive patients aged under 55yrs: offer an ACE inhibitor or a low-cost ARB (if ACE inhibitor not tolerated)

Drug	Compelling indications	Possible indications	Compelling contraindications	Possible contraindications
ACE inhibitor	Heart failure Left ventricular dysfunction Acute MI Diabetes		Pregnancy Hyperkalaemia Bilateral renal artery stenosis	
ARBs	ACE inhibitor cough Diabetes mellitus	Heart failure	Pregnancy Hyperkalaemia Bilateral renal artery stenosis	

STEP 2. If BP not controlled, offer a CCB (or thiazide-like diuretic if CCB not suitable) in combination with an ACE inhibitor or ARB (if an ACE inhibitor is not tolerated). Consider adding an ARB in preference to an ACE inhibitor in black patients

STEP 3. Review medications, ensure treatment is optimal. Combine an ACE inhibitor (or ARB), CCB, and thiazide-like diuretic

STEP 4. If BP still not controlled on three drugs at optimal doses consider adding a fourth drug either low dose spironolactone or a higher dose thiazide-like diuretic. Alternatively consider an α-blocker or β-blocker

Drug	Compelling indications	Possible indications	Compelling contraindications	Possible contraindications
β-blockers	Angina Acute myocardial infarct Tachyarrhythmias Heart failure	Pregnancy Diabetes mellitus	Asthma and COPD Heart block	Dyslipidaemia Athletes and physically active patients Peripheral vascular disease
α-blockers	Prostatic hypertrophy	Glucose intolerance Dyslipidaemia	Orthostatic hypotension	

ACE inhibitors and ARBs can cause an ↑ in creatinine clearance and hyperkalaemia. Serum potassium and creatinine clearance should be monitored at the start of treatment and then at regular intervals, especially after dose changes and in patients with renal impairment.

ACE inhibitors can cause a dry irritating cough due to an excess of bradykinins. They are also not recommended in patients of black African and Caribbean origin due to the ↑ risk of angio-oedema. ARBs are generally better tolerated than ACE inhibitors and can be used as an alternative, especially in patients who cannot tolerate the dry cough caused by ACE inhibitors.

The combination of ACE inhibitors and ARBs for treatment of hypertension is no longer recommended due to the ↑ incidence of side effects particularly renal dysfunction and hyperkalaemia.

Calcium channel blockers

CCBs inhibit L-type calcium channels in vascular smooth muscle, the myocardium, and cardiac conduction tissues causing vasodilation and a reduction in contractility and HR.

The CCBs are first-line antihypertensive agents in patients aged 55yrs or over (step 1).

The dihydropyridine CCBs (e.g. amlodipine, felodipine, or modified-release nifedipine), have greater selectivity for vascular smooth muscle and are preferred for treatment of hypertension. The non-selective CCBs diltiazem and verapamil may be used in patients with hypertension and concurrent angina or certain arrhythmias (e.g. AF) due to their additional effects on the myocardium and HR. However, these agents should not be used in patients with heart failure or in those taking β-blockers. The main side effects of CCBs include headaches, facial flushing (both usually self-limiting), and ankle swelling.

Diuretics

Diuretics reduce salt and water retention, the resulting diuresis reduces circulating volume and cardiac output which reduces BP. Thiazides and thiazide-like diuretics are also vasodilators. Thiazide-type diuretics can cause hypokalaemia, hyponatraemia (rarely), as well as dehydration. Serum electrolytes and renal function should be monitored regularly during treatment. Thiazides can be used instead of CCBs in patients with heart failure (step 1 and step 2) or in addition to CCBs and ACE inhibitors or ARBs (step 3). Avoid thiazides in patients with diabetes, gout, and renal impairment. Low-dose thiazide-like diuretics (e.g. indapamide and chlortalidone) should be used in preference to the traditional thiazide diuretics such as bendroflumethiazide and hydrochlorothiazide.

Beta-blockers

β-blockers are no longer recommended as first-line therapy for hypertension. However, they may be considered as initial therapy in younger patients who cannot tolerate ACE inhibitors or ARBs, in ♀ of child-bearing age, or in people with ↑ sympathetic drive. β-blockers are also considered at step 4 in patients with resistant hypertension (see **◗** 'Resistant hypertension', p. 339).

Target blood pressure for treatment

Patients aged younger than 80yrs of age
- Clinic BP <140/90mmHg.
- ABPM or HBPM during waking hours <135/85mmHg.
- In patients with co-morbidities such as diabetes or CKD, achievement of target BP is particularly important and patients may require more aggressive BP lowering.

Patient aged older than 80yrs
- Clinic BP <150/90mmHg.
- ABPM or HBPM during waking hours <145/85mmHg.
- In the elderly, more aggressive treatment may be associated with poorer outcomes, especially due to treatment side effects.

Resistant hypertension
Hypertension is considered resistant if clinic BP remains persistently >140/90mmHg at step 3 of treatment. Addition of a fourth agent can be considered (step 4):
- Low-dose spironolactone in patients with serum potassium <4.5mmol/L. Monitor serum electrolytes and renal function regularly.
- Higher-dose thiazide-like diuretic in patients with hyperkalaemia.
- Consider α-blocker or β-blocker in patients who cannot tolerate diuretic therapy (e.g. those with renal impairment).

If BP still remains uncontrolled, refer to a specialist for further advice (if not already obtained).

Further reading
'British Hypertension Society' website, ℘ www.bhsoc.org

NICE (2009). 'Type 2 diabetes: the management of type 2 diabetes (CG87)', ℘ www.nice.org.uk/guidance/cg87

NICE (2010). 'Hypertension in pregnancy: the management of hypertensive disorders during pregnancy (CG107)', ℘ www.nice.org.uk/guidance/cg107

NICE (2011). 'Hypertension in adults: diagnosis and management (CG127)', ℘ www.nice.org.uk/guidance/cg127

NICE (2014). 'Chronic kidney disease in adults: assessment and management (CG182)', ℘ www.nice.org.uk/guidance/cg182

Understanding anticoagulation

After injury, three separate mechanisms are activated to ↓/halt bleeding: vasoconstriction, gap plugging by platelets, and the coagulation cascade. These mechanisms can be activated inappropriately and predispose patients to stroke.

The endothelial surface cells of blood vessels are involved in the balance between clotting and bleeding by secreting compounds such as von Willebrand factor, tissue plasminogen activator (t-PA), and prostaglandins (e.g. prostacyclin). The surface cells are also involved in the balance between fibrinolysis and fibrin formation.

Platelet response
- Adhesion
- Secretion
- Aggregation
- Propagation of procoagulant activity.

Regulation of coagulation and fibrinolysis
The coagulation factors consist of 12 plasma proteins that circulate in their inactive form. Coagulation of blood causes a cascading series of proteolytic reactions that result in an active protease which activates (in an enzymatic way) the next clotting factor until a fibrin clot is formed.

Coagulation factors
- Vitamin-K-dependent factors (II, VII, IX, and X).
- Contact activation factors (XI, XII, prekallikrein, and high-molecular-weight kininogen).
- Thrombin-sensitive factors (V, VIII, XIII, and fibrinogen).
- Clotting begins at either an intrinsic or an extrinsic pathway, with activation cascading to the common pathway.
- Tissue injury releases either of the following factors (see Fig. 16.1):
  - Tissue factor (extrinsic to blood), which activates the extrinsic pathway through factor VII.
  - Subendothelial membrane contact with factor XII initiates intrinsic pathway (intrinsic—all necessary coagulation factors are present in blood).

Fibrinolysis
Formation of a fibrin clot occurs as a result of the coagulation system. The fibrinolytic system opposes coagulation, dissolving the developing clot and restoring blood flow. The process starts by the release of t-PA from endothelial cells. In response to thrombin or venous stasis, t-PA is incorporated into the forming clot by binding to fibrin. t-PA converts inactive plasminogen into plasmin, which digests fibrin and dissolves the clot.

Laboratory tests
Bleeding time
Bleeding time measures the length of time to the cessation of bleeding following a standardized skin cut.

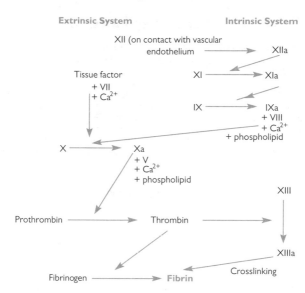

Extrinsic System   **Intrinsic System**

Fig. 16.1 The intrinsic and extrinsic pathways of blood coagulation. Reproduced with permission from Longmore M, Wilkinson IB, Baldwin A, and Wallin E. (2014). *Oxford Handbook of Clinical Medicine* (9th edn). Oxford: Oxford University Press.

Factors that prolong bleeding time include:
- thrombocytopenia
- platelet dysfunction
- aspirin/NSAIDs
- SSRIs.

Prothrombin time (PT)

Thromboplastin is added to test the extrinsic system. PT is expressed as a ratio compared with control (INR) and has a normal range of 0.9–1.2. The INR is prolonged by warfarin, vitamin K deficiency, and liver disease.

Thrombin time

Thrombin is added to plasma to convert fibrinogen to fibrin (normal range, 10–15s). The thrombin time is ↑ by heparin therapy, disseminated intravascular coagulation (DIC), and fibrinogen deficiency.

Kaolin cephalin clotting time (KCCT) APTT = PTT
(partial thromboplastin time)

Kaolin activates the intrinsic system (normal range, 26–34s). KCCT is prolonged by heparin therapy or haemophilia.

Clinical use of anticoagulants

Prevention of venous thromboembolism

Venous thromboembolism (VTE) is the collective term for deep vein thrombosis (DVT) and pulmonary embolism (PE). VTE is a common complication of hospital admission, All patients must be assessed for their risk of VTE on admission to hospital, 24h after admission, and again whenever the clinical situation changes. Each risk assessment needs to be documented in the patient's medical notes. The risk of developing VTE during hospitalization, immobilization at home, or in a nursing home depends on factors related to the individual patient and the features of any predisposing medical illness, or surgical procedure performed. Patients must also be assessed for their risk of bleeding (Table 16.3 and Box 16.1).

Types of thromboprophylaxis
Pharmacological and non-pharmacological methods of prophylaxis are both effective in preventing VTE, and their use in combination is additive.

Pharmacological prophylaxis
- Unfractionated heparin (UFH) was the first pharmacological agent to be used for thromboprophylaxis. Because of its presentation in multiple concentrations, it is generally reserved for second- or third-line choice for those patients unable to use low-molecular-weight heparin (LMWH) or fondaparinux.
- LMWH has been shown to be clearly superior to UFH in preventing DVT in patients undergoing orthopaedic surgery and should be used in that situation. Its efficacy in other high- and moderate-risk situations is at least that of UFH, and it is considered a reasonable alternative first-line choice.
- Fondaparinux is a selective anti-Xa inhibitor which, unlike UFH and LMWH, has no antithrombin activity. Fondaparinux may be more effective at DVT prevention than LMWH in patients undergoing hip and knee arthroplasty and hip fracture surgery, and is a suitable option for those procedures. Fondaparinux is also a treatment option for many patients who have a history of heparin-induced thrombocytopenia (HIT), although it is not licensed for all patient groups—check product literature.
- Aspirin has only a weak effect in preventing venous thrombosis and should not be considered adequate as sole prophylaxis.
- DVT prophylaxis should continue until the patient is fully ambulant and fit for hospital discharge. In particularly high-risk clinical situations, including hip and knee arthroplasty and oncology surgery, prolonged prophylaxis should be strongly considered.
- In situations where the slightest risk of local bleeding is unacceptable (e.g. after neurosurgery, ophthalmic surgery, some plastic surgery, head injury, or haemorrhagic stroke), anticoagulant therapy should be avoided and mechanical preventive methods should be used.

Table 16.3 Risk factors for VTE

Medical patients	Surgical patients and patients with trauma
If mobility significantly reduced for 3 days or	If total anaesthetic + surgical time >90 min or
If expected to have ongoing reduced mobility relative to normal state plus any VTE risk factor	If surgery involves pelvis or lower limb and total anaesthetic + surgical time >60min or
	If acute surgical admission with inflammatory or intra-abdominal condition or
	If expected to have significant reduction in mobility or
	If any VTE risk factor present

VTE risk factors
Active cancer or cancer treatment
Age >60yrs
Critical care admission
Dehydration
Known thrombophilias
Obesity (BMI >30kg/m^2)
One or more significant medical co-morbidities (e.g. heart disease, metabolic, endocrine, or respiratory pathologies, acute infectious diseases, inflammatory conditions)
Personal history or first-degree relative with a history of VTE
Use of HRT
Use of oestrogen-containing contraceptive therapy
Varicose veins with phlebitis
Pregnancy or < 6wks postpartum (refer to NICE guidance for specific risk factors)
Hip or knee replacement or hip fracture

Mechanical prophylaxis
Methods of mechanical prophylaxis include graduated compression stockings providing 16–20mmHg pressure at the ankle, sequential pneumatic compression devices, and pneumatic foot compression. These should be applied the evening before surgery and continued until the patient is fully ambulant.

Prophylaxis treatment
The type of prophylaxis recommended depends on the patient's risk category. However, in all patients it is advisable to avoid dehydration and to commence mobilization as soon as possible.

Effective regimens for prophylaxis include the following:
- UFH 5000 units SC every 8–12h.
- Enoxaparin 40mg or dalteparin 5000 units SC daily, or other LMWH (commencing ≥6h postoperatively in surgical patients) for high- and moderate-risk surgical and medical patients.

Box 16.1 Risk factors for bleeding

All patients who have any of the following:
- Active bleeding
- Acquired bleeding disorders (such as acute liver failure)
- Concurrent use of anticoagulants known to ↑ the risk of bleeding (such as warfarin with INR >2.0)
- Lumbar puncture/epidural/spinal anaesthesia within the previous 4h or expected within the next 12h
- Acute stroke
- Thrombocytopenia (platelets <75 × 10^9/L)
- Uncontrolled systolic hypertension (230/120mmHg)
- Untreated inherited bleeding disorders (such as haemophilia or von Willebrand disease)
- Neurosurgery, spinal surgery, or eye surgery
- Other procedures with high bleeding risk.

- Enoxaparin 20mg or dalteparin 2500 units SC daily, commencing ≥6h postoperatively, for low-risk surgical patients (or for patients with a very low body weight or if significant renal impairment is present).
- Fondaparinux 2.5mg SC daily (commencing ≥6h postoperatively in surgical patients).

Treatment of acute DVT

The aim of treatment for established venous thrombosis is to prevent thrombus extension, PE, the post-thrombotic syndrome, and recurrent VTE. The type of therapy employed depends on the anatomical extent of the thrombus (Table 16.4).

Anticoagulation

Before anticoagulant therapy is instituted, blood should be collected for determination of APTT, PT, and platelet count. A thrombophilia screen should be considered if there is a family history of VTE, recurrent VTE, and possibly if there is spontaneous VTE. This should include activated protein C resistance, fasting plasma homocysteine, prothrombin, protein C, protein S, antithrombin III, lupus anticoagulant, blood count, and anticardiolipin antibody tests. More specialized testing is occasionally indicated.

LMWH has been shown to be at least as effective and safe as an IV UFH infusion in the initial management of DVT. LMWH has the advantages of not requiring routine laboratory monitoring and enabling management in a hospital out-patient or general practice setting in selected cases, and is now the treatment of choice.

Any of the following regimens are recommended:
- Enoxaparin 1.5mg/kg body weight SC daily (up to a maximum dose of 150mg daily).
- Dalteparin once-daily dose graduated to weight (see *BNF*) or 100 units/kg body weight SC twice daily (for patients at higher risk of bleeding or obese patients).
- Tinzaparin 175 units/kg body weight SC daily.

Table 16.4 Overview of the treatment of deep vein thrombosis (DVT)

Extent of DVT	Therapy
Proximal veins (the popliteal or more proximal veins	Anticoagulation
Distal veins	Anticoagulation or ultrasound surveillance programme

- In the presence of renal impairment LMWH requires factor Xa monitoring and possible dose adjustment (calculated creatinine clearance ≤30mL/min).
- Oral anticoagulation can be commenced as soon as the diagnosis is confirmed.
- A normal loading dose of warfarin is 15–30mg, divided between 3 days (it is vital to follow local protocol as determination of the first INR will differ for different loading regimens).
- The INR should be monitored daily and the dose adjusted according to the INR until a therapeutic level is achieved. The initial dose of warfarin should be ↓ in the elderly.
- LMWH should be given for a minimum of 5 days or until the INR has been >2 on two consecutive days, whichever is the longer.
- An infusion of UFH or treatment-dose fondaparinux is a suitable alternative for patients who cannot be treated with LMWH.
- Warfarin should not be commenced alone (i.e. without a LMWH) because this is associated with a high rate of DVT recurrence.
- The duration of anticoagulation depends on the risk of both recurrent VTE and bleeding.
- Recent evidence suggests that graduated compression stockings do not ↓ the incidence and severity of post-thrombotic syndrome. Stockings should no longer be prescribed routinely but only used selectively in patients to treat symptoms.

Warfarin dosing

Loading dose

A normal loading dose of warfarin is 15–30mg, divided over 3 days—see Table 16.5 for a suggested loading regimen. The individual response is unpredictable and factors that particularly influence first doses should be considered:

- Age and weight—consider ↓ loading dose if patient >60yrs old or weight <60kg.
- Pathophysiological changes—consider ↓ loading dose in the following conditions:
  - Liver disease
  - Cardiac failure
  - Nutritional deficiency.
- Drug interactions—check *BNF* (Appendix 1). Remember over-the-counter medicines and complementary therapies.

Maintenance dose

The response to the loading dose can be used to predict the maintenance dose. Aim for an INR of 2–4, depending on the indication (Table 16.6). If the loading regimen has been followed and INRs are determined at the correct intervals, the dose for day 4 in Table 16.5 is a good predictor of maintenance dose in the majority of patients. For those patients who are particularly sensitive or resistant to the effects of warfarin, your local anti-coagulation service can be contacted for advice.

Monitoring therapy

It is important to take account of trends rather than single results. If a patient has an unusual individual result, consider whether recent changes in behaviour (e.g. diet, alcohol consumption) could have affected it. If so, these changes should be 'corrected' rather than correcting the warfarin dose.

Table 16.5 Suggested loading regimen for warfarin

Days 1 and 2	Day 3		Day4	
	INR	Dose (mg)	INR	Dose (mg)
Give 5mg each evening if baseline INR is ≤1.3 (PT <17s)	<1.5	10	<1.6	10
	1.5–2.0	5	1.6–1.7	7
	2.1–2.5	3	1.8–1.9	6
	2.6–3.0	1	2.0–2.3	5
	>3.0	0	2.4–2.7	4
			2.8–3.0	3
			3.1–3.5	2
			3.6–4.0	1
			>4.0	0

Table 16.6 INR targets and durations for anticoagulant therapy

Indication	Target INR (range)	Duration
Antiphospholipid syndrome	2.5 (2.0–3.0)	Consider long term
Arterial thromboembolism	2.5 (2.0–3.0)	Discuss with haematologist
AF	2.5 (2.0–3.0)	Long term
Calf DVT	2.5 (2.0–3.0)	3 months
Cardiomyopathy	2.5 (2.0–3.0)	Long term
Cardioversion	2.5 (2.0–3.0)	3wks before and 4wks after
Mechanical prosthetic heart valve (MHV)	varies according to position and type of valve	Long term
Mural thrombosis	2.5 (2.0–3.0)	3 months
Proximal DVT	2.5 (2.0–3.0)	3 months
Pulmonary embolus	2.5 (2.0–3.0)	3 months
Recurrence of VTE (if no longer on oral anticoagulants)	2.5 (2.0–3.0)	Consider long term
Recurrence of VTE (while on oral anticoagulants)	3.5 (3.0–4.0)	Consider long term

Factors that can affect response to warfarin include the following:
- Compliance—including timing of dose.
- Changes in kinetic parameters—e.g. weight change and fluid balance.
- Diseases—e.g. infection, congestive cardiac failure, malabsorption, liver disease, renal impairment, and GI disturbances.
- Changes in social behaviour—e.g. smoking and, alcohol.
- Diet (green vegetables contain significant amounts of vitamin K).
- Stress.
- Drug interactions—consult BNF (Appendix 1) or Stockley's Drug Interactions.[1]

Reference

1. Baxter K, Preston CL (eds) (2013). Stockley's Drug Interactions (10th edn). London: Pharmaceutical Press.

Counselling patients treated with warfarin

After the decision has been made to initiate anticoagulation therapy, the ward pharmacist should counsel the patient about the risks associated with warfarin.

Counselling

All patients, whether initiated within the hospital setting or in the community should ideally be given written information on anticoagulants. The following points should be covered:

- Dose—how much, how often, and how long?
- The colour of tablets corresponds to strength. (Imperative to check the patient's understanding on how to work out which tablet(s) to take to allow for the correct dose. This can be done by getting them to explain what they would take for a selection of doses.)
- Missed doses—what to do?
- Importance of compliance.
- How warfarin works—might need to be simplistic for certain patients (i.e. makes the blood take longer than usual to clot; ↓ the risk of clot extending).
- Need for blood tests.
- Importance of telling or reminding healthcare professionals (dentist, community pharmacist, and practice nurse) about their warfarin treatment.
- Signs of overdose/underdose and what to do.
- Recognition of drug interactions, including over-the-counter medicines and herbal preparations.
- Alcohol and diet.
- Pregnancy (if appropriate).
- Record detail of dose and INR result.
- Follow-up and duration of therapy, including arrangements for further monitoring (e.g. need to attend GP practice or out-patient clinic).

Patients should be informed that the dose of warfarin might need to be changed from time to time, and that monitoring their blood is necessary for as long as the therapy is administered. The therapeutic range is narrow and varies according to the indication. It is measured as the ratio to the standard PT.

Each patient should have an explanation of intended duration of therapy, indication for therapy, concurrent medical problems, other medication that must be continued, and target coagulation laboratory values for the patient's condition. This information also needs to be communicated to the patient's primary care team.

Thereafter, there should be a mechanism to ensure that the patient's therapy is monitored in terms of efficacy and risk during the duration of anticoagulation therapy.

Ideally, discharged patients should be reviewed within 48h of discharge (for new patients), but certainly no later than 1wk (stable patients). Each condition requires a specific range of INR values. Therefore adjusting the oral anticoagulant loading dose and maintenance doses is very necessary. Some patients could be particularly sensitive to warfarin—e.g. the elderly, those with high-risk factors, such as liver disease, heart failure, or diabetes mellitus, those who regularly consume alcohol, those on drug therapy that is known to ↑ or ↓ the effect of oral anticoagulation, and those with poor compliance. Knowledge of concomitant medical problems and medication is essential for the safe management of anticoagulation.

Reversing the effects of warfarin (or other vitamin K antagonists)

Because of the unpredictable nature of warfarin dosing, or when an anticoagulated patient needs to go for an invasive procedure, it may be necessary to reverse the anticoagulant effects of warfarin.

Reversal of over-anticoagulation

In all cases of over-anticoagulation proceed as follows:

- Identify the precipitating cause.
- Establish whether it is temporary (e.g. other medications) or permanent (e.g. liver failure).
- Review the need for ongoing anticoagulation.
- If the patient is to continue with anticoagulation therapy, the degree of reversal must be decided. For example, patients with metallic heart valves will need to continue their anticoagulation after the event, so complete reversal may not be indicated (except in the case of severe bleeding).

The risk of bleeding on warfarin ↑ significantly when the INR is ≥5.0. Therapeutic decisions regarding reversal depend on the INR level and the degree of bleeding.

Major/life-threatening bleeding requiring immediate/ complete reversal

This relates to patients with intracranial or rapid-onset neurological signs, intraocular (not conjunctival) bleeds, compartment syndrome, pericardial bleeds, or active bleeding and shock. These patients need urgent assessment of clotting.

Patients on warfarin may be haemorrhagic for reasons other than the effect of the anticoagulant, such as DIC or factor VIII inhibitor. An urgent FBC should be requested as well as APTT and INR.

- Stop warfarin and reverse anticoagulation with prothrombin complex concentrate (PCC) *and* IV phytomenadione (vitamin K).
- Anticoagulation can be effectively reversed with PCC (maximum 3000 units) *and* 5mg phytomenadione.
- As soon as PCC has been given, another clotting screen should be performed to assess the degree of correction of INR. If not corrected, advice should be sought from a haematologist.
- All patients with bleeding should be evaluated to see if there is a local anatomical reason for bleeding.

Minor bleeding

INR ≥5.0

- Omit warfarin.
- Give IV phytomenadione 1–3mg (or 5–10mg if anticoagulation is to be stopped).

INR <5.0
- A clinical decision needs to be made as to whether lowering the INR is required. If this is the case, consider giving IV phytomenadione 0.5–1mg and modifying the warfarin dose.

No bleeding

INR 5.0–7.9
- Omit warfarin.
- Restart at a lower dose when INR <5.0.

INR 8.0–12.0
- Omit warfarin.
- Give 2mg oral phytomenadione.

INR >12.0
- Omit warfarin.
- Give 5mg oral phytomenadione.

Product details

Phytomenadione
- For administration guidelines, see local or national injectables monographs.
- Oral phytomenadione will work within 16–24h of administration; IV phytomenadione will work within 6–8h.

Prothrombin complex concentrate
- Examples of PCCs are Beriplex® and Octaplex®.
- PCCs are derived from human plasma which has been virally inactivated, and they contain coagulation factors II, VII, IX, and X.
- The dose should be rounded to the nearest complete vial.
- Doses stated are based on factor IX content.
- Administration of PCC more rapidly than is stated in the product literature is a clinical decision based on risk versus benefit.

Safe medication practice

- Fresh frozen plasma (FFP) is not recommended for warfarin reversal. In non-urgent situations, phytomenadione is sufficient, and in urgent situations PCC is more effective.
- Anticoagulated patients should not be given IM injections.
- Oral phytomenadione should generally be measured in multiples of 1mg so that doses can be accurately measured using the oral syringes provided with the licensed preparation.
- The effects of PCC will wear off relatively quickly, so IV phytomenadione must be given as well if the reversal is to be sustained.

Out-patient anticoagulation clinics

Anticoagulation management is a good example of an area in which patient care is undertaken by a multidisciplinary team of physicians, nurses, and pharmacists. Although warfarin is an effective anticoagulant, its use is complicated in clinical practice by its narrow therapeutic index, with a relatively small margin between safety and toxicity, dietary fluctuations in vitamin K, the effects of certain disease states, and physiological, genetic, and patient-specific factors (e.g. compliance with therapy).

The major implications of long-term therapy with anticoagulants are a tendency to bleeding, haemorrhage, and other factors, such as interaction between warfarin and other drugs, which make it difficult to maintain anticoagulant control in the therapeutic range.

The anticoagulation clinic provides ongoing monitoring of the INR and continual recommendations for warfarin dose adjustment, including management of drug interactions involving warfarin and out-of-range INRs. The goal is to provide follow-up and dose adjustment adequate to maintain the INR within designated therapeutic ranges specific to the conditions for which the anticoagulation is indicated.

Hospital-based clinics

Oral anticoagulation monitoring has traditionally taken place in secondary care because of the need for laboratory testing. The need for frequent monitoring and close patient follow-up introduced the need for coordinated warfarin management by means of an organized system of clinical follow-up. Anticoagulation clinics have historically fulfilled this role. The patients attend the hospital for venepuncture; blood is then sent to the laboratory for testing. The pharmacist, doctor, or nurse is informed of the results and can then discuss dosage adjustment and arrange a further appointment for blood test and review. The healthcare professional also discusses whether any changes in the patient's diet or recent change in alcohol consumption, for example, might have been the reason for the INR being outside the patient's therapeutic range.

GP surgery-based clinics

The development of reliable near-patient testing systems for INR estimation has facilitated the ability to manage patients within primary care. With the introduction of finger-prick testing services, there is no longer a reliance on the hospital pathology laboratory for INR measurement. The GP discusses compliance with patients and recommends dose and the follow-up date for INR recheck.

Outreach DVT service

In some cases, coordination between primary and secondary care is established. Patients attend their local surgery for blood sampling, the samples for laboratory analysis are collected, and subsequent dosing and patient management are undertaken within the secondary-care anticoagulation clinic.

Domiciliary service

This service is only suitable for patients who are on the telephone and whose anticoagulation is reasonably well controlled. The patient's GP sends a district nurse to the patient's home to collect blood samples.

Alternative oral anticoagulants

- The emergence of direct acting anticoagulant therapies has started to dramatically change the options available for many patients who require oral anticoagulation. Currently, two groups of agents are available: direct thrombin inhibitors (dabigatran) and factor Xa inhibitors (rivaroxaban, apixaban, and edoxaban).
- Both these groups have several advantages over warfarin. They have a wider therapeutic index, a predictable dose–response profile, quick onset of action, and fewer drug and food interactions. These advantages may make them easier and more convenient to administer than warfarin therapy.
- These drugs should be used with caution or avoided in patients with liver and renal impairment (see product information sheet).
- The licensed indications for these drugs currently include prevention of VTE post elective hip and knee replacement surgery, treatment of acute VTE and long-term secondary prevention, and non-valvular AF. They are currently contraindicated in patients with prosthetic heart valves.
- It is still important that patients are counselled on these drugs to minimize harm and promote safe practice. Without monitoring, compliance is essential and patient understanding of this is vital for effective outcomes.
- Currently no antidotes to reverse the effects of these agents are available. However, clinical trials are underway. As such, it is important that all health professionals are made aware of these newer anticoagulants and local guidelines on managing bleeding are available.

Further reading

Baglin TP, Barrowcliffe TW, Cohen A, et al. (2006). Guidelines on the use and monitoring of heparin. Br J Haematol 133: 19–34.

Heidbuchel H, Verhamme P, Alings M, et al. (2013) European Heart Rhythm Association Practical Guide on the use of new oral anticoagulants in patients with non-valvular atrial fibrillation. Europace 15: 625–51. ℗ www.escardio.org/communities/EHRA/publications/novel-oral-anticoagulants-for-atrial-fibrillation/Documents/EHRA-NOAC-Practical-Full-EPEuropace-2013.pdf

Keeling D, Baglin T, Tait C, et al. (2011). Guidelines on oral anticoagulation (warfarin): fourth edition – 2011 update. Br J Haematol 154: 311–24.

National Patient Safety Agency (2007). Safety Alert 18. Actions That Can Make Anticoagulation Therapy Safer. London: NPSA.

NICE (2010, updated 2015). 'Venous thromboembolism: reducing the risk for patients in hospital (CG92)', ℗ www.nice.org.uk/guidance/cg92

NICE (2014). 'Atrial fibrillation: the management of atrial fibrillation (CG180)', ℗ www.nice.org.uk/guidance/cg180.

Acute coronary syndrome

- Acute coronary syndromes (ACS) are attributable to myocardial ischaemia due to an unstable atheromatous plaque, caused by plaque erosion or rupture, associated with thrombus formation, arterial wall inflammation, and significant narrowing of the affected artery.
- The syndromes cover a spectrum of conditions ranging from unstable angina to transmural MI.
- The clinical presentation of ACS depends on the extent of thrombosis, distal platelet and thrombus embolization, and resultant myocardial necrosis. If the artery is completely occluded, myocardial damage will occur, the extent and severity depending on the duration and site of the occlusion.
- Most patients present with chest pain, of ↑ severity which occurs at rest or with minimal exertion. Prompt investigation is crucial to aid diagnosis and guide subsequent treatment.

Diagnosis of ACS is based on:
- prolonged or new anginal chest pain
- 12-lead ECG showing ischaemic changes—e.g. ST-segment elevation or depression and/or T-wave changes
- raised troponin level.

The cardiac muscle proteins troponin I and T are released within hours of myocardial cell damage and are highly sensitive for MI. They have replaced other biomarkers as a diagnostic tool (see Fig. 16.2).
 ACS can be classified as follows:
- ST-segment elevation MI (STEMI)—ST elevation on the ECG, troponin rise and chest pain.
- Non-ST-segment elevation MI (NSTEMI)—ST depression or transient elevation and/or T-wave changes on the ECG, troponin rise, and chest pain.
- Unstable angina (UA)—normal or undetermined ECG, normal troponin level and chest pain. If troponin levels remain normal more than 6h after the onset of chest pain and the ECG is normal, the risk of MI is small.

Note: not all patients will present with typical chest pain symptoms.

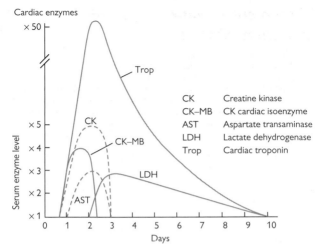

Fig. 16.2 Enzyme changes following acute MI. Reproduced with permission from Longmore M, Wilkinson IB, Rajagopalan S (2004). *Oxford Handbook of Clinical Medicine*, 6th edn. Oxford: Oxford University Press.

ST-segment elevation myocardial infarction (STEMI)

- Following atherosclerotic plaque rupture or erosion, if the resultant thrombus completely occludes the coronary artery, so that there is no flow beyond it, severe transmural myocardial ischaemia and necrosis occurs.
- Patients usually present with severe chest pain, lasting >20min, which is not relieved by GTN, the pain radiates to the neck, lower jaw, or left arm. Patients can also present with atypical symptoms such as nausea, sweating, fatigue, and syncope (common in elderly, in ♀, and in diabetics).
- The presence of ST-segment elevation on the ECG correlates with an occluded coronary artery and is used as a primary diagnostic aid.
- The diagnosis is confirmed by a raised troponin level.
- Patients diagnosed with STEMI are at high risk of death due to ventricular fibrillation and undergo reperfusion treatment.
- If the coronary perfusion is not restored, myocardial damage develops progressively over the next 6–12h with further risks of arrhythmias and development of heart failure.

The aim of emergency treatment of STEMI is as follows:
- Prevent and treat cardiac arrest:
  - Relieve pain.
  - Reperfusion of the myocardium urgently to minimize infarct size.
- It is important to reopen the artery and re-establish myocardial perfusion as soon as possible. This can be achieved by using fibrinolysis therapy or by primary percutaneous coronary intervention (PCI).
- Reperfusion therapy should be delivered as soon as feasible. Current standards indicate that if thrombolytic therapy is chosen, it should be given within 30min of arrival in hospital.
- If primary PCI is the selected therapy, the aim should be to have the artery reopened within 60min of arrival at hospital.

STEMI: pre-hospital management

- The patient should be advised to call the ambulance directly and rest until it arrives.
- If the patient has previously had angina they should be advised to take a short-acting nitrate to aid pain relief, if available:
  - GTN spray 400 micrograms sublingually. Repeat after 5min if pain persists (up to a maximum of two metered doses).
  - GTN tablet 500 micrograms sublingually. Repeat every 3–5min (up to a maximum dose of 1500 micrograms, three tablets).

STEMI: immediate ambulance/early hospital management

- A 12-lead ECG should be performed immediately. If on the basis of clinical and ECG assessment, a diagnosis of STEMI is suspected give the following treatment and supportive therapy:
  - Aspirin 300mg chewed or dissolved before swallowing unless contraindicated.
- Monitor oxygen saturation and offer oxygen therapy as appropriate (caution in COPD patients who are at risk of hypercapnic failure).

- GTN sublingually either 500-microgram tablet or 400-microgram spray. Repeat after 5min if pain persists, providing systolic BP >95mmHg.
- For severe pain consider IV morphine by slow injection titrated to the pain, the usual dose is 1–10mg, with respiratory monitoring.
- Antiemetics if patient is nauseous/vomiting.

STEMI: reperfusion therapy

Reperfusion therapy should be performed as early as possible due to the high mortality risk and to limit myocardial damage and long-term complications. Patient selection for reperfusion therapy does not rely on waiting for the troponin result as this may delay treatment; it is based on clinical presentation and ECG changes. The extent of troponin rise, usually measured at initial presentation and then at 6h, will provide information on the extent of myocardial damage.

Patient selection for reperfusion therapy

Reperfusion therapy is indicated in the following circumstances:
- Ischaemic/infarction symptoms for >20min.
- Patient's symptoms commenced within 12h.
- Persistent ST-segment elevation or new left bundle branch block on the ECG.
- No contraindications to reperfusion therapy.

Percutaneous coronary intervention

Coronary angiography with follow-on PCI is the preferred reperfusion strategy for people with acute STEMI if presentation is within 12h of symptoms and primary PCI can be performed within 120min. The main contraindication to PCI treatment is hypersensitivity to X-ray contrast agents which are used during the procedure. Only the infarcted artery should be treated during PCI.

Prior to PCI patients should receive dual antiplatelet therapy, this is often in the pre-hospital setting, upon the instruction of the primary PCI centre, once the diagnosis of STEMI is made. Early administration ensures efficacy of the antiplatelet agent at the time of the PCI. Aspirin 300mg should be given, if not already given and continued at a dose of 75mg daily. The choice of the second agent is dependent on local protocol. Either ticagrelor 180mg oral loading dose followed by 90mg orally twice daily or prasugrel 60mg oral loading dose followed by 10mg orally once daily (use 5mg daily in patient aged >75yrs or with a low body weight <60kg) should be given. These newer $P2Y_{12}$ receptor inhibitors have a more rapid onset of action and have been shown to be superior to clopidogrel in patients with ACS including STEMI patients in large randomized controlled trials (RCTs). However, they may ↑ the bleeding risk and should not be used in patients with a history of intracranial bleeding and/or haemorrhagic stroke or in patients with moderate to severe liver disease. Prasugrel is also contraindicated in patients with a history of stroke or TIA, and is not recommended in those aged >75yrs or <60kg body weight.

Alternatively, clopidogrel 600mg orally may be given as a loading dose followed by 75mg daily, if the newer agents are contraindicated or not available. As clopidogrel requires a two-step metabolism to the active drug, a higher loading dose is used to achieve a more rapid inhibition of the $P2Y_{12}$ receptor to ensure antiplatelet activity at the time of the PCI.

The PCI procedure involves either radial or femoral arterial access (radial access is preferred as less risk of bleeding) and insertion of a catheter to administer a contrast agent to assess coronary artery circulation and occlusion using contrast imaging. Once the culprit occluded coronary artery has been identified, the thrombus may be aspirated from the artery. Angioplasty is then performed to open the vessel, usually followed by insertion of one or more stents (either bare-metal stents or drug-eluting stents) to support the artery wall and maintain patency.

During the PCI procedure further IV antiplatelet agents and anticoagulants are given to prevent procedure-related thrombosis and ischaemic complications during PCI. However, use of these agents ↑ the risk of bleeding and thrombocytopenia. Current practice varies widely between primary PCI centres and is likely to change further in the future. Ultimately the cardiac interventionalist will have a variety of agents from which they can choose to ensure antiplatelet and anticoagulant therapy is optimized for each individual depending on the size of the clot within the occluded artery, location of occluded artery and other patient factors such as bleeding risk, renal function, cardiac history, and co-morbidities.

The following agents are used either in combination or individually started either pre-PCI or during PCI depending on local protocols:

- IV bolus dose of UFH given pre-procedure and repeated as necessary during the PCI to maintain activated clotting time within required range. In some UK centres, heparin is the only anticoagulant used during the PCI procedure.
- Bivalirudin, a direct thrombin inhibitor, is given in conjunction with aspirin and clopidogrel. It is given as an initial IV bolus at a dose of 0.75mg/kg body weight followed by an IV infusion of 1.75mg/kg body weight/h for at least the duration of the PCI procedure but may be continued post PCI, especially in patients with a large clot burden or failed PCI. Bivalirudin has a short half-life (25min) in patients with normal renal function. It has been shown to have a net clinical benefit when compared to abciximab therapy in patients with STEMI undergoing primary PCI in a large RCT.
- Abciximab, a monoclonal antibody to the glycoprotein (GP) IIb/IIIa platelet receptor, inhibits platelet aggregation. It is used in conjunction with heparin and is given as an initial IV bolus dose of 0.25mg/kg body weight, ideally 10–60min prior to PCI, followed by an IV infusion of 0.125 micrograms/kg body weight/min (to a maximum of 10 micrograms/min) for 12h. It is more expensive than bivalirudin, and some centres reserve use of abciximab for patients who have ongoing ischaemic complications during PCI despite receiving bivalirudin treatment, often termed 'bail out' therapy. Abciximab has a long duration of action and can affect platelet function for at least 48h and remains in the circulation for 15 days or more which ↑ bleeding risk.
- Tirofiban is an alternative non-peptide (small molecule) GP IIb/IIIa receptor antagonist which may be administered in conjunction with heparin and oral antiplatelet therapy in patients diagnosed with STEMI who are planned to undergo a PCI. It is administered as an initial IV bolus of 25 micrograms/kg body weight over 3min, followed by a continuous infusion of 0.15 micrograms/kg body weight/min usually for

12–24h (maximum 48h). Tirofiban is less expensive than abciximab and may be used first line by some centres.
- Eptifibatide is another small-molecule GP IIb/IIIa inhibitor but is only licensed for prevention of MI in patients with unstable angina/NSTEMI. However, as it is the least expensive GP IIb/IIIa inhibitor it is used first line in some primary PCI centres as a cost-effective agent. Although use in this context is unlicensed it is accepted practice.

Fibrinolysis therapy

Fibrinolysis (also termed thrombolysis) is no longer routinely used, it is only indicated if PCI is not available, e.g. transfer to primary PCI centre is not possible within an acceptable time frame (120min) or if PCI is contraindicated, e.g. severe hypersensitivity to contrast agents. The decision whether or not to give thrombolysis requires analysis of risk versus benefit. Patients likely to gain most benefit present early with a large MI, usually anterior, especially if there is any evidence of heart failure. As with primary PCI, the importance of quick access to fibrinolysis is crucial to restore perfusion before irreversible myocardial damage occurs. Those with a small MI, often inferior, benefit less. After 24h, the chances of benefit are very small and there is ↑ risk of cardiac rupture.

Contraindications to fibrinolytic therapy can be absolute or relative.

Absolute contraindications
- Risk of bleeding:
  - Active bleeding.
  - Recent history, within 1 month, of major surgery or trauma.
- Risk of intracranial haemorrhage:
  - Any history of haemorrhagic stroke or ischaemic stroke within the past 2–6 months.
  - Anatomical abnormalities, intracerebral neoplasms, and arteriovenous malformation.

Relative contraindications
- Risk of bleeding:
  - Previous use of anticoagulants or INR >2.0.
  - Non-compressible vascular punctures.
  - Prolonged cardiopulmonary resuscitation (for >10min).
- Risk of intracranial haemorrhage:
  - Previous stroke at any time.
  - Previous TIA.
- Other:
  - Pregnancy
  - Severe hypertension that cannot be controlled (systolic BP >180mmHg and/or diastolic BP >110mmHg diastolic BP).

Use one of the following thrombolytic agents:
- Alteplase 15mg bolus IV, followed by an IV infusion of 0.75mg/kg body weight over a period of 30min (up to a maximum of 50mg); then 0.5mg/kg body weight over a period of 60min up to 35mg (the total dose should not exceed 100mg).
- Reteplase 10 units IV bolus over 2min, followed by a second IV bolus dose of 10 units 30min later.

- Streptokinase 1.5 million units by IV infusion over a period of 60min.
- Tenecteplase 500 micrograms/kg body weight as an IV bolus over 10 seconds (up to a maximum dose of 50 mg).

The plasminogen activators alteplase, reteplase, and tenecteplase are superior to streptokinase but are considerably more expensive. Streptokinase is no longer the drug of choice, antibodies are produced against streptokinase and repeat treatment should not be given between 5 days and 12 months after the initial treatment due to reduced effectiveness. It can also cause hypotension. Allergic reactions are also common with streptokinase and include bronchospasm, periorbital swelling, angio-oedema, urticaria, itching, flushing, nausea, headache, and musculoskeletal pain. Delayed hypersensitivity reactions, such as vasculitis and interstitial nephritis, have also been observed. Anaphylactic shock is rare. If allergic reactions occur, treatment should be discontinued and managed with IV antihistamine and/or corticosteroid. If severe anaphylactic reactions occur, administer IV adrenaline (epinephrine).

The bolus agents reteplase (double bolus) and tenecteplase (single bolus) have major advantages in terms of convenience and can be used in the pre-hospital setting, usually by suitably trained paramedic staff.

In general, most patients who receive fibrinolysis should have a follow-up angiography with PCI if indicated.

Antithrombin therapy with fibrinolysis
Antithrombin therapy should be given at the same time as fibrinolysis:
- IV UFH 60 units/kg body weight initially (maximum of 5000 units), followed by an infusion, initial rate according to local protocol and adjust according to the APTT.
- LMWHs have also been used in conjunction with fibrinolytic agents. Particular care is needed in patients >75yrs old due to ↑ risk of excess bleeding, including intracranial haemorrhage.
- The use of heparin with streptokinase is debatable, there seems to be a small but significant benefit.

Occasionally, bleeding can occur following treatment with fibrinolytic therapy and heparin. Intracranial haemorrhages are devastating and life-threatening. Systemic bleeding and GI bleeding can also occur.

Heparin should be reversed with IV protamine and FFP and/or other supportive treatment as advised by haematology should be given.

Other therapy
- An IV β-blocker should be considered for patients with persistent pain and tachycardia that is not related to heart failure, those with hypertension, and those with a large MI:
  - Atenolol 5–10mg IV slow bolus at a rate of 1mg/min or metoprolol 5mg IV slow bolus at a rate of 1–2mg/min and repeated as necessary up to a maximum of 15mg.
- Repeat doses should only be given provided that systolic BP does not fall below 95mmHg and HR does not fall below 55 beats/min.
- β-blockers are contraindicated in patients with a significant history of bronchospasm or symptomatic bradycardia.
- The routine use of magnesium in the management of patients with acute MI is not recommended. Electrolyte abnormalities should be corrected appropriately.

Secondary prevention therapy following STEMI

Following initial reperfusion therapy patients should receive long-term treatment to reduce cardiovascular risk. Patients should also be enrolled on a cardiac rehabilitation programme to provide the following information and support:

- Lifestyle changes including diet, smoking cessation, alcohol consumption, weight management, and physical activity.
- Advice on driving.
- Health education.
- Psychological and social support.
- Information on drug therapy and importance of long-term adherence.

Antiplatelet therapy

- Aspirin 75mg orally daily for life unless patient is aspirin intolerant or has a clinical indication for anticoagulation.
- A second antiplatelet agent should be continued post reperfusion therapy or as part of medical management if patient did not undergo reperfusion therapy. The newer antiplatelet agents ticagrelor and prasugrel are used in preference to clopidogrel as they have been shown to be superior to clopidogrel in large RCTs, despite a small ↑ bleeding risk:
  - Ticagrelor 90mg orally twice a day for up to 12 months.
  - Prasugrel 10mg orally once a day (use 5mg daily in patients over 75yrs of age or those weighing <60mg) for up to 12 months.
  - Clopidogrel 75mg daily for up to 12 months.

In some patients, the second antiplatelet agent may be used for a shorter duration (e.g. for 1 month) depending on individual patient factors, especially if there is a high risk of bleeding, concomitant anticoagulant therapy, multiple co-morbidities, or if use of bare-metal stents during PCI or if patient has received medical management only.

If a patient is intolerant of aspirin, the antiplatelet regimen will vary according to local protocol. Some centres may use an aspirin desensitization protocol. Alternatives include monotherapy with ticagrelor or dual therapy with clopidogrel and dipyridamole. However, there is little evidence to support any particular regimen. For lifelong antiplatelet therapy, clopidogrel may be used instead of aspirin at a dose of 75mg orally daily.

Beta-blocker therapy

β-blockers should be started as soon as possible post MI once patients are haemodynamically stable, unless contraindicated. β-blockers offer prognostic benefit following MI, especially in high-risk patients such as those with significant left ventricular dysfunction and/or ongoing ischaemia. Any of the following regimens is recommended:

- Atenolol 25–100mg orally daily.
- Bisoprolol initially 1.25mg to 2.5mg orally daily and ↑ up to 10mg daily (unlicensed but widely used in practice).
- Metoprolol initially 25–50mg orally two to three times daily and ↑ up to 100mg orally twice daily.
- Timolol initially 5mg orally twice daily and ↑ up to 10mg twice daily.
- Propranolol initially 40mg orally four times a day for 2–3 days then 80mg twice daily.

- Start at a low dose and titrate upwards to the maximum tolerated dose within the recommended range, provided that systolic BP does not fall below 95mmHg and HR does not fall below 55 beats/min.
- The benefit of β-blocker therapy persists long term. In patients with left ventricular systolic dysfunction, continue β-blocker indefinitely.
- In patients without left ventricular systolic dysfunction, continue β-blocker for at least 1yr.
- The usual contraindications to the use of β-blockers apply.
- Patients with significant left ventricular dysfunction should be observed closely for the development of congestive heart failure.

ACE inhibitor therapy

ACE inhibitors improve outcome after acute MI. Start ACE inhibitor therapy as soon as possible once patients are haemodynamically stable and continue indefinitely. An ACE inhibitor which is licensed for use post MI should be used:

- Ramipril start at 1.25mg to 2.5mg orally once or twice daily and ↑ up to 5mg twice daily
- Trandolapril 500 micrograms orally daily and ↑ up to 4mg daily
- Perindopril 2–4mg orally daily and ↑ up to 8mg daily
- Lisinopril 2.5–5mg orally once daily and ↑ up to 10mg once daily
- Complications of early ACE inhibitor therapy include persistent hypotension and renal dysfunction.
- BP should be closely monitored, and renal function and plasma electrolytes should be monitored frequently, e.g. on alternate days while the patient is in hospital.
- Start at a low dose and titrate upwards at short intervals, e.g. every 12 to 24h as tolerated to the maximum tolerated dose or target dose during the in-patient hospital stay or within 4–6wks of hospital discharge. If the maintenance dose has not been achieved at discharge, the dose must be ↑ more slowly as an out-patient (e.g. weekly), with renal function and plasma electrolytes determined before each ↑ in dose.
- ARBs should be reserved for patients who are intolerant to ACE inhibitors.

Aldosterone antagonists

For patients who develop heart failure and left ventricular dysfunction following a STEMI, treatment with an aldosterone antagonist should be offered after initiation of ACE inhibitor therapy:

- Eplerenone (licensed for post-MI treatment) or spironolactone 25mg orally daily and ↑ to 50mg orally daily as tolerated.

Monitor renal function and serum potassium before and during treatment and if hyperkalaemia develops, reduce the dose of aldosterone antagonist or stop treatment.

Statin therapy

Statin therapy reduces premature death, MI, and other adverse outcomes, such as stroke and revascularization post-MI. Statin therapy should initiated at a high dose for secondary prevention of CAD (e.g. atorvastatin 80mg daily). Consider a lower dose in patients with potential drug interactions, a high risk of side effects, or if strong patient preference for a lower dose. Measure lipid profile (total cholesterol, HDL cholesterol, and non-HDL cholesterol) 3 months after starting high-dose therapy and assess response to treatment (aim for a 40% in non HDL cholesterol).

Calcium channel blocker therapy

CCBs should not be routinely used in patients post STEMI to reduce cardiovascular risk. If β-blockers are contraindicated, diltiazem or verapamil may be used for secondary prevention, but only in patients who do not show any signs of heart failure (e.g. those without pulmonary congestion or left systolic dysfunction). CCBs may be used to treat hypertension and/or angina in patients who are stable post STEMI. For patients with heart failure, use a long-acting dihydropyridine CCB (e.g. amlodipine).

Oral anticoagulant therapy

Rivaroxaban, an oral anti Xa inhibitor, has recently been licensed for prevention of atherothrombotic events in patients who have had ACS with raised cardiac biomarkers, e.g. troponin, in conjunction with aspirin and clopidogrel. It is given at a dose of 2.5mg orally twice daily, usually for 12 months. Currently the use of rivaroxaban for this indication is not in widespread within the UK.

Drug treatment in acute coronary syndromes

ACS without ST elevation on the ECG, also termed non-ST-elevation ACS (NSTE-ACS), is classified as unstable angina or NSTEMI depending on whether there are ischaemic changes on the ECG and/or a rise in troponin level. Initial presentation may be similar but with NSTEMI, the myocardial ischaemia is severe enough to cause myocardial damage and troponin release.

Unstable angina and NSTEMI represent a continuum and patients should have a formal assessment of their future cardiovascular risk using an established scoring system such as GRACE 2.0 (Global Registry of Acute Coronary Events), which predicts in-hospital and future mortality (at 6 months, 1yr, and 3yrs). Patients can be assessed as low, intermediate, and high risk depending on their % mortality risk which is calculated using various factors, e.g. age, HR, systolic BP, presence of heart failure and renal failure, creatinine level, ST deviation, troponin level, and cardiac arrest at presentation. Based on current NICE guidance (2010) treatment is then stratified depending on mortality risk. Intermediate risk is defined as a 3–6% 6-month mortality and high risk is defined as greater than a 6% 6-month mortality.

Patients usually present with severe, prolonged chest pain at rest, lasting for >20min. The pain usually radiates to the jaw and left arm and may be accompanied by nausea, syncope, and shortness of breath. Atypical symptoms, which are more common in the elderly, in ♀, and those with diabetes, include epigastric pain, indigestion, ↑ shortness of breath, as well as absence of chest pain.

Initial supportive therapy

- Administer oxygen if patient is hypoxic or if there is evidence of pulmonary oedema. Hyperoxia should be avoided in patients with chronic obstructive airways disease.
- Give sublingual GTN to relieve ischaemic chest pain. If pain continues, consider IV GTN titrated upwards to achieve pain relief provided systolic BP is maintained >95–100mmHg.

- For severe pain consider IV morphine by slow injection titrated to the pain, the usual dose is 1–10mg, with respiratory monitoring.
- An antiemetic such as metoclopramide should also be given if patient is nauseous/vomiting.

Once a diagnosis of unstable angina or NSTEMI has been made, the following treatments, based on cardiovascular risk, should be initiated (based on NICE guidance 2010).

Oral antiplatelet agents

- Aspirin 300mg oral loading dose to all patients unless contraindicated. Aspirin should be continued life-long at maintenance dose of 75mg oral daily.

For patients at intermediate to high risk a second oral antiplatelet agent should be initiated. Choice of antiplatelet agent depends on local guidelines and risk stratification for treatment. Prasugrel is only licensed for use in ACS if patients are undergoing a PCI and is contraindicated in patients with a history of stroke. Ticagrelor is licensed for use in ACS in patients that are managed medically or undergo reperfusion therapy (either PCI or coronary artery bypass graft). Doses of available agents are as follows:

- Clopidogrel 300mg oral loading dose and continued for up to 12 months at a dose of 75mg daily.
- Prasugrel 60mg oral loading dose and continued for up to 12 months at a dose of 10mg daily (5mg daily if aged >75yrs or body weight <60kg) if patients are undergoing a PCI.
- Ticagrelor 180mg oral loading dose and continued for up to 12 months at a dose of 90mg orally twice daily.

Antithrombin therapy

- NICE guidance recommends the use of fondaparinux 2.5mg SC daily (for a maximum of 8 days) following a diagnosis of unstable angina/NSTEMI. Fondaparinux, a factor Xa inhibitor, was shown to be as efficacious as the LMWH enoxaparin (1mg/kg body weight SC twice daily) but with significantly less bleeding.
- IV infusion of UFH is recommended for patients with renal impairment (creatinine clearance <20mL/min or creatinine >265 micromoles/L) or if PCI is planned or likely within 24h. An IV bolus dose of up to 5000 units should be followed by an infusion, usually initiated at around 1000 units/h and titrated according to local protocol with monitoring of APTT.
- Bivalirudin may also be considered as an alternative antithrombin agent in patients who are not already receiving heparin plus GP inhibitor. It may be used in patients undergoing PCI or in those who are scheduled to undergo angiography with follow-on PCI if indicated, within 24h in combination with aspirin and clopidogrel. Bivalirudin is initiated with an IV bolus dose of 0.1mg/kg body weight, followed by an infusion of 0.25mg/kg body weight/h for up to 72h if the patient does not undergo PCI. If the patient proceeds to PCI an additional loading dose of 0.5mg/kg body weight is given and the infusion ↑ to 1.75mg/kg body weight/h. The bivalirudin infusion is usually continued until the end of the PCI

procedure. If bivalirudin is initiated at the time of PCI then the dosing regimen as per primary PCI should be followed (see ➔ pp. 357–9).

Glycoprotein IIb/IIIa inhibitors

These agents inhibit the glycoprotein IIb/IIIa receptor on platelets and prevent the binding of fibrinogen and platelet aggregation. The use of eptifibatide or tirofiban with IV UFH may be considered in intermediate-to high-risk patients if angiography is planned within 96h of admission. Abciximab in conjunction with heparin may be used as an adjunct to PCI in patients who are not already receiving a small molecule GP inhibitor (eptifibatide or tirofiban) and UFH. The following doses are used:

- Tirofiban: an IV loading infusion dose of 400 nanograms/kg body weight/min for 30min, followed by a maintenance infusion of 100 nanograms/kg body weight/min if planned PCI is within 48h of diagnosis. Duration of infusion will depend on timing of angiography and PCI, maximum infusion time should not exceed 108h. If planned PCI is within 4h of diagnosis a higher dosing regimen is used—refer to STEMI section for information (➔ pp. 357–9).
- Eptifibatide: an IV bolus of 180 micrograms/kg body weight followed by a continuous infusion of 2 micrograms/kg body weight/min for up to 72h. If patients proceed to PCI then continue eptifibatide for at least 20–24h post PCI (maximum duration of therapy 96h).
- Abciximab may be used in patients undergoing a PCI—refer to STEMI section for dosing information (➔ pp. 357–9).

Revascularization

Coronary angiography with follow-on PCI, if indicated, should be considered in all patients at intermediate to high risk, within 96h of admission, unless contraindicated. Clinical trials have demonstrated the benefit of an early invasive strategy and PCI should be performed as early as possible if patient is clinically unstable or at high ischaemic risk.

During PCI antithrombin therapy (bivalirudin) or heparin plus GP inhibitor (tirofiban or eptifibatide) or GP inhibitor abciximab may be used (see ➔ pp. 357–9 for dosing details). If a patient has been receiving fondaparinux prior to PCI, an additional IV dose of heparin (50–100 units/kg) is needed to prevent procedure-related thrombosis

Depending on angiography findings (e.g. multivessel disease) and patient co-morbidities, revascularization using coronary artery bypass grafting may be preferable. This decision is made between the interventional cardiologist and cardiac surgeon.

Drug treatment of low-risk unstable angina/NSTEMI

Patients who have a <1.5% 6-month cardiovascular mortality (classified as lowest risk) should be managed conservatively with a single antiplatelet agent (e.g. aspirin 75mg oral daily). If a patient's 6-month mortality is between 1.5% and 3% (classified as low risk) then a second antiplatelet agent, usually clopidogrel 300mg oral loading dose followed by 75mg oral daily, should be added. Further cardiac assessment should be undertaken, usually as an out-patient to rule out coronary disease. This involves stress testing, which could be exercise testing with an ECG, stress echocardiography, or a nuclear stress study. Patients proved to have coronary disease should proceed to further investigation and management, e.g. coronary angiography and revascularization if necessary.

Long-term drug treatment of patients diagnosed with unstable angina/NSTEMI

Once the patient is stabilized, secondary prevention treatment with β-blockers, ACE inhibitors, and statins should be offered to all patients diagnosed with an NSTEMI and those with unstable angina with intermediate to high cardiovascular mortality risk (see ➔ 'Secondary prevention therapy following STEMI', pp. 361–4).

For patients with low cardiovascular risk, the use of secondary prevention treatment will depend on the results of cardiac assessment and patient co-morbidities. If CAD is identified, patients should be offered secondary prevention therapy.

Further reading

European Society of Cardiology (2012). '2012 ESC guidelines for the management of acute myocardial infarction in patients presenting with ST-segment elevation' ℜ www.escardio.org/Guidelines/Clinical-Practice-Guidelines/Acute-Myocardial-Infarction-in-patients-presenting-with-ST-segment-elevation-Ma

European Society of Cardiology (2015). '2015 ESC guidelines for the management of acute coronary syndromes in patients without persistent ST-segment elevation', ℜ www.escardio.org/Guidelines/Clinical-Practice-Guidelines/Acute-Coronary-Syndromes-ACS-in-patients-presenting-without-persistent-ST-segm

NICE (2010). 'Unstable angina and NSTEMI (CG94)', ℜ www.nice.org.uk/guidance/CG94NICE (2011). 'Ticagrelor for the treatment of acute coronary syndromes (TA236)', ℜ www.nice.org.uk/guidance/ta236

NICE (2011). 'Bivalirudin for the treatment of ST-segment elevation myocardial infarction (TA230)', ℜ www.nice.org.uk/guidance/ta230

NICE (2013). 'Myocardial infarction: cardiac rehabilitation and prevention of further cardiovascular disease (CG172)', ℜ www.nice.org.uk/guidance/CG172

NICE (2014). Lipid modification: risk assessment and reduction, including lipid modification (CG181)', ℜ www.nice.org.uk/guidance/CG181

NICE (2014). 'Prasugrel with percutaneous coronary intervention for treating acute coronary syndromes (TA317)', ℜ www.nice.org.uk/guidance/ta317

Cardiopulmonary resuscitation

Cardiac arrest in adults: what the pharmacist needs to know

The management of cardiopulmonary arrest can be divided into two categories: basic and advanced life support. Note that this advice applies to *adults only*.

Basic life support

Basic life support is the 'first-responder' phase of the chain of survival. It can be carried out by anyone who has the relevant knowledge or training (Fig. 16.3).

Before approaching the patient, the first responder must always check that it is safe to do so. The patient should then be assessed to check consciousness (e.g. by calling the patient's name or gentle shaking). If no response, *shout for help*.

- Confirm whether an arrest has occurred by checking the airway, breathing, and circulation (ABC):
  - Tilt head (if no spine injury) and lift chin/jaw thrust. Clear the mouth. If this does not restore breathing, check for signs of circulation, taking no longer than 10 seconds.
  - Ask someone to call the arrest team and to bring the automated external defibrillator (AED) if available. Note the time.
- Start cardiopulmonary resuscitation (CPR):
  - Give 30 compressions to 2 breaths (30:2). *Chest compressions* work to promote the forward flow of blood. (Allow the chest to recoil completely between each compression.) Cardiopulmonary resuscitation (CPR) should not be interrupted, except to give shocks or intubate.
  - Use the heel of the hand with the other hand placed on top and straight elbows in the middle of the lower half of the sternum, which should be depressed by 5–6cm. Compressions should be fairly fast (100–120/min).
  - After 30 compressions, open airway again using head tilt and chin lift. Pinch the patient's nose shut and give two breaths (each inflation should be 1 second long), ideally using a pocket mask or bag mask device. Otherwise give mouth-to-mouth ventilation (unless poisoning is suspected).
  - Resume chest compressions. Do not interrupt CPR to check on patient unless they display clear signs of recovery (e.g. opening eyes, purposeful moves, speaking) and are breathing normally. If possible, the person providing chest compressions should change about every 2min to avoid fatigue and maintain good-quality compressions.
- If an AED is available, switch it on and follow instructions while aiming to minimize interruption of chest compressions.

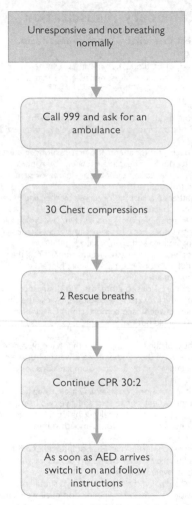

Fig. 16.3 UK adult basic life support algorithm. Reproduced with permission from the Resuscitation Council (UK) Guidelines 2015.

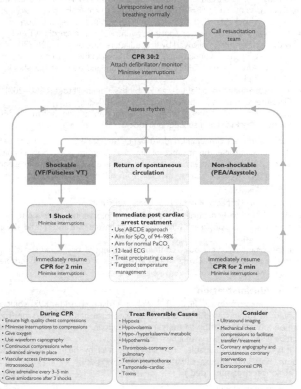

Fig. 16.4 UK adult advanced life support algorithm. Reproduced with permission from the Resuscitation Council (UK) Guidelines 2015.

Advanced life support

Advanced life support starts when trained personnel arrive, and is usually provided by the cardiac arrest team (Fig. 16.4):
- Basic life support maintained.
- The patient's airway is secured and O_2 is administered.
- IV access is obtained (in hospital, blood is taken for urgent blood gas analysis and determination of electrolyte levels).
- The patient is attached to the cardiac monitor on the defibrillator to allow diagnosis of the arrhythmia. Further management depends on whether or not the type of arrhythmia present responds to defibrillation.

The most common cause of cardiac arrest is an arrhythmia—ventricular fibrillation. Ventricular fibrillation and pulseless ventricular tachycardia are known as 'shockable rhythms' because they respond to defibrillation.

- Treat ventricular fibrillation/pulseless ventricular tachycardia (VF/VT) with a single shock, followed by immediate resumption of CPR (30 compressions to 2 ventilations). Do not reassess the rhythm or feel for a pulse. After 2min of CPR, check the rhythm and give another shock (if indicated).
- The recommended initial energy for biphasic defibrillators is 150–200J. Give the second and subsequent shocks at 150–360J.
- The recommended energy when using a monophasic defibrillator is 360J for both the initial and subsequent shocks.

Asystole and electromechanical disturbance cannot be corrected using defibrillation. Asystole is the absence of any heart rhythm. Electro-mechanical disturbance (also known as pulseless electrical activity, PEA) is the presence of organized electrical activity that fails to result in mechanical contraction of the heart.

Pharmaceutical aspects of cardiopulmonary resuscitation

Basic CPR and early defibrillation are the only interventions proved to benefit survival in cardiac arrest. However, drugs have a role and should always be considered.

In hospital, an 'arrest box', containing a variety of drugs, is usually kept with the arrest trolley. Drugs in the arrest box should be pre-assembled syringes wherever feasible.

Drug administration

For IV administration, a flush of 20mL of sodium chloride 0.9% solution should be administered after each drug dose to enhance its passage from the peripheral circulation to the central circulation. Alternatively, the dose can be given in tandem with a fast-flowing IV fluid.

If IV access is unattainable, drugs should be given by the intraosseous (IO) route (tibial and humeral sites preferred). (Giving drugs via a tracheal tube is no longer recommended.)

Adrenaline (epinephrine)

When treating VF/VT cardiac arrest, current guidelines recommend the administration of 1mg of adrenaline (epinephrine) IV (i.e. 10mL of 1 in 10 000 pre-filled syringe) after the third shock once chest compressions have restarted and then every 3–5min during resuscitation. For PEA/asystole, give adrenaline as soon as IV access is established, then every 3–5min. IV doses >1mg are no longer considered to be of benefit and should not be used.

Atropine

- Doses of 0.5–1mg IV can be given in bradycardia, up to a maximum total of 3mg. Atropine was often used in the management of asystole or bradycardia to block any excessive vagal activity that might be contributing to a ↓ in HR but it is no longer recommended for asystole and slow PEA (<60/min).
- *Amiodarone* is the antiarrhythmic of choice in resistant ventricular fibrillation or pulseless ventricular tachycardia. If VF/VT persists after

three shocks, a dose of 300mg in 20mL glucose 5% solution is given as a slow bolus over a period of at least 3min before delivery of the fourth shock. Remember that amiodarone is incompatible with normal saline, and bags of glucose 5% solution should be available to enable prompt setting up of the infusion and for flushing after dose(s). A further 150mg can be given, followed by an infusion of 1mg/min for 6h, and then 0.5mg/min for 6h. It is recommended that, if possible, amiodarone is administered using a volumetric control infusion pump rather than drip-counting technique because of the drug's effect on drip size.

- *Lidocaine* 1mg/kg can be used as an alternative, if amiodarone is not available. Do not give lidocaine if amiodarone has already been given. Do not exceed a total dose of 3mg/kg during the first hour.
- *Magnesium sulfate* is the agent of choice in torsades de pointes, a type of arrhythmia that is often drug induced. It can also be useful in resistant arrhythmias, especially if they are associated with hypo-magnesaemia (more common in patients taking diuretics). A bolus of 8mmol (4mL of a 50% w/v preparation) is usually given.
- *Sodium bicarbonate*—give sodium bicarbonate (50mmol) only if cardiac arrest is associated with hyperkalaemia or tricyclic antidepressant overdose. Repeat the dose according to the clinical condition of the patient and the results of repeated blood gas analysis. Should only be administered after arterial blood gas analysis where pH has fallen below 7.1. A 50mmol dose (50mL of the 8.4% solution) would normally be given as a slow IV bolus.
- *Oxygen*—once return of spontaneous circulation is achieved and oxygen saturation of arterial blood can be monitored (by pulse oximetry and/or arterial blood gas analysis), inspired oxygen should be titrated to achieve SaO_2 of 94–98%.
- *Calcium chloride*—10mL of the 10% preparation (equivalent to 6.8mmol of calcium ions) is administered in suspected or actual CCB overdose or in magnesium-induced heart block. Calcium can slow the HR and precipitate arrhythmias. *Do not give calcium solutions and sodium bicarbonate simultaneously by the same route.*

After successful resuscitation, perform the following:
- 12-lead ECG, CXR, U&Es, glucose, blood gases, FBC, creatinine kinase/troponin levels.
- Transfer to coronary care unit.
- Monitor vital signs.
- Communicate to relatives.

Resuscitation in out of hospital situations is generally stopped after 20min if there is refractory asystole or electromechanical dissociation.

Suggested contents of the adult emergency drug box used in pre-arrest and arrest situations
- 5 × adrenaline (epinephrine) 1:10 000 solution, 1mg in 10mL pre-filled syringe (pre-assembled syringe).
- 1 × amiodarone 300mg in 10mL pre-filled syringe (pre-assembled syringe).
- 1 × 5% glucose, 50mL to flush amiodarone.

Suggested contents of back-up emergency box, containing the following drugs

- 6 × adenosine, 6mg in 2mL vial.
- 5 × adrenaline (epinephrine) 1:1000 solution, 1mg in 1mL ampoule.
- 2 × amiodarone 150mg in 3mL ampoule.
- 5 × atropine 600 micrograms in 1mL ampoule
- 1 × calcium chloride 6.8mmol in 10mL (10%) pre-filled syringe (pre-assembled syringe).
- 1 × 50% glucose solution in 50mL vial.
- 1 × magnesium sulfate 10mmol in 5mL (50% solution) ampoule.
- 1 × sodium bicarbonate 8.4% in 50mL pre-filled syringe (pre-assembled syringe).

It is envisaged that back-up emergency boxes are issued only to wards and departments with manual defibrillators. This reduces waste but ensures the medicines are promptly available when required.

Therapy-related issues: respiratory system

Asthma management in adults

The British Thoracic Society/Scottish Intercollegiate Guidelines Network (BTS/SIGN) 'British Guideline on the Management of Asthma' (2014)[1] recommends that all adults with asthma (and/or their parents or carers) should be offered self-management education which should include a written personalized asthma action plan (PAAP) and be supported by regular professional review. These written PAAPs may be based on symptoms and/or peak flows and should be used alongside the pharmacological management.

PAAPs can help patients recognize the deterioration of their asthma control and provide an individualized plan on treating an exacerbation in the early stages. The recognition of deterioration of a patient's symptoms requires interpretation of both subjective and objective measures in line with the patient's asthma severity.

A PAAP should inform the patient about when and how they modify their medications in response to worsening of their condition and when to see a healthcare professional.

Pharmacological management

The aim of asthma management is control of the disease. Complete control is defined as:

- no daytime symptoms
- no night-time awakening due to asthma
- no need for rescue medication
- no asthma attacks
- no exacerbations
- no limitations on activity, including exercise
- normal lung function (in practical terms forced expiratory volume in 1 second (FEV_1) and/or peak expiratory flow >80% predicted or best)
- minimal side effects from medication.

A stepwise approach aims to abolish symptoms as soon as possible and optimize peak flow by starting treatment at the level most likely to achieve this. Patients should start treatment at the step most appropriate to the initial severity of their asthma. The aim is to achieve early control and to maintain it by stepping up treatment as necessary and stepping down treatment when good control is achieved.

Before initiating a new drug therapy, practitioners should check adherence with existing therapies and inhaler technique, and eliminating trigger factors (such as aeroallergen and food avoidance).

The management of chronic asthma in adults is split into five steps:

Step 1: mild intermittent asthma

- An inhaled short-acting β_2-agonist (SABA) should be prescribed as a short-term reliever for all patients with symptomatic asthma.
- SABAs act on β_2 adrenoceptors on bronchial muscle causing bronchodilation and temporary relief of symptoms. Examples include salbutamol and terbutaline.

- Good control is associated with little or no need for the SABA.
- Stepping up to the next treatment step should be considered when the patient is:
  - using a SABA three times a week or more *and/or*
  - symptomatic three times a week or more *and/or*
  - waking one night a week or more with symptoms.
- Anyone prescribed with more than one SABA inhaler device a month should be identified and have an urgent appointment to undergo a review to determine if measures are required to improve asthma control if this is poor.

Step 2: regular preventer therapy

- Inhaled corticosteroids (ICSs) are the recommended preventer drug for adults for achieving overall treatment goals.
- ICSs work to reduce both inflammation in the airways and airway hyper-responsiveness. Regular use of ICSs can reduce the severity and frequency of exacerbations, improve quality of life, improve lung function, and reduce mortality.
- In adults, a reasonable starting dose of ICS will usually be 400 micrograms of beclometasone dipropionate (BDP) equivalence per day (see Table 17.1 for BDP equivalence ratio of ICSS). The dose should be titrated to the lowest dose at which effective control of asthma is maintained.
- There is little evidence of long-term side effects of ICS therapy (such as diabetes and skin thinning) at doses of <800 micrograms of BDP equivalence per day; however, therapy adherence may be limited due to local side effects, such as dysphonia and oral candidiasis.
- Counselling patients to use spacer devices when using pressurized metered-dose inhalers (pMDIs) and rinsing the mouth with water after each dose should minimize any local side effects.

Table 17.1 Beclometasone dipropionate (BDP) equivalence ratio of inhaled corticosteroids

Drug	BDP equivalence ratio
Beclometasone dipropionate CFC (non-proprietary and Clenil Modulite®)	1:1
Beclometasone dipropionate CFC (QVAR® and Fostair®)	2:1
Beclometasone dipropionate dry powder (Asmabec Clickhaler®)	2:1
Budesonide	1:1
Ciclesonide	2:1
Fluticasone propionate	2:1
Mometasone furoate	2:1

Before stepping up therapy, remember to check the patient's adherence, inhaler technique, and ensure trigger factors have been reduced/eliminated.

Option 1

In adult patients taking ICSs at doses of 200–800 micrograms of BDP per day, the first choice is an inhaled long-acting β_2-agonist (LABA)—if a good response is achieved, continue using the LABA.

Many patients benefit more from adding a LABA to therapy at this stage (step 3) rather than ↑ the dose of the ICS.

LABAs produce a longer duration of bronchodilation compared to SABAs. They should, however, always be used in conjunction with an ICS and not as lone therapy. It has been found that the use of LABAs alone is associated with ↑ asthma morbidity and possible mortality.

Option 2

If asthma control remains suboptimal after the addition of an inhaled LABA, the dose of ICS should be ↑ to 800 micrograms of BDP equivalence per day in adults if the patient is not already on this dose.

High doses of ICSs (>800 micrograms of BDP equivalence per day) have the potential to induce adrenal suppression. These patients should therefore be provided with a 'steroid card'.

Option 3

If there appears to be no response to the addition of LABA, the LABA should be stopped and the dose of ICS should be ↑ to 800 micrograms of BDP equivalence per day in adults (if not already on this dose) and sequential trials of the following add-on therapies should be tried:

- Leukotriene receptor antagonists (LTRAs)
- Theophyllines
- Slow-release β_2-agonist tablets.

Information regarding add-on therapies

Leukotriene receptor antagonists

This group of medicines may improve lung function, reduce exacerbations, and improve asthma symptoms. They work by blocking the pathway of leukotriene mediators which are released from mast cells, eosinophils, and basophils.

Examples of LTRAs include montelukast and zafirlukast, which are of benefit in patients with exercised-induced asthma, patients with aspirin intolerance, or those with concomitant rhinitis.

Side effects of LTRAs include headaches, nausea and vomiting, GI disturbances, and skin rashes. Zafirlukast may also affect the liver.

Theophylline

Theophylline belongs to a group of drugs called methylxanthines and is less potent but much more toxic than inhaled LABAs.

The mechanism of action of methylxanthines is uncertain, with several modes of action having been proposed, including inhibition of phosphodiesterase (an adenosine receptor antagonist), causing the stimulation of catecholamine release, and the inhibition of intracellular calcium release.

Methylxanthines promote bronchial smooth muscle relaxation, an ↑ in mucociliary transport, ↑ diaphragmatic contractility, and stimulate central respiratory drive.

Side effects can be a problem with theophylline and can include tachycardia, palpitations, headaches, insomnia, nausea, and other GI disturbances. Some of these side effects may be dose related, so it is important that patients have their dose adjusted to ensure their plasma level of theophylline is within the safe narrow therapeutic range (10–20mg/L or 55–110mmol/L).

Care should also be taken to ensure that drug–drug interactions are minimized.

Slow-release β₂-agonist tablets
Slow-release formulations of β₂-agonists may improve symptoms and lung function, but are now rarely used in practice. Side effects are more common with the oral formulations as opposed to the inhaled formulations which can include tremor, cramps, palpitations, and headache.

Long-acting muscarinic antagonists (LAMAs)
This group of medication is commonly used in chronic obstructive pulmonary disease (COPD) but is not currently recommended within the BTS/SIGN 'British Guideline on the Management of Asthma' (2014).[1]

Anecdotally, LAMAs do appear to be as effective as salmeterol in the short-term control of asthma, and may be more effective in some patients than doubling the dose of ICS in patients with fixed airways obstruction.

In 2014, tiotropium (in the Respimat® device) became the first LAMA licensed for use in asthma; however, longer-term studies are required to confirm its place in asthma therapy.

Step 4: persistent poor control
- In a small proportion of patients, asthma is not adequately controlled when prescribed with a combination of SABA, ICS (800 micrograms of BDP equivalence per day), and an additional drug (usually a LABA). In these patients, the addition of a fourth drug should be considered.
- Before stepping up therapy, check the patient's adherence, inhaler technique, and ensure trigger factors have been reduced/eliminated.
- The following medications can be considered as the additional intervention:
  - ↑ ICS to 2000 micrograms of BDP equivalence per day
  - LTRAs
  - Theophyllines
  - Slow-release β₂-agonist tablets, although caution needs to be used in patients already prescribed with LABAs.

Step 5: Continuous or frequent use of oral steroids
- The aim of treatment is to control asthma using the lowest possible doses of medication. Some patients with very severe asthma who are not controlled at step 4 with a high-dose ICS and who are also still taking LABAs, leukotriene antagonists, or theophyllines, require regular long-term steroid tablets.

- Before stepping up therapy, remember to check the patient's adherence, inhaler technique, and ensure trigger factors have been reduced/ eliminated.
- Prednisolone is the most widely used steroid for maintenance therapy in patients with chronic asthma.
- The lowest maintenance dose possible that controls symptoms should be ascertained and prescribed.
- It should always be considered that patients who are on long-term steroid tablets (i.e. >3 months) or requiring frequent courses of steroid tablets (e.g. three to four courses per year) will be at risk of systemic side effects. Patients should be monitored closely for any changes in BP, plasma, or urine glucose levels, cholesterol, and bone mineral density. Other adverse effects of long-term oral corticosteroids include obesity, cataracts, glaucoma, skin thinning and bruising, and muscle weakness. Patients in this risk category must therefore receive regular review appointments in order to ensure supplementary management of any risks/side effects as required.

Stepping down treatment

Discontinuation of therapy can worsen clinical outcomes quickly, in some cases within weeks. NICE developed guidance that was published in 2012 to support clinicians in stepping down patients' treatment when needed, specifically identifying when high doses of ICSs should be reviewed.

These guidelines advise that patients who are on an equivalent of 800 micrograms of BDP equivalence per day or higher should have their dose reviewed if they have been stable for 3 months or more. At this stage, if clinically appropriate, the dose can be reduced by 25–50%.

Other medications and potential steroid tablet-sparing treatments

Omalizumab

- Omalizumab is a humanized monoclonal antibody which binds to circulating immunoglobulin E (IgE), reducing levels of free serum IgE available to bind to mast cells and initiate the allergic cascade that often results in asthma exacerbations.
- The NICE technology appraisal (TA278),[2] published in 2013, recommends omalizumab 'as an option for treating severe persistent confirmed allergic IgE-mediated asthma as an add-on to optimised standard therapy in people aged 6 years and over who need continuous or frequent treatment with oral corticosteroids (defined as 4 or more courses in the previous year)'.
- Omalizumab is approved in England through a patient access scheme provided by the manufacturer.
- Omalizumab is given by SC injection every 2–4wks. The administered dose is based upon the patient's weight and total IgE prior to starting treatment.
- This treatment has been shown to reduce severe exacerbations, reduce reliever use, and improve the patient's quality of life.

- Omalizumab treatment should only be initiated in specialist clinics that have been designated 'difficult asthma centres' who have experience of evaluation and management of patients with severe and difficult asthma.
- Side effects may occur, such as local skin reactions or anaphylaxis presenting as bronchospasm, hypotension, syncope, urticaria, and/or angio-oedema of the throat or tongue.
- It should be noted that anaphylaxis has been reported to occur after administration of omalizumab as early as the first dose, but has also occurred after 1yr. Due to the risk of anaphylaxis, omalizumab should only be administered to patients in a healthcare setting under direct medical supervision.

Potential steroid tablet-sparing treatments

- Immunosuppressants (such as methotrexate, ciclosporin, and oral gold) ↓ long-term steroid tablet requirements, but all have significant side effects. There is no available evidence to support persisting beneficial effect after stopping them, with marked patient variability in response.
- For patients who require frequent courses or long-term daily dosing of oral corticosteroids to control their asthma, an immunosuppressant may be given as a 3-month trial once other drug treatments have proved unsuccessful.
- Treatment should be initiated in a specialist asthma centre with experience of using these medicines, where risks and benefits should be discussed with the patient, with their treatment effects carefully monitored.

References

1. British Thoracic Society/Scottish Intercollegiate Guidelines Network (BTS/SIGN) (2014). 'British Guideline on the Management of Asthma – A National Clinical Guideline', ℘ www.brit-thoracic.org.uk/guidelines-and-quality-standards/asthma-guideline
2. NICE (2013). 'Omalizumab for treating severe persistent allergic asthma (review of technology appraisal guidance 133 and 201) (TA 278)', ℘ www.nice.org.uk/guidance/TA278

Inhalers and technique

Delivery through inhalation is the preferred method of delivering medication for respiratory conditions such as asthma and COPD. This method of application ensures that the drug is delivered directly to the lungs, allowing a lower dose of drug to be used.

Both the BTS/SIGN 'British Guideline on the Management of Asthma' (2014)[3] and the NICE COPD clinical guideline (2010)[4] recommend that inhalers should only be prescribed after patients have received training in the use of the chosen device and are able to demonstrate a satisfactory technique.

To support this recommendation, a large body of evidence from randomized clinical trials has shown that the inhaler technique of a patient can be improved by education from a health professional or other person trained in the correct techniques, with the amount of instruction on inhaler technique given being shown to influence the likelihood of correct use.

Unfortunately, many clinical studies available state that a large proportion of patients who are prescribed with inhaled medications do not use their inhalers correctly, with up to 90% of patients with either standard pMDIs or dry-powder inhalers (DPIs) showing incorrect technique. Reassessment and education of correct inhaler technique is therefore advised during every clinical encounter in order to ensure optimum efficacy of use.

Education

When inhaled medication is prescribed, the choice of inhaler for stable asthma and COPD should be mainly based on patient preference, where assessment of use to ensure that the individual is capable of using the relevant inhaler correctly prior to prescription is highly recommended.

Published studies from around the world suggest that as many as 25% of patients with asthma or COPD have never received verbal inhaler technique instruction. When given, instruction is often rushed, of poor quality, and not reinforced. Only an estimated 11% of patients receive follow-up assessment and education on their inhaler technique.

Incorrect technique when taking inhaled medications frequently prevents patients from receiving the maximal benefit from their medications, with associated poor asthma control due to SABAs not being effectively delivered (leading to loss of bronchodilator effect).

Although the newer DPI inhalers were designed to improve ease of use, significant rates of incorrect use among patients have been reported for all currently used inhaler designs, even among regular users.

Recent studies confirm the following:

- Regardless of the type of inhaler device prescribed, patients are unlikely to use inhalers correctly unless they receive clear instruction, including a physical demonstration
- The risk of misusing inhalers is particularly high in older patients and those with multiple co-morbidities
- Brief verbal instruction on correct technique, with a physical demonstration, is effective when repeated over time and can improve clinical outcomes.

- With all inhaler types, error rates are seen to ↑ in correlation to age and the severity of airflow obstruction.
- Even after training is provided, some patients will continue to have difficulties using inhalers properly.

It cannot be stressed highly enough that incorrect use of pMDIs for ICSs has been associated with ↑ reliever use, ↑ use of emergency medical services, worsening asthma, and higher rates of asthma instability as assessed by a GO. These outcomes are most pronounced among patients with poor inspiration–actuation coordination.

Inefficient technique with DPIs may also lead to insufficient drug delivery and deposition within the lungs.

Common issues encountered with inhaler use

The most frequently prescribed inhaler is the pMDI. The following incorrect techniques are often seen when patients using this type of device are reviewed:

- Not shaking the inhaler before use—if the contents of the canister (propellant and medication) are not mixed thoroughly, too much or too little of one component will be released leading to inconsistent dosing and poorly functioning inhalers.
- Not breathing out before inhaling—for the medication to work as effectively as possible, it is important that the medication reaches the correct areas of the lungs. The patient should breathe out fully (or as comfortably as possible) prior to inhaling the medication.
- Inhaling too early before pressing the canister—breathing in too early can mean that little or no medication gets into the lungs and instead resides in the mouth/back of the throat resulting in local side effects.
- Inhaling too late after pressing the canister—starting to breathe in too late can mean that little or no medication gets to the lungs and instead resides in the mouth/back of the throat resulting in local side effects.
- Inhaling too fast—a reduction in the amount of medication that reaches the lungs is seen, with the medication leaving the pMDI at an accelerated rate. The majority of the dose hits the back of the throat, giving rise to local side effects, instead of going into the lungs.
- Not continuing to breathe in after the canister is pressed—inhaled medication is likely to penetrate deeper into the lungs if the inhalation is full.
- The patient not holding their breath after inhalation—holding the breath for 10sec after inhalation, if possible, ↑ lung deposition through the process of sedimentation.
- Patients frequently fail to detect when the inhaler is empty or nearly empty, particularly when using reliever pMDIs as these do not have built-in dosage counters. This problem can result in patients continuing to use the inhaler when it may no longer be delivering the required dose.
- Patients with osteoarthritis may be unable to activate a pMDI easily and may benefit from the use of a Haleraid® or a breath-activated inhaler.

Mechanical difficulties can usually be overcome by checking the technique of each individual and helping them identify which inhaler they can use best before a prescription is written.

Even with training, some will be unable to overcome these problems and may do better with a pMDI with the inclusion of a spacer.

A substantial body of evidence has shown that incorrect inhaler technique is particularly common among older people with asthma or COPD, whether using a pMDI or a DPI. A study using Accuhalers® and Turbohalers® showed that patients with severe COPD were less likely to achieve a high enough inspiratory rate to activate the inhaler, even after instruction. These patients might achieve a better and more effective technique using a breath-activated inhaler, where possible. Some older patients with advanced COPD may benefit from the use of a spacer with a pMDI; however, evidence available suggests that this patient group may also have difficulties connecting the inhaler to the spacer.

Regardless of the type of inhaler prescribed, the following issues are also encountered:

- An inability to achieve a firm seal around the mouthpiece—often seen in the elderly or those with cognitive impairment. A spacer face mask can often overcome this problem.
- Difficulty retaining skills after instruction in the use of an inhaler.
- Lower education levels have been associated with an ↑ rate of incorrect technique.
- Built-in dose counters in preventer inhalers may not overcome this problem for patients with poor eyesight.
- Poor maintenance of inhalers or failure to replace an inhaler when necessary, resulting in suboptimal drug delivery.
- The concurrent use of multiple inhaler types with different techniques can confuse patients.[1]

Spacer

For those patients who find the pMDI technique difficult or need a high dose of corticosteroid, a large-volume spacer and education from a health professional (rather than simply changing inhaler type) might be the best initial strategy for achieving an effective technique.

The use of these devices, which are attached to the prescribed inhaler, help overcome the problem of coordinating inspiration with actuation: after the canister is pressed, the medication remains in suspension in the spacer for a short time allowing the user to inhale the drug by drawing in one deep breath or though tidal breathing (inhale and exhale at a normal, resting rate—usually at a rate of one press of the inhaler to five tidal breaths).

The aerosol medication only stays suspended for a short time, so if patients fail to take each dose without delay immediately after loading the spacer, a proportion of the dose is deposited onto the inner surface of the spacer and therefore lost.

---

[1] Prescribing mixed inhaler types may cause confusion and potentially lead to an ↑ in errors of use. Using the same type of device to deliver preventative and relieving medication(s) may improve outcomes.

It is recommended that patients with pMDIs should use a spacer:
- whenever ICS medications are used
- if they have poor inspiration–activation coordination
- when taking a reliever during acute asthma episodes (if available).

A spacer with a mask attached is available for children and adults who have difficulty sealing their lips around a mouthpiece (NB: the mask must be closely applied to the face while the pMDI is activated).

Spacer care and hygiene
- Spacers should be cleaned before first use and then monthly by washing in warm water with kitchen detergent and allowing to air dry. The mouthpiece should be wiped clean of detergent before use.
- Drying with a cloth or paper towel can result in electrostatic charge ('static') on the inside of the spacer, which can reduce availability of dose, therefore this is not recommended.
- Spacers should be reviewed every 6–12 months to check the structure is intact (e.g. no cracks) and the valve is functioning. Plastic spacers should be replaced at least every 12 months.
- Among patients taking ICSs, failure to maintain meticulous oral hygiene (rinse, gargle, and spit) after each dose ↑ the risk of oropharyngeal candidiasis ('thrush') and hoarseness as a result of medication being deposited in the mouth and pharynx. For those using a pMDI, the risk of these local side effects can be reduced by using a spacer.
- Poor maintenance of spacers, or failure to replace a spacer when necessary, can also result in suboptimal drug delivery.

Even when patients are able to demonstrate correct technique during consultation with a health professional, it should be noted that they may not maintain this standard at other times. Those patients prescribed with and instructed to use a spacer may subsequently revert to using their pMDI alone, therefore continual review and re-education is recommended.

How healthcare professionals can help patients use their inhalers correctly

Make sure your own knowledge of correct technique is up to date
It should never be assumed that your own technique is correct. A high proportion (31–85%) of health professionals have been seen to show incorrect technique when tested objectively—these rates are similar between doctors, nurses, and community pharmacists.

It is important to learn how to use each inhaler type correctly, including new devices, along with knowing the rationale for each step of the instructions, so that the importance of compliance in use can be clearly explained and the technique of use can be confidently demonstrated to patients.

The common errors with different types (shown in Tables 17.2–17.7) should also be known.

Ensure the inhaler is appropriate for the patient

Clinicians and practitioners who see patients with asthma and COPD should be aware of common errors encountered, resulting in poor inhaler technique. In the case of patients prescribed with a pMDI, the addition of a large-volume spacer and education from a health professional (rather than simply changing inhalers) might be the best initial strategy for improving inhaler technique.

Where possible, the prescription of multiple inhaler types should be avoided, as this may lead to confusion and errors.

Give verbal instructions, not just a product leaflet

The manufacturer's instruction sheet alone is ineffective in achieving correct technique. Patients with asthma or COPD using an inhaler for the first time are more likely to show correct technique after receiving verbal instruction rather than reading the manufacturer's leaflet.

Give a physical demonstration

Correct education regarding inhaler technique sees verbal instructions accompanied with a physical demonstration of the technique by a skilled educator, which can help overcome potential language barriers or issues regarding interpretation.

Those providing education need to ensure they have a range of placebo inhalers to demonstrate the correct technique—these are available from the manufactures of the inhalers and are for single-use only.

Following education, it should be ensured that the patient is able to understand the instructions and be able to demonstrate the correct technique.

Other devices are available which are helpful when choosing an inhaler and follow-up checks:
- The In-Check DIAL® device for checking the patient's inspiratory flow rate through different inhalers
- The 2-Tone® inhaler device which helps train the patient to inhale through the pMDI at the correct speed.

Ask patients to show you how they use their inhaler during every clinical attendance/encounter

The technique employed by the patient should be actively checked and reviewed against the appropriate checklist for the specific inhaler type prescribed.

It is not considered good practice to rely on the patient's assurance that they know how to use their inhaler because patients are unlikely to ask for advice, with most being unaware that their inhaler technique is faulty.

Repeat instruction/education regularly

Inhaler technique must be checked and education reinforced regularly (ideally during every clinical attendance) in order to maintain correct technique. It has been documented that inhaler technique deteriorates after education, with a loss of skill associated with a deterioration in some asthma outcomes within 3 months after training is given.

Suggested checklists to follow for the most commonly prescribed inhaler devices

The following tables list the suggested checklists to follow for the five inhalers which are most frequently prescribed to patients with asthma and COPD: pMDIs (both with and without a spacer device) are presented in Tables 17.2 and 17.3, and DPIs in Tables 17.4–17.7. Common errors and advice are also included in these tables.

Table 17.2 Pressurized metered-dose inhaler (pMDI)

Suggested checklist of steps*	Problems and common errors	Tips
1. Remove cap	• Inability to coordinate activation with inhalation	• All patients using a pMDI for an ICS medication should use a spacer
2. Hold inhaler upright and shake well		
3. Breathe out gently	• Failure to hold breath for a sufficient time	• Patients with weak hands or osteoarthritis who have difficulty using a pMDI may benefit from a Haleraid® device
4. Put mouthpiece between teeth without biting and close lips to form good seal	• Multiple actuations without waiting or shaking in between doses	
5. Start to breathe in slowly through mouth and press down firmly on canister	• Incorrect position of inhaler	• Keep chin up and inhaler upright (not aimed at roof of mouth or tongue)
	• Difficult for people with osteoarthritis affecting hands	
6. Continue to breathe in slowly and deeply	• May be unsuitable for patients with severe COPD with poor inspiratory flow rate	
7. Hold breath for about 10sec or as long as comfortable		
8. While holding breath, remove inhaler from mouth		
9. Breathe out gently away from mouthpiece		
10. If an extra dose is needed, wait 1min and then repeat steps 2–9		
11. Replace cap		

* Check the package insert for any specific instructions relating to an individual prescribed inhaler.

Table 17.3 Pressurized metered-dose inhaler (pMDI) plus spacer

Suggested checklist of steps	Problems and common errors	Tips
1. Assemble spacer 2. Remove inhaler cap 3. Hold inhaler upright and shake well 4. Insert inhaler upright into spacer 5. Put mouthpiece between teeth without biting and close lips to form good seal 6. Breathe out gently 7. Hold spacer level and press down firmly on canister once 8. Breathe in slowly and deeply then hold breath for about 10sec or as long as comfortable *Or* Breathe in and out normally for 4 breaths* 9. Remove spacer from mouth 10. Breathe out gently 11. Remove inhaler from spacer 12. If an extra dose is needed, wait 1min and then repeat steps 3–11 13. Replace cap and disassemble spacer	● Compromised drug delivery to lungs due to build-up of electrostatic charge, damaged or sticky valves, or by multiple actuations ● Multiple actuations without waiting or shaking in between doses ● Delay between actuation and inhalation leading to no medication being inhaled ● Patients with cognitive impairment may be unable to form adequate lip seal	● Overcomes errors with pMDI alone for many patients ● Good spacer care and hygiene can improve efficacy ● Use a facemask for infants and patients unable to form a good lip seal

* Multiple breaths (tidal breathing) is used for young children and during acute exacerbations where a single deep breath cannot be managed.

Table 17.4 Easi-Breathe® inhaler

Suggested checklist of steps*	Problems and common errors	Tips
1. Remove cap 2. Hold inhaler upright and shake well* 3. Push lever up 4. Breathe out gently away from mouthpiece 5. Put mouthpiece between teeth without biting and close lips to form good seal	● Incorrect position of inhaler ● Multiple actuations without shaking in between doses* ● Stopping breathing in when the click is heard ● Excess moisture from humidity or breathing into device	● Keep chin up and inhaler upright (not aimed at roof of mouth or tongue) ● Always lift the lever before using the inhaler ● Always put the cover back on the inhaler after use

Table 17.4 (*Contd.*)

Suggested checklist of steps*	Problems and common errors	Tips
6. Breathe in slowly and deeply. Keep breathing in after click is heard		
7. Hold breath for about 10sec or as long as comfortable		
8. While holding breath, remove inhaler from mouth		
9. Breathe out gently away from mouthpiece		
10. Push lever down		
11. If an extra dose is needed, repeat steps 2–10		
12. Replace cap		

* QVAR® Autohaler does not need to be shaken before use

Table 17.5 Accuhaler® inhaler

Suggested checklist of steps	Problems and common errors	Tips
1. Check dose counter	• Not loading dose before inhaling	• Never hold the inhaler with the mouthpiece pointing downwards during or after loading a dose, as the medication can dislodge. Always keep it horizontal.
2. Open using thumb grip		
3. Holding horizontally, load dose by sliding lever until it clicks	• Failure to breathe in deeply and with enough force to deliver medication	
4. Breathe out gently away from mouthpiece		
5. Place mouthpiece in mouth and seal lips	• Failure to hold breath for a sufficient time after inhalation	• Always close the inhaler after use
6. Breathe in steadily and deeply	• Excess moisture from humidity or breathing into device	
7. Hold breath for about 10sec or as long as comfortable		
8. While holding breath, remove inhaler from mouth		
9. Breathe out gently away from mouthpiece		
10. If an extra dose is needed, repeat steps 3–9		
11. Close cover to click shut		

Table 17.6 HandiHaler® inhaler

Suggested checklist of steps	Problems and common errors	Tips
1. Open cap 2. Open mouthpiece 3. Remove capsule from blister and place in chamber 4. Close mouthpiece until it clicks 5. Press green piercing button in once and release 6. Breathe out gently away from mouthpiece 7. Put mouthpiece between teeth without biting and close lips to form good seal 8. Breathe in slowly and deeply, so capsule vibrates 9. Continue to breathe in as long as comfortable 10. While holding breath, remove inhaler from mouth 11. Breathe out gently away from mouthpiece 12. Put mouthpiece back between teeth without biting and close lips to form good seal 13. Breathe in slowly and deeply, so capsule vibrates 14. Continue to breathe in as long as comfortable 15. While holding breath, remove inhaler from mouth 16. Breathe out gently away from mouthpiece 17. Open mouthpiece and remove used capsule 18. If an extra dose is needed, repeat steps 3–17 19. Close mouthpiece and cap	• Not piercing capsule or, conversely, piercing capsule multiple times • Not using a new capsule for each dose • Failure to breathe in deeply and with enough force to deliver medication • Not taking second breath to receive full dose from capsule • Swallowing capsule instead of inhaling it through the HandiHaler®	• When dispensing a new device to a patient with weak hands, work the cover back and forth several times to loosen up • Always close the inhaler after use

Table 17.7 Turbohaler® inhaler

Suggested checklist of steps	Problems and common errors	Tips
1. Unscrew and remove cover	• Incorrect positioning of inhaler during loading of a dose	• Place inhaler on a flat surface
2. Check dose counter		(e.g. table) for loading dose to ensure it remains upright
3. Keep inhaler upright while twisting grip around and then back until click is heard	• Failing to complete both steps of loading manoeuvre (around and then back)	• Read the dose counter in the middle of the window
4. Breathe out gently away from mouthpiece	• Failure to breathe in deeply and with enough force to deliver medication	• Always replace the cover back on the inhaler after use
5. Place mouthpiece between teeth without biting and close lips to form a good seal	• Excess moisture from humidity or breathing into device	
6. Breathe in strongly and deeply		
7. Remove inhaler from mouth		
8. Breathe out gently away from mouthpiece		
9. If an extra dose is needed, repeat steps 3–9		
10. Replace cover		

References

3. British Thoracic Society/Scottish Intercollegiate Guidelines Network (BTS/SIGN) (2014). 'British Guideline on the Management of Asthma – A National Clinical Guideline', ℜ www.brit-thoracic. org.uk/guidelines-and-quality-standards/asthma-guideline
4. NICE. 'Chronic Obstructive Pulmonary Disease—Management of Chronic Obstructive Pulmonary Disease in Adults and Primary and Secondary Care (CG101)', ℜ www.nice.org.uk/ guidance/cg101

Management of stable chronic obstructive pulmonary disease

Chronic obstructive pulmonary disease (COPD) is now the preferred term for the conditions in patients with airflow obstruction who were previously diagnosed as having chronic bronchitis or emphysema. The definition of COPD documented in the NICE 2010 guidelines (CG101)[5] is as follows:

'COPD is characterised by airflow obstruction that is not fully reversible. The airflow obstruction does not change markedly over several months and is usually progressive in the long term. COPD is predominantly caused by smoking. Other factors, particularly occupational exposures, may also contribute to the development of COPD. Exacerbations often occur, where there is a rapid and sustained worsening of symptoms beyond normal day-to-day variations.'

The following should be also be used as a definition of COPD:

• Airflow obstruction is defined as a reduced FEV_1/forced vital capacity (FVC) ratio, such that FEV_1/FVC is <0.7.
• If FEV_1 is >80% of predicted normal, a diagnosis of COPD should only be made in the presence of respiratory symptoms, e.g. breathlessness or cough.

It is estimated that 3 million people in the UK have COPD, with ~900 000 people having a diagnosis and ~2 million people remaining undiagnosed. Most patients are not clinically diagnosed until they are in their fifties.

The airflow obstruction is present because of a combination of airway and parenchymal damage resulting from chronic inflammation and is usually the result of tobacco smoke.

Significant airflow obstruction may be present before the person is aware of it. The symptoms, disability, and impaired quality of life associated with COPD may respond to pharmacological and other therapies that have limited or no impact on the airflow obstruction.

The Global Initiative for Obstructive Lung disease (GOLD) 2016 guidelines[6] and the NICE 2010 guidelines[5] also define COPD according to the severity of airflow obstruction in four stages. Pharmacological management is based on these stages, which are outlined in Table 17.8.

Table 17.8 Pharmacological management of COPD

Post-bronchodilator FEV_1/FVC	FEV_1 % predicted	Severity of airflow obstruction
<0.7	>80%	Stage 1—mild
<0.7	50–79%	Stage 2—moderate
<0.7	30–49%	Stage 3—severe
<0.7	<30%	Stage 4—very severe

Pharmacological management

Pharmacological treatment is used to manage the patient's symptoms, maintain quality of life, and reduce both the frequency and severity of exacerbations. Treatments should be monitored closely and adjusted accordingly, the effectiveness of which should be assessed by the following: patient symptoms, activities of daily living, exercise tolerance, exacerbation rate, as well as lung function.

If the treatment has no impact on the symptoms of a patient, then the medication should be reviewed with the aim of stopping.

Smoking cessation

This is the single most important intervention that can be undertaken in patients with COPD who smoke and is the only pharmacological method of reducing the rate of decline in lung function.

Smoking cessation advice is an essential part of the management of COPD and should be offered to patients at every opportunity. This action can improve symptoms of cough and sputum production as well as survival rates; however, it does not restore lung function that has already been lost.

The most successful smoking cessation interventions are those that include advice and support along with pharmacological intervention, such as nicotine replacement therapy (NRT) or oral therapy (varenicline or bupropion). These should only be prescribed when the smoker has made a commitment to stop smoking on or before a particular date.

The choice of smoking cessation product should be chosen after discussions have been held with the patient in order to deduce which method is most appropriate.

Inhaled therapy

Bronchodilators

Although characterized by irreversible airflow obstruction, many patients with COPD show clinical benefits from bronchodilators. These are noted to alleviate breathlessness by their direct effect on the airway by alleviating airway smooth muscle tone and ↑ airway calibre. These drugs can also lead to a ↓ in pulmonary hyperinflation, ↑ mucociliary clearance, and improve respiratory muscle function.

There are three classes of bronchodilator:

- β_2-agonists—short and long acting
- Antimuscarinics—short and long acting
- Methylxanthines.

Short-acting β_2-agonists

SABAs are the most widely used bronchodilators in the management of COPD. The onset of action is slower than that seen in patients with asthma. They act on β_2-adrenergic receptors within the smooth muscle of the airway, mimicking the effects of the sympathetic nervous system. They relax airway smooth muscle, enhance mucociliary clearance, and ↓ vascular permeability. Inhalation of β_2-agonists is more effective than oral administration in producing bronchodilation, giving a more rapid onset of action and fewer side effects.

Adverse effects of SABAs include tremor, tachycardia, and ↑ anxiety, but these effects are considered minimal when the drugs are taken by inhalation and at the recommended dose. Hypokalaemia is observed following inhaled and systemic administration of β_2-agonists, but is minimal during stable management and is more likely to occur during the treatment of acute exacerbations when higher doses are clinically indicated.

Examples: salbutamol, terbutaline

Long-acting β_2-agonists

The advantage of the LABAs is that they produce a sustained relaxation of the airways for ~12h. The degree of bronchodilation is similar to SABAs, with much of the same side effects, and similarly few when the inhaled route is used and at recommended doses.

Examples: salmeterol, formoterol.

Short-acting antimuscarinics

Short-acting muscarinic antagonists (SAMAs) act by reducing reflex cholinergic bronchoconstriction, vagal airway tone, and airway mucus secretion. The onset of action is slower than that seen with SABAs, with the bronchodilation being more sustained and at least as effective.

In practice, many COPD patients benefit from antimuscarinics. Side effects may include dry mouth, blurred vision, and paradoxical bronchospasm.

Example: ipratropium.

Long-acting antimuscarinics

The majority of long-acting muscarinic antagonists (LAMAs) are once-daily products and act for 24h. The exception to this is aclidinium bromide which works over a 12h period and therefore needs to be administered twice daily.

Compared to SAMAs, LAMAs have the advantages of producing improvements in lung function, health status, exercise tolerance, and reduced breathlessness.

Examples: tiotropium, glycopyrronium, aclidinium bromide.

Methylxanthines

Methylxanthines have a small bronchodilator effect in COPD and may ↑ diaphragmatic strength in patients, as well as affecting mucociliary clearance.

Due to the potential toxicity and significant interactions with other drugs, methylxanthines are only recommended for use when other treatments have failed or when a patient remains symptomatic, despite a trial of optimal bronchodilator therapy.

In order to reduce possible adverse effects (such as nausea, headaches, and GI reflux), a low dose of oral methylxanthine should be introduced, ensuring plasma levels are monitored after the initiation of therapy.

Examples: theophylline, aminophylline.

Inhaled corticosteroids

Although inflammatory changes are present in the airways of COPD patients, the inflammation is mediated by neutrophils, which are relatively insensitive to the effects of corticosteroids, even in high doses. This is different to the inflammation in asthma which is mediated by eosinophils and responds very well to corticosteroids.

ICSs appear to reduce exacerbations in COPD patients with stage 2 disease and should be prescribed in combination with a LABA.

The following are current examples of combined ICS and LABA inhalers that are licensed for use in COPD:

- Seretide 500 Accuhaler® (fluticasone propionate 500 micrograms/ salmeterol 50 micrograms per dose)—1 puff twice daily
- Symbicort 400/12 Turbohaler® (budesonide 400 micrograms/ formoterol fumarate 12 micrograms per dose)—1 puff twice daily
- Fostair® 100/6 metered dose inhaler (100 micrograms of BDP/ formoterol fumarate 6 micrograms per dose)—2 puffs twice daily
- Relvar 92/22 Ellipta® (92 micrograms of fluticasone furoate/22 micrograms of vilanterol trifenatate)—1 puff once daily.

When are inhaled therapies used in COPD?

The NICE COPD guidelines (2010)[5] recommend that inhalers should only be prescribed after patients have received training and are able to demonstrate a satisfactory technique with the most appropriate device, with the inhaler of choice being largely based on patient preference.

It is highly recommended that the reassessment of inhaler technique is carried out at every clinical encounter to ensure optimum efficacy.

The NICE COPD guidelines[5] also recommend the following sequence for inhaled therapies for people with stable COPD:

- A once-daily LAMA should be started in preference to a four-times-daily SAMA in patients with stable COPD who remain breathless or have exacerbations despite using short-acting bronchodilators as required, and in whom a decision has been made to commence regular maintenance bronchodilator therapy with a muscarinic antagonist.
- For patients with stable COPD who remain breathless or have exacerbations despite using short-acting bronchodilators as required, the following should be offered as maintenance therapy:
  - Either LABA or LAMA if FEV_1 is ≥50% predicted, or
  - Either LABA with ICS in a combination inhaler, or a LAMA if FEV_1 is <50% predicted.
- In people with stable COPD and an FEV_1 of ≥50% who remain breathless or have exacerbations despite maintenance therapy with a LABA:
  - Consider LABA + ICS in a combination inhaler, or
  - Consider LAMA in addition to LABA where ICS is declined or not tolerated.
- A LAMA should be considered in addition to LABA + ICS to people with COPD who remain breathless or have exacerbations despite taking LABA + ICS alone, irrespective of their FEV_1.
- Consider LABA + ICS in a combination inhaler in addition to a LAMA for those patients with stable COPD who remain breathless or have exacerbations despite maintenance therapy with a LAMA alone, irrespective of their FEV_1.

Other medications used in stable COPD therapy

Oral corticosteroids

Maintenance use of oral corticosteroids in COPD is not normally recommended; however, some patients with severe disease may require maintenance therapy when oral corticosteroids cannot be withdrawn following an exacerbation. In these cases, the dose should be kept as low as possible, with the patient being regularly reviewed.

It should be remembered that patients on long-term steroid tablets (i.e. >3 months) or requiring frequent courses of steroid tablets (e.g. three to four per year) will be at risk of systemic side effects. Patients should be monitored closely for any changes in BP, plasma or urine glucose levels, cholesterol, and bone mineral density. Other adverse effects of long-term oral corticosteroids include obesity, cataracts, glaucoma, skin thinning and bruising, and muscle weakness.

Patients treated with long-term oral corticosteroid therapy should be monitored for the development of osteoporosis and given appropriate prophylaxis. Patients over the age of 65 should be started on prophylactic treatment without monitoring.

Secondary adrenal insufficiency

This disorder typically results from abrupt withdrawal from chronic steroid use. This is because the exogenous administration of steroids has resulted in suppression of the hypothalamus–pituitary–adrenal (HPA) axis, causing a reduction in cortisol and androgen levels as well as plasma adrenocorticotropic hormone (ACTH) levels.

Patients with adrenal insufficiency generally present with flu-like symptoms such as fever, shaking, chills, headache, diarrhoea, cramping, vomiting, weakness, and fatigue. Other symptoms include vertigo, hypotension, depression, salt craving, and vitiligo (depigmented patches of skin). Patients with secondary adrenal insufficiency have low levels of ACTH and generally do not experience hyperpigmentation.

To avoid the development of secondary adrenal insufficiency, patients treated with chronic steroids, usually for >14 days of consecutive therapy, should undergo a taper of the glucocorticoid. In patients receiving chronic steroid administration, alternate-day dosing is preferred to reduce the risk of HPA axis suppression, once the patient has been stabilized.

Mucolytics

Many patients with COPD cough up sputum. Mucolytics are believed to ↑ the expectoration of sputum by reducing its viscosity and should be considered in patients with a chronic, productive cough. Therapy should be continued beyond 1 month if the patient reports an improvement in their cough, sputum production, or expectoration and does not report experiencing any unacceptable side effects.

Caution is advised in patients with a history of peptic ulceration as mucolytics may disrupt the gastric mucosal layer.

Examples: carbocisteine, erdosteine, mecysteine.

Oxygen therapy

Severe COPD leads to chronic hypoxia and an associated decline in the health and prognosis of a patient. If left untreated, the 5yr survival rate is <50%. The administration of supplemental oxygen has been shown to prolong life in people diagnosed with COPD.

According to the 2010 NICE guidelines,[5] long-term oxygen therapy (LTOT) is indicated in patients with COPD who have:

- a PaO_2 of <7.3kPa when stable *or*
- a PaO_2 >7.3kPa and <8kPa when stable along with one of the following:
  - secondary polycythaemia
  - nocturnal hypoxaemia (oxygen saturation of arterial blood (SaO_2) <90% for >30% of the time)
  - peripheral oedema
  - pulmonary hypertension.

For the benefits of LTOT to be noted, patients should breathe supplemental oxygen for at least 15h per day. Greater benefits are seen in patients receiving oxygen for 20h per day.

The need for oxygen therapy should be assessed in:

- all patients with very severe airflow obstruction (FEV_1 <30% predicted)
- patients with cyanosis
- patients with polycythaemia
- patients with peripheral oedema
- patients with a raised jugular venous pressure
- patients with oxygen saturations ≤92% breathing air.

Assessment should also be considered for patients diagnosed with a severe airflow obstruction (FEV_1 30–49% predicted) as well as those patients who have a confident diagnosis of COPD who are receiving optimum medical management and whose COPD is stable. Oxygen therapy is contraindicated in patients who continue to smoke.

References

5. NICE (2010). 'Chronic obstructive pulmonary disease—management of chronic obstructive pulmonary disease in adults and primary and secondary care (CG101)', ℘ www.nice.org.uk/guidance/cg101
6. Global Initiative for Chronic Obstructive Lung Disease (GOLD) (2016). 'Global strategy for the diagnosis, management and prevention of COPD', ℘ www.goldcopd.org

Therapy-related issues: central nervous system

Pain: a definition

The International Association for the Study of Pain defines pain as 'an unpleasant sensory and emotional experience associated with actual or potential tissue damage, or described in terms of such damage'.[1]

Pain is always subjective. Each individual learns the application of the word through experiences related to injury in early life. Accordingly, pain is that experience we associate with actual or potential tissue damage. It is unquestionably a sensation in a part or parts of the body, but it is always unpleasant and therefore is also an emotional experience.

Many people report pain in the absence of tissue damage or any likely pathophysiological cause. Usually this happens for psychological reasons. There is usually no way to distinguish their experience from that caused by tissue damage if we take the subjective report. If they regard their experience as pain and if they report it in the same ways as pain caused by tissue damage, it should be accepted as pain. This definition avoids tying pain to the stimulus.[1] In view of this, pharmacists should be wary of expressing opinions about whether a particular patient is in pain or not.

Types of pain

Nociceptive pain

'Nociceptive pain' is pain that occurs when nociceptors (pain receptors) are stimulated. This is normal pain in response to injury of the body. The purpose of this type of pain is to discourage the use of injured body parts, which could potentially extend the injury further. This pain normally responds to conventional analgesics, such as paracetamol, NSAIDs, and opioids (Fig. 18.1).

Neuropathic pain

'Neuropathic pain' is pain initiated or caused by a primary lesion or dysfunction in the nervous system. The pain is often triggered by an injury, but this injury might or might not involve actual damage to the nervous system. It seems to have no physiological purpose. The pain frequently has burning, lancinating (stabbing), or electric-shock qualities. Persistent allodynia, pain resulting from a non-painful stimulus such as a light touch, is also a common characteristic of neuropathic pain. The pain can persist for months or years beyond the apparent healing of any damaged tissues. This pain might not respond to standard analgesics but might respond to unconventional analgesic treatments, such as antidepressants, anticonvulsants, and various other therapies, such as clonidine or capsaicin (Fig. 18.1).

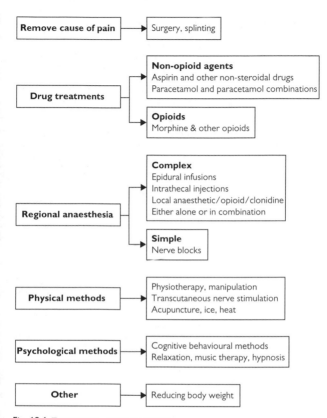

Fig. 18.1 Treating pain—methods available.

Reference

1. 'International Association for the Study of Pain' website, ℰ www.iasp-pain.org

Assessment of pain

There are good validated scales for assessing pain. These are usually derived from assessment of both pain intensity and pain relief when analgesics are used. Both visual analogue scales (VASs), a line moving from 'no pain' to 'worst possible pain', and categorical scales, using words such as 'none', 'slight', 'moderate', or 'severe', are employed, often together. They can be useful to monitor progress in patients who are suffering from pain.

Categorical scales

Categorical scales use words to describe the magnitude of the pain. The patient picks the most appropriate word; most research groups use four words (none, mild, moderate, and severe). Scales to measure pain relief were developed later. The most common is the five-category scale (none, slight, moderate, good, and complete).

For analysis, numbers are given to the verbal categories (for pain intensity, none = 0, mild = 1, moderate = 2, and severe = 3, and for relief, none = 0, slight = 1, moderate = 2, good or lots = 3, and complete = 4).

The main advantages of categorical scales are that they are quick and simple. However, the small number of descriptors could force the scorer to choose a particular category when none describes the pain satisfactorily.

Visual analogue scales

VASs, lines with the left end labelled 'no relief of pain' and the right end labelled 'complete relief of pain', seem to overcome this limitation. The standard VAS is 100mm long. Patients mark the line at the point that corresponds to their pain. The scores are obtained by measuring the distance between the 'no relief' end and the patient's mark, usually in millimetres. The main advantages of VASs are that they are simple and quick to score, avoid imprecise descriptive terms, and provide many points from which to choose. More concentration and coordination are needed, which can be difficult postoperatively or with neurological disorders.

Pain relief scales are perceived as more convenient than pain intensity scales (Fig. 18.2), probably because patients have the same baseline relief (zero), whereas they could start with different baseline intensities (usually moderate or severe). They are based on the same approach of a 100mm scale but are asked to rate the amount of relief from 0 to 100mm. Relief scale results are then easier to compare. They can also be more sensitive than intensity scales. A theoretical drawback of relief scales is that the patient has to remember what the pain was like to begin with.

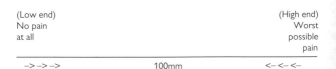

(Low end)	(High end)
No pain	Worst
at all	possible
	pain

–> –> –>   100mm   <– <– <–

Fig. **18.2** Example of a VAS for pain intensity.

Global subjective efficacy ratings, or simply 'global scales', are designed to measure overall treatment performance. Patients are asked questions such as 'How effective do you think the treatment was?' and answer using a labelled numerical or categorical scale. Although these judgements probably include adverse effects, they can be the most sensitive way to discriminate between treatments.

Judgement of pain by the patient, rather than by a carer, is the ideal. Carers tend to overestimate the pain relief compared with the patient's version (Fig. 18.2).

Instructions

It is important that the use of the scale is explained to each patient. Patients are instructed to place a mark on the line to report the intensity or quality of the sensation experienced. Instructions should be written above the scale, e.g. INSTRUCTION: Put a mark on the line at the point that best describes HOW MUCH PAIN YOU ARE HAVING RIGHT NOW. Notice that what is measured is 'the perception right now', not a comparison such as: 'What is your pain compared with what you had before?'

Fig 18.3 can be completed to show changes in pain intensity and/or pain relief across time. This can be valuable when introducing changes to analgesia and provides an ongoing assessment of progress.

A range of pain assessment tools including those in a range of languages and some for children, can be found at the Partners Against pain website.[2]

An example of a chart for patients with chronic pain is presented in Fig. 18.3. Patients are asked to assess their pain on a weekly basis and to bring their charts when attending clinics.

Reference

2. 'Partners Against Pain' website, 🔊 www.partnersagainstpain.com

1. Please choose a suitable time and day of the week, and complete the chart on the same day and time every week.
2. Stop when the chart is full, or when the pain returns to the same intensity as it was before the treatment started.
3. If you have more than one pain (e.g. back pain and leg pain) we may ask you to complete a separate chart for each pain.

Type of treatment: . . . .
Date of treatment: . . . .

Patient's name

Main Area of Pain:

	Weeks	0	1	2	3	4	5	6	7	8	9	10	11	12	13	14	15	16
How bad has your pain been today?	None																	
	Mild																	
	Moderate																	
	Severe																	
	V Severe																	
How much pain relief have you had today from the injection?	Complete																	
	Good																	
	Moderate																	
	Slight																	
	None																	
Please record the name and number of pain killing tablets taken per week																		
How effective was the treatment this week?	Excellent																	
	Very Good																	
	Good																	
	Fair																	
	Poor																	

Date when full pain returned . . . .

Used with permission

Fig. 18.3 Oxford chronic pain record chart.

Acute pain: incidence

Acute pain is common. A survey of >3000 patients newly discharged from hospital revealed the results shown in Table 18.1.

Not all of the patients in the survey had undergone surgery, so this is not just a problem for surgical wards.

Pain can be a problem after operations, dental procedures, and wound dressings. Some types of surgery have a less painful recovery than others, so analgesia must be tailored.

The need for pain relief in medical settings such as MI, sickle cell crisis, musculoskeletal disease, and renal colic must be considered along with the needs of cancer, trauma, burns, and obstetric patients.

Table 18.1 Responses to questions on pain by 3163 in-patients

	Proportion of patients (%)
Pain was present all or most of the time	33
Pain was severe or moderate	87
Pain was worse than expected	17
Had to ask for drugs	42
Drugs did not arrive immediately	41
Pain was present all or most of the time	33

Acute pain

NSAIDs and non-opioids

Effective relief can be achieved with oral non-opioids and NSAIDs. It is clear from the NNT chart (Fig. 18.4) that NSAIDs are superior to paracetamol and to paracetamol combined with codeine. Combining paracetamol with an NSAID can enhance pain relief for a number of patients in the acute phase post surgery. The current vogue of supplying separate paracetamol and codeine is to be discouraged (as a cost-saving exercise) because it leads to confusion in some patients, and there have been cases of (inadvertent) codeine overdosing leading to hospitalization.

There is wisdom in the saying that if patients can swallow, they should receive medicines by mouth. There is no evidence that NSAIDs given rectally or by injection work better or faster than the same oral dose. They do not ↓ the risk of GI damage either. Gastric upset and bleeding are important

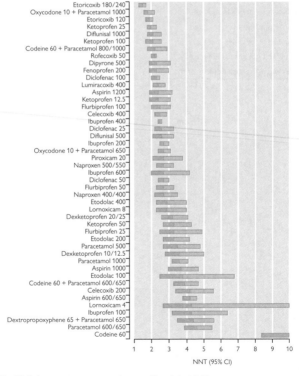

Fig. 18.4 Acute pain treatments: league table of the NNT.

adverse effects. Ibuprofen is probably the safest in this respect; however, long-term NSAID treatment should be covered with a gastric-protecting agent such as a PPI. Beware also of using NSAIDs in patients with pre-existing kidney problems; an NSAID can precipitate acute kidney injury, requiring dialysis.

The belief that NSAIDs should not be used after orthopaedic surgery because they inhibit healing is a myth.

Opioids

- These are first-line treatment for acute pain. Intermittent doses might provide effective relief, but patient-controlled analgesia is the preferred method. There are many stories of adequate doses being withheld because of misconceptions, fear, and ignorance.
- Dependence is not a problem in acute pain, and respiratory depression is only a problem if the patient is either not in pain or given doses larger than those needed to treat the pain.
- The key principle is to titrate the analgesic until either pain relief is obtained or unacceptable side effects are experienced.
- There is no evidence that one opioid is better than another, although pethidine (meperidine) should be avoided because of its toxic metabolites, which can accumulate, acting as a CNS irritant and eventually inducing convulsions, particularly if underlying renal failure is present. There is no evidence for the view that pethidine is best for renal colic pains.
- The metabolite of morphine (morphine-6-glucuronide) can accumulate in renal disease, with the effect of prolonging the action of morphine. Provided that the dose is titrated carefully, this should not be a problem.
- It makes good sense to select one opioid for the treatment of acute pain, so that everyone is familiar with its profile. In most settings, morphine does the job.

Regional anaesthesia

- Regional anaesthesia works by interrupting pain transmission from a localized area. The risk of neurological damage is the main concern.
- Pharmacists should be aware of the compatibility issues surrounding medicines for epidural or intrathecal use, in addition to careful monitoring of the doses used. Preservative-free morphine should be used as a rule (because of the potential neurotoxicity of preservatives), unless patients are in the terminal phase of illness.

Topical agents

- Topical agents can be useful in treating acute injuries, such as strains, sprains, and soft tissue trauma. There is limited evidence for the benefits of rubefacients, which work by producing a counter-irritation to relieve musculoskeletal pains. The NNT is ~2, but this is based on three small trials (with 180 participants).
- There is good systematic review evidence to show that topical NSAIDs are effective in acute pain. The NNT for pain relief is 2–4 based on 37 placebo-controlled trials with a range of NSAIDs. Ketoprofen, felbinac, ibuprofen, and piroxicam are superior to placebo, but indometacin and benzydamine are no better than placebo. Adverse events for NSAIDs were no different than placebo.

Treating cancer pain

Since the introduction of the WHO three-step ladder (Fig. 18.5), potent opioids (usually morphine) have been the analgesics of choice for managing cancer pain.

Morphine is still considered the benchmark by the European Association for Palliative Care mainly because it is available in a number of different dose forms, it has extensive clinical experience, and it has an ability to provide analgesia. However, it is not always ideal, with wide individual variation in dose needs and active metabolites that can accumulate, particularly in renal failure. There is no maximum dose for morphine, but a systematic review showed that mean daily doses range from 25 to 300mg and, in unusual cases, can reach 2000mg daily. The adverse effects of morphine are not tolerated in ~4% of patients.

Drugs such as hydromorphone and oxycodone can be substituted, but these offer no real advantages. Transdermal fentanyl has become popular in recent years and can offer less constipation and daytime drowsiness.

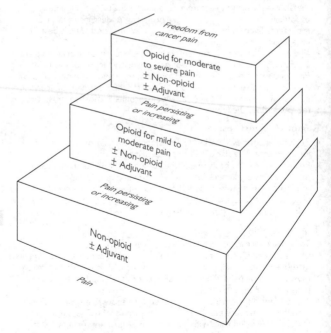

Fig. 18.5 WHO analgesic ladder.

Methadone can produce similar analgesia to morphine and has similar side effects, but it has a narrower dose range. It is the safest in renal failure; it also has a long and unpredictable half-life and its potency is often underestimated.

Spinal opioids

A few patients benefit from spinal opioids if they are unable to tolerate oral morphine. Spinal morphine in combination with a local anaesthetic is helpful for incident pain, and the addition of clonidine can help neuropathic pain. Spinal opioids are associated with greater risks, especially of epidural abscesses, CSF leaks, and catheter problems.

Dealing with breakthrough pain

Cancer pain often presents as a continuous pain, with intermittent more serious pain breaking through. This can arise in up to 80% of patients with cancer pain. Four episodes daily is about the average, with each pain lasting ~30min. There are several dose strategies to manage breakthrough pain, with the usual 4h dose every 1–2h as needed (as an instant-release formulation). With transmucosal fentanyl, there seems to be little relationship between the rescue dose and the daily dose.

Use of NSAIDs with opioids

There is good evidence that NSAIDs can ↓ the total dose of opioids and ↓ their adverse effects. Gastric protective agents are needed for chronic long-term dosing.

Equianalgesic doses for opioids

Calculating equivalent doses is not an exact science, so care is needed. The literature contains much conflicting information, so key points are listed in the next section together with some external sources for suggested conversion factors.

Key points to consider when converting patients from one opioid to another

- Ratios for acute pain might not be the same as those for chronic pain.
- Ratio tables are for guidance only—they can be useful, but there can be wide variation between individuals. Therefore the dose needs to be started cautiously and titrated to effect.
- Monitor pain and pain relief—use of pain-assessment tools and adverse-effect monitoring should be considered.
- Tolerance to one opioid might not be carried over to another—this can lead to greater potency than expected. This can be anticipated by ↓ the equianalgesic dose by a further 30–50% and providing further analgesic rescue in the early stages.
- Be careful if treating patients with renal impairment—certain metabolites accumulate in renal impairment, so caution is needed. Fentanyl probably does not produce active metabolites in renal impairment, but caution is still advised.

Further reading

There is an opioid conversion software program for use on a handheld computer (and now a desktop version) at the Johns Hopkins Center for Cancer Pain Research. You can download the program free. Free registration is required, ℘ www.hopweb.org

Department of Anesthesiology and Critical Care Medicine at Johns Hopkins Medical Center has a useful website with additional suggested resources, ℘ www.hopkinsmedicine.org/anesthesiology/index.shtml

Pereira J, Lawlor P, Vigano A, et al. (2001). Equianalgesic dose ratios for opioids. *J Pain Symptom Manage* 22: 672–87.

Regnard C (1998). Conversion ratios for transdermal fentanyl. *Eur J Palliat Care* 5: 204.

Compatibility of drugs in pain and palliative care

There are a number of mixtures in common use, including opioids combined with drugs such as baclofen, midazolam, or local anaesthetics.

It is common to differentiate between chemical and physical compatibilities. Ideally, information for the former would be available for all mixtures, but in practice this is often hard to find. Some information is available in the peer-reviewed pharmacy literature and a search of international pharmaceutical abstracts can be helpful.

Time and temperature are two key components affecting chemical reactions, so it is wise not to leave mixtures sitting in syringe drivers for many hours in a warm room. An ↑ number of a drugs mixed together and the greater the concentration will ↑ the risk of incompatibility.

The majority of recommendations are desired from on physical compatibility, i.e. drugs are mixed and no obvious colour change or precipitation occurs, even when examined microscopically. Additionally, no change in pharmacological effect is seen when the drugs are administered.

Further reading

There are several useful sources for information on common opioid mixtures:

Dickman A, Schneider J (2016). *The Syringe Driver: Continuous Subcutaneous Infusions in Palliative Care* (4th ed). Oxford: Oxford University Press.

Trissel L (2012). *Handbook of Injectable Drugs* (17th ed). Bethesda, MD: American Society of Health System Pharmacists.

Trissell LA (2012). *Trissel's Stability of Compounded Formulations* (5th ed). Washington, DC: American Pharmacists' Association.

Twycross R, Wilcock A (2014). *Palliative Care Formulary* (5th ed). Nottingham: Palliativedrugs. com Ltd.

Chronic pain

Overview

Chronic pain is a major under-treated illness. The Pain in Europe study interviewed >46 000 people and it makes grim reading.

Chronic pain is a widespread problem in Europe, affecting 1 in 5 adults. More than one-third of European households contain a pain sufferer. Two-thirds of chronic pain sufferers experience moderate pain, whereas one-third experience severe pain. The most common pain is back pain, and the most common cause of this is arthritis.

People with chronic pain have been suffering on average for 7yrs, with one-fifth of sufferers reporting a >20yr history. One-third of sufferers have pain all the time. Adequate pain control took >2yrs to achieve in >50% of sufferers. Pain has a huge social impact. One in five sufferers have lost their job as a result of their pain. A similar number have been diagnosed with depression as a result of their pain. Generally, patients are satisfied with their care, but only 23% of sufferers have seen a pain management specialist and only 1 in 10 have been evaluated using pain scales.

In terms of treatment, two-thirds of sufferers report that their pain control is inadequate at times, and one-third of sufferers believe that their doctor does not know how to control their pain.

What about the UK?

Almost 1 in 7 people in the UK suffer from chronic pain (~7.8 million people).

One-third of UK households are affected by chronic pain. 50% of chronic pain sufferers report the following:

- Feel tired all the time
- Feel helpless
- Feel older than they really are
- Do not remember what it feels like not to be in pain.

In addition, the following statistics here been reported.

- One in five sufferers say the pain is sometimes so bad that they want to die.
- Two-thirds of sufferers are *always* willing to try new treatments, but almost as many sufferers are worried about potential side effects of pain medication.
- Pain sufferers are proactive, with 80% of chronic pain sufferers treating their pain in some way, mainly with prescription medications.
- More than 1 in 5 (22%) sufferers have tried, and then stopped taking, prescription pain medication.
- Weak opioids are the most used class (50%) of pain medication.
- Other commonly prescribed drugs are paracetamol (38%) and NSAIDs (23%).
- The mean number of tablets taken every day is 5.7.

Despite this, much can be done to alleviate the suffering of patients with of chronic pain. The approach to treatment is the same as for acute pain, i.e. to titrate with analgesics until either pain relief or unacceptable side effects occur. In addition, there is a wide range of medicines other than analgesics that can provide relief.

Analgesics

In treating chronic pain, it is important to start with the simplest and most obvious treatments first, rather than move directly to unconventional analgesics. NSAIDs and/or paracetamol should be tried early. The combination of NSAIDs and paracetamol can be effective and can ↓ the dose of NSAID needed. The addition of a weak opioid can help in chronic pain. Patients on long-term NSAIDs should be given gastric protection and informed of the reasons for this. ~1 in 120 patients who take an NSAID for >2 months without gastric protection develop a bleeding ulcer, and ~1 in 1200 patients die of a bleeding ulcer.

If simple analgesics are insufficient, there are other choices including so-called 'unconventional analgesics', such as antidepressants and anticonvulsant drugs. A strong opioid can be justified for some patients, provided that adequate steps are taken to screen patients before initiating treatment.

Non-pharmacological interventions can also help. Weight loss in overweight patients who suffer with arthritis can have a real benefit. Transcutaneous electronic nerve stimulation (TENS) can also be a useful addition. Radiotherapy can be effective in dealing with painful bony metastases. In specialist clinics, nerve blocks and epidural injections can also be helpful. A list of unconventional analgesics that can be effective in chronic neuropathic pain follows. It is usual to start at low doses and titrate the dose upwards until pain relief, unacceptable adverse effects, or the maximum dose is reached:

- Amitriptyline 50–150mg at night, or similar tricyclic antidepressants.
- Carbamazepine 100mg three times daily initially, ↑ slowly up to a maximum of 1200mg daily.
- Gabapentin, doses up to 3.6g daily.
- Clonazepam 0.5mg twice daily, ↑ to 1mg three times daily.
- Baclofen 5mg three times daily, ↑ to 10mg three times daily.
- Pyridoxine 100mg up to five times daily.
- Capsaicin cream.
- Other anticonvulsants, such as pregabalin, lamotrigine, phenytoin, and sodium valproate.
- SSRIs can also be beneficial, but evidence for their use is very limited.

Antidepressant drugs for neuropathic pain

- Neuropathic pain refers to a group of painful disorders characterized by pain caused by dysfunction or disease of the nervous system at a peripheral or central level, or both. It is a complex entity, with many symptoms and signs that fluctuate in number and intensity over time. The three common components of neuropathic pain are steady and neuralgic pain paroxysmal spontaneous attacks and hypersensitivity.

- This type of pain can be very disabling, severe, and intractable, causing distress and suffering for individuals, including dysaesthesia and paraesthesia. Sensory deficits, such as partial or complex loss of sensation, are also commonly seen.
- The clinical impression is that both antidepressants and anticonvulsants are useful for neuropathic pain, but there are unanswered questions, including the following.
  - Which drug class should be the first-line choice?
  - Is one antidepressant drug superior to another?
  - Is there any difference in response to antidepressants in different neuropathic syndromes?
- The mechanisms of action of antidepressant drugs in the treatment of neuropathic pain are uncertain. Analgesia is often achieved at lower dosage and faster (usually within a few days) than the onset of any antidepressant effect, which can take up to 6wks. In addition, there is no correlation between the effect of antidepressants on mood and pain. Furthermore, antidepressants produce analgesia in patients with and without depression.
- Two main groups of antidepressants are in common use: the older tricyclic antidepressants, such as amitriptyline, imipramine, and many others, and a newer group of SSRIs. The clinical impression was that tricyclic antidepressants are more effective in treating neuropathic pain. However, SSRIs are gaining acceptance for pain relief.
- Tricyclic antidepressants exhibit more significant adverse effects which limit clinical use, particularly in the elderly. The most serious adverse effects of tricyclic antidepressants occur within the cardiovascular system:
  - Postural hypotension
  - Heart block
  - Arrhythmias.
- The most common adverse effects are:
  - sedation
  - anticholinergic effects (e.g. dry mouth, constipation, and urinary retention).
- SSRIs are better tolerated. They are free from cardiovascular side effects, are less sedative, and have fewer anticholinergic effects than tricyclic antidepressants.

Depression

Background and prevalence

Depression is very common—>350 million people worldwide suffer with depression and it affects all ages.[3] There is a particularly high prevalence in those with long-term physical conditions such as cardiovascular disease, cancer, diabetes, Parkinson's disease, and stroke as well as a high prevalence in the elderly; 10–15% of women having a baby will suffer with depression.

A depressive episode is classed as mild, moderate, or severe depending on the number and severity of symptoms and the impact on daily living. Those with severe depression may be completely unable to function. Symptoms can vary significantly between people but in general, low mood, hopelessness, and loss of pleasure in activities that were once enjoyed are present. Other psychological symptoms include feelings of guilt, anxiety, low self-esteem, and suicidal thoughts. Physical symptoms such as changes in appetite, weight loss, fatigue, aches and pains, loss of libido, and disturbed sleep (e.g. early morning wakening) are also often present. A diagnosis of depression is only made if symptoms have been present for 2wks or more. Depression often relapses and remits but the aim of treatment is complete resolution of symptoms and maintenance of remission.

Severe depression may also present with psychotic symptoms (hallucinations or delusions) which may or may not be mood congruent, psychomotor retardation, or stupor.

Certain medicines can cause depression as a side effect and this should always be considered during an assessment, or where depressive symptoms have worsened. Examples include:

- anticonvulsants—e.g. levetiracetam, zonisamide, pregabalin, gabapentin
- antihypertensives—e.g. β-blockers, calcium channel blockers, ACE inhibitors
- corticosteroids
- opiates
- contraceptives.

Treatment

A stepped care model is used to manage depression in the UK.[4]

Psychological therapies are usually sufficient to treat mild depressive episodes.

Medication (in combination with psychological therapy) is usually necessary for moderate to severe depressive episodes. Classifications for antidepressants are shown in Table 18.2.

Serotonin reuptake inhibitors (SSRIs) are usually recommended first line.[4] It is generally accepted that no antidepressant is significantly more effective than any other, however there is some evidence that sertraline and escitalopram are the most effective and the best tolerated antidepressants.[5]

Table 18.2 Classification of antidepressants

SSRIs	Serotonin and noradrenaline (norepinephrine) reuptake inhibitors (SNRIs)	Tricyclic antidepressants (TCAs)	Monoamine oxidase inhibitors (MAOI and RIMA***)	Noradrenaline (norepinephrine) reuptake inhibitors	Others
Citalopram	Duloxetine	Amitriptyline	Isocarboxazid	Reboxetine	Agomelatine
Escitalopram	Venlafaxine	Imipramine	Phenelzine		Flupentixol****
Fluoxetine		Lofepramine*	Tranylcypromine		Mirtazapine
Fluvoxamine		Clomipramine**	Moclobemide***		Trazodone
Paroxetine					
Sertraline					

* Lofepramine is a TCA but predominantly inhibits the reuptake of noradrenaline.

** Clomipramine is a TCA, but predominantly inhibits the reuptake of serotonin.

*** Moclobemide is a reversible inhibitor of monoamine oxidase A.

**** Flupentixol is a thioxanthene antipsychotic with antidepressant properties at low doses.

Initiating an antidepressant

Doses should start low and be ↑ slowly according to response and tolerability.

The following advice should be given:[5]

- The likelihood of developing adverse effects (see Table 18.3).
- Response is achieved gradually and may take several weeks for the best effect from a dose to become apparent.
- Treatment will need to be continued for 6 months after remission of symptoms (for a first episode) but may need to continue indefinitely if there have been recurrent episodes.
- Antidepressants are not addictive but may be associated with discontinuation symptoms if stopped suddenly.
- There may be an ↑ risk of suicidal thoughts in the early stages of treatment, particularly in younger people.

If response to an initial antidepressant is inadequate at the maximum tolerated dose for an appropriate length of time—usually 3 or 4wks—or if it is not tolerated, switch to a different antidepressant. NICE recommends a different SSRI or a better tolerated newer-generation antidepressant. Antidepressants from other pharmacological groups can be considered if response from this strategy is insufficient, but tolerability may not be as good.

Adverse effects

Most antidepressants are usually well tolerated but all may be associated with some adverse effects, particularly at the start of treatment. TCAs are generally associated with a greater side effect burden than newer antidepressants, such as the SSRIs and SNRIs. MAOIs are not so commonly used and are usually reserved for the treatment of depression that has not responded to other antidepressants. They have a high side effect burden and their use is complicated by the dietary restrictions that are required (see Table 18.3 for more detail).

Serotonin syndrome

All antidepressants that raise serotonin levels can potentially cause serotonin syndrome, however it is more common with the SSRIs and SNRIs (and the predominantly serotonergic TCA clomipramine). Serotonin syndrome is a potentially life-threatening adverse effect. Symptoms initially may be mild and include tachycardia, shivering, sweating, mydriasis, diarrhoea, and tremor but if not treated can quickly escalate to life-threatening delirium, neuromuscular rigidity, and hyperthermia. Serotonin syndrome is more likely with higher doses or when used in combination with other drugs that ↑ serotonin levels (e.g. other antidepressants, lithium, triptans, and tramadol). Care should also be taken when switching between antidepressants, particularly from those with long half-lives such as fluoxetine. Anticholinergic poisoning, malignant hyperthermia, and neuroleptic malignant syndrome should be excluded. Removal of the precipitating drug usually results in quick resolution; however, supportive symptomatic treatment may be necessary in hospital.

Table 18.3 Adverse effects of antidepressants

Adverse effect	Incidence	Advice and management
SSRIs and SNRIs		
Nausea	Common, particularly at the start of treatment. It is related to dose and is usually transient	Minimize by starting with low doses and taking with food. In severe cases, nausea can be alleviated with a short course of an antiemetic
Anxiety	Occasionally anxiety may be exacerbated, particularly at the start of treatment, but SSRIs are anxiolytic in the long term	Advice and reassurance may be all that is necessary
Bleeding	There is an ↑ risk of bruising, nose bleeds, GI bleeding, and prolonged bleeding time. The absolute risk is very small and comparable to the relative risk with aspirin or other NSAIDs	Monitor. If bleeding occurs withdraw the antidepressant and switch to one with a lower risk, e.g. mirtazapine
Insomnia	Common	Can be helped by taking the dose in the morning or a dose reduction NB: insomnia is also a common symptom of depression and treating the depression with an antidepressant may improve the insomnia
Sexual dysfunction and loss of libido	Common and not usually transient	Switch to a lower-risk antidepressant, e.g. mirtazapine or moclobemide
Hyponatraemia	See below	Switch to an antidepressant with a different mode of action
Suicidal thoughts and self-harm	There may be an ↑ risk of suicidal thoughts in the early stages of treatment, particularly in younger people	Advise the patient and monitor closely, particularly during the first few weeks of treatment
Serotonin syndrome	See below	Stop antidepressant and treat serotonin syndrome accordingly
TCAs		
Nausea	Common, particularly at the start of treatment. It is related to dose and is usually transient	Minimize by starting with low doses and taking with food. In severe cases, nausea can be alleviated with a short course of an antiemetic

Table 18.3 (*Contd.*)

Adverse effect	Incidence	Advice and management
Anticholinergic effects, e.g. dry mouth, nausea, constipation, blurred vision	Very common	Usually transient If persistent, treat appropriately, e.g. treat constipation by ↑ fibre/use laxative, or consider lower-risk antidepressant
Cardiovascular effects, e.g. postural hypotension, tachycardia	Common	Advise patients who feel dizzy on standing to stand up slowly A fast pulse is usually transient. Persistent tachycardia may need to be treated—or switch antidepressant
Weight gain/ appetite ↑	Very common	Recommend healthy eating and ↑ exercise. Switch to lower-risk antidepressant if appropriate
Drowsiness	Very common with sedating TCAs (e.g. amitriptyline, clomipramine, trimipramine)	Sedative properties may be beneficial for some people. If drowsiness becomes a problem switch to a non-sedating TCA (e.g. imipramine, lofepramine, nortriptyline) or a different class of antidepressant
Sexual dysfunction	Common and not usually transient	Switch to a lower-risk antidepressant, e.g. mirtazapine or moclobemide
Hyponatraemia	See below	Switch to an antidepressant with a different mode of action
Serotonin syndrome	See below	Stop antidepressant and treat serotonin syndrome accordingly
MAOIs		
Anticholinergic effects, e.g. dry mouth, nausea, constipation, blurred vision	Very common	Usually transient If persistent, treat appropriately, e.g. treat constipation by ↑ fibre/use laxative, or consider lower-risk antidepressant
Postural hypotension	Very common	Advise patients who feel dizzy on standing to stand up slowly

(Continued)

Table 18.3 (*Contd.*)

Adverse effect	Incidence	Advice and management
Hypertensive crisis	Rare	MAOIs prevent the breakdown of tyramine, and a build-up of tyramine can result in dangerous ↑ in BP (hypertensive crisis). Tyramine is present if foods such as cheese, hung game, processed meat, paté, avocados, sauerkraut, yeast extracts such as Marmite®, and red wine
Weight gain	Uncommon	Recommend healthy eating and ↑ exercise. Switch to lower-risk antidepressant if appropriate
Insomnia	Common	Take the last dose of the day no later than early afternoon
Hyponatraemia	See below	Switch to an antidepressant with a different mode of action
Serotonin syndrome	See below	Stop antidepressant and treat serotonin syndrome accordingly
Others—mirtazapine		
Drowsiness	Very common	May be more of a problem at the start of treatment. Lower doses are more likely to cause drowsiness than higher doses. Usually a transient effect. Take before bedtime
Weight gain	Very common	Recommend healthy eating and ↑ exercise. Switch to lower-risk antidepressant if appropriate

Hyponatraemia

Hyponatraemia is a relatively uncommon, but potentially serious problem that can occur as a result of antidepressant treatment. It is usually seen early on in treatment—often within a few days to weeks, but it can occur at any time. Risk factors include being elderly, ♀, and being a smoker. Antidepressants affecting serotonin reuptake may be more likely to cause hyponatraemia than those that predominantly affect noradrenaline reuptake (e.g. lofepramine and reboxetine).

If hyponatraemia occurs stop the antidepressant, monitor sodium levels daily until levels normalize—this could take a few days, but has in some cases taken several weeks. Mild hyponatraemia (sodium >125mmol/L) may respond to fluid restriction but very low levels (<125mmol/L) or sympto-matic patients should receive appropriate treatment urgently.

Once the sodium has returned to normal, antidepressant treatment can be restarted. This should usually be with an antidepressant from a different class. Monitor sodium levels weekly for the first few weeks. Re-challenge with the same antidepressant or one from the same class often results in return of low sodium levels, but may in some cases be necessary. Take into account the following when selecting an alternative:

• Response to previously tried antidepressants.
• The condition being treated.
• Other adverse effects.
• Risks in overdose (is the patient suicidal?).

Notes on specific antidepressants are displayed in Table 18.4.

Discontinuation symptoms

All antidepressants have the potential to cause discontinuation symptoms when they are stopped if taken for longer than about 6–8wks. Symptoms are more likely to occur if the antidepressant is stopped suddenly or if it has a short half-life (e.g. paroxetine, venlafaxine) but not everyone will experience a problem. Symptoms are generally mild and transient but for some people they can be unpleasant and not well tolerated. To help reduce the likelihood of them occurring, antidepressants should be stopped gradually—usually over several weeks.

Discontinuing TCAs, SSRIs, and SNRIs can commonly result in flu-like symptoms and can affect sleep by causing vivid dreams or insomnia. Other symptoms vary depending on the antidepressant being stopped but may include nausea, anxiety, and irritability.

Treatment-resistant depression

Different strategies may be employed to help treat resistant depression. The most common strategies include the following:

• Combining antidepressants with different modes of action.
• Augmenting the existing antidepressant with lithium (see ➌ p. 431). For recurrent unipolar depression, aim for a minimum lithium level of 0.5mmol/L. Some people may require higher levels in the range of 0.5–1mmol/L.
• Augmenting with an antipsychotic such as aripiprazole, olanzapine, quetiapine, or risperidone (see ➌ p. 423).

Other strategies include the use of liothyronine, bupropion, tryptophan, or electroconvulsive therapy (ECT).

St John's wort

St John's wort is a herbal treatment that can be bought over the counter in many pharmacies and health food shops. It may be beneficial in mild to moderate depression[6] but it is unclear if it is effective in severe depression. St John's wort may weakly inhibit MAO-A and MAO-B, inhibit reuptake of serotonin, dopamine and noradrenaline, and upregulate 5-HT_2 recep-tors.[7] As St John's wort products are not regulated or standardized, their content (and effects) can differ significantly. NICE advises practitioners not

Table 18.4 Important notes about specific antidepressants

Fluoxetine	Fluoxetine and its metabolite are strong CYP2D6 and CYP3A4 inhibitors and are therefore associated with a large number of drug interactions. Fluoxetine (and its active metabolite) has a long half-life and takes several weeks to clear from the body
Citalopram and escitalopram	Citalopram and escitalopram are associated with dose-dependent QT interval prolongation. Both are contraindicated in patients with known QT interval prolongation or congenital long QT syndrome and in anyone taking another other medicines known to prolong the QT interval (e.g. antipsychotics, TCAs, methadone, some antimicrobials, lithium, some antihistamines, antimalarials)
	Combined use may not always be possible to avoid:
	• E.g. citalopram plus an antipsychotic—if other treatments have been ineffective/not tolerated and relapse is considered a greater risk than continuing with the combination, ensure regular ECG monitoring is in place (e.g. 6–12-monthly) and any other risk factors are reduced and monitored
	• E.g. in otherwise healthy patients with an infection that has sensitivities to a contraindicated antimicrobial (macrolides, pentamidine, 4-quinolones), where another antimicrobial that is not contraindicated cannot be used, combined treatment could be justified, as the risk from the infection is likely to be greater than the possible ↑ in risk of prolonging the QT interval from adding a short course of antimicrobial treatment
	NB: both these examples constitute off-label use
Paroxetine Venlafaxine	Due to the very short half-lives of these antidepressants they are associated with a high incidence of discontinuation symptoms (see below)
Mirtazapine	Mirtazapine is one of the most sedating antidepressants. It is also associated with a high incidence of weight gain
Agomelatine	Agomelatine may cause liver toxicity. The risk is greatest earlier on in treatment. LFTs are required at baseline and at 3, 6, 12, and 24wks after starting treatment. Agomelatine should be stopped if transaminases ↑ >3 × upper limit of normal. Advise patients to watch for signs and symptoms that may suggest liver damage such as bruising, jaundice, and dark urine
Tricyclic antidepressants	Tricyclic antidepressants are associated with the greatest risk in overdose (with the exception of lofepramine) and should be avoided in anyone who is suicidal
Moclobemide	Moclobemide is a reversible inhibitor of MAO-A. For most people there is not an issue with moclobemide and tyramine (see MAOIs and hypertensive crises earlier in this table), however some people may be particularly sensitive and it is generally recommended that large quantities of tyramine-rich food should be avoided. If patients are taking more than the licensed dose of moclobemide, the full dietary restrictions of a MAOI should be followed

to prescribe it or to recommend that it is used by people with depression because of uncertainty about appropriate doses, persistence of effect, variation in the nature of preparations and potential serious interactions with other drugs.[4] St John's wort causes pharmacokinetic interactions with other medicines by inducing CYP3A4 and through effects on P-glycoprotein.[7] Medicines that may be affected include oral contraceptives, anticoagulants, certain anticonvulsants, antiretrovirals, digoxin, verapamil, and ciclosporin. There is also the potential for a pharmacodynamic interaction with other antidepressants and triptans resulting in serotonin syndrome (see 'Serotonin syndrome', p. 415).

References
3. World Health Organization (2016). 'Depression. Fact sheet no 369', ℘ www.who.int/mediacentre/factsheets/fs369/en/
4. NICE (2009, updated 2016). 'Depression in adults: recognition and management (CG90)', ℘ www.nice.org.uk/guidance/cg90
5. Cipriani A, Furukawa TA, Salanti G, et al. (2009). Comparative efficacy and acceptability of 12 new-generation antidepressants: a multiple treatments meta-analysis. *Lancet* 373:746–58.
6. Linde K, Berner MM, Kriston L (2008). St John's wort for major depression. *Cochrane Database Syst Rev* 4: CD000448.
7. Driver S (Ed) 'Herbal Medicines', ℘ www.medicinescomplete.com/about/publications.htm

Schizophrenia and psychosis

There are numerous causes for psychosis, which can be best described as a loss of contact with reality. Hallucinations, delusions, and thought disorder may be present.

The following may cause psychosis:

- Infections, particularly in the elderly
- Seizures
- Parkinson's disease
- Dementia
- Stroke
- Stressful life events
- Certain medicines (e.g. cabergoline, levodopa, steroids, methylphenidate)
- Substance misuse or withdrawal
- Mental disorders such as schizophrenia, mania, severe depression (see ➜ 'Depression', pp. 413–21), and some personality disorders
- Autoimmune process—antibody screening should take place in all patients with an acute psychotic presentation if not previously tested.

Management of psychosis depends on the cause.

Schizophrenia

Schizophrenia is a serious mental illness with a prevalence of ~1%. There is often (but not always) a prodromal phase, where a change in behaviour, thoughts, and perceptions are experienced before the onset of clear psychotic symptoms. This phase varies in duration from a few days to a few years. A first psychotic episode often occurs in late adolescence or early adulthood, but can occur at any time, and the condition affects more ♂ than ♀. Schizophrenia is a lifelong illness and often associated with poor levels of functioning, high levels of unemployment, and poor quality of life. There is considerable stigma associated with schizophrenia and there remains a disparity in the level of healthcare that people with a diagnosis of schizophrenia receive. Schizophrenia is associated with higher levels of morbidity and mortality than in the rest of the population. People with schizophrenia die on average ~15–20yrs earlier than the general population, with suicide being one of the major causes of death. Cardiovascular disease is also a significant cause. Demographically there more are smokers and higher levels of obesity and type 2 diabetes. People with schizophrenia not only need appropriate treatment of their psychotic symptoms but also need a high level of input to, and aggressive treatment of, their physical health. Physical health screening for patients with schizophrenia is essential.

Symptoms of schizophrenia are often divided into positive and negative symptoms.

Positive symptoms:

- Delusions—these may be:
  - paranoid—e.g. believing that someone is watching them through hidden cameras
  - of reference—e.g. believing that someone on the TV is specifically sending them a message
  - of grandeur—e.g. believing that they are Jesus
  - of control—e.g. believing that an alien force is controlling their actions.

- Hallucinations—e.g. hearing voices discussing them or talking about what they are doing.
- Thought disorder—e.g. disorganized thinking which may present as garbled speech.

Negative symptoms:
- Marked apathy
- Paucity of speech
- Blunting or incongruity of affect.

A diagnosis of schizophrenia is made when certain symptoms have been present for most of the time during a period of at least 1 month.[8]

Psychotic episodes are treated with antipsychotics (APs), which may be combined with cognitive behavioural therapy. APs are often divided into two groups—the 'typicals' or 'first-generation' and the 'atypicals' or 'second-generation' (see Table 18.5).

The precise mode of action of APs is unknown. First-generation APs are dopamine antagonists, resulting in reduced dopaminergic neurotransmission in the brain. With the exception of aripiprazole, second-generation APs are dopamine and serotonin (5-HT$_{2a}$) antagonists. Aripiprazole is different as it reduces dopaminergic neurotransmission by partial agonism at D$_2$ receptors, as well as being a 5-HT$_{2a}$ antagonist. APs also bind to other various receptors, some of which may contribute to their efficacy and some (e.g. histamine-1, muscarinic, alpha-1) contribute to their side effect profiles.

Table 18.5 Classification of antipsychotics

First-generation APs	Second-generation APs
Chlorpromazine	Amisulpride
Fluphenazine	Aripiprazole
Flupentixol	Asenapine*
Levomepromazine	Clozapine
Haloperidol	Lurasidone
Perphenazine	Olanzapine
Pericyazine	Paliperidone
Pimozide	Quetiapine
Prochlorperazine	Risperidone
Promazine	
Sulpiride	
Trifluoperazine	
Zuclopenthixol	

* UK licence for acute mania only.

The grouping into first and second generation is not usually helpful, particularly when considering the second-generation antipsychotics, which all differ significantly in their receptor pharmacology and notably in their side effect profiles. The first-generation APs are associated with a higher incidence of movement disorders than the second-generation Aps; however, the second-generation APs are associated with varying degrees of numerous other serious adverse effects. With the exception of clozapine all antipsychotics are equally efficacious; however, there is some evidence to suggest that amisulpride may have better efficacy[9] than other APs (not including clozapine). Antipsychotic choice is therefore guided by relative risk of side effects and by patient preference.

Starting treatment with antipsychotics

Baseline physical monitoring should be carried out prior to starting antipsychotics wherever possible. Initial doses should be low and ↑ according to response and tolerability. Many side effects are dose related. APs should be trialled for 4–6wks at a therapeutic dose. If there is a poor response following an adequate trial, a second AP should be trialled. If there has been an inadequate response to two APs clozapine is indicated (see Table 18.6).

Depots and long-acting injections

For some people, compliance with medication can be a significant problem, resulting in frequent relapses. APs in depot or long-acting injection form may be appropriate. Almost 100% of people with schizophrenia who stop their oral antipsychotic will eventually relapse. First-generation depot APs are formulated in oil and they are given every 1–4wks depending on the AP and the level of symptom control achieved and administered into the gluteal muscle.

In the UK, there are currently four second-generation long-acting injection (LAI) formulations available: risperidone, paliperidone, aripiprazole, and olanzapine (see Table 18.8)

Monitoring

Baseline monitoring[10] prior to the initiation of an AP:

- Weight, waist circumference.
- Pulse and BP.
- Fasting blood glucose and HbA1c.
- Blood lipid profile.
- Prolactin level (for APs that raise prolactin).
- Assessment of any movement disorders.
- Assessment of nutritional status, diet, and level of physical activity.
- ECG in all in-patients, or if stated in the SPC or if there is a cardiovascular disease or cardiovascular risk factors.

Subsequent monitoring:

- Weight—weekly for the first 6wks, then at 12wks, at 1yr and then annually.
- Waist circumference annually.
- Pulse and BP at 12wks and then annually.
- Fasting blood glucose, HbA1c, and blood lipids at 12wks, at 1yr and then annually.
- Emergence of movement disorders.

Table 18.6 Antipsychotic adverse effects and their management

Sedation and somnolence	Usually more of a problem at the start of treatment and often resolves, however it may persist. Manipulate the dose if possible (take the dose at night if once daily, or take a larger dose at night if twice-daily dosing)
Weight gain	Diet, exercise, switch to lower risk AP if appropriate*
Blood glucose dysregulation, diabetes, and lipid abnormalities	Switch to a lower-risk AP if appropriate* as metabolic adverse effects have significant long-term implications. If switching is not possible, monitor more closely, minimize other risks, and treat complications following standard guidance
Cardiovascular complications	ECG abnormalities—QTc prolongation; changes in BP, tachycardia, longer-term indirect cardiac complications associated with obesity and diabetes. Monitor and switch to lower-risk drug if appropriate*

Movement disorders, also called extrapyramidal side effects (EPSEs), include:

Parkinsonian-like symptoms such as tremor and rigidity.	Treat with an anticholinergic or switch to a lower-risk AP*
Akathisia—a feeling of inner restlessness.	Anticholinergics do not help. A dose reduction may help or consider switching to a lower-risk AP*
Dystonias (muscular spasms affecting the face and body)	Spasms can occur acutely on initiation of antipsychotics (within hours to a few days) causing spasms in the neck resulting in a twisted head (torticollis) and/or an oculogyric crisis (eyes rolling upwards) and requires prompt treatment with anticholinergic drugs (IV or IM administration may be necessary)
Tardive dyskinesia (TD)	Usually associated with longer-term use of antipsychotics and often presents as abnormal mouth and tongue movements. Anticholinergics should be stopped. Withdrawal of the AP or switching to a lower-risk AP* usually results in resolution; however, TD can be irreversible
Hyperprolactinaemia	Raised prolactin can cause sexual dysfunction, gynaecomastia, galactorrhoea, and in the longer term osteoporosis as a result of hypogonadism. Most antipsychotics can raise prolactin. However, aripiprazole, lurasidone, quetiapine, and olanzapine do not generally cause a sustained rise in prolactin and are alternatives to switch to if appropriate*

(Continued)

Table 18.6 (*Contd.*)

Sexual dysfunction	May be related to raised prolactin but various other mechanisms, including the effect of antipsychotics on alpha-1 and cholinergic receptors, can also contribute. It is a significant reason for poor compliance
Photosensitivity	This is a listed side effect of many antipsychotics; however, the only AP that specifically requires an alert to be included in the labelling is chlorpromazine. Patients should be advised to avoid sun exposure and to use a high factor sunscreen.
Neuroleptic malignant syndrome (NMS)	This is a rare side effect of all APs. NMS has a variable onset but can develop very quickly. Early features often include rigidity and an altered mental state, and these are then followed by autonomic changes and hyperthermia. If not identified and treated, NMS can be fatal

* Switching may result in relapse therefore should be done with care and with close monitoring for signs of relapse. See Table 18.7 or alternatives when an AP is poorly tolerated.

Table 18.7 Lower-risk AP treatment options (based on relative risk for side effects)

Side effect	Best choice (alphabetical)	Other choices (alphabetical)
Sedation	Amisulpride, aripiprazole, sulpiride	Haloperidol, risperidone, trifluoperazine
Weight gain/ metabolic effects (raised lipids, raised glucose)	Amisulpride, aripiprazole, haloperidol, lurasidone, trifluoperazine	Quetiapine, risperidone
QT prolongation	Aripiprazole, lurasidone	Olanzapine
Dystonias and parkinsonian-like side effects	Aripiprazole, lurasidone, olanzapine, quetiapine	Risperidone (<4mg/day), clozapine (third-line only)
Akathisia	Quetiapine	Clozapine (third-line only)
Tardive dyskinesia	Clozapine	Quetiapine
Hyperprolactinaemia	Aripiprazole, lurasidone, quetiapine	Olanzapine, clozapine (third-line only)

- Side effects and impact on functioning.
- Overall physical health.
- Once on a stable dose for 3–6 months enquire about potential symptoms of hyperprolactinaemia—check prolactin if symptoms are present. If it is normal there is no need for further measurements unless symptoms indicate a need, if doses change, or if the AP is switched to a different prolactin raising AP.

Table 18.8 Comparison of long-acting injection (LAI) antipsychotics

AP LAI	Formulation	Dose frequency	Administration site	Notes
Risperidone	Extended-release microspheres in an aqueous solution	Fortnightly	Deltoid or gluteal	Requires a minimum of 3 but often 5 or 6wks of oral supplementation on initiation due to the LAI's release characteristics. Refrigeration required
Paliperidone	Nanoparticles suspended in an aqueous solution	Monthly	Doses 1 and 2 = deltoid Third dose onward = either the deltoid or gluteal	Loading dose required—day 1 and day 8 followed by monthly thereafter
Aripiprazole	Aqueous suspension	Monthly	Gluteal	Requires 14 days of oral supplementation
Olanzapine	Aqueous suspension	4 weekly	Gluteal	3h of post-injection observation in a healthcare facility is required after every dose to monitor for post-injection syndrome

Clozapine

Clozapine is the most effective antipsychotic and is associated with a lower mortality rate than other APs; however, due to its risk of causing agranulocytosis it is licensed only for treatment-resistant schizophrenia.

- Indicated only when a trial of two APs (including a second-generation AP) have been ineffective or not tolerated.
- Requires the patient, prescriber, and dispensing pharmacy to be registered with a clozapine monitoring service.
- FBCs (specifically for WBCs, neutrophils, and platelets) are required weekly for first 18wks, then fortnightly between weeks 18 and 52, then monthly thereafter. If clozapine is discontinued, monthly monitoring should continue for 4wks.
- Clozapine requires a very gradual dose titration phase which lasts at least 2wks.
- A break in treatment may require a re-titration (see p. 428).
- Clozapine can only be given if the most recent blood result is green (or amber).
- Clozapine must be stopped if the blood result is red.

- Advise the patient to be aware of signs and symptoms that might indicate neutropenia such as a sore throat/flu-like illnesses.
- Do not use with other medicines that carry a significant risk of neutropenia (e.g. carbamazepine).

Clozapine monitoring

- Baseline:
  - FBC, temperature, BP and pulse.
- On initiation:
  - temperature, BP and pulse hourly for the first 6h and then twice a day until the titration is complete—if parameters are abnormal: closely monitor; if normal: monitor, but determine the frequency on an individual basis.
- Carry out monitoring recommended by NICE.
- Additional ongoing monitoring:
  - FBCs.
  - Plasma level—this is usually only recommended where compliance or toxicity is a concern. However it is sometimes used as an aid to finding the safest and most effective dose for a patient, but remember to treat the patient and not the level. Recommended range = 0.35–0.6mg/L.
  - Ask about smoking status, see ❯ 'Clozapine and smoking', p. 429.

Clozapine adverse effects

See Table 18.6 (p. 425) and Table 18.9, but clozapine has a low risk for movement disorders and for hyperprolactinaemia.
  Also:

- *Neutropenia*—risk is greatest during the first 18wks and is unpredictable.
- *Hypotension*—common particularly during the initial titration and may require a slower titration or a dose reduction; advise the patient to stand slowly from lying or sitting.
- *Hypertension*—can occur during initiation and may require a slower titration or a dose reduction.
- *Tachycardia*—very common particularly during titration. It is usually not clinically significant (but may be a symptom of myocarditis). Symptoms may resolve on slower titration or a dose reduction. Sometimes it can persist and treatment with a β-blocker may be necessary.
- *Fever*—most common in the early weeks of treatment and usually clinically insignificant, but check FBC, give paracetamol, and consider myocarditis.
- *Myocarditis*—this is rare but the greatest risk is during the first couple of months of treatment. Tachycardia if persistent at rest and associated with fever, hypotension, or chest pain may indicate myocarditis. Other symptoms include flu-like symptoms, fatigue, dyspnoea, and arrhythmias. Clozapine should be stopped if myocarditis is suspected.
- *Constipation*—a very common and important side effect but often overlooked. It is usually not clinically significant and can be easily treated. However, rarely constipation can result in serious complications and fatalities.
- *Hypersalivation*—very common and related to dose/plasma level. Often worse at night but can occur during the day. A dose reduction may help (but care as may compromise efficacy). Non-drug measures include using

Table 18.9 Green, amber, and red FBC results (×10⁹/L)

Green	Amber	Red
WBC >3.5	WBC 3–3.5	WBC <3.0
and	or	or
neutrophils >2	neutrophils 1.5–2	neutrophils <1.5
and		or
no ↓ of >10% or repeatedly ↓ values in previous test(s)		platelets <50

absorbent pillows at night and/or chewing gum during the day. Hyoscine (sucked or chewed) is commonly used, but other treatments may also help, e.g. pirenzepine, atropine eye drops as a mouth wash, ipratropium nasal spray sprayed under the tongue (all are off-label or unlicensed uses).

• *Seizures*—clozapine is the most epileptogenic AP. The risk is dose/plasma-level related. If response is only achieved with high plasma levels, prophylactic seizure cover should be started—usually this is with valproate, and sometimes with lamotrigine particularly if augmentation is necessary (but never with carbamazepine due to additive risk if neutropenia). Take great care with or avoid concomitant use with other medicines that lower the seizure threshold.

Missed doses

It is important that clozapine is taken regularly. Treatment breaks of >48h require re-titration. A FBC should be taken and the clozapine monitoring service contacted. The frequency of FBC monitoring is ↑ to weekly for 6wks if the treatment break has been >72h.

Clozapine and smoking

Smoking significantly reduces clozapine levels. The polyaromatic hydrocarbons in smoke (not the nicotine) induce CYP1A2, which is responsible for metabolizing clozapine. If a patient wants to stop smoking this should ideally be planned so that baseline clozapine levels can be taken, the patient monitored, gradual dose reductions made, and further level monitoring carried out.

If smoking cessation is unplanned (e.g. on admission to hospital), clozapine levels will ↑ and serious adverse effects could occur as the plasma level rises. Patients should be very carefully monitored and the dose amended accordingly. It is estimated that it may take 4 days to 1wk for enzymes to return to pre-smoking levels, it will then take a few more days for clozapine to reach a new steady state level and complications may take up to 3wks before being seen, so continued vigilance is necessary. The use of nicotine replacement therapy does not prevent this interaction from happening. Timely plasma level monitoring may be useful.

References

8. Cooper JE (Ed) (1994). *Pocket Guide to the ICD-10 Classification of Mental and Behavioural Disorders*. Edinburgh: Churchill Livingstone.
9. Leucht S, Cipriani A, Spineli L, et al. (2013). Comparative efficacy and tolerability of 15 antipsychotic drugs in schizophrenia: a multiple-treatments meta-analysis. *Lancet* 382: 951–62.
10. NICE (2013, updated 2016). 'Psychosis and schizophrenia in children and young people: recognition and management (CG155)', ℘ www.nice.org.uk/guidance/cg155

Bipolar disorder

Background and prevalence

Bipolar disorder is a serious mental illness characterized by episodes of elevated or irritable mood (manic or hypomanic episodes) and episodes of low mood and loss of energy (depressive episodes). A diagnosis should only be made after a definite episode of hypomania, mania, or a mixed episode.

Hypomania

At least 4 days of elevated or irritable mood along with at least three of the following signs that are interfering with daily functioning:[11]

- ↑ activity; ↑ talkativeness, concentration difficulties, reduced need for sleep, ↑ sexual energy, overfamiliarity, mildly irresponsible behaviour.

Mania

Usually at least a week of elevated, expansive or irritable mood along with at least three of the following signs that are severely interfering with daily functioning:[11]

- ↑ activity, ↑ talkativeness, flight of ideas or racing thoughts, socially disinhibited leading to inappropriate behaviour, reduced need for sleep, grandiosity, highly distractable, reckless behaviour, marked sexual energy.

Mania may also present with psychotic symptoms:

- Mixed episode—either a mixture of, or a rapid alteration between, manic and depressive symptoms for a period of at least 2wks.
- Bipolar depression—depression occurring in someone who has had at least one manic, hypomanic, or mixed episode.
- Rapid cycling—at least four episodes within a 12-month period.
- Bipolar I disorder—episodes of mania and depression.
- Bipolar II disorder—episodes of hypomania and depression.

In the general population, the lifetime prevalence of bipolar I disorder is 1% and bipolar II disorder is 0.4%. The condition is associated with a high mortality, primarily from suicide.

Treatment of the different phases of the illness

Mania/hypomania

- For patients with mania/hypomania, the initial aim is to achieve rapid control of agitation, aggression, and dangerous behaviour and the first-line treatment is with medication.[12]
- Antidepressants can precipitate mania/hypomania and should be reviewed and stopped if appropriate.
- If an antipsychotic or mood stabilizer is not already being taken, the patient should be offered haloperidol, olanzapine, quetiapine, or risperidone.
- If an antipsychotic or mood stabilizer is already being taken, check compliance. Plasma levels should be checked for those taking lithium (see ➔ p. 431) and the dose optimized accordingly. An antipsychotic may need to be added to existing mood stabilizer treatment.

Bipolar depression

Initial management should be with a psychological intervention. However if symptoms are moderate or severe, medication should be offered:

- First line—quetiapine monotherapy or a combination of fluoxetine and olanzapine.
- Alternative options—olanzapine monotherapy, lamotrigine monotherapy.
- If lithium is already being taken—check levels and optimize the dose. If response is inadequate, add one of the options previously listed.

Maintenance/relapse prevention

Psychological intervention should be offered alongside medication:

- First line—lithium.
- When lithium is ineffective—valproate.
- When lithium is poorly tolerated—valproate, olanzapine or quetiapine (if it has been effective during the acute phase).

Recommended yearly physical monitoring for people with bipolar disorder

Weight/BMI, diet, nutritional status, physical activity level, cardiovascular status (including pulse and BP), metabolic status (including fasting blood glucose, HbA1c, and lipid profile), and LFTs.[12]

Commonly used medicines for bipolar disorder

- Antipsychotics—see ➔ p. 423. NB: not all antipsychotics are licensed to treat bipolar disorder.
- Lithium:
  - Response in mania is delayed, therefore it is not often used for acute mania.
  - Mainly used for prophylaxis, but more effective at preventing relapse to mania than to depression.
  - Relapse risk following discontinuation is high.
  - Should be stopped very gradually over a number of weeks to reduce relapse risk (unless stopping because of serious side effects).
  - Significantly reduces suicide risk.
  - Narrow therapeutic index.
  - Plasma levels can be severely affected by changes in fluid and electrolyte balance.

Other specific physical monitoring

- Baseline—eGFR, TSH, pregnancy test, weight, ECG (if cardiac risk factors).
- At 3 months and then 6 monthly thereafter—eGFR, TSH.
- Yearly—calcium levels.

Therapeutic drug monitoring

- 12h post-dose trough samples 5–7 days following initiation and after all dose changes, then weekly until dose has remained constant for 4wks, then 3-monthly thereafter.
- Recommended range for bipolar disorder—0.6–0.8mmol/L or if the patient has relapsed previously on lithium or if there are sub-syndromal symptoms aim for 0.8–1.0mmol/L

Drug interactions

- Due to lithium's narrow therapeutic index, drugs which ↑ lithium concentrations should be avoided or used with great care. These include NSAIDs, COX-2 inhibitors, diuretics, and ACE inhibitors.

Adverse effects

- Most adverse effects are dose related.
- Fine tremor, nausea, polyuria, and polydipsia are all very common.
- Hypothyroidism can occur but it can be treated with levothyroxine without the need to discontinue the lithium.
- Skin conditions such as acne and psoriasis can occur or worsen.
- Cardiac effects can include bradycardia and QTc prolongation.
- Nephrogenic diabetes insipidus is usually reversible.
- Renal impairment—seek nephrology advice and consider stopping lithium if any of the following occur:[3]
  - A fall in eGFR to <45mL/min/1.73m^2, a rapidly falling rate or heavy proteinuria.
  - A steady or persistent fall in eGFR (rather than a single measurement).
- Stage 4 and 5 chronic kidney disease.

Toxicity

Signs of toxicity can occur with levels >1.5mmol/L (see Table 18.10).

Mild toxicity can often be successfully managed by interrupting lithium treatment for a short period of time or by reducing the dose, whilst closely monitoring levels and symptoms. However, if more significant signs and symptoms of toxicity are present, lithium should be withheld and the patient assessed in hospital.

Valproate/valproic acid

- Used to treat acute mania.
- For prophylaxis it is more effective at preventing relapse to mania than relapse to depression.
- Should be avoided in ♀ of child-bearing potential as it is teratogenic.
- Valproate should be stopped very gradually over a number of weeks to reduce relapse risk (unless stopping because of serious side effects).

Table 18.10 Toxic signs and symptoms of lithium

Mild	Moderate	Severe
Nausea, diarrhoea, blurred vision, polyuria, light headedness, fine resting tremor, muscular weakness, drowsiness	↑ confusion, blackouts, fasciculation, and ↑ deep tendon reflexes, myoclonic twitches and jerks, choreoathetoid movements, urinary or faecal incontinence, ↑ restlessness followed by stupor, hypernatraemia	Coma, convulsions, cerebellar signs, cardiac dysrhythmias including sinoatrial block, sinus and junctional bradycardia and first-degree heart block, hypotension or rarely hypertension, circulatory collapse and renal failure

Other specific physical monitoring
- Baseline—FBC including PTT, LFTs, weight, pregnancy test.
- Follow up within 6 months—LFTs, FBC including PTT, weight.

Therapeutic drug monitoring
- No specific therapeutic levels established for mood stabilization.
- Not carried out routinely.
- May be useful to check compliance or if toxicity is suspected.

Drug interactions
- Lamotrigine metabolism is significantly reduced and if used concomitantly with valproate/valproic acid, the titration and maintenance doses of lamotrigine should be reduced by half.
- Levels can be ↑ by cimetidine, erythromycin, and aspirin.
- Avoid the use of carbapenem antibacterials if possible due to the significant reduction in valproic acid levels that occur.
- Mefloquine, chloroquine, and rifampicin use may result in the need to ↑ the valproate/valproic acid dose.

Adverse effects
- Nausea and tremor are very common and related to dose.
- Significant weight gain can occur—monitor weight and BMI.
- Be alert for signs of infection—leucopenia and pancytopenia have been reported.
- Hair loss can occur. Regrowth begins within about 6 months but is often curly.
- ↑ liver enzymes are common, particularly at (but not confined to) the beginning of treatment, but they are usually transient. Severe liver damage is very rare.
- Reduced bone mineral density can occur with long-term use.
- ↑ suicidal behaviour with antiepileptics has been highlighted as a risk by the MHRA; however, it is possible that this may not be the case when they are used in bipolar patients. Nonetheless, patients should be closely monitored and asked about suicidal thoughts, particularly as suicidal thoughts and behaviour commonly occur anyway in people with bipolar disorder (regardless of whether they are taking medication or not).

Lamotrigine
- Used for bipolar depression as a second-line treatment.
- Used for relapse prevention, but more effective against relapse to depression than mania.
- Requires slow titration to reduce the risk of rash.

Drug interactions
- Valproate/valproic acid—combined use is associated with a higher risk of rash.
- Hormonal contraception—lamotrigine levels are significantly reduced.
- Medicines such as phenytoin, carbamazepine, primidone, phenobarbital, and rifampicin can significantly reduce lamotrigine levels.

Adverse effects

- Rashes very commonly occur, particularly during the initiation of lamotrigine and are associated with high initial doses or escalating the dose too quickly. Rash is usually mild and self-limiting but serious rashes can occur such as Stevens–Johnson syndrome and toxic epidermal necrolysis. The incidence of serious rash in bipolar patients is ~1 in 1000. Lamotrigine should be stopped if rash occurs.
- Headache is very common.
- GI upset (diarrhoea, nausea, and vomiting), somnolence, dizziness, and tremor are common.
- Suicidal thoughts and behaviour—see ➲ 'Valproate', pp. 432–3.

Antidepressants

- Avoid where possible.
- Do not use TCAs as they carry a high risk for precipitating mania.
- SSRIs may also precipitate mania and should be used cautiously and only with cover from a mood stabilizer that protects against manic relapse.

References

11. Cooper JE (Ed) (1994). *Pocket Guide to the ICD-10 Classification of Mental and Behavioural Disorders*. Edinburgh: Churchill Livingstone.
12. NICE (2014, updated 2016). 'Bipolar disorder: assessment and management (CG185)', ℳ www.nice.org.uk/guidance/cg185
13. Kripalani M, Shawcross J, Reilly J, *et al*. (2009). Lithium and chronic kidney disease. *BMJ* 339: b2452.

Obsessive–compulsive disorder

Background and prevalence

Obsessive–compulsive disorder (OCD) is estimated to affect ~1–2% of the population.[14] ICD-10 classification requires either obsessions or compulsions (or both) to be present on most days for a period of 2wks.[15] Obsessional thoughts are ideas, images, and beliefs that intrude into a person's mind. They are recognized as their own but usually cause significant distress. Compulsions are rituals that are repeated over and over again. They may be visible to others, e.g. checking something is locked or hand-washing, or they may be performed in the mind e.g. counting or repeating phrases.[14] A peak of incidence for OCD appears to occur in preadolescence and another one in early adulthood (mean age 21yrs).[16]

Treatment

- A stepped care model is used for treatment of OCD in the UK.[14]
- Psychological interventions (low intensity) are usually offered to people with mild OCD (e.g. group cognitive behavioural therapy (CBT), CBT with exposure and response prevention (ERP) by telephone)
- Treatment with a more intensive CBT (with ERP) or with medication is recommended if low-intensity interventions have been ineffective or if OCD is more severe.
- SSRIs are usually recommended first line (see ➜ p. 414).
- All SSRIs are likely to be equally efficacious but not all are licensed for this indication.
- If symptoms remain after an adequate length of treatment at the highest tolerated dose, check compliance and switch to a different SSRI or to clomipramine.
- Clomipramine is more effective than SSRIs for OCD, but it is not usually used first line due to a greater burden of adverse effects and its cardiac toxicity. Doses up to 250mg may be required.
- Response to antidepressant treatment is often delayed—it can take up to 12wks for the best effect from a dose to become apparent.
- High doses are usually required to effectively treat symptoms (e.g. sertraline 200mg, fluoxetine 60mg, clomipramine 250mg).
- Treatment should continue for 12 months following remission.
- If OCD does not respond to trials of antidepressant monotherapy, or this is poorly tolerated treatment options include antipsychotic augmentation (see ➜ p. 423) or the combined use of an SSRI and clomipramine. Great care should be taken with the latter strategy due to the ↑ risk of serotonin syndrome (see ➜ 'Serotonin syndrome', p. 415).

References

14. NICE (2005). 'Obsessive-compulsive disorder and body dysmorphic disorder: treatment (CG31)'. ℜ www.nice.org.uk/guidance/cg31
15. Cooper JE (Ed) (1994). *Pocket Guide to the ICD-10 Classification of Mental and Behavioural Disorders*. Edinburgh: Churchill Livingstone.
16. Geller DA, March J, AACAP Committee on Quality Issues (2012). AACAP practice parameter for the assessment and treatment of children and adolescents with obsessive compulsive disorder 2012. *J Am Acad Child Adolesc Psychiatry* 51(1): 98–113.

Multiple sclerosis

Multiple sclerosis (MS) is a chronic immune-mediated inflammatory disease of the CNS.

In MS, the immune system attacks and damages myelin, oligodendrocytes (myelin-producing cells), and underlying nerve fibres (axons). This in turn interferes with conduction of impulses along the nerve fibre, resulting in a range of disabling neurological symptoms which vary from one person to another depending on where the damage has occurred. The CNS can restore function by remyelinating the axons. After remyelination, function is restored but may not be as quick or as efficient. Permanent loss of function in MS is caused by failure to remyelinate which in turn leads to axonal loss and neuronal death.

Approximately 2.3 million people worldwide (100 000 people in the UK) are affected by MS. It is the most common cause of non-traumatic disability in young adults. Most people are diagnosed between the ages of 20 and 50yrs.

The exact cause of MS is unknown, but is thought to be a combination of environmental and genetic factors.

Symptoms of MS

- Balance impairment
- Motor symptoms—muscle cramping secondary to spasticity, muscle weakness, paralysis
- Autonomic symptoms—bladder, bowel and sexual dysfunction
- Cerebellar symptoms – dysarthria, ataxia, tremor
- Optic neuritis
- Trigeminal neuralgia
- Fatigue
- Dizziness
- Pain
- Depression
- Cognitive impairment.

Diagnosis of MS

A diagnosis of MS should be made by a consultant neurologist on the basis of established criteria such as the 2010 revised McDonald criteria (see Table 18.11) after:

- assessing that clinical attacks are consistent with an inflammatory demyelinating process
- eliminating alternative diagnoses
- establishing that CNS lesions have developed at different times (dissemination in time) and are in different locations (dissemination in space) for a diagnosis of relapsing–remitting MS
- establishing that progressive neurological deterioration has occurred over 1 or more years for a diagnosis of primary progressive MS.

Table 18.11 2010 Revised McDonald criteria for diagnosing MS

Number of clinical attacks	CNS lesions	Additional data needed for MS diagnosis
Two or more	Objective clinical evidence of two or more lesions *or* Objective clinical evidence of one lesion with reasonable historical clinical evidence of a prior attack	None
Two or more	Objective clinical evidence of one lesion	Dissemination in space demonstrated by: • One or more T2 lesions detected in at least two of four MS-typical regions of the CNS (periventricular, juxtacortical, infratentorial, or spinal cord), or • Await a further clinical attack implicating a different part of the CNS
One	Objective clinical evidence of two or more lesions	Dissemination in time demonstrated by: • Simultaneous presence of asymptomatic gadolinium-enhancing and non-enhancing lesions at any time, or • A new T2 and/or gadolinium-enhancing lesion(s) on follow-up MRI or • Await a second clinical attack

One	Objective clinical evidence of one lesion (known as a clinically isolated syndrome)	Dissemination in space and time demonstrated by:
		• For dissemination in space:
		  • One or more T2 lesions detected in at least two of four MS-typical regions of the CNS (periventricular, juxtacortical, infratentorial, or spinal cord) or
		  • Await a further clinical attack implicating a different part of the CNS
		• For dissemination in time:
		  • Simultaneous presence of asymptomatic gadolinium-enhancing and non-enhancing lesions at any time or
		  • A new T2 and/or gadolinium-enhancing lesion(s) on follow-up MRI or
		  • Await a second clinical attack

(Continued)

Table 18.11   (Contd.)

Number of clinical attacks	CNS lesions	Additional data needed for MS diagnosis
	Insidious neurological progression suggestive of primary progressive MS	1yr of disease progression (determined retrospectively or prospectively) plus two of three of the following criteria: • Evidence of dissemination in space in the brain based on one or more T2 lesions in the MS characteristic regions of the CNS (periventricular, juxtacortical, infratentorial, or spinal cord) • Evidence of dissemination in space in the spinal cord based on two or more T2 lesions in the cord • Positive CSF (isoelectric focusing evidence of oligoclonal bands and/or elevated immunoglobulin G index)

Notes:

• T2 lesions are detected with T2-weighted MRI imaging. T2 sequences provide good contrast between CSF and brain tissue. Water such as CSF appears bright whilst fat such as lipids in the white matter appears dark. Pathological processes such as demyelination and inflammation ↑ water content in tissues. These areas appear as brighter images, making subtle changes easier to detect.

• IV gadolinium contrast medium is used to enhance clarity of MRI images.

Four disease courses have been identified in MS

Relapsing–remitting MS (RRMS)
RRMS is characterized by clearly defined periods of worsening neurological function (relapse) which are followed by periods of partial or complete recovery (remission) without apparent disease progression. Around 85% of patients with MS have RRMS at the time of diagnosis.

Secondary progressive MS (SPMS)
SPMS is characterized by gradual disease progression with or without relapses. It occurs in around 60–70% of patients with RRMS, typically 10–30yrs after initial onset.

Primary progressive MS (PPMS)
PPMS is characterized by steady disease progression and worsening neurological function from onset, with no distinct periods of relapse or remission. Around 10% of patients have PPMS.

Progressive-relapsing MS (PRMS)
PRMS characterized by steadily worsening neurological function from the onset with occasional relapses. Around 5% of people with MS have PRMS.

Management of relapse episodes

MS relapses are defined as new symptoms (or worsening of existing symptoms) that last for >24h in the absence of infection or any other cause, after a stable period of at least 1 month.

Relapses occur as a result of immune-mediated inflammatory attacks that cause damage to CNS myelin. Resulting symptoms are usually related to the area(s) of the CNS affected

Triggers for relapse include:

- Infections
- live vaccines
- stress
- post-partum period.

The severity of relapse can range from very mild exacerbations that do not significantly impact daily activities to severe exacerbations that interfere with mobility and overall ability to function, such as poor balance, severe muscle weakness, and loss of vision.

Mild exacerbations often do not require treatment.

For severe exacerbations, high-dose corticosteroids are used to reduce inflammation and limit the duration of the relapse. Treatment options include oral methylprednisolone 500mg once daily for 5 days or IV methylprednisolone 1g daily for 3–5 days if a relapse is severe enough to warrant in-patient treatment.

Corticosteroids have no impact on disease progression.

Management of MS symptoms

A range of pharmacological and non-pharmacological options are used to manage MS symptoms, depending on which symptoms affect the patient (see Table 18.12).

Non-pharmacological options include physiotherapy, exercise, rehabilitation, occupational therapy and CBT.

Table 18.12 Pharmacological management of MS symptoms

Symptom	Treatment options
Spasticity	Baclofen, benzodiazepines (e.g. diazepam and clonazepam), dantrolene, gabapentin, tizanidine
	Patients with severe symptoms may be managed by specialist centres with botulinum toxin injections or baclofen intrathecal infusions administered through an implanted pump
	Sativex®, a cannabinoid oral spray, is not considered cost-effective by NICE
Fatigue	Amantadine
Bladder dysfunction	Antimuscarinics, e.g. oxybutynin, solifenacin, tolterodine
	Botulinum toxin type A can be considered where antimuscarinics are not effective or are poorly tolerated
Difficulty in walking	Fampridine (not considered cost-effective BY NICE)
Oscillopsia	Gabapentin, memantine
Emotional lability	Amitriptyline
Neuropathic pain	Amitriptyline, carbamazepine, duloxetine, gabapentin, pregabalin
Constipation	Combination of stimulant, osmotic and bulk forming laxatives

Table 18.13 Pre-treatment screening conducted prior to starting DMTs

All DMTs	Additional tests
FBC	Teriflunomide : BP, active and latent TB screening
U&Es	Dimethyl fumarate: urinalysis with microscopy
LFTs	Fingolimod: ECG with first dose, ophthalmologic evaluation for those with history of diabetics or uveitis
Pregnancy test if appropriate	Natalizumab: John Cunningham virus (JCV) serology
Varicella zoster immunoglobulin	Alemtuzumab: HIV, hepatitis B and C, urinalysis with microscopy, thyroid function tests, active and latent TB screening

Disease-modifying treatments (DMTs)
- Reduce the frequency and severity of MS relapses.
- Reduce the accumulation of CNS inflammatory lesions.
- May slow the development of disabling symptoms.

Most DMTs are indicated for relapsing forms of MS. Despite the wide range of treatment options for relapsing-remitting MS, almost no effective DMT options are available for people with progressive MS. See pre-treatment screening in Table 18.13.

DMTs are available as self-injectable therapies, oral dose forms, and IV infusions.

Prescribing and monitoring of DMT is undertaken by specialist MS multidisciplinary teams. Factors that are taken into account when deciding on the choice of DMT include patient preference, disease stage, contraindications, adverse effects, route of administration, treatment frequency, and funding arrangements.

Interferon betas
Interferon betas are immunomodulatory drugs indicated for relapsing MS. Interferon beta is thought to act by reducing blood–brain barrier disruption and by modulating T-cell, B-cell and cytokine functions. Treatment options include:
- interferon beta-1a as once-a-week IM injections (Avonex®) or three-times-a-week SC injections (Rebif®)
- interferon beta-1b as alternate-day SC injections (Betaferon® and Extavia®)
- peginterferon beta-1a, a pegylated form of beta interferon that has a longer duration of action, which is administered once every 2wks by SC injection (Plegridy®).

Adverse effects associated with interferon beta include:
- injection site reactions
- flu-like symptoms
- elevated liver enzymes
- ↓ WCC
- low mood and leg stiffness.

Monitoring of patients on treatment with interferon beta:
- LFTs
- FBC.

(Typically conducted at 2wks, 1 month, 3 months and 6 months after starting therapy, and every 6 months thereafter.)

Some patients receiving interferon beta develop neutralizing antibodies that may limit the efficacy of treatment. Plegridy® is associated with the lowest incidence (<1%) of interferon beta neutralizing antibodies, compared with around 30% of people receiving Betaferon® and Extavia®, 25% receiving Rebif® and 5% receiving Avonex®.

Glatiramer

Glatiramer is indicated for relapsing MS. It is thought to act by stimulating regulatory T cells. Glatiramer is administered three times a week as a SC injection.

Adverse effects include:
- injection site reactions
- lipoatrophy
- chest pain
- palpitations
- anxiety.

No ongoing blood monitoring is required for patients on glatiramer.

Teriflunomide

Teriflunomide is indicated for relapsing MS. It works by inhibiting dihydroorotate dehydrogenase, an enzyme required for pyrimidine synthesis in proliferating cells. It is taken orally as one 14mg tablet once a day.

Adverse effects include:
- elevated liver transaminases
- liver toxicity
- hypertension
- nausea
- diarrhoea
- alopecia
- interstitial lung inflammation.

Monitoring of patients on teriflunomide:
- FBC
- LFTs.

(Typically every 2wks for 6 months after starting treatment, and every 8wks thereafter.)

Teriflunomide is teratogenic and has a long half-life (18–19 days) due to enterohepatic recirculation; it takes an average of 8 months, or up to 2yrs to eliminate after discontinuation. Colestyramine or activated charcoal may be used to facilitate accelerated elimination if patients become pregnant while on therapy or experience a serious adverse effect such as liver toxicity. The *BNF* recommends stopping treatment with teriflunomide and giving either colestyramine 8g three times a day for 11 days or activated powdered charcoal 50g every 12h for 11 days. This accelerated procedure can also be used if the patient wishes to become pregnant, although a post-accelerated elimination teriflunomide plasma concentration of <20 micrograms/L and a waiting period of at least 1.5 months before conception is necessary.

Dimethyl fumarate

Dimethyl fumarate is indicated for relapsing MS. It promotes a shift of cytokine secretion patterns from predominantly pro-inflammatory cytokines (i.e. interleukin-6, interleukin-12, interferon gamma, and tumour necrosis factor alpha) to predominantly anti-inflammatory cytokines (i.e. interleukin-4, interleukin-5, interleukin-10). Dimethyl fumarate is metabolized to monomethyl fumarate, an active metabolite which is eliminated through respiration.

Patients initially start dimethyl fumarate on 120mg orally twice a day, which is ↑ after 7 days to 240mg twice a day.

The most frequently reported side effects are flushing and hot flushes, and GI adverse effects (e.g. abdominal pain, diarrhoea, nausea and vomiting). These effects are most common during the first month of treatment. Flushing is thought to be a result of dimethyl fumarate's agonist effect on nicotinic acid receptors, and effects of monomethyl fumarate mediated by prostaglandin E2.

Flushing and GI adverse effects may be improved by temporary dose reduction to 120mg twice a day (within the first month) or taking dimethyl fumarate with food. The incidence and severity of flushing can also be reduced by taking low-dose aspirin (e.g. 75mg) 30min before taking dimethyl fumarate.

Dimethyl fumarate may also cause elevated hepatic transaminases (alanine aminotransferase (ALT) ≥3 × the upper limit of normal), primarily during the first 6 months of treatment, and a ↓ lymphocyte count.

Monitoring of patients on dimethyl fumarate:
- FBC
- Renal function tests
- LFTs.

(Typically at 1 month, 3 months, and 6 months, then every 6 months.)

Fingolimod

Fingolimod is indicated for relapsing MS. It is a sphygosine-1-phosphate (S1P) receptor modulator. Fingolimod interferes with a key mechanism that lymphocytes use to exit lymph nodes. This leaves lymphocytes unavailable for entering the CNS to initiate MS lesions. Treatment with fingolimod should be initiated and supervised by a specialist. It is taken as one 500-microgram oral tablet once a day.

Fingolimod is contraindicated in patients with known immunodeficiency, severe active infection, active chronic infections (hepatitis, tuberculosis), severe liver impairment, and active malignancies.

Adverse effects of fingolimod reflect the fact that subtypes of S1P receptors are expressed on various other tissues. These include:
- elevated liver transaminases
- macular oedema
- reduced WCC

- bradycardia
- ↑ risk of infection (notably from varicella zoster and herpes simplex)
- minor reduction in forced expiratory volume (fingolimod should be used with caution in patients with severe respiratory disease, pulmonary fibrosis, and COPD)
- haemophygocytic syndrome (HPS)—a rare but potentially fatal disease of normal but overactive histiocytes and lymphocytes (signs and symptoms of HPS include fever, hepatosplenomegaly, rash, hepatic failure and respiratory distress cytopenia, elevated serum-ferritin concentrations, hypertriglyceridaemia, hypofibrinogenaemia, coagulopathy, hepatic cytolysis, hyponatraemia).

Fingolimod affects cardiac smooth muscle and is known to cause bradycardia and heart block after the first dose. It is not recommended in patients with the following:

- Second-degree Mobitz type II or higher-degree arteriovenous block, sick sinus syndrome, or sinoatrial heart block.
- Significant QT prolongation (>470ms in ♀, >450ms in ♂).
- History of symptomatic bradycardia, recurrent syncope, ischaemic heart disease, cerebrovascular disease, history of myocardial infarction, congestive heart failure, cardiac arrest, uncontrolled hypertension, or severe sleep apnoea.

Fingolimod is contraindicated in patients taking class 1a or class III antiarrhythmic medicines; β-blockers, heart rate-lowering calcium channel blockers; and other medicines that may ↓ heart rate.

First dose monitoring:
- When starting treatment with fingolimod, patients require continuous cardiac monitoring for at least 6h following their first dose.
- Cardiac monitoring should be repeated in all patients whose treatment is interrupted for at least 1 day during the first 2wks of treatment, for >7 days during weeks 3 and 4 of treatment, or for >2wks after 1 month of treatment.

LFT treatment monitoring:
- FBC and LFTs, typically 2wks after starting treatment, then at months 1, 2, 3, 6, 9, and 12, then every 6 months.
- Due to risk of macular oedema, eye examinations are recommended 3–4 months after initiation of treatment.

Natalizumab
Natalizumab is a humanized monoclonal antibody indicated for relapsing MS. It selectively targets alpha-4, a cell adhesion molecule expressed on the surface of lymphocytes and monocytes, preventing migration of immune cells across the blood–brain barrier into the CNS.

Natalizumab 300mg is administered by IV infusion once every 4wks.

Adverse effects include:
- infusion-related hypersensitivity reactions
- raised LFTs
- reduced WCC
- ↑ risk of infection.

Around 6% of people receiving natalizumab develop neutralizing antibodies that may limit efficacy of the drug.

Natalizumab ↑ the risk of progressive multifocal leucoencephalopathy (PML), a CNS infection with the JCV, which may lead to irreversible neurological disability or death. Risk factors for PML include prior exposure to JCV, previous treatment with immunosuppressants, and use of natalizumab for >2yrs. Early signs of PML include progressive speech deficits, hemiparesis, or seizures.

Patients on natalizumab require routine monitoring. This typically involves a FBC, U&Es, and LFTs monthly for 3 months then every 3 months, JCV serological testing (if JCV seronegative) every 6 months, and a MRI scan for evidence of PML every 6 months (if JCV seropositive), or every 12 months (if JCV seronegative).

Alemtuzumab

Alemtuzumab (indicated for relapsing MS) is a humanized monoclonal antibody which targets the surface molecule of CD52 on T lymphocytes, B lymphocytes, monocytes and other immune cells. When administered IV, alemtuzumab depletes T- and B-lymphocyte populations for extended periods.

Alemtuzumab is administered as a once-daily 12mg infusion for 5 consecutive days in year 1, followed by a 12mg once-daily infusion for 3 consecutive days 12 months later.

Alemtuzumab is licensed for only two treatment courses. Interim results from the second year of an extension study for patients who were previously treated with alemtuzumab in the 2yr pivotal MS studies (CARE-MS I and CARE-MS II) indicated that 70% of patients did not require a third treatment course during years 3 and 4. These patients were eligible to receive additional treatment with alemtuzumab if they experienced at least one relapse or at least two new or enlarging brain or spinal cord lesions.

Adverse effects include:
• infusion-related hypersensitivity reactions (rash, pruritus, headache, nausea, diarrhoea, chills, flushing, dizziness, dyspnoea and pyrexia)
• autoimmune conditions (thyroid disorders, idiopathic thrombocytopenia purpura, nephropathies)
• lowered blood cell counts
• infections.

Patients are prescribed herpes prophylactic treatment with oral aciclovir 200mg twice a day or equivalent starting on the first day of each treatment course and continued for at least 1 month.

The risk of infusion-related hypersensitivity reactions is reduced by administering corticosteroids and antihistamines prior to starting each alemtuzumab infusion.

Monitoring:
• Monthly FBC with differential, serum creatinine, and urinalysis with microscopy for 48 months after the last infusion.
• LFTs are monitored every 3 months for 48 months after the last infusion.

Treatment with alemtuzumab is not recommended during pregnancy. Women of child-bearing potential are advised to use effective contraception during and for 4 months after treatment. Autoimmune thyroid disease (which is a potential adverse effect of alemtuzumab) ↑ the risk of miscarriage and fetal defects.

Treatments that are currently being developed for MS include:

Anti-LINGO-1 is under investigation as an experimental drug treatment to promote remyelination. It is thought to promote the development of oligodendrocytes, the cells which maintain myelin coating around nerves.

Daclizumab is a monoclonal antibody that binds to CD25 on the surface of activated immune cells and reduces the number of them in the body. Activated immune cells are responsible for some of the damage to the myelin sheath in relapsing–remitting MS.

Laquinimod affects the levels of certain cytokines and reduces the passage of immune cells into the brain and spinal cord. Laboratory investigations have suggested it may have both neuroprotective and anti-inflammatory actions.

Ofatumumab reduces the number of B-cell lymphocytes which are thought to influence the abnormal immune response that causes the attack on the myelin coating of nerves.

Ocrelizumab targets lymphocytes. This helps to supress the immune response and the subsequent damage to myelin that occurs in MS.

Siponimod belongs to the same class of drugs as fingolimod. It binds to sphingosine-1-phosphate receptors (S1P-R) on the surface of the lymphocytes. This causes a larger proportion of lymphocytes to be retained in the lymph glands. The number of activated lymphocytes reaching the brain is ↓, resulting in reduced immune attack on nerve cells in the brain and spinal cord.

Therapy-related issues: infections

Basic microbiology

Micro-organisms are classified in many ways. The most important classifications are as follows:

- Category—e.g. viruses, bacteria, and protozoa
- Genus—i.e. the 'family' that the micro-organism belongs to, such as *Staphylococcus*
- Species—i.e. the specific name, such as *aureus*
- To name a micro-organism correctly, both the genus and the species name must be used—e.g. *Staphylococcus aureus, Haemophilus influenzae*.

Identifying micro-organisms

To diagnose and treat an infection correctly, the micro-organism must be identified. This is usually done by examining samples of faeces, blood, and sputum in various ways.

Microscopy

The sample is examined under the microscope. Sometimes the organism can easily be seen and identified—e.g. some helminths (worms) and their ova (eggs).

Dyes are used to stain cells so that they can be seen more easily. Differential staining uses the fact that cells with different properties stain differently and therefore can be distinguished. Bacteria are divided into two groups according to whether they stain with the Gram stain. The difference between Gram-positive and Gram-negative bacteria is in the permeability of the cell wall when treated with a purple dye followed by a decolorizing agent. Gram-positive cells retain the stain, whereas Gram-negative cells lose the purple stain and appear colourless, until stained with a pink counterstain (Fig. 19.1).

Mycobacteria have waxy cell walls and do not readily take up the Gram stain. A different staining technique is used, and then the sample is tested to see if it withstands decolorization with acid and alcohol. Mycobacteria retain the stain and thus are known as acid-fast bacilli (AFB), whereas other bacteria lose the stain.

Examination of stained films allows the shape of the cells to be seen, which can aid identification.

Bacteria are classified as follows:

- Cocci (spherical, rounded)—e.g. streptococci
- Bacilli (straight rod)—e.g. *Pseudomonas* species
- Spirochaetes (spiral rod)—e.g. *Treponema* species
- Vibrios (curved, comma-shaped)—e.g. *Vibrio cholerae*.

Culture

Bacteria and fungi can be grown on the surface of solid nutrient media. Colonies of many thousands of the micro-organism can be produced from a single cell. Colonies of different species often have characteristic appearances, which aids identification. For most species, it takes 12–48h for a colony to develop that is visible to the naked eye. Some organisms (e.g. mycobacteria) multiply much more slowly and can take several weeks to develop.

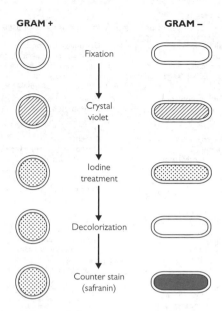

Fig. 19.1 Gram-staining procedure.

Samples can be grown in an environment from which O_2 has been excluded. Bacteria that grow in the absence of O_2 are known as 'anaerobes' and bacteria that need O_2 to grow are 'aerobes'. Bacteria are often described as a combination of their Gram staining, shape, and anaerobic/aerobic characteristics. This helps to narrow the range of bacteria under consideration before lengthier tests identify the individual organism (Table 19.1). Other tests that can be used to identify the organism include the following:
- Detection of microbial antigen
- Detection of microbial products—e.g. toxin produced by *Clostridium difficile*
- Using gene probes
- Polymerase chain reaction.

Discussion of these tests is beyond the scope of this topic. For further information the reader is referred to microbiology texts.

Table 19.1 Examples of pathogens from various types of bacteria

Gram-positive cocci Staphylococci: Coagulase +ve, e.g. *Staph. aureus* Coagulase −ve, e.g. *Staph. epidermidis* Streptococci:* β-haemolytic streptococci: *Strep. pyogenes (Lancefield group A)* α-haemolytic streptococci: *Strep. mitior* *Strep. pneumoniae (pneumococcus)* *Strep. sanguis* Enterococci (non-haemolytic):† *E. mutans, E. faecalis* Anaerobic streptococci **Gram-positive bacilli (rods)** Aerobes: *Bacillus anthracis (anthrax)* *Corynebacterium diphtheriae* *Listeria monocytogenes* *Nocardia* spp. Anaerobes: *Clostridium:* *C. botulinum* (botulism) *C. perfringens* (gas gangrene) *C. tetani* (tetanus) *C. difficile* (diarrhoea) *Actinomyces:* *A. israeli, A. naeslundii* *A. odontolyticus, A. viscosus*	**Gram-negative cocci** *Neisseria, N. meningitidis* (meningitis, septicaemia), *N. gonorrhoeae* (gonorrhoea) *Moraxella, M. catarrhalis* (pneumonia) **Gram-negative bacilli (rods)** Enterobacteriaceae: *Escherichia coli* *Shigella* spp. *Salmonella* spp. *Citrobacter freundii, C. koser* *Klebsiella pneumoniae, K. oxytoca* *Enterobacter aerogenes, E. cloacae* *Serratia morascens* *Proteus mirabilis/vulgaris* *Morganella morganii* *Providencia* spp. *Yersinia, Y. enterocolitica, Y. pestis,* *Y. paratuberculosis* *Pseudomonas aeruginosa* *Haemophilus influenzae* *Brucella* spp. *Bordetella pertussis* *Pasterurella multocida* *Vibrio cholerae* *Campylobacter jejuni*
Obligate intracellular bacteria *Chlamydia, C. trachomatis, C. psittaci,* *C. pneumoniae* *Coxiella burnetii* *Bartonella, Ehrlichia* *Rickettsia* (typhus) *Legionella pneumophilia* *Mycoplasma pneumoniae*	**Anaerobes** *Bacteroides* (wound infections) *Fusobacterium* *Helicobacter pylori* **Mycobacteria** *Mycobacterium tuberculosis, M. bovis,* *M. leprae* (leprosy) 'Atypical' mycobacteria: *M. avium intracellulare* *M. scrofulaceum, M. kansasii* *M. marinum, M. malmoense* *M. ulcerans, M. xenopi, M. gordonae* *M. fortuitum, M. chelonae,* *M. flaverscens* *M. smegmatis-phlei* Spirochaetes: *Treponema* (syphilis. yaws, pinta) *Leptospira* (Weil's disease, canicola fever) *Borrelia* (relapsing fever; Lyme disease)

* Streps are classified according to haemolytic pattern: (α–β or non-haemolytic) or by Lancefield antigen (A–G), or by species (e.g. *Strep. pyogenes*). There is crossover among these groups; this table is a generalization for the chief pathogens.

† Clinically, epidemiologically, and in terms of treatment, enterococci behave unlike other streps.

Reproduced with permission from Longmore M, Wilkinson IB, and Rajagopalan S (2014). *Oxford Handbook of Clinical Medicine*, 9th edn. Oxford: Oxford University Press.

Modes of action of antibacterials

To avoid unwanted toxic effects on human cells, most antibacterials have a mode of action that affects bacterial but not mammalian cells.

There are many possible sites of action of antimicrobial agents. However, the most common mechanisms are as follows:

* Inhibition of cell wall synthesis
* Alteration of the cell membrane (usually antifungals)
* Inhibition of protein synthesis
* Inhibition of nucleic acid synthesis.

Inhibition of cell wall synthesis

Mammalian cells do not have a cell wall (only a cell membrane) so this mode of action does not affect mammalian cells.

Penicillins, cephalosporins, and other β-lactam antibacterials interfere with the synthesis of a substance called peptidoglycan. Peptidoglycan is an essential component of bacterial cell walls. If synthesis of peptidoglycan is inhibited, it is unable to support the cell wall and thus the bacteria lose their structure and eventually lyse (disintegrate) and die.

Isoniazid also acts on the cell wall. It inhibits enzymes that are essential for synthesis of mycolic acids and the mycobacterial cell wall. The mode of action of ethambutol is not completely known, but it also inhibits the action of enzymes involved in cell wall synthesis.

Inhibition of protein synthesis

The mechanism of protein synthesis is similar in bacterial and mammalian cells, but there are differences in ribosome structure (involved in protein synthesis) and other target sites, which ↓ the risk of toxicity to mammalian cells.

Tetracyclines, aminoglycosides, macrolides, and chloramphenicol all work by inhibiting synthesis of proteins essential to the growth and reproduction of bacteria.

Tetracyclines, macrolides, and chloramphenicol interfere with the binding of new amino acids onto peptide chains.

Aminoglycosides prevent initiation of protein synthesis and cause non-functional proteins to be created.

Inhibition of nucleic acid synthesis

Sulfonamides are structural analogues of para-amino benzoic acid (PABA). PABA is an essential precursor in bacterial synthesis of folic acid, which is necessary for the synthesis of nucleic acids. Mammalian cells are not affected as they use exogenous folic acid.

Trimethoprim is an inhibitor of dihydrofolic acid reductase, an enzyme that reduces dihydrofolic acid to tetrahydrofolic acid. This is one of the stages in bacterial synthesis of purines and thus DNA. Trimethoprim inhibits dihydrofolic acid reductase 50 000 times more efficiently in bacterial cells than in mammalian cells.

Sulfonamides and trimethoprim produce sequential blocking of folate metabolism and therefore are synergistic.

Bacteria use an enzyme called DNA gyrase to make the DNA into a small enough package to fit into the cell. This is called supercoiling. The quinolones inhibit DNA gyrase and supercoiling.

Rifampicin inhibits bacterial RNA synthesis by binding to RNA polymerase. Mammalian RNA polymerase is not affected.

Nitro-imidazoles (e.g. metronidazole) cause the DNA strand to break (cleavage).

Selection and use of antimicrobials

To treat or not to treat

The presence of micro-organisms does not necessarily mean that there is infection. The human body hosts a wide range of micro-organisms (mostly bacteria), but these rarely cause infection in an immuno-competent host. These organisms are known as 'commensals' and some have an important role in host defences. For example, *Clostridium difficile* is a pathogen that is normally suppressed by normal bowel flora. Eradication of the bowel flora (e.g. by broad-spectrum antibacterials) allows overgrowth of *C. difficile*, leading to diarrhoea and, sometimes, pseudomembranous colitis. Indiscriminate drug therapy can thus ↑ the risk of other infection.

Some organisms might be commensals in one part of the body and pathogens in another—e.g. *Escherichia coli* is part of the normal bowel flora but if it gets into the bladder it can cause urinary tract infection.

Some pathogenic organisms can reside on the host without causing infection. This is known as 'colonization', and signs and symptoms of infection are absent. A skin or nasal swab positive for meticillin-resistant *Staphylococcus aureus* (MRSA) does not usually require treatment except where elimination of MRSA carriage is required—e.g. prior to surgery.

Some infections are self-limiting and resolve without treatment. Many common viral infections resolve without treatment, and in any case most do not have specific antiviral drugs.

Choice of therapy

If infection is confirmed or is strongly suspected, appropriate therapy must be selected. Ideally, the pathogen is identified before antimicrobial therapy is started. However, identification of an organism by the laboratory usually takes a minimum of 24h and antimicrobial sensitivity tests can take a further 24h. For some slow-growing organisms, such as mycobacteria, culture and sensitivity results can take several weeks. Thus, in most cases, therapy will be started using 'best guess' (empirical) antimicrobials and tailored after culture and sensitivity results are known (Table 19.2).

Whenever possible, samples for culture and sensitivity tests should be taken before starting antimicrobial therapy so that growth is not inhibited. However, this delay might not be possible in very sick patients—e.g. those with suspected bacterial meningitis.

Factors that should be taken into account when selecting an antimicrobial are described as follows:

Clinical

- Does the patient have an infection that needs treating?
- Is there an infection diagnosis/likely source of infection?
- Anatomical site of infection.
- Severity or potential severity of infection (and possible consequences—e.g. loss of prosthetic joint).
- Patient's underlying condition (if any) and vulnerability to infection—e.g. neutropenic patients more susceptible to sepsis.
- Patient-specific factors—e.g. allergies and renal function.

- Does the infection require empirical therapy or can antimicrobials be delayed until culture and sensitivity results are available?
- Foreign material, necrotic tissue, and abscesses are relatively impervious to antimicrobials. Abscesses should be drained and necrotic tissue debrided. If possible, foreign material should be removed.

Microbiology
- What are the pathogens?
  - Identified by microscopy or culture.
  - Presumed, according to epidemiology and knowledge of probable infecting organisms for the site of infection.
- Sensitivity of organisms to antimicrobial agents (Table A12):[1]
  - National and local resistance patterns
  - Culture and sensitivity data.

Pharmaceutical
- Is there evidence of clinical efficacy:
  - against the organism?
  - at the site of infection?
- Bactericidal versus bacteriostatic agents:
  - Bactericidal drugs generally give more rapid resolution of infection.
  - Bacteriostatic drugs rely on phagocytes to eliminate the organisms and therefore are not suitable for infection in which phagocytes are impaired (e.g. granulocytopenia) or do not penetrate the site of infection (e.g. infective endocarditis).
- Spectrum of activity:
  - Narrow-spectrum antimicrobials are preferred if the organism has been identified.
  - Broad-spectrum antimicrobials might be required in empirical therapy or mixed infection.
  - Indiscriminate use of broad-spectrum antimicrobials ↑ the risk of development of drug resistance and super-infection, e.g. *C. difficile*.
- Appropriate route of administration:
  - Topical antimicrobials should be avoided, except where specifically indicated—e.g. eye or ear infection or metronidazole gel for fungating tumours.
  - Oral therapy is preferred and most antimicrobials have good bioavailability.
  - IV therapy might be necessary in the following circumstances:
    —If the infection is serious
    —If the drug has poor oral bioavailability
    —If the patient is unconscious or unable to take oral drugs (e.g. perioperatively).
  - Possible side effects or drug interactions.
- Pharmacokinetics:
  - Tissue penetration—will the antimicrobial reach the site of infection?
  - Clearance in liver/kidney impairment.
- Dose and frequency must be sufficient to give adequate blood levels but avoid unacceptable toxicity. Serum levels four to eight times the minimum inhibitory concentration (MIC) are considered adequate.

Table 19.2 Diseases, potential causative bacteria, and typical treatment choices*

Specific condition	Potential bacterial pathogens	Typical empirical treatment
Meningitis	*Streptococcus pneumoniae, Neisseria meningitidis, Haemophilus influenzae.* Group B streptococci (seen in neonates). Less commonly, *Escherichia coli* and *Listeria monocytogenes.* Other Gram-negative bacteria and *Staphylococcus* spp. usually associated with neurosurgery	Cefotaxime and ceftriaxone provide broad cover and good CNS penetration. Ampicillin or amoxicillin is required to cover *Listeria* spp. (elderly and neonates). Causative agents can also be mycobacterial, viral, or, rarely, fungal and these will require appropriate therapy
Brain abscess	*S. aureus,* anaerobic streptococci, *Bacteroides* spp., Gram-negatives, such as *Escherichia, Proteus, Klebsiella* spp.	Cefotaxime or ceftriaxone, meropenem if broader cover required (avoid imipenem due to CNS side effects). The condition can occasionally be fungal or parasitic
Otitis media	*Strep. pneumoniae, H. influenzae, Moraxella catarrhalis, S. aureus,* mixed anaerobes	Antibacterial therapy not always necessary as most uncomplicated cases resolve. Amoxicillin or co-amoxiclav. Can also be viral (e.g. influenza, respiratory syncytial virus, enteroviruses)
Otitis externa	*Pseudomonas aeruginosa* ('swimmer's ear'), *S. aureus* (pustule)	Topical gentamicin. Less commonly fungal (*Candida albicans, Aspergillus* spp.)
Upper respiratory tract infections:		
Pharyngitis/ tonsillitis	*Strep. pyogenes* (group A)	Phenoxymethylpenicillin but note that approx. 50% of sore throats are viral in origin
Epiglottitis	*H. influenzae, Strep. pyogenes* (group A)	Ceftriaxone or cefotaxime
Sinusitis	*Strep. pneumoniae, H. influenzae,* mixed anaerobes, *S. aureus, M. catarrhalis*	Co-amoxiclav. Sinusitis may be viral (e.g. rhinovirus, influenza) or, occasionally, fungal
Lower respiratory tract infections‡		
Community acquired	*Strep. pneumoniae, H. influenzae, M. catarrhalis,* atypical organisms (*Mycoplasma pneumoniae, Chlamydia pneumoniae,* and, rarely, *Legionella pneumophila*)	Amoxicillin or doxycycline oral or ceftriaxone IV (depending on severity) ± macrolide if atypical organisms are suspected (clarithromycin for *Legionella*)

(*Continued*)

Table 19.2 (Contd.)

Specific condition	Potential bacterial pathogens	Typical empirical treatment
Hospital acquired	E. coli, Ps. aeruginosa, and other Gram-negative organisms, MRSA	Broad-spectrum antibacterials are required until a definitive diagnosis is made, e.g. meropenem/ imipenem/piperacillin + tazobactam, vancomycin + quinolone if MRSA suspected. Infection can be viral. Fungal infection is more likely in immunocompromised patients
Endocarditis	Enterococcus spp., Viridans group streptococci, S. aureus, coagulase-negative staphylococci	Benzylpenicillin and gentamicin (synergistic action) or flucloxacillin and gentamicin if staphylococci are suspected (often seen in injecting drug users)
Gastrointestinal infections	E. coli, Shigella spp., Campylobacter jejuni, Salmonella spp., S. aureus, Bacillus cereus (toxin mediated)	GI infections are generally self-limiting and often viral. Fluid replacement may be all that is required. Expert advice should be sought if antibacterials are considered necessary. In severe disease, ciprofloxacin is used for Salmonella spp. and erythromycin for Campylobacter
Urinary tract infections	E. coli, enterococci, Klebsiella spp., Enterobacter spp., Pseudomonas spp. (UTI)/Pyelonephritis Proteus spp.	For UTI use amoxicillin, cefradine/ cefalexin, trimethoprim, or nitrofurantoin depending on local resistance patterns. For uncomplicated UTI in a young ♀, 3 days of treatment should be sufficient. A longer course may be required in ♂. Recurrent or complicated UTIs require further investigation, consideration of resistant organisms, and use of second-line agents. Co-amoxiclav or ceftriaxone (± single dose of gentamicin) are often used for pyelonephritis
Skin and soft tissue infection (cellulitis)	S. aureus, Strep. pyogenes (group A)	Flucloxacillin (oral or IV depending on severity). Always check (and treat) for co-existing athlete's foot which can be an entry point for organisms
Septic arthritis	S. aureus, Strep. pneumoniae, occasionally Gram-negatives guided by culture results	Flucloxacillin or ceftriaxone empirically, but therapy should be guided by culture results

Table 19.2 (Contd.)

Specific condition	Potential bacterial pathogens	Typical empirical treatment
Osteomyelitis	S. aureus, Strep. pneumoniae, coagulase-negative staphylococci (usually associated with implanted material). Many other organisms infrequently cause disease	Flucloxacillin or ceftriaxone empirically, but therapy should be guided by culture results. Infections involving prostheses will require longer therapy
Sepsis Neutropenic	S. aureus (MRSA), Strep. viridans, coagulase-negative staphylococci, E. coli, Klebsiella spp., Ps aeruginosa or Pneumocystis jirovecii (carinii) pneumonia (PCP)	Meropenem/imipenem/ piperacillin + tazobactam ± gentamicin. Vancomycin if Staphylococcus spp. (including MRSA) suspected. Co-trimoxazole for PCP. If fever persists, consider fungal or viral infections
Non-neutropenic	S. aureus (MRSA), Streptococcus spp., E. coli, Pseudomonas spp.	Therapy depends on source of infection. Empirically— flucloxacillin/ceftriaxone ± gentamicin. Vancomycin if MRSA suspected. Meropenem/ imipenem/piperacillin + tazobactam initially in septic shock

* Pathogens/therapy may differ in children and neonates—seek specialist advice.

† Patients with MRSA or high risk of MRSA, add vancomycin or teicoplanin.

‡ See also British Thoracic Society Guidelines for the management of community acquired pneumonia in adults.[2]

- Duration of treatment:
  - Not too long—e.g. uncomplicated urinary tract infection only requires 3–5 days of therapy.
  - Not too short—e.g. bone infection might require therapy for several weeks or months.
- Local policies/restrictions on antimicrobial use:
  - Cost.

Combined antimicrobial therapy

- Combined antimicrobial therapy may be prescribed for certain indications.
- To give a broad spectrum of activity in empirical therapy, especially in high-risk situations such as neutropenic sepsis.
- To treat mixed infection if one drug does not cover all possible pathogens.
- To achieve a synergistic effect, thus ↑ efficacy but ↓ the dose required of each drug (and thus ↓ the risk of side effects)—e.g. penicillin and gentamicin in the treatment of streptococcal endocarditis. Relatively low doses of gentamicin are used, ↓ the risk of nephrotoxicity.

- To ↓ the probability of the emergence of drug resistance—e.g. treatment of TB requires a minimum of two drugs and antiretroviral therapy requires a minimum of three drugs.
- To restore or extend the spectrum of activity by including an enzyme inhibitor—e.g. co-amoxiclav.

Penicillin and cephalosporin hypersensitivity

Up to 10% of people are allergic to penicillins and up to 7% of these people are also allergic to cephalosporins. This can range from mild rash to fever to a serious anaphylactic reaction. Penicillins and cephalosporins should never be used again in a patient who has had a severe (type 1) hypersensitivity reaction including anaphylaxis, wheezing/bronchospasm, angio-oedema, immediate rash, or laryngeal oedema

If a patient has had a severe hypersensitivity reaction to penicillins, it is advisable to avoid cephalosporins unless there is no alternative. It may be advisable to seek advice from a specialist (e.g. microbiologist). If the penicillin allergy is relatively mild (e.g. delayed rash), cephalosporins can be prescribed cautiously.

Some patients state that they have had an allergic reaction when they have really only had nausea or a headache. This is not drug allergy and therefore it is safe to use penicillins and cephalosporins in these patients.

Ampicillin and amoxicillin can cause rashes in patients who have had glandular fever or leukaemia, or who are HIV positive. This is not a true allergic reaction and penicillins can be used again in these patients.

A careful review of allergy status with the patient is important to establish specific symptoms were present and the onset of the reaction.

Monitoring therapy

It is essential to monitor and review antimicrobial therapy regularly, both to ensure that treatment is working and to avoid inappropriate continuation of therapy (Fig. 19.2). The pharmacist should monitor the following parameters:

- Temperature should ↓ to normal (36.8°C). (Note: drug hypersensitivity is a possible cause of persistent pyrexia.)
- Pulse, BP, and respiratory rate revert to normal.
- Raised white cell count ↓.
- Raised C-reactive protein ↓ (normal <8).
- Symptoms such as local inflammation, pain, malaise, GI upset, headache, and confusion resolve.

Reasons for treatment failure

- Wrong antimicrobial
- Drug resistance
- The isolated organism is not the cause of the disease
- Treatment started too late
- The wrong dose, duration, or route of administration
- Lack of patient compliance
- Difficulty getting the drug to the site of infection
- ↓ immunity of the patient.

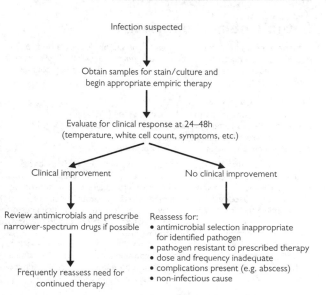

Infection suspected

↓

Obtain samples for stain/culture and
begin appropriate empiric therapy

↓

Evaluate for clinical response at 24–48h
(temperature, white cell count, symptoms, etc.)

Clinical improvement   No clinical improvement

Review antimicrobials and prescribe   Reassess for:
narrower-spectrum drugs if possible   • antimicrobial selection inappropriate
                                               for identified pathogen
                                             • pathogen resistant to prescribed therapy
                                             • dose and frequency inadequate
Frequently reassess need for   • complications present (e.g. abscess)
continued therapy   • non-infectious cause

Fig. 19.2 Flowchart of selection and use of antimicrobials.

Further reading

Wickens H, Wade P (2005). How pharmacists can promote the sensible use of antimicrobials. *Pharm J* 274: 427–30.

Wickens H, Wade P (2005). The right drug for the right bug. *Pharm J* 274: 365–8.

References

1. Wickens H, Wade P (2005). The right drug for the right bug. *Pharm J* 274: 365–8.
2. Lim WS, Baudouin SV, George RC, *et al.* (2009). BTS guidelines for the management of community acquired pneumonia in adults: update 2009. *Thorax* 64(Suppl III):iii1–iii55. ℬ www.thorax.bmj.com/content/64/Suppl_3/iii1.full.pdf+html

Antimicrobial prophylaxis

Indiscriminate and prolonged courses of antimicrobials should be avoided, but in some situations short- or long-term antimicrobial prophylaxis might be appropriate to prevent infection (and thus further courses of antimicrobials).

Surgical prophylaxis

Antibacterial drugs are given to ↓ the risk of the following:
• Wound infection after potentially contaminated surgery—e.g. GI or genitourinary surgery and trauma.
• Losing implanted material—e.g. joint prosthesis.

It is important that there are adequate concentrations of antibacterials in the blood at the time of incision ('knife-to-skin time') and throughout surgery. Thus it is important to administer antibacterials at an appropriate time (usually 30–60min) before surgery starts and repeat doses of short-acting antibacterials if surgery is delayed or prolonged. It is rarely necessary to continue antibacterials after wound closure. More prolonged therapy is effectively treatment rather than prophylaxis.

The choice of antibacterial depends on the type of surgery and local bacterial sensitivities. Vancomycin or teicoplanin should be used for patients with proven or suspected MRSA colonization. Drugs are usually administered by IV infusion to ensure adequate levels at the critical time.

Medical prophylaxis

Medical prophylaxis is appropriate for specific infections and for high-risk patients, as follows:
• Contacts of sick patients—e.g. meningitis and TB
• Immunosuppressed patients—e.g. organ-transplant recipients, HIV-positive patients, and splenectomy patients
• Malaria
• Post-exposure prophylaxis, following exposure to HIV or hepatitis B.

Further reading

General principles on antimicrobial prophylaxis: see SIGN and NICE guidelines, ℔ www.sign.ac.uk/ guidelines/fulltext/104/index.html, ℔ www.nice.org.uk/guidance/cg74
Rahman MH, Anson J (2004). Peri-operative antibacterial prophylaxis. *Pharm J* **272**: 743–5.
Prophylaxis regimens can be found in the *British National Formulary*, ℔ www.bnf.org

Antimicrobial stewardship

↓ antimicrobial use might not actually ↓ the rate of resistance, but it might limit the rate at which new resistance emerges. Pharmacists have an important role in optimizing antimicrobial use—often known as 'antimicrobial stewardship'. In the UK, the Department of Health has specifically promoted the role of pharmacists in monitoring and optimizing antimicrobial use. In most UK hospitals, specialist antimicrobial pharmacists work alongside microbiologists and infectious diseases doctors, as well as infection control teams, to promote good antimicrobial stewardship through education, audit, and production of prescribing policies. However, all pharmacists, whether in hospitals or the community, have a role in ensuring 'prudent use' of antimicrobials.

Strategies for antimicrobial stewardship

- Use of non-antimicrobial treatment as appropriate—e.g. draining abscesses and removing infected invasive devices such as catheters.
- Improved systems for resistance testing and better communication of resistance data in the hospital and community settings to enable better-directed therapy:
  - Avoid continued use of ineffective drugs.
  - Enable switching from broad-spectrum to narrower-spectrum antimicrobials.
- Faster diagnosis of infection to ↓ the amount of unnecessary empirical therapy:
  - Obtain cultures in a timely manner.
  - Review all prescriptions within 48h and then daily to review diagnosis and continuing need for antibacterials.
- Ensuring that empirical therapy considers the following adjustments, as necessary:
  - Therapy is stopped if infection is ruled out.
  - Therapy is changed, as necessary, when culture results are available.
- Production of antimicrobial prescribing policies and promoting adherence to evidence-based guidelines.
- Documentation of the indication and proposed duration on the prescription by the prescriber.
- Ensuring choice, dose, and duration of therapy, including the following:
  - Monitoring serum levels and adjusting doses for antimicrobials that require TDM.
  - Ensuring that kinetic factors are taken into account—e.g. nitrofurantoin is not excreted into the urine in adequate concentrations to be effective in patients with renal impairment.
  - Community pharmacists should ask patients the reason for the antimicrobial prescription to ensure prescription is appropriate.
  - Ensure individual patient factors are taken into account including previous antimicrobial history, infection previously with multi-resistant organisms, allergy status.
  - Most antimicrobials do not need a duration >7 days.
- Avoiding unnecessary/overlong use of broad-spectrum antimicrobials.

- Promotion of good prescribing practice including daily review of IV antibacterials, and IV to oral switches in cases where:
  - the pathogen and sensitivities are known
  - the patient is clinically improving and is haemodynamically stable with no signs of fever
  - patient is able to absorb oral medicines
  - the oral alternative is suitable for the patient—e.g. co-morbidities or interactions with other medicines.
- Appropriate use of antimicrobials for surgical prophylaxis, including avoiding prolonged courses (usually only one dose is needed).
- Use of combination therapy if there is a high risk of resistance emerging—e.g. rifampicin should never be used alone for TB or other infections.
- Avoiding co-prescribing of antimicrobials that have the same or an overlapping spectrum of activity—e.g. co-amoxiclav and metronidazole.
- Considering rotational use of antimicrobials (cycling) in some circumstances.
- Review of prescribing patterns of antibacterials—e.g. through point prevalence audits.
- Educating patients to take antimicrobials correctly and that some infections do not require antimicrobial therapy.

Points to consider when reviewing a prescription for an antimicrobial

- Is it the right choice for the infection (or appropriate empirical therapy)?
- Does it comply with local policies/restrictive practices?
- Could a narrower-spectrum antimicrobial be used?
- Should it be used in combination with another antimicrobial?
- Is more than one antimicrobial with an overlapping spectrum of activity being used, and if so, why?
- Will the antimicrobial be distributed to the target (infected) organ?
- Is the dose correct taking into account the following?
  - Renal impairment.
  - Severity of infection.
  - Patient weight.
- Is TDM and subsequent dose adjustment required?
- Is the route of administration appropriate?
- Is the duration of therapy appropriate?
- Does the patient understand the dosing instructions and importance of completing the course?

Further reading

Frost K (2014). Improving antimicrobial stewardship. *Pharm J* 293: 525–7.
NICE (2014). 'Infection prevention and control [QS61]', ℳ www.nice.org.uk/guidance/qs61
Public Health England (2011, updated 2015). 'Antimicrobial stewardship: Start smart – then focus',
    ℳ www.gov.uk/government/publications/antimicrobial-stewardship-start-smart-then-focus
Wicken H, Wade P (2005). Understanding antibiotic resistance. *Pharm J* 274: 501–4.

Antimicrobial prescribing guidelines

Antimicrobials are the second most frequently prescribed class of drugs, after analgesics. ~80% of antimicrobial prescribing is in the UK is in the community, and although the emergence of 'superbugs' is less of a problem than in hospitals, resistance and cost are still an issue. Education of patients and GPs to reduce pressure to prescribe has contributed to a reduction in antimicrobial usage in the community.

The remaining 20% of antimicrobial prescribing is in hospitals. However, this class represents some of the more expensive drugs used in secondary care and antimicrobial resistance in the hospital setting is an ↑ problem. ↑ in resistant bacteria have been seen with selection of extended spectrum beta-lactamase (ESBL)-producing Gram-negative bacteria, as well as acquisition of MRSA as inpatients in hospital.

Both WHO and the UK Department of Health have emphasized the need for 'prudent use' of antimicrobials. WHO defines this as:

'the cost-effective use of antimicrobials which maximises their clinical therapeutic effect, while minimising both drug-related toxicity and the development of antimicrobial resistance'.

A good antimicrobial prescribing policy or guidelines will contribute to prudent (and thus cost-effective) use of antimicrobials.

Type and format of guidance

Antimicrobial prescribing guidelines come in many formats. Before starting to write guidelines, both the format and the intent must be decided:
- Advisory or mandatory
- Policy, guidelines, restricted list
- Educational.

It has been shown that prescribers prefer an educational approach and this may have the best long-term impact. However, it may be necessary to give mandatory advice on the use of certain high-cost/sensitive drugs.

The format must be easily accessible to prescribers at the time of prescribing. Computer-based guidelines offer the opportunity to provide additional educational material and may be linked to a computerized prescribing package. This may be the best approach in the community where most GP practices use electronic prescribing. Apps are increasingly being used to provide information and education in many therapeutic areas and are an effective way to produce widely held (via smartphones) but easy to update guidelines. The Microguide® app is specifically designed for antimicrobial guidelines and is being increasingly used by UK hospitals.

The amount of detail will be determined by the presentation. As a minimum the recommended drug and an alternative (if needed) due to allergy, (adult) dose, route, and duration should be included. More detailed policies might also include side effects, contraindications, use in children, in the elderly, in renal impairment, and in pregnancy, etc.

Style and layout must be clear and easy to follow. In lengthier guidelines an index or contents list should be provided. Use plain English throughout and avoid Latin abbreviations such as 'TDS' (if space permits). Note that different countries use different abbreviations, which may cause confusion for visiting staff—e.g. the US abbreviation 'QD' means once a day but may be misinterpreted as the UK 'QDS' or four times a day. During the drafting process it is advisable to 'pilot' the guidelines to ensure that potential users interpret them in the way intended.

Target audience

This should be identified. Are restrictions just applicable to junior doctors or to senior medical staff as well? Write the guidelines as if they are aimed at a doctor who has newly joined the hospital/GP practice and who needs to find what to prescribe in a situation quickly and easily.

Authors

Hospital antimicrobial guidelines are usually produced as a collaboration between microbiology and pharmacy. To ensure local ownership, consultants in the relevant specialities should be invited to contribute or comment—e.g. surgeons for surgical prophylaxis. In the community, guidelines may be produced by a committee of GPs from one or more practices, usually with the assistance of the prescribing adviser. Ideally, local primary and secondary care policies should be linked and certainly should not contain conflicting advice.

Content

Guidelines should:
- be evidence based and recommendations referenced as appropriate, including typical course length if appropriate
- advise on when *not* to prescribe, as this is as valid as advice on when and what antimicrobial to prescribe
- emphasize the need to urgently commence (within 1h) empirical broad-spectrum antibacterials in significant infection
- discourage unnecessary use of the parenteral route
- include contact numbers for microbiology, pharmacy medicines information service, etc.
- be cross-referenced to other relevant hospital/practice guidelines
- take into account local antibacterial resistance patterns and indicate any deviation from national guidelines
- suggest alternative antibacterials for patients with allergies
- suggest alternative oral choices when IV to oral switch is appropriate
- list antimicrobials available in the institution including those which are restricted to certain specialties/prescribers or to certain conditions (e.g. for use in cystic fibrosis patients only).

Cost may be included but may become outdated before the guidelines are due for revision.

An extensive list of what might be included in local guidelines is available in the Department of Health Advisory Committee on Antimicrobial Resistance and Healthcare Associated Infection (ARHAI) pack 'Start Smart—Then Focus'.[3]

As a minimum, the following areas should be covered:
- Surgical prophylaxis.
- Empirical treatment (first and second choice) for infections including:
  - meningitis
  - urinary tract infection
  - lower respiratory tract infection
  - sepsis
  - CNS infection (e.g. bacterial meningitis).

Other areas which should be included are as follows:
- Prophylaxis in asplenic patients
- Empirical treatment for:
  - GI infection
  - MRSA
  - C. difficile infection
  - upper respiratory tract infection
  - skin infection.

Updating

The guidelines should state the issue date and frequency of review. As a minimum, guidelines should be reviewed and updated as necessary every 2yrs.

Monitoring and audit

Adherence to the guidelines should be monitored. For example, a specific area such as vascular surgery prophylaxis can be audited. If there is significant non-adherence, the reasons should be established and addressed, and if necessary the guidelines adjusted accordingly.

Reference

3. Public Health England (2011, updated 2015). 'Antimicrobial stewardship: Start smart – then focus', ℘ www.gov.uk/government/publications/antimicrobial-stewardship-start-smart-then-focus

Antimicrobial resistance

Resistance is an almost inevitable consequence of antimicrobial use. As bacteria, viruses, or other micro-organisms reproduce, mutations can spontaneously occur. These mutations might provide some protection against the action of certain antimicrobials. 'Survival of the fittest' means that when these micro-organisms are exposed to antimicrobials, the fully sensitive ones are suppressed but resistant ones survive, reproduce, and become the dominant strain. Most attention has been focused on bacterial resistance, but the principles discussed here apply to all micro-organisms. As the problem with antimicrobial resistance continues to grow, there is ↑ use of antibiotics which were once considered last-line therapy (e.g. IV colistin).

Mechanisms of resistance

- Change in cell wall permeability, thus ↓ drug access to intracellular target sites. The relatively simple cell wall of Gram-positive bacteria makes them inherently more permeable and therefore this resistance mechanism is more common in Gram-negative than Gram-positive bacteria.
- Enzyme degradation of the drug—the best known is breakdown of the β-lactam ring of penicillins, cephalosporins, and carbapenems by β-lactamases.
- Efflux pumps actively remove the drug from the cell.
- Mutation at the target site:
  - Alteration of penicillin-binding proteins leads to resistance to β-lactam antibiotics.
  - Changes in the structure of the enzyme reverse transcriptase lead to resistance to reverse transcriptase inhibitors.
- Some organisms can develop multiple resistance mechanisms—e.g. *Pseudomonas aeruginosa* manifests resistance to carbapenems through production of β-lactamase, ↑ in efflux pumps, and changes to the bacterial cell wall.

Implications of antimicrobial resistance

Antimicrobial resistance leads to ↑ in the following:
- Morbidity:
  - Patients might be sicker for longer
  - Hospital stays are ↑
  - Alternative antimicrobials might be more toxic
  - Residential placements might be difficult
  - Isolation and institutionalization
  - Multiple resistant organisms with limited options for effective treatment
- Mortality
- Cost:
  - Newer, potentially more expensive antimicrobials might have to be used
  - Extended hospital stay
  - More nursing time
  - ↑ use of disposables (e.g. aprons and gloves)
  - In some cases, equipment might have to be discarded.

New strains of resistant bacteria are appearing at an alarming rate. Within the hospital environment, MRSA has been a problem for many years but the emergence of vancomycin-resistant MRSA (VRSA) and community-acquired MRSA (C-MRSA) is of significant concern. Other increasingly problematic resistant organisms are as follows:

- Vancomycin-resistant enterococci (VRE)
- Extended-spectrum β-lactamases (ESBLs)
- *Acinetobacter baumanii*
- Carbapenemase-producing Enterobacteriaceae (CPE).

At present, agents to treat these resistant organisms are available, but they tend to be expensive, with a higher risk of side effects. However, the production of new drugs is not keeping up with development of new resistant bacteria, and the possibility of resistant species emerging for which there is no antibacterial therapy available is very real. In the case of CPE, there are very few treatment choices and monotherapy is not recommended.

Measuring resistance

In vitro resistance tests generally require the organism to be cultured in the presence of antimicrobials.

Disk diffusion

Disk diffusion involves culturing bacteria on an agar plate that has had samples (impregnated disks) of an antibacterial placed on it. If there is no growth around the antibacterial, the bacteria are sensitive to the antibacterial, but if the bacteria grow around the sample, this means that they are resistant. Partial growth represents intermediate susceptibility.

E-test

The E-test is based on similar principles to disk diffusion, but here an impregnated strip containing a single antibacterial at ↑ concentrations is placed on the agar plate. Bacterial growth is inhibited around the strip after it reaches a certain concentration. This is equivalent to the MIC.

These tests can be problematic for slow-growing bacteria, such as mycobacteria, and for organisms that are difficult to culture, such as viruses. Newer tests involve amplifying and examining the genetic material of the organism to look for mutations that are known to be associated with resistance. This technique is used for HIV-resistance testing.

Risk factors for antimicrobial resistance

Excessive and inappropriate antimicrobial use results in selective pressures that facilitate the emergence of resistant micro-organisms. It is estimated that up to 50% of antimicrobial use is inappropriate. Unnecessary antimicrobial use contributes to resistance without any clinical gain. This includes the following:

- Use of antimicrobials for infections that are trivial or self-limiting.
- Use of antibacterials to treat infection of viral origin—e.g. the common cold.
- Over-long antimicrobial prophylaxis or treatment courses.

Even appropriate antimicrobial therapy is ↑ worldwide, in addition to ↑ use of broad-spectrum antibacterials and prolonged courses. This is due to the following reasons:

- ↑ numbers of severely ill hospital patients.
- Ageing population with increasingly complex medical needs
- More frequent use of invasive devices and procedures.
- Presence of more severely immunocompromised patients in hospitals and the community. ↑ opportunity for dissemination of infection ↑ the possibility of spread of resistant organisms between patients. This is facilitated by the following:
  - Overcrowding in hospital and community healthcare facilities
  - ↑ hospital throughput
  - Poor cleaning and disinfection of rooms, equipment, and hands.

Strategies to ↓ or contain antimicrobial resistance

- Multiple strategies on both local and national or international levels are required to ↓ or contain antimicrobial resistance.
- Prevention of infection through the following mechanisms:
  - Vaccines
  - Prophylaxis
  - ↓ use of invasive devices
  - Good hygiene.
- ↓ dissemination of antimicrobial-resistant organisms (see ➜ 'Infection control', pp. 469–71).
- Limiting or modifying antimicrobial use.
- Improvement in the knowledge and understanding of the problem (both amongst healthcare professionals and also the public).
- Development of new agents to ↑ treatment options.
- Worldwide and local surveillance strategies to identify patterns of resistance.

Further reading

Department of Health, Public Health England (2013). 'Antimicrobial prescribing and stewardship competencies', ✍www.gov.uk/government/publications/antimicrobial-prescribing-and-stewardship-competencies

'European Antibiotic Awareness Day' website, ✍ www.ecdc.europa.eu/en/EAAD/Pages/Home.aspx

Infection control

Infection control is important in hospital and community residential facilities for the following reasons:

- To prevent cross-transmission of infection.
- To prevent the spread of resistant micro-organisms.

Special attention should be paid to infection control in areas where patients are most vulnerable:

- Intensive care units
- Neonatal units
- Burns wards
- Vascular wards
- Units treating immunocompromised patients.

Special attention should also be paid to infection control where procedures or devices make patients more vulnerable:

- Urinary catheters
- Intravascular devices
- Surgical procedures
- Respiratory care equipment
- Enteral or parenteral feeding.

Infection control should be an integral part of the culture of any institution. This requires the following considerations:

- There is an infection control lead clinician or nurse.
- There are written procedures for infection control.
- Staff (including temporary staff and locums) receive education and training on infection control procedures.
- There are adequate supplies and facilities—e.g. availability of aprons and gloves.
- There is documentation of additional infection control requirements, as necessary, for individual patients.
- Healthcare staff are immunized, as needed, for hepatitis B, TB, chickenpox, and influenza.
- There are written procedures for managing occupational exposure to blood-borne viruses, and staff are made aware of these procedures.

Universal precautions

Strict attention to hygiene is essential. All body fluids and contaminated equipment, including linen, from all patients should be handled as if infected. This is known as 'universal precautions' and includes taking appropriate measures to ensure the following:

- Prevent contamination—e.g. wearing apron and gloves and bagging dirty linen.
- Dispose of waste safely—e.g. use of clinical waste bins and sharps boxes.
- Protect staff against occupational exposure to blood-borne viruses—e.g. hepatitis B and C, and HIV.

Isolation of patients

It might be necessary to nurse patients in isolation in the following circumstances:

- They are a potential source of infection—e.g. MRSA, *C. difficile*-associated diarrhoea, and TB.
- They are particularly vulnerable to infection ('reverse barrier nursing')—e.g. severely neutropenic patients.

Isolation procedures include the following:

- Nursing patients in a side room or, if more than one patient has the same infection, in a cordoned-off area.
- Wearing protective clothing when in contact with the patient. This includes staff who might be in contact with the patient elsewhere in the hospital (e.g. hospital porters).
- Ensuring that equipment is disinfected immediately after use.
- Ensuring that aprons, gloves, and other disposables are disposed of safely (usually bagged within the room).
- Ensuring that visitors take appropriate measures to prevent cross-contamination—e.g. handwashing and wearing protective clothing for particularly vulnerable patients.

Handwashing or decontamination

Hand hygiene is an essential part of infection control. It is effective for prevention of cross-contamination, but unfortunately compliance is often poor—particularly if staff are overworked and stressed.

Education of all staff (clinical and non-clinical) on hand hygiene is essential, in addition to ensuring adequate facilities for washing or decontamination. The usual procedures include the following:

- Staff 'bare below the elbows' in clinical areas (i.e. wearing short or rolled-up sleeves, no wrist watches or bracelets, no rings except wedding rings) in order to facilitate hand hygiene.
- Hands must be decontaminated before and after any episode of patient contact, including handling patients' possessions at the bedside—e.g. when checking patients' own drugs.
- Visibly soiled or potentially grossly contaminated hands should be washed with soap and water; otherwise alcohol gel can be used (with the exception of potential exposure to *C. difficile* as the spores are resistant to alcohol).
- Attention should be paid to ensuring the whole of the hand is decontaminated, including the following:
  - Wrists
  - Thumbs
  - Between the fingers
  - Backs of hands.

Pharmacists and infection control

To avoid contamination of medicines, in addition to presenting a professional appearance, a high standard of cleanliness should be maintained in pharmacy shops and dispensaries. Special attention should be paid to ensuring that the following areas are kept clean and tidy:

• Dispensing benches—especially areas where extemporaneous
  dispensing is carried out
• Drug refrigerators
• Toilets
• Storage areas (often neglected).

Pharmacy staff should have access to handwashing facilities with soap and hot water. Aprons, gloves, and (as appropriate) masks should be used when preparing extemporaneous preparations. Tablets and capsules should not be handled—use counting trays and tweezers or a spatula, and disinfect these frequently.

Note that the type of patient contact experienced in a community pharmacy is extremely unlikely to lead to transmission of infection, including MRSA and TB.

Pharmacists do not often have 'hands-on' contact with patients but they should still observe infection-control procedures. These include the following:

• Decontaminating hands on entering and leaving clinical areas, and before
  and after direct patient contact.
• Wearing gloves and an apron when in close or prolonged contact with
  high-risk patients—e.g. those with MRSA.
• Wearing gloves, as appropriate, for 'hands-on' patient contact—e.g.
  wound care.
• Checking that new staff, trainees and locums, or temporary staff, if
  necessary, have immunity to chickenpox, TB, and hepatitis B.

In the UK, NICE[4] has published guidelines on infection control in primary and community care (including antimicrobial treatment and prophylaxis) in the following areas:

• Standard principles
• Care of patients with long-term urinary catheters
• Care during enteral feeding
• Care of patients with central venous catheters.

Reference

4. NICE (2012). 'Healthcare-associated infections: prevention and control in primary and community care [CG139]', ℳ www.nice.org.uk/guidance/cg139

Management of patients with HIV

HIV stands for human immunodeficiency virus and belongs to a group of viruses known as 'retroviruses'. HIV attacks the immune system and if left untreated it can cause damage to the immune system leading to a variety of potentially lethal illnesses which are known as acquired immunodeficiency syndrome (AIDS). Patients with HIV will not necessarily develop AIDS-related illnesses if given the proper treatment. The number of patients with an AIDS diagnosis has fallen thanks to effective treatments for HIV.

In 2012, ~35.3 million people were living with HIV, with >9.7 million people receiving antiretroviral (ARV) treatment. In the UK, in 2013, an estimated 107 800 patients were living with HIV with an estimated 25% of patients being unaware of their status.

Transmission

HIV is present in blood, genital fluids, and breast milk, and can therefore be transmitted through the following ways:
- Direct contact with infected blood—blood transfusions, blood derived products, sharing needles (IVDU)
- Sexual contact (unprotected anal or vaginal, possibly oral)
- Direct contact with seminal and vaginal secretions
- Mother-to-child transmission (MTCT)—during pregnancy, delivery, or through breastfeeding.

The risk of HIV transmission is:
- ↑ if mucosal linings are damaged—e.g. patients with sexually transmitted infections or ulceration
- is greatly reduced when patients are on the correct treatment and their viral load is undetectable.

Table 19.3 shows stages following the transmission of HIV.

Diagnosis

Diagnosis of HIV is a key priority to ensure infected patients are treated appropriately and also to prevent the spread of the disease (Box 19.1):
- Testing is offered in sexual health clinics, doctors' surgeries, and in some community pharmacies across the UK.
- HIV tests currently detect the presence of antibodies to HIV and p24 antigen in the blood.
- Fourth-generation HIV tests can detect infection as little as 2wks after infection. However, if this is negative a retest may be recommended 1 month later to cover the minority of people who have a delayed antibody response.
- Many people who have been recently infected will not have any symptoms of the illness. Some people may experience flu-like symptoms when they start to produce antibodies—known as seroconversion.

Treatment

Treatment of HIV has greatly improved over the last 20yrs and the disease is now a chronic illness with patients expected to have a near normal life expectancy. Treatment is relatively easy to take and tolerability has greatly

Table 19.3 Stages following HIV transmission

1. Seroconversion	• Person is infected with HIV and antibodies develop to the virus
	• The HIV virus replicates rapidly and viral load in blood ↑ rapidly
	• May get some symptoms (80% patients) e.g. fever, headache, rash, general flu-like symptoms
2. Asymptomatic stages	• Immune system controls HIV but replication of virus continues
	• Viral load ↓ and CD4 T cells reduce over time
	• No symptoms
3. Symptomatic stages	• Some physical signs of HIV due to reduced immune functioning (reduced CD4 count)
	• ↑ in viral load
	• Minor infections—e.g. oral candida/skin problems/weight loss/fever
4. AIDS stage	• CD4 count is low (usually <200) and viral load is likely to be high
	• Opportunistic infections e.g. *Pneumocystis jirovecii* pneumonia (PCP)
	• HIV-related cancers

Box 19.1 Promotion of prevention
- Condom use associated with 85% reduction in risk of transmission
- ↑ testing available for HIV
- Counselling and education relating to risks
- Medical male circumcision
- Using ARV medications (pre- and post-exposure prophylaxis as well as treatment and treatment as prevention)
- Needle exchange schemes
- Elimination of MTCT.

improved allowing patients with HIV to have a normal lifestyle. Treatment is lifelong and patients should not stop taking their medicines.

HIV treatment can be referred to as:
- anti-HIV medicines
- highly active antiretroviral treatment (HAART)
- ARVs
- combination therapy
- triple therapy.

The main aim of treatment is to reduce the amount of HIV in the body to allow the immune system to function properly. Current treatment does not allow full eradication of HIV from the system, so if a patient stops taking their medicines the virus will start to replicate again. Research into a cure for

HIV is ongoing and promising, but currently there is no cure available. The virus easily mutates to produce resistant versions so triple therapy using two classes of ARV is necessary to fully suppress the virus and avoid resistant strains emerging. National or international guidelines should be followed for when to initiate treatment and choice of therapy.

Treatment as prevention

If a person is on ARV treatment and their viral load is suppressed or undetectable they are much less likely to transmit to another person. This is currently being used in the following ways:

- Prevention of mother-to-child transmission (PMTCT):
  - Mother receives ARVs during (at least) the last trimester regardless of CD4 count
  - Infant is given 4wks of treatment after delivery
  - Mother and/or the infant continue ARVs if breastfeeding.
- Pre-exposure prophylaxis (PrEP):
  - ARVs are taken before risk of exposure to HIV
  - Not widely used but may be targeted for men who have sex with men (MSM), sex workers, or prior to conception.
- Post-exposure prophylaxis (PEP/PEPSE):
  - Short-term treatment (usually 1 month) after possible exposure to HIV
  - Must be started with 72h of potential exposure
  - May be exposure through occupation causes (e.g. needlestick injuries) or via sexual exposure (e.g. unprotected sex, sexual assault).
- Treatment as prevention (TasP):
  - Treatment regardless of CD4 count to prevent transmission to others
  - Discordant couples (i.e. one HIV+ve, one –ve), patients with multiple (casual) partners especially if not consistently using condoms
  - HIV+ve healthcare workers carrying out exposure prone procedures to prevent transmission to patients.

In all these scenarios, the preventative effect of ARVs is only as good as patient adherence. For effective PMTCT or TasP the aim is an undetectable viral load (<50 copies/mL).

ARV classes and mechanisms of action are shown in Table 19.4.

New medicines are continually being added to the market with the aims of:
- improving viral control
- reducing the potential risk of resistance occurring
- ↓ pill burden
- improving tolerability
- reducing the degree of monitoring required
- improving the safety profile including minimizing interactions with other medicines and food.

Table 19.4 Antiretroviral classes and mechanism of action

Class	Mechanism of action	Common examples
Nucleoside analogue reverse transcriptase inhibitors (NRTIs)	The inhibitor binds to the evolving DNA chain produced by reverse transcriptase and terminates production of viral DNA	Abacavir Emtricitabine Lamivudine Tenofovir Zidovudine Combinations include: Kivexa®, Truvada®, Combivir® (now generic available)
Non-nucleoside analogue reverse transcriptase inhibitors (NNRTIs)	The inhibitor binds to the reverse transcriptase enzyme, changing the configuration of the molecule so that it is no longer functional	Efavirenz Etravirine Nevirapine Rilpivirine
Protease inhibitors (PI)*	The protease enzyme cleaves the newly made polypeptides, creating mature protein particles for the new virus. PIs bind to this enzyme to inhibit this process and prevent maturation of the virus	Atazanavir/ritonavir Darunavir/ritonavir Lopinavir/ritonavir (Kaletra®)
Integrase inhibitors	Inhibition of the enzyme integrase which prevents integration of the viral DNA into the host DNA	Dolutegravir Elvitegravir Raltegravir
CCR5 receptor antagonists	Block the entry of the HIV virus into the CD4 cell by preventing the virus from binding to CCR5 receptors	Maraviroc

*The commonly used PIs are always used with ritonavir which inhibits metabolism of the PI, so boosting blood levels and extending the half-life.

Monitoring

Before a patient commences HIV therapy, the following factors need to be considered:

• Viral load level (copies/mL)—a baseline figure is necessary to indicate success of the treatment once started. If the viral load is too high, with some medicines there may be a higher risk of treatment failure (e.g. if viral load is >100 000 copies/mL then the patient is potentially less likely to achieve viral load suppression when taking certain ARVs such as rilpivirine).

- CD4 count—a baseline figure is required for monitoring purposes. It is also necessary for some medicines (nevirapine), as if the CD4 count is above a certain level the likelihood for adverse effects is greater.
- Baseline resistance test—to identify any resistance mutations which might exclude use of certain ARVs or classes.
- HLA-B*5701 status—this test is conducted as patients who test positive to this test are likely to have a hypersensitivity reaction to abacavir and therefore abacavir must be avoided as this could be life-threatening.
- Past medical history—e.g. Cardiac disease, renal and liver function, psychological history.
- Allergies
- Drug history (including over-the-counter, herbal, and recreational drugs)—to avoid or manage drug interactions.
- Investigations—including FBC, creatinine, eGFR, liver function tests, glucose, lipid profile, bone profile, urinalysis, urine protein:creatinine ratio, BP.
- Hepatitis B and C status.
- Sexual history/sexually transmitted infections.
- Weight.
- Adherence potential.

These factors will then be monitored with ongoing therapy depending on the medicines prescribed.

Effect of triple-therapy regimens

- Viral load will ↓ with the aim of becoming undetectable. This is the threshold at which standard blood tests will not detect a virus which can be as low as 20 copies/mL, though <50 is usually considered as the threshold for undetectable virus.
- The CD4 count should also ↑ as the viral load reduces. This will vary depending on when treatment was started in relation to CD4 count and there is great inter-patient variability.

Adherence

Adherence is one of the most important aspects of HIV treatment. Poor adherence will lead to treatment failure due to resistance of the HIV medicines. Pharmacists play a key role in helping patients to understand their illness, the medications being used, and try to tailor the regimen to the patient, as well as being supportive throughout their treatment and responding to queries including side effects and interactions with other medicines.

Patient involvement in the choice of therapy is vital to ensure the patient is on a regimen which suits them (see also ➲ Chapter 1, pp. 1–16):

- Reasons for non-adherence can often be more complex than in other illnesses, due to the stigma which is often still attached to the disease.
- In HIV, adherence can be specifically assessed using the viral load. If adherence is poor, the viral load will ↑.
- It is recommended that patients should be 95% adherent to their ARV treatment. For a once-a-day regimen this means not missing or significantly delaying more than two to three doses each month. Poor adherence will ↑ the risk of developing resistance and can lead to treatment failure.

Resistance

Resistance with HIV medicines occurs if patients do not adhere to their medication regimen. HIV replicates rapidly, making billions of new virus daily, some of which may mutate and be spontaneously resistant to ARVs. For example, the reverse transcription enzyme which makes DNA is very error prone. When a patient is not on ARV treatment, the mutated viruses will be the minority and overwhelmed by 'wild-type' (fully sensitive) virus. However, if a patient is poorly adherent to therapy the wild-type virus load will ↓, allowing the resistant viruses to predominate. The viral load will ↑, CD4 count will drop, and HIV complications may develop (e.g. opportunistic infections). Adherence to ARVs should then be checked as well as investigating likely drug interactions and history of vomiting or diarrhoea which may result in poor absorption.

If no other cause for the viral load ↑ is found then resistance should be suspected and a resistance test done to determine which ARVs the virus is resistant to. Note that if the patient has not been taking ARVs at all and/or the viral load is high then it is likely that wild-type virus has become the predominant species again and the resistance test may not pick up resistant virus. BHIVA recommends that patients should have been consistently taking their ARV regimen for at least 2wks before performing a resistance test. The ARV regimen should be changed as soon as possible based on the resistance test. Continuing a partially effective ARV regimen can allow further mutations to evolve.

Interactions

(See also ➔ 'Drug interactions', pp. 23–5.)

Interactions with HIV medicines are increasingly common and complex as patients are on triple therapy and with ↑ life expectancy are often receiving medicines for other illnesses. A thorough medication history is required including over-the-counter, herbal, and recreational medicines. Interactions can occur due to the ARVs affecting other medicines or other medicines can affect the effectiveness of the ARVs themselves.

The most common interactions occur with the PIs and NNRTIs (mainly metabolized by the CYP450 enzyme system), but it is important to be vigilant with all of the medicines. Some ARVs (e.g. efavirenz) can act as inhibitors and inducers of the CYP450 enzyme system.

All potential drug interactions must be checked before administration of another medicine—℘ www.hiv-druginteractions.org is a useful resource.

Another important aspect of interactions with HIV medicines is consideration of absorption of the medicine related to food. For example, rilpivirine absorption is ↑ by food (with a requirement to take it with a minimum number of calories) or ↑ the risk of side effects (efavirenz).

Counselling points for patient on ARVs:
- Aim to take ARVs at roughly same time each day—emphasize adherence and the risk of resistance.
- Do not miss a dose.
- Never run out of supplies of ARVs.
- Information about whether the ARV needs to be taken with food/ empty stomach.

- Interactions with other medicines including herbal, recreational, and over-the-counter medicines (should keep the clinic and pharmacist up to date on any changes).
- What to expect from side effects and how to manage them, when to contact the clinic, etc.
- Treatment is currently lifelong.
- Healthy living advice including reducing cardiovascular risk, stopping smoking due to ↑ risk of cardiovascular disease, and certain cancers in patients with HIV.
- Advise that the patient should inform their GP of their HIV diagnosis if they have not already done so.

The HIV Pharmacist Association (HIVPA) produce patient information leaflets on all the antiretrovirals which are available on their website.

Further reading

'British HIV Association' website, ℘ www.bhiva.org
HIV Pharmacist Association (HIVPA)' website, ℘ www.hivpa.org

Tuberculosis: treatment considerations

Mycobacteria represent a genus of >100 species of which a number are pathogenic in man. For clinical purposes they are generally divided into three groups:

- *Mycobacterium tuberculosis* (MTB) and MTB complex (*M. bovis*, *M. africanum*, *M. canetti*, *M. africanum*) which cause tuberculosis (TB)
- *M. leprae* which causes leprosy
- Non-tuberculosis mycobacteria (NTM) such as *M. avium intracellular* (MAI) or *M. abcessus* which generally only cause disease in patients with underlying conditions such as HIV and cystic fibrosis.

Mycobacteria are mostly environmental pathogens though MTB complex and leprosy require a living organism as host. Typically they will colonize the host without causing active disease. It is thought that up to a third of the world population is colonized with TB. Most commonly (but not always) active disease is associated with co-morbidities such as poor health and hygiene conditions. ~1% of the world's population has active TB at any time, mostly in developing countries. However, TB, including drug-resistant TB, is being seen increasingly in the UK.

TB is predominantly transmitted as an airborne infection and consequently most commonly presents as pulmonary TB. Due to the risk of transmission, pulmonary TB is regarded as a public health risk and consequently contact tracing is done and every effort is made to ensure the patient adheres to treatment and doesn't infect others. In addition to the lungs, TB can affect other organs (e.g. CNS, bone, abscesses, and lymph nodes). These extrapulmonary presentations of TB are not regarded as a risk to public health.

Treatment

All forms of drug-sensitive TB and MTB complex are treated with standard four-drug therapy of rifampicin, isoniazid, pyrazinamide, and ethambutol initially for 2 months, and then rifampicin and isoniazid alone for a further 4 months (occasionally longer for non-pulmonary TB). Pyridoxine is usually added to reduce the risk of isoniazid-induced peripheral neuropathy.

Multi-drug resistant TB (MDRTB) is defined as TB infection resistant to isoniazid and rifampicin and extremely-drug resistant TB (XDRTB) is also resistant to quinolones and injectable anti-TB drugs. These infections represent a significant public health risk and ↑ costs both financially and to the patient in terms of treatment burden and potential side effects. The WHO guidelines[5] should be followed using at least four drugs for which there is sensitivity and for a year or more.

Role of the pharmacist

Pharmacists have an important role to play in the management of TB. While many TB clinics will employ specialist nurses to support patients, do contact tracing, etc., pharmacists also have much to contribute. Non-specialist pharmacists need to be especially alert if a patient on TB drugs is admitted or seen in the community pharmacy due to the multiple drug interactions and complex side effects of TB drugs. An invaluable source of

information on TB therapy including drugs used to treat MDRTB and XDRTB is
℘ www.tbdrugmonographs.co.uk. This resource includes recommendations on dose, therapeutic drug monitoring, and monitoring for side effects.

Adherence

Adherence is particularly important as treatment failure can lead to recurrence and resistance. It is important to make sure that this is fully understood and the patient is aware of the consequences of poor adherence.
Patients who are unable to swallow the tablets/capsules may need a liquid
formulation for a period of time. Those nil by mouth will need parenteral
formulations. Part of adherence relies on maintaining continuity of supplies
and this may need to be communicated to the patient's preferred pharmacy. The majority of TB clinics in the UK will supply the drugs for the
full treatment course but community pharmacies may need to be aware
of availability issues for second-line (unlicensed) agents. As TB is a public
health risk, in most countries TB treatment is provided free. It is advisable
to provide both written and verbal information. Patient information leaflets
(including in many other languages) can be found on the TB Alert website
(℘ www.tbalert.org). WHO has recommended that to ensure adherence
directly observed therapy (DOTS) is used. This usually involves the patient
attending a clinic or pharmacy to be observed taking their medicines, or a
specialist healthcare professional visiting the patient to administer the drugs.
In the UK, DOTS is usually only used under exceptional circumstances but
pharmacists may be asked to facilitate this, e.g. observing the TB drugs being
taken for patients who are also on supervised opioid replacement therapy.

Adverse effects

Be aware and warn patients that their body fluids may become orange or
red (due to rifampicin) but that this is harmless. Advise patients of the signs
of potential hypersensitivity, visual disturbance, hepatotoxicity, and neurotoxicity and to seek medical advice if these occur. Monitor for side effects.

Drug interactions

Rifampicin is a potent CYP450 enzyme inducer and is also metabolized by
CYP450. This can be especially challenging in patients with co-morbidities
such as seizures or HIV where significant drug interactions may occur.
Check for potential drug interactions with all other TB drugs especially isoniazid (which is a mild inhibitor of MAOIs) and second-line agents.

Dose adjustments

Many patients with TB are underweight and as their health improves, weight
gain may occur and doses will need to be adjusted to compensate for this.
Dose adjustment is required in renal impairment for many TB drugs, notably
ethambutol. A number of the second-line TB drugs require TDM—check
that levels are being taken at the right time and dose adjustments made as
needed.

Pregnancy and breastfeeding

Ideally ♀ patients should avoid becoming pregnant while on TB treatment as the debilitating nature of the disease can lead to poor pregnancy
outcomes (e.g. low birth weight). However, many patients will already be
pregnant at diagnosis. There is no evidence of congenital abnormalities

associated with first-line TB drugs and the benefit of improved maternal health far outweighs any risks. Some of the second-line agents have known risks in pregnancy (e.g. aminoglycosides) but for some there will be little or no information. For patients with MDRTB and XDRTB, there is often little choice of drug and it may be necessary to use a drug which is linked to congenital abnormalities or has little or no information on safety in pregnancy. Again, the benefit of improving maternal health likely far outweighs any risks as TB is potentially life-threatening to the mother and fetus but pregnant ♀ should be fully informed and involved in decision-making. First-line TB drugs are excreted into breast milk but in quantities that are not considered a risk to the infant, though supplementation with additional pyridoxine for the infant is usually advised. Due to limited evidence on second-line drugs and breastfeeding, ideally the mother should be advised to formula feed if at all possible.

Reference

5. WHO (2011). 'Guidelines for the programmatic management of drug-resistant tuberculosis: 2011 update', ℹ http://apps.who.int/iris/bitstream/10665/44597/1/9789241501583_eng.pdf

Therapy-related issues: endocrine

Diabetes mellitus

Diabetes is a common, life-long health condition. According to Diabetes UK, in 2014 there were 3.2 million people diagnosed with diabetes in the UK and an estimated 630 000 people who had the condition, but were unaware of it.

Diabetes is a condition in which the concentration of glucose in the blood is too high because the body cannot use it properly. This is because the pancreas doesn't produce any insulin, or not enough insulin, to help glucose enter the body's cells or when the insulin that is produced does not work properly (known as insulin resistance).

There are two main types of diabetes—type 1 and type 2.

Type 1 diabetes develops when the insulin-producing cells in the body have been destroyed and the body is unable to produce any insulin. This is secondary to autoimmune dysfunction. Type 1 diabetes accounts for about 10% of all adults with diabetes and is treated by daily insulin injections, a healthy diet, and regular physical activity. Type 1 diabetes can develop at any age but usually appears before the age of 40, and especially in childhood. It is the most common type of diabetes found in childhood.

Type 2 diabetes develops when the insulin that is produced does not work properly (insulin resistance), or when the insulin-producing cells in the body (pancreatic β-cells) are unable to produce enough insulin. Type 2 diabetes usually appears in people over the age of 40, though in South Asian people, who are at greater risk, it often appears from the age of 25. It is also increasingly becoming more common in children, adolescents, and young people of all ethnicities. Type 2 diabetes accounts for between 85% and 95% of all people with diabetes and is initially treated with a healthy diet and ↑ physical activity. In addition to this, medication and/or insulin are often required.

Diabetic risk factors

The number of people with diabetes in the UK is growing. By 2025, it is estimated that 5 million people will have diabetes—risking all the serious secondary complications that are associated with it.

At the moment, there is nothing that can be done to prevent type 1 diabetes. But around 80% of cases of type 2 diabetes can be prevented or delayed by maintaining a healthy weight, eating well, and being active.

Type 2 diabetes can come on slowly, usually in people over the age of 40. The symptoms may not be obvious, or there may be no symptoms at all. Therefore it might be up to 10yrs before a person has a diagnosis.

People are more at risk of type 2 diabetes if they:
- are overweight or have a high BMI
- have a large waist (>80cm/31.5 inches in ♀, 94 cm/37 inches in ♂, or 90cm/35 inches in South Asian ♂)
- are from an African-Caribbean, Black African, Chinese, or South Asian background and >25yrs old
- are from another ethnic background and >40yrs old
- have a parent, brother, or sister with diabetes
- have ever had high BP, a heart attack, or a stroke
- have a history of polycystic ovaries, gestational diabetes, or have given birth to a baby >10 pounds/4.5kg
- suffer from schizophrenia, bipolar illness, or depression, or are taking antipsychotic medication
- have impaired glucose regulation.

Diabetes symptoms and diagnosis

Symptoms occur because some or all of the glucose stays in the blood and is not being used as fuel for energy. The body tries to reduce blood glucose levels by flushing the excess glucose out of the body in the urine.

The main signs and symptoms of diabetes are:
- passing urine more often than usual (polyuria), especially at night (nocturia)
- ↑ thirst (polydipsia)
- extreme tiredness
- unexplained weight loss
- genital itching or regular episodes of thrush
- slow healing of cuts and wounds
- blurred vision.

Together with these symptoms, a diagnosis of diabetes can be confirmed when any of the following results are noted:
- A random plasma glucose level of >11mmol/L
- A fasting plasma glucose of >7mmol/L
- A 2h plasma glucose of >11mmol/L.

The second and third results are measured during an oral glucose tolerance test (OGTT). The patient will have been asked to not eat or drink certain fluids for 8–12h. They then have a blood sample taken at the start of the test, after which they drink 75g of glucose, then a second blood sample is taken after 2h.

In type 1 diabetes, the signs and symptoms are usually very obvious and develop very quickly, typically over a few weeks. The symptoms are quickly relieved once the diabetes is treated and under control.

In type 2 diabetes, the signs and symptoms may not be so obvious as the condition develops slowly over a period of years and may only be picked up in a routine medical check-up. Symptoms are quickly relieved once diagnosis is confirmed and the diabetes is treated and under control.

Pharmaceutical management of diabetes

As well as making lifestyle changes, people with diabetes often need additional treatments, such as medication, to control their diabetes. Patients must understand that medication is not a substitute for following a healthy diet and taking regular physical activity.

Pharmaceutical management of diabetes is through:
- oral or SC medication
- insulin.

Diabetes medication lowers blood glucose levels. There are a number of different types of medication which work in different ways. People with type 2 diabetes may need medication including insulin. It should be noted and patients informed that diabetes medication cannot cure diabetes, and most people will have to take it for the rest of their lives.

The type of medication required will depend on the individual needs and situation of each patient. Despite keeping to a healthy diet, physical activity, and taking diabetes medication regularly, diabetes control may deteriorate with time. This is because type 2 diabetes is a progressive condition and, over time, the medication may need to be changed in order to manage the blood glucose levels.

NICE published a clinical guideline for the management of type 2 diabetes in adults in December 2015 (updated in July 2016).[1] This guideline should be followed when the combination of medications is being considered for individual patients.

Types of oral or subcutaneous diabetes medication

There are several different types of diabetes medication:
- Biguanide
- Sulfonylureas
- α-glucosidase inhibitor
- Meglitinides
- Thiazolidinediones (glitazones)
- Incretin mimetics
- DPP-4 inhibitors (gliptins).
- SGLT2 inhibitors.

These groups may contain more than one medication.

Biguanide
- The only biguanide used is metformin.
- It is available in different forms—tablets for immediate release (up to three times per day) or prolonged release (usually once per day), and oral solution and powder for oral solution for immediate release.
- Mechanism:
  - ↓ gluconeogenesis
  - ↑ peripheral utilization of glucose.
- Metformin is often the first-line treatment if management by a healthy diet and physical activity alone has not sufficiently controlled blood glucose levels.
- Often used for people who are overweight because it generally does not encourage weight gain and can reduce the risk of cardiovascular complications.
- Can lead to a reduction in HbA_{1c}: 1–1.3%.
- The initial dose is 500mg daily, which can be ↑ by 500mg/day weekly and has a maximum effective dose of 2000mg/day.
- Lactic acidosis is rare (<0.3%). However, it can be fatal in up to 50% of these instances.
- Metformin does not cause hypoglycaemia.
- Contraindicated with serum creatinine >133μmol/L in ♂ and 124μmol/L in ♀.
- Use with caution in patients aged >80yrs (should have normal renal clearance) and in those with hepatic dysfunction, alcoholism, unstable congestive heart failure (CHF), or dehydration.
- GI side effects (nausea, vomiting, diarrhoea) are noted to occur in up to 50% of patients with this medication. In these cases, advice can be given for the patient to take this with food, maintaining a 'Start low and go slow' method.
- Improves lipid profile; weight neutral or weight loss.
- ↓ macrovascular events.

Sulfonylureas
- Mechanism: stimulates insulin release from binding to sulfonylurea β-cell site, targeting post-prandial glucose (short acting).
- Place in therapy: monotherapy, combination therapy, can be first line.
- Sulfonylureas are most suitable for people who are not overweight, as they may encourage weight gain.
- Taken once or twice daily with or shortly before a meal.
- Can lead to a reduction in HbA_{1c}: 0.9–2.5%.
- Examples: gliclazide, glibenclamide, tolbutamide
- Risks: hypoglycaemia, weight gain.
- No additional benefit has been noted at doses of >50% of maximum dose.

Alpha-glucosidase inhibitors
- Mechanism: slows carbohydrate absorption in gut, targeting post-prandial glucose.
- Place in therapy: monotherapy or combination therapy with metformin
- Can lead to a reduction in HbA_{1c}: 0.6–1.3%.
- Only one α-glucosidase inhibitor available: acarbose. As this medication ↓ post-prandial glucose, it must be taken with the first bite of a carbohydrate-containing meal.
- Patients prescribed this medication should 'Start low and go slow' in order to avoid GI intolerance.
- If hypoglycaemia occurs (risk if on insulin or sulfonylurea), patients must be treated with glucose (not sucrose) as acarbose interferes with sucrose absorption.

Meglitinides
- Mechanism: stimulates insulin release from binding to sulfonylurea β-cell site, targeting post-prandial glucose (short acting).
- Place in therapy: monotherapy or combination therapy.
- Can lead to a reduction in HbA_{1c}: 0.6–0.8%.
- Examples: repaglinide, nateglinide.
- Risks: hypoglycaemia, weight gain.
- The need for frequent dosing may adversely affect compliance.

Thiazolidinediones (glitazones)
- Mechanism: activates PPAR-G (peroxisome proliferator-activated receptor-γ), ↑ peripheral insulin sensitivity in skeletal muscle cells, targeting fasting blood glucose.
- Place in therapy: considered second line, but could be monotherapy in patients with lower HbA_{1c} range (6.5–8%), combination therapy.
- Can lead to a reduction in HbA_{1c}: 1.5–1.6%.
- Example: pioglitazone, which may have positive effects on lipids (↑ HDL, ↓ TG).
- A delayed onset of action is usually seen, which may be 6–8wks or as much as 12wks.
- Oedema and weight gain are noted to occur more if thiazolidinediones are used in combination with insulin.
- Thiazolidinediones are contraindicated in patients with NYHA class III and IV heart failure, nor should it be used in patients who are diagnosed with underlying liver dysfunction.

- An ↑ in bone fracture rates has been reported in ♀who are prescribed with this medication.
- Following a Europe-wide review of available data on the risks and benefits of rosiglitazone in September 2010, the UK Commission on Human Medicine (CHM) withdrew this product from clinical use in the UK because of an ↑ risk of cardiovascular disorders including MI and cardiac failure.
- Restrictions on pioglitazone—please check with the *BNF*.

Incretin mimetics
- Glucagon-like peptide-1 (GLP-1) incretin mimetic; mimics incretin hormone given by injection.
- Mechanism: stimulates insulin secretion in response to glucose load; inhibits release of glucagon following a meal; ↑ satiety; slows absorption of nutrients through delayed gastric emptying.
- Place in therapy: adjunct therapy for use in combination with sulfonylureas, metformin, or a combination of these.
- Can lead to a reduction in HbA_{1c} of 0.8–0.9%.
- Examples include: exenatide, liraglutide, and lixisenatide.
- Common side effects of incretin mimetics include nausea and vomiting (dose-related), with recent reports arising of possible exenatide pancreatitis.
- Currently its use is not recommended in patients with a history of pancreatitis.
- NICE guidance for the use of exenatide and liraglutide in the management of type 2 diabetes is available.[1]

DPP-4 inhibitors (gliptins)
- Mechanism: slows inactivation of incretin hormone GLP-4, suppressing glucagon secretion and ↑ glucose-dependent insulin release and targeting post-prandial blood glucose.
- Place in therapy: monotherapy or combination therapy.
- Can lead to a reduction in HbA_{1c} of 0.8%.
- Examples: sitagliptin, vildagliptin.
- Dosage adjustment is necessary for patients diagnosed with renal dysfunction.
- ↑ satiety has been noted, along with a delay in gastric emptying and patient's weight maintaining neutral.

SGLT2 (sodium-glucose co-transporter 2) inhibitors (gliflozins)
- Mechanism: lowers blood glucose in people with type 2 diabetes by blocking the reabsorption of glucose in the kidneys and promoting excretion of excess glucose in the urine.
- Place in therapy: monotherapy or combined therapy.
- Can lead to a reduction in HbA_{1c} of 0.2–0.5%.
- Examples: canagliflozin and dapagliflozin
- Known risks for SGLT2s include hypoglycaemia.
- Canagliflozin should not be recommended to patients with an estimated glomerular filtration rate (eGFR) which is persistently <45mL/min/1.73 m^2, and dapagliflozin is not recommended when a patient's eGFR is persistently <60mL/min/1.73 m^2
- Weight loss has been noted for patients on this medication.
- Additional NICE guidance is available for canagliflozin in combination therapy for treating type 2 diabetes.[2]

Insulin

The three groups of insulin

There are three groups of insulin: animal, human, and analogues. Most patients use human insulin and insulin analogues, although a small number of people still use animal insulin because they have some evidence/experience that they may otherwise lose their awareness of hypos, or they find animal insulin works better for them.

Main types of insulin

There are six main types of insulin:

- Rapid-acting analogues:
  - These can be injected just before, with, or after food and have a peak action at between 0h and 3h and only last long enough for the meal at which they are taken. They tend to last between 2h and 5h and are clear in appearance.
  - Examples: insulin glulisine, insulin lispro, insulin aspart.
- Long-acting analogues:
  - This type of insulin tends to be injected once a day to provide background insulin and lasts ~24h. Long-acting analogues don't need to be taken with food because they don't have a peak action and are clear in appearance.
  - Examples: insulin glargine, insulin detemir, insulin degludec.
- Short-acting insulins:
  - Short-acting insulins need to be injected 15–30min before a meal to cover the rise in blood glucose levels that occurs after eating. They have a peak action of 2–6h and can last for up to 8h. They are clear in appearance.
  - Example: insulin Actrapid®.
- Medium- and long-acting insulins:
  - These insulins are to be taken once or twice a day in order to provide background insulin, or in combination with short-acting insulins/rapid-acting analogues. Their peak activity is between 4h and 12h and can last up to 30h. They are cloudy in appearance.
  - Example: isophane insulin.
- Mixed insulin:
  - A combination of medium- and short-acting insulin.
- Mixed analogue:
  - Comprises a combination of medium-acting insulin and rapid-acting analogue.

References

1. NICE (2015, updated 2016). 'Type 2 diabetes in adults: management (NG28)', ℘ www.nice.org.uk/guidance/ng28
2. NICE (2014). 'Canagliflozin in combination therapy for treating type 2 diabetes (TA315)', ℘ www.nice.org.uk/guidance/ta315

Monitoring and control of diabetes

Monitoring diabetes is important in preventing some of the possible short- and long-term complications associated with diabetes.

There are two aspects to monitoring diabetes:
- Monitoring which the patient carries out themselves at home:
  - blood glucose
  - urine glucose (in some patients)
  - blood ketones (in some patients)
- Monitoring which should be carried out by the patient's diabetes team at least yearly to screen for complications—see ➔ 'Care from healthcare professionals' pp. 493–4.

This section will mainly focus on the monitoring that adult patients carry out themselves.

Blood glucose levels

Self-monitoring of blood glucose can be a beneficial part of diabetes management. As part of the day-to-day routine it can help with necessary lifestyle and treatment choices as well as help to monitor symptoms of hypo- or hyperglycaemia. Monitoring can also help the patient and healthcare team to adjust treatment, which in turn can help prevent any long-term complications from developing.

Some patients with diabetes (but not all) will test their blood glucose levels at home. Home blood glucose testing gives an accurate picture of the blood glucose level at the time of the test. It involves pricking the side of the finger (as opposed to the pad) with a finger-pricking device and putting a drop of blood on a testing strip.

Patients should be informed by their diabetes healthcare team regarding the frequency with which monitoring should be carried out.

Blood glucose targets

It is important to aim for blood glucose levels which are as near normal as possible (i.e. in the range seen in a non-diabetic), which are:
- 3.5–5.5mmol/L before meals
- <8mmol/L, 2h after meals.

There are many different opinions about the ideal range to aim for. This is so individual to each patient that the target levels must be specifically agreed between the patient and the diabetes team.

The following target blood glucose ranges are indicated as a guide.
Adults with type 1 diabetes:[3,4]
- A fasting plasma glucose level of 5–7mmol/L on waking *and*
- A plasma glucose level of 4–7mmol/L before meals at other times of the day.

Type 2 diabetes:[5]
- Before meals: 4–7mmol/L
- 2h after meals: <8.5mmol/L.

Blood glucose meters

Choosing a meter can be quite complex as new products are coming on to the market all the time. Some manufacturers have also produced computer software packages that enable the patient to look at trends in their blood glucose levels. Members of the patient's diabetes team (usually the diabetes nurse) should help the patient to choose a meter that suits their individual needs. It's essential that the patient is taught how to carry out a test properly—poor technique may lead to incorrect results which could lead to inaccurate medication dosing.

Test strips

The strips used with meters are nearly always provided in batches of 50. The Monthly Index of Medical Specialities (MIMS) has a monthly up-to-date table to help healthcare professionals ensure that the correct testing strips are chosen for the meter which the patient owns—care has to be taken in matching the correct strips to the individual patient's monitor as there are many different monitors and strips on the market.

Finger-pricking devices and lancets

Finger-pricking devices are automatic devices that pierce the skin so that a drop of blood can be extracted for testing. The devices insert a lancet (a very short, fine needle) into the skin using a spring mechanism. The depth at which the needle is inserted can be adjusted depending on the thickness of the skin. Lancets are available in different sizes, or gauges. A higher-gauge lancet is generally less painful; however, the patient may not get enough blood to test with the higher-gauge needles.

It is important to let the patient know that lancets are designed to be used only once. If they are used more than once they become blunt and painful to use.

Patients should be made aware of the following steps to make the process of blood glucose testing easier:
• Washing the hands in warm water and shaking the hand to ↑ blood flow before testing.
• Always using the sides of the fingers rather than the more sensitive fleshy pulp at the tips.

Recording blood glucose results

It is important that patients record their blood glucose tests as it will help them to adjust treatment if they have been taught how to adjust medication in conjunction with their blood glucose readings. It also helps the healthcare team to assess how well the patient's diabetes is being managed.

Although the majority of the blood glucose meters which are on the market now store a specific number of previous readings, it is best that patients record their readings in a more permanent long-term form. Some patients choose to record their results in a diary and others use a computer software package provided by the meter manufacturer or use the Diabetes UK Tracker smartphone app. The Diabetes UK Tracker app, launched in 2013, was designed by a team that included user experience professionals, clinical specialists, and people with diabetes.

Urine testing

Urine testing involves holding a test strip under a stream of urine for a few seconds and comparing the colour change on the strip, after a set amount of time, with the chart on the strip container. This form of glucose testing tends to be used by patients who do not like using lancets/have needle phobias.

Testing is best carried out in the morning before breakfast. The patient should empty their bladder once they have got up, then test a sample of urine passed 30min later. Tests done at this time should be negative for glucose. Patients can also test 2–3h after a meal, when their blood glucose will have been at its highest.

- Urine testing gives a less accurate picture of diabetes control than blood testing, due to the fact that there is usually no glucose in the urine unless the glucose levels have risen to 10mmol/L or above, which is considered quite high.
- Urine testing does not give an indication of what the blood glucose level is at the time of the test, because the urine being tested may have been produced several hours before the test.
- Urine tests also cannot tell if blood glucose is too low—which is important for patients on insulin.
- Older patients may develop a high renal threshold, this means glucose does not appear in the urine until the level in the blood is much higher than 10mmol/L.
- Because urine testing involves comparing a colour change on the urine testing strip, it is not suitable for patients who are visually impaired.

Ketone monitoring

The presence of high levels of ketones in the bloodstream is a serious complication of diabetes, leading to the clinical state of diabetic ketoacidosis.

Ketones are acids remaining when the body burns its own fat. When the body has insufficient insulin, it cannot take glucose from the blood into the body's cells to use as energy, and will instead begin to burn fat. When the body is burning too much fat, it may cause ketones to become present in the bloodstream.

High levels of ketones are more common in people with type 1 diabetes, particularly when the patient is unwell and/or when patients are having difficulties controlling their diabetes and the blood glucose level is 13.9mmol/L (250mg/dL) or above for two consecutive tests.

Historically, ketones could only be tested in a hospital. However, there are a few home blood ketone meters which measure levels in a similar way to blood glucose testing. A member of the diabetes healthcare team will recommend when a patient should have these meters for home use.

Blood ketone levels

Blood ketone readings should be taken in conjunction with blood glucose readings and not used on their own. Interpretation of levels for home readings is as follows:

- <0.6mmol/L—a normal blood ketone value
- 0.6–1.5mmol/L—more ketones are being produced than normal; retest 2h later to see if the value has lowered

- 1.6–3.0mmol/L—a high level of ketones which could present a risk of ketoacidosis. The patient should contact their GP or diabetes nurse
- >3.0mmol/L—a dangerous level of ketones which requires immediate medical attention.

Glycated haemoglobin (HbA1c)

The most common annual blood test carried out in diabetic patients is the HbA1c test, which indicates the blood glucose levels for the previous 2–3 months.

The term HbA1c refers to glycated haemoglobin. This is formed when haemoglobin, a protein within red blood cells that carries oxygen throughout the body, joins with glucose in the blood, thus becoming 'glycated'. By measuring HbA1c, clinicians are able to get an overall picture of that patient's average blood glucose levels over the previous 2–3 months.

The amount of glucose that combines with the haemoglobin is directly proportional to the total amount of glucose that is in the patient's bloodstream at that time.

Because red blood cells in the human body survive for 8–12wks before renewal, measuring HbA1c can be used to reflect average blood glucose levels over that duration, thus providing a useful longer-term gauge of blood glucose control.

For patients with diabetes this measure is important, as the higher the HbA1c, the greater the risk of developing diabetes-related complications.

HbA1c targets

For adults *without diabetes*, the range is 20–41mmol/mol (4–5.9%), For most adults *with diabetes*, the HbA1c target is <48mmol/mol (6.5%),[3,4] since evidence shows that this can reduce the risk of developing complications, such as nerve damage, eye disease, and kidney disease. Individuals at risk of severe hypoglycaemia should aim for a less stringent HbA1c of <53mmol/mol (7%).[4] However, any reduction in HbA1c levels (and therefore, any improvement in control), is still considered to have beneficial effects on reducing the onset and progression of complications.

HbA1c results

HbA1c results are now reported using the IFCC (International Federation of Clinical Chemistry) reference measurement procedure of mmol/mol. HbA1c can be expressed as a percentage (DCCT unit) or as a value in mmol/mol (IFCC unit). Since 2009, mmol/mol has been the default unit to use in the UK. Table 20.1 equates the HbA1c as expressed as a percentage (DCCT unit) with the equivalent as a value in mmol/mol (IFCC unit).

Note that the HbA1c value, which is measured in mmol/mol, should not be confused with a blood glucose level which is measured in mmol/L.

Care from healthcare professionals

Whether patients have just been diagnosed or have had diabetes for some time, it is important that they get the right support for managing their diabetes.

Table 20.1 HbA1c results: equivalence table

DCCT unit (%)	IFCC unit (mmol/mol)
6.0	42
6.5	48
7.0	53
7.5	58
8.0	64
9.0	75

This check is referred to as an annual diabetes review: its purpose is to examine for early signs of complications and enable the patient to lead a healthy life. The annual review consists of a few tests, often on different days, and with different healthcare professionals.

The main tests that patients should have are:

- HbA1c blood test
- BP measured and recorded
- lipid blood test
- eyes screen for retinopathy
- feet check
- kidney function test
- care plan review—a discussion between the patient and healthcare team to agree goals.

NICE have clinical guidance on all aspects of care within diabetes, which is important to follow in patients with diabetes to allow best possible care for this condition.

References

3. NICE (2015). 'Type 1 diabetes in adults: diagnosis and management (NG17)', ℘ www.nice.org.uk/guidance/ng17
4. NICE (2015). 'Diabetes (type 1 and type 2) in children and young people: diagnosis and management (NG18)', ℘ www.nice.org.uk/guidance/ng18
5. NICE (2015, updated 2016). 'Type 2 diabetes in adults: management' NICE guideline [NG28], ℘ www.nice.org.uk/guidance/ng28

Thyroid disorders

The thyroid gland is the only endocrine gland to store large quantities of preformed hormones. Found anterior to the trachea in the lower neck, it is the largest endocrine organ of the human body and regulates the body's metabolism through the release of thyroid hormones in response to thyroid stimulating hormone (TSH) formed by the anterior pituitary gland.

Cells are arranged within the gland in spherical follicles that surround a thyroid hormone store and release two hormones:
- Thyroxine (T_4)—a pro-hormone that acts as a plasma reservoir
- Tri-iodothyronine (T_3)—the active hormone.

These hormones are derived from two molecules of iodine and the amino acid tyrosine, with T_3 containing three iodine atoms and T_4 containing four. The iodine required is acquired mainly from iodized salt, meat, and vegetables in the diet. The recommended daily intake of iodine is 150mg/day, though only a fraction of this amount is absorbed as the thyroid gland cells are the only cells in the body that can actively absorb and utilize plasma iodine. Iodine is then returned to plasma by the breakdown of these hormones and excreted from the body mainly via the kidneys.

The T_3 and T_4 hormones released by the thyroid gland regulate the rate of metabolism in almost every cell in the body, oxygen consumption, and heat production. They also have a role in growth and development, as well as sensitizing the cardiovascular and nervous system to catecholamines.

Regulation of thyroid hormones

Hypothalamic thyrotropin-releasing hormone (TRH) stimulates the release of TSH from the anterior pituitary gland which, in turn, acts on extracellular receptors on the surface of the thyroid follicular cells to stimulate the synthesis and secretion of T_3 and T_4. TSH also has long-term actions on the thyroid gland in ↑ its size and vascularity to improve hormone synthesis.

Thyroid hormone release is inhibited by excess thyroid hormones being in the bloodstream and glucocorticoids (e.g. cortisol) by acting on the anterior pituitary to suppress TSH release.

T_3, the active hormone, has its effect on almost every cell in the body. Peripheral tissues can regulate the amount of T_3 levels in circulation by ↑ or ↓ the amount of T_3 synthesis. Most of the deiodination is carried out by the liver and kidney. T_4, a relatively inactive molecule, is converted to T_3 by deiodination. It is important to note the following:
- The majority of plasma T_3 is formed by deiodination of T_4 and not directly from the thyroid gland.
- The concentration of T_4 in circulation is much higher than that of T_3 by a ratio of 50:1, respectively.
- T_4 has a longer half-life than T_3 (7 days:1 day, respectively).

A number of factors affect T_3 and T_4 release, the three foremost being:
- long-term exposure to cold temperatures on the anterior pituitary gland
- oestrogens acting on the anterior pituitary gland
- adrenaline (epinephrine) acting directly on the thyroid gland.

Transport of the thyroid hormones

T_3 and T_4 hormones are carried in circulation bound to plasma proteins produced in the liver thereby protecting them from enzymic attack, with 70% bound to thyroid-binding globulin (TBG) and 30% bound to albumin.

Only 0.1% of T_4 and 1% of T_3 are carried unbound. It is this free (unbound) fraction which is responsible for their hormonal activities.

Disorders of the thyroid gland

The thyroid gland is prone to a number of diseases that can alter its function and structure. As nearly all body tissues are affected by thyroid hormones, an alteration in their level of secretion affects the activity of virtually all body systems, giving rise to a wide range of presenting symptoms. The main categories of disease are:
- hyperthyroidism
- hypothyroidism
- goitre formation
- adenoma of the thyroid
- carcinoma of the thyroid.

Thyroid function tests

First-line diagnosis of primary hyper- and hypothyroidism is made from examination of serum TSH concentrations; however, this test alone is misleading in patients with secondary thyroid dysfunction.

Free hormone concentrations are unaffected by changes in binding protein concentration or affinity and usually correlate better with the metabolic state than do total hormone concentrations, therefore measurements of serum T_3 and T_4 concentrations is made through highly specific and sensitive radioimmunoassay.

As the presenting symptoms of thyroid disorders can be varied and non-specific, biochemical confirmation is necessary, yet it is important to remember that these tests should never be used alone to diagnose and decide whether treatment is necessary as clinical features need to be taken into account. Indeed, abnormalities are noted in thyroid function tests during systemic illnesses, therefore a diagnosis of hyper- or hypothyroidism should not be made in the presence of any recognized concurrent systemic illness, with the tests repeated once the illness has resolved to ensure an accurate representation of a patient's thyroid function. In instances where abnormal test results are detected in the absence of any signs or symptoms, close monitoring of the patient is required but no treatment.

Table 20.2 shows thyroid hormone concentrations seen with various thyroid abnormalities, with Table 20.3 showing the reference ranges used against which variances are determined.

When interpreting the results of thyroid function tests, the effects of drugs that the patient is taking should be borne in mind. Table 20.4 shows how the processes of the thyroid gland can be affected with certain medications.

Table 20.2 Table showing thyroid hormone concentrations associated with various thyroid abnormalities

Condition	TSH	Free T$_4$	Free T$_3$
Primary hyperthyroidism	Undetectable	↑↑	↑
T$_3$ toxicosis	Undetectable	Normal	↑↑
Thyrotoxicosis	↓	↑	↑
Subclinical hyperthyroidism	↓	Normal	Normal
Secondary hyperthyroidism (TSHoma)	↑ or normal	↑	↑
Thyroid hormone resistance or consider adherence to treatment	↑ or normal	↑	↑
Primary hypothyroidism	↑	↓	↓ or normal
Secondary hypothyroidism	↓ or normal	↓	↓ or normal
Subclinical hypothyroidism	↑	Normal	Normal
Pituitary disease/sick euthyroidism	↓	↓	↓

Table 20.3 Table showing the typical reference ranges used in thyroid function tests

Test	From	To	Units
TSH	0.4	4.5	mU/L
Free T$_3$	3.5	7.8	pmol/L
Free T$_4$	9.0	25.0	pmol/L

Table 20.4 Table showing the influence of drugs on thyroid function tests

Metabolic process	Increased	Decreased
TSH secretion	Amiodarone (transiently: becomes normal after 2–3 months)	Glucocorticoids, dopamine agonists, phenytoin, dopamine
T$_4$ synthesis/release	Iodide	Iodide, lithium
Binding proteins	Oestrogen, clofibrate, heroin	Glucocorticoids, androgens, phenytoin, carbamazepine
T$_4$ metabolism	Anticonvulsants; rifampicin	
T$_4$/T$_3$ binding in serum		Salicylates, furosemide, glucocorticoids, mefenamic acid, amiodarone, β-blockers

Hyperthyroidism

Hyperthyroidism affects ~1% of the UK population and is six times more common in women. It is defined as overactivity of the thyroid gland leading to the release of excess T_3 and T_4 hormones which, when symptomatic, is called thyrotoxicosis. The two main causes in the UK, which account for >90% of cases, are:

- Graves' disease—an autoimmune disease which is the most common cause of hyperthyroidism in the 20–50yrs age group. It is characterized by the presence of thyroid-stimulating antibodies in the blood which bind to TSH receptors in the thyroid and stimulate them to produce excess thyroid hormones in the same way as TSH stimulates the receptors
- solitary toxic nodule/toxic multinodular goitre (depending on number of nodules).

Other causes include:

- solitary toxic adenoma
- thyroiditis—due to viral infection, pregnancy, or some drugs such as amiodarone or interferon—usually transient
- exogenous iodine and iodine-containing drugs
- excessive T_3 and T_4 ingestion.

Clinical features

The presenting features in mild cases are often noted to mimic an anxiety state. The most common clinical features of hyperthyroidism are as follows:

- Weight loss (but normal appetite)
- Sweating, heat intolerance
- ↑ rate and depth of respiration
- Diarrhoea/↑ frequency of defecation
- Fatigue
- Generalized muscle weakness and muscle tremor
- Cardiac symptoms: palpitations, sinus tachycardia or atrial fibrillation, angina, heart failure.

Other symptoms include the following:

- Agitation
- Hyperkinesis
- Insomnia
- Oligomenorrhoea; infertility
- Goitre
- Eyelid retraction; lid lag.

Features specific to Graves' disease include periorbital oedema, proptosis, diplopia, ophthalmoplegia, corneal ulceration, and loss of visual acuity, with pretibial myxoedema occurring in one-third of these patients. Untreated Graves' disease has a natural history of remission and relapse, with 30–40% of patients only ever having a single episode of hyperthyroidism.

On rare occasions, patients with thyrotoxicosis present with a thyroid storm or crisis, which is considered a medical emergency as features include hyperpyrexia, dehydration, and cardiac failure.

Treatment of Graves' disease and nodular thyrotoxicosis

Antithyroid drugs

Carbimazole (the first choice of antithyroid drug in the UK) and propylthiouracil are both thionamides which inhibit thyroid peroxidase-catalysed iodination of T_4 residues and the coupling of iodotryosyl residues to reduce the synthesis of T_4 from iodine. These drugs are the first choice of therapy in younger patients with Graves' disease and are usually given for a period of 1–2yrs, monitoring thyroid status during this time and after. A delay in effect of up to 4wks from initial administration is often seen due to the preformed hormones still being released from the thyroid gland when using this prescription.

Once thyroid function tests have revealed that the patient has reached a state of normal gland function (i.e. of a euthyroid state), the prescribed dose can usually be reduced to a lower maintenance dose, the actual dose being determined by regular monitoring of thyroid function tests.

30–40% of patients treated with these drugs stay euthyroid 10yrs after discontinuation of therapy, with a further course of the same or alternative treatment given if the patient relapses,

NB: 5mg of carbimazole is roughly equivalent to 50mg of propylthiouracil, with propylthiouracil being the drug of choice during pregnancy and lactation because of its lower concentration in breast milk and the possible association of carbimazole with aplasia cutis.

There are two alternative treatment regimens practised:

Dose-titration regimen

As mentioned previously, the primary aim is to achieve a euthyroid state with high doses and then maintain euthyroidism with a low stable dose for ~18 months. The dose of thionamides is titrated according to the thyroid function tests performed every 4–8wks, aiming for a serum free T_4 in the normal range and a detectable TSH. A high serum TSH indicates a need for a dose reduction. TSH may remain suppressed for weeks or months.

The typical starting dose of carbimazole is 20–30mg daily and the treatment is continued for 18 months

Block-and-replace regimen

After achieving a euthyroid state on carbimazole alone, carbimazole at a dose of 40mg daily together with levothyroxine at a dose of 100 micrograms daily can be prescribed. The main advantage of this regimen is that fewer hospital visits are required and the duration of treatment is often reduced to 6 months. During treatment, free T_4 levels are measured 4wks after starting levothyroxine and the dose of levothyroxine altered, if necessary in increments of 25 micrograms to maintain free T_4 in the normal range. Most patients do not require dose adjustments.

NB: relapses are common after either regimen within the first year and are most likely in patients with large goitres and high T_4 levels at the time of diagnosis.

Side effects

Potential side effects of carbimazole and propylthiouracil are as follows:

- Pruritus and maculopapular rash—these can be treated with antihistamines without discontinuing treatment.
- Sensitivity reaction (e.g. arthralgia, jaundice, lymphadenopathy, vomiting, pyrexia)—withdrawal from treatment is required in this instance. There is rarely cross-sensitivity between the two drugs, therefore, once the patient has recovered, the other drug can be tried.
- Agranulocytosis—characterized by fever, systemic upset, mouth ulceration, and sore throat. This rare but serious side effect of both drugs is seen in 0.1–0.5% of patients and occurs very suddenly (usually within the first 3 months of therapy) in equal frequency with both antithyroid drugs. All patients prescribed these drugs should be told to report these symptoms to their GP or hospital consultant and the drug stopped immediately. The patient should have a full blood count to confirm diagnosis should this condition arise.

NB: one drug should not be substituted for the other after this reaction has been diagnosed.

Compliance with these drugs can be a problem as the patient may initially feel worse in terms of their presenting symptoms, with women often concerned about weight gain. Patients should be counselled that they will have adjusted to the change in metabolic rate after a few months, with a general improvement to symptoms seen.

Beta-blockers

β-blockers (e.g. propranolol at a dose of 20–80mg, three times a day), may provide effective temporary relief of cardiac symptoms, particularly palpitations and tremor as well as anxiety, while the antithyroid drugs (thionamides) take effect, but should be avoided in patients with asthma. It is important to consider, however, that many of the symptoms of hyperthyroidism have a β2 component, therefore contraindicating the use of cardioselective β-blockers.

Surgery

Thyroid surgery, a total or sub-total thyroidectomy, is rarely performed as a primary course of action as the thyroid overactivity needs to be controlled, usually with antithyroid drugs, prior to such a procedure to make the use of anaesthetic safe and reducing the risk of precipitating a dangerous hyperthyroid crisis or 'thyrotoxic storm'. To this end, β-blockers, usually propranolol at a dose of 20mg three times a day, can be prescribed to provide temporary symptomatic relief prior to surgery.

A recognized side effect of surgery is hypothyroidism, for which levothyroxine replacement will be needed lifelong.

Radioactive iodine

This is the primary choice of treatment for toxic nodular hyperthyroidism, if the goitre is not large, and for Graves' disease especially if there is a relapse after medical treatment or subtotal thyroidectomy, with further doses given at 2–4 months to patients who have not responded.

Radioactive iodine-131 causes necrosis of the overactive gland with minimal local or systemic side effects to the patient and minimal radiation hazard and is administered as a tasteless oral liquid after ensuring that antithyroid drugs are stopped 1wk prior to commencement of this treatment, with β-blockers able to be maintained throughout. The thyroid gland may be tender for a few days after treatment.

Precautions

Careful evaluation of the risks and benefits of this treatment option is needed as patients with thyroid eye disease are more likely to worsen with this therapy; however, worsening of eye symptoms may be prevented with a short course of corticosteroids.

Although fertility is not affected by this treatment, it is advised that ♀ should avoid getting pregnant for 6 months following treatment and ♂ should avoid fathering a child within 4 months of treatment. This treatment is contraindicated during pregnancy and it is advised not to breastfeed after therapy.

Treatment of thyroiditis

Many forms of thyroid inflammation (thyroiditis) are described as 'self-limiting'. In instances where thyroiditis is painful or prolonged, anti-inflammatory agents or corticosteroids may be helpful, with patients suffering from severe symptoms of thyrotoxicosis finding potential benefit from β-blockers.

Subclinical hyperthyroidism

In cases of subclinical hyperthyroidism, the TSH level is suppressed but the free T_3 and T_4 levels are seen as being normal. This condition, regarded as a precursor of clinical hyperthyroidism, is currently under debate as to whether or not it should be treated. Although treatment may be worthwhile in the elderly, particularly if the heart rhythm becomes abnormal or there is thinning of the bones, the decision of prescribed treatment is a matter for individual clinical assessment and evaluation.

Thyroid crisis

Thyroid crisis, or 'thyrotoxic storm', is a rare but life-threatening exacerbation of the manifestations of thyrotoxicosis and is associated with significant mortality. It is characterized by:

- severe hyperthyroidism associated with fever
- disproportionate tachycardia
- CNS dysfunction—especially confusion or severe irritability
- GI dysfunction—diarrhoea, vomiting, and jaundice.

Treatment is needed immediately under intensive care, which is beyond the remit of this chapter.

Hypothyroidism

Hypothyroidism, defined as an underactivity of the thyroid gland leading to deficient levels of serum T_3 and T_4, affects ~2% of the population in the UK and is 10 times more common in ♀ than ♂. When this becomes symptomatic, it is called myxoedema. The two main causes in the UK, which account for >90% of cases, are:

- autoimmune hypothyroidism (Hashimoto's thyroiditis) which typically affects middle aged and elderly ♀ where the thyroid cells are destroyed by lymphocytes and is usually accompanied by the presence of thyroid peroxidase (TPO) antibodies, which can be detected in the blood and are therefore a useful tool for diagnosis.
- post-surgery, radioactive iodine, and antithyroid drugs.

Other causes include:
- viral agents (De Quervain's thyroiditis)
- idiopathic atrophic hypothyroidism
- congenital factors
- dyshormonogenic hypothyroidism
- secondary to pituitary or hypothalamic disease
- iodine deficiency
- drugs—reversible caused mainly by amiodarone, lithium, and iodine.

Clinical features
The presentation of hypothyroidism is more gradual than hyperthyroidism, with many symptoms often being ignored. The onset may be insidious, with occasional symptoms noted. The clinical signs and symptoms reflect the diverse action that thyroid hormones have on the body, the most common being:
- lethargy
- cold intolerance
- dryness and coarsening of skin and hair and subcutaneous swelling (myxoedema)
- hoarseness
- weight gain
- hyperlipidaemia.

Other clinical signs and symptoms include:
- anaemia—usually macrocytic
- depression, dementia, psychosis
- constipation
- bradycardia, angina, heart failure, pericardial effusion
- muscle stiffness, carpal tunnel syndrome
- infertility, menorrhagia, galactorrhoea
- vitiligo.

Children with hypothyroidism may present with growth failure, delayed pubertal development, or deterioration in academic performance.

Goitre can occur in patients who are hypothyroid, particularly in the presence of Hashimoto's thyroiditis due to the accumulation of lymphocytes in the thyroid gland. In many recorded cases, however, there is no goitre present and the thyroid is destroyed by the time diagnosis is confirmed.

Treatment
Thyroid hormone replacement, usually with T_4 (levothyroxine), is the treatment of choice for hypothyroidism whereby the metabolic rate and demand for oxygen is ↑; however, angina or MI may be precipitated if the

latter occurs too quickly. Treatment with levothyroxine is preferable to replacement with T_3 for most patients due to its slower onset of action, with T_3 used occasionally where a more rapid response is indicated.

The required dose of levothyroxine ranges between 25 and 200 micrograms daily; the initial dose usually being 50 micrograms, ↑ in increments of 50 micrograms every 3–4wks. Elderly patients and those with ischaemic heart disease, however, are prescribed an initial dose of 25 micrograms daily or on alternate days as indicated as higher doses may cause or precipitate cardiac complications such as angina, infarction, or arrhythmias. The dose should be taken at least 30min before breakfast as food can reduce its absorption.

Although symptomatic improvement is often seen within 2–3wks, it may take up to 6wks before TSH levels respond fully. As a result, TSH levels should be checked after 6wks of commencement of levothyroxine therapy and adjusted accordingly by increments of 25–50 micrograms.

Once TSH and T_4 levels return to normal and the patient is symptom free, the adequacy of continuing treatment should be assessed by conducting annual thyroid function tests.

Most patients prescribed with levothyroxine therapy require lifelong treatment. Dose requirements rarely change once the TSH and T_4 levels are stable, with the exceptions of a dose ↑ which may be necessary during pregnancy and a dose ↓ which is sometimes indicated in the elderly. Advice is given to patients not to stop taking the treatment without consulting their doctor as the symptoms would reoccur. Patients in the UK issued with this prescription can obtain a medical exemption certificate from having to pay for this medication from the NHS Business Services Authority, having filled out a FP92A form available from GP surgeries.

NB: if under-treated, hypothyroidism can progress to a life-threatening myxoedema coma—a medical emergency with high mortality rate where T_3 (oral or injection) is the main treatment advised; however, this may be precipitated by infection, therapy with sedative drugs, or hypothermia, particularly in the elderly population.

Further reading

'British Thyroid Association' website, ℜ www.btf-thyroid.org

Daniels GH, Dayan CM (2006). *Fast Facts: Thyroid Disorders*. Abingdon: Health Press Limited.

Lazarus JH, Obuobie K (2002). Graves disease. In: Robinson S, Meeran K (eds) *Endocrinology: Specialist Handbook*, pp. 233–42. London: Martin Dunitz Limited.

The Association of Clinical Biochemistry, The British Thyroid Association, The British Thyroid Foundation (2006). 'UK Guidelines for the Use of Thyroid Function Tests', ℜ www.british-thyroid-association.org/info-for-patients/Docs/TFT_guideline_final_version_July_2006.pdf

Toft AD (2002). Hyperthyroidism. In: Robinson S, Meeran K (eds) *Endocrinology: Specialist Handbook*, pp. 211–32. London: Martin Dunitz Limited.

Turner HE, Wass JAH (2014). Thyroid. In: *Oxford Handbook of Endocrinology and Diabetes* (3rd ed), pp.1–106. Oxford: Oxford University Press.

Wahid ST, Robinson ACJ (2002). Hypothyroidism. In: Robinson S, Meeran K (eds) *Endocrinology: Specialist Handbook*, pp. 243–55. London: Martin Dunitz Limited.

Therapy-related issues: obstetrics and gynaecology

Hormonal contraception

Contraception has been an important part of human lives since the time of the early Egyptians. While methods have changed dramatically over the years, the purpose remains the same—to control fertility.

Most methods used today are female-driven and involve hormones. These methods are very effective in preventing pregnancy when taken or used as directed. Barrier methods rely on their availability at the time of intercourse and are more efficacious when used with spermicides.

Factors that need to be considered when selecting a method of contraception include the woman's potential ability to adhere to treatment, the age of the patient, medical history, personal history, and reversibility of the agent.

Failure rates for methods include the *perfect rate*, when the method is used perfectly all of the time, and the *typical rate*, which is more consistent with normal use.

Oral contraceptive pills

- Combined oral contraceptives (COCs)—containing an oestrogen and a progestogen. These are the most reliable in general use.
- Progestogen-only pills (POPs)—these are a suitable alternative where oestrogens are contraindicated or not tolerated but they have a higher failure rate than COCs as good adherence is essential.
- The perfect-use failure rates for COCs and POPs are 0.1% and 0.5%, respectively.
- The typical failure rate is 5% for both pill types.
- Healthcare professionals should ensure that women are counselled on what to do if a pill is missed—because of either forgetting to take it or a GI upset (Box 21.1).

Transdermal patch

- The patch is changed every week for 3wks, with the fourth week being hormone free.
- The failure rate is 1% for both perfect and typical use.
- ~60% more oestrogen is absorbed into the bloodstream than with traditional 35-microgram pills. This places women at higher risk for thrombosis and myocardial infarctions.
- The patch is less effective in women weighing >90kg, and other methods should be considered.

If a patch change is forgotten in the first week, change the patch-change day and use alternative contraception for the first week of the new cycle. Patch changes forgotten in the second and third week do not need alternative contraception as long as the duration was <48h. Apply a new patch and keep the same day for the next patch-change day. If it was >48h, restart the entire cycle and use alternative contraception for the first week. Patches should not be stuck on with adhesives or bandages, if they are no longer sticky use a new patch.

Box 21.1 Advice to women who have missed an oral contraceptive pill

A pill counts as missed:
- If you have completely forgotten to take it
- If you vomit within 2h of taking a pill or have severe diarrhoea.

Combined oral contraceptives

If you miss ONE pill (for 20-microgram pills) or ONE or TWO pills (for 30–35-microgram pills) anywhere in the pack:
- Take a pill as soon as possible and continue to take the pills in the pack (even if it means taking two pills in 1 day).
- Use condoms or abstain from sex until you have taken pills for 7 days in a row.
- Emergency contraception is not required. Any pills missed in the last week of the previous pack should be taken into consideration when deciding on emergency contraception.

If you miss TWO or more pills (for 20-microgram pills) or THREE or more pills (for 30–35-microgram pills)
- Take the most recent pill as soon as possible and then continue taking pills daily at the usual time.
- Also use condoms or abstain from sex until pills have been taken for 7 days in a row.
- If pills are missed in week 1 (pills 1–7) and unprotected sex occurs in week 1 or the preceding pill-free interval (PFI), consider the use of emergency contraception.
- If pills are missed in week 2 (pills 8–14), no emergency contraception is needed.
- If pills are missed in week 3 (pills 15–21), finish the pills in your current pack and start a new pack the next day. If you miss out the PFI, no emergency contraception is needed.
- Remember: it is extending the pill-free interval that is risky.
- Take into account any pills missed in the last week of your previous pack when deciding about emergency contraception.

For every-day pill regimens

If you miss any inactive pills, discard the missed pills and then continue taking the pills daily, one each day.

Progesterone-only pill
- Take it as soon as you remember and take the next pill at the usual time.
- If the pill was 3h late (12h for desogestrel), use alternative contraception for the next 2 days.
- If you have unprotected sex before two further tablets are taken correctly, consider the use of emergency contraception.

Vaginal ring

The vaginal ring is a small plastic ring that is placed inside the vagina and releases oestrogen and progestogen.

- The ring remains in place for 3wks and is removed for the fourth. A new ring is used each month. It can be removed for up to 3h.
- Side effects include ↑ vaginal discharge, irritation, or infection.
- The perfect-use failure rate is <0.3% and the typical-use failure rate is 2%.
- The ring can be dislodged with bowel movements.
- If the ring is removed for <3h it should be rinsed and reinserted—no alternative contraception is required. If it is removed for >3h:
  - During weeks 1 or 2, rinse and reinsert, and use alternative contraception for 7 days.
  - During week 3, insert a new ring or allow a withdrawal bleed and insert a new ring no later than 7 days after the old ring was removed. No alternative contraception is required provided that a new ring is inserted within 7 days.

Intrauterine system (IUS)

An IUS is a small, T-shaped plastic device that is inserted into the uterus by a specially trained doctor or nurse. The IUS releases levonorgestrel and is a long-acting, reversible form of contraception.

- The device can remain in place for 5yrs.
- Suitable for women taking drugs which are potent enzyme inducers (e.g. phenytoin).
- The failure rate is 0.1% for both perfect and typical use.

Note: the IUS is not the same as an intrauterine device (IUD), also known as 'the coil' and which releases copper, not hormones.

Injection

Depot injection containing:

- Medroxyprogesterone 150mg:
  - Given by IM injection every 3 months. First dose must be given within 5 days of the beginning of the cycle, or pregnancy must be ruled out if >5 days.
  - Suitable for women taking drugs which are potent enzyme inducers (e.g. phenytoin).
  - The failure rate is 0.3% for both perfect and typical use.
  - Risk of reduction in bone mineral density and, rarely, osteoporosis. Avoid in adolescents or women with risk factors for osteoporosis unless other forms of contraception are unsuitable.

or:

- Norethisterone 200mg:
  - Given by deep IM within 5 days of the beginning of the cycle
  - For short-term contraception only—may be repeated once only after 8wks.

Implantable

Single-rod implant containing etonogestrel:

- Implanted within first 5 days of cycle
- Has a 3yr duration
- Requires a specially trained professional for placement and removal
- Failure rate is <0.1% for both perfect and typical use.

Risk of venous thromboembolism

The risk of VTE is ↑ by oestrogen-containing hormonal contraception, though it is lower than the risk of VTE in pregnancy (Table 21.1). Progestogen-only methods appear not to be associated with ↑ risk of VTE (although evidence is limited). Factors which ↑ the risk are as follows:

- First year of use
- Increasing age
- Higher doses of oestrogen
- Third-generation progestogen
- Possible higher risk with transdermal patches than with COCs
- Presence of other risk factors (e.g. ↑ BMI).

Women should be counselled on the relative risks before starting hormonal contraception, and women on COCs, transdermal patches, and the vaginal ring should be advised that they have an ↑ risk of VTE associated with long periods of immobility (e.g. long-haul travel). Women on oestrogen-containing contraception should be advised to stop their contraceptive 4wks before major elective surgery or any surgery involving immobilization of a lower limb. The contraceptive can be restarted at the beginning of the next cycle at least 2wks after mobility is restored. For non-elective surgery, where it has not been possible to stop the contraceptive in advance, VTE prophylaxis should be given.

Drug interactions

Enzyme-inducing drugs such as rifampicin (including 2-day course for meningitis prophylaxis), some anticonvulsants, St John's wort, and some antiretrovirals can significantly reduce the effectiveness of COCs, POPs, transdermal patches, and vaginal rings. Women should be counselled to use an alternative form of contraception while taking these drugs and until enzyme induction has completely resolved (4–8wks). Women on long-term therapy with enzyme-inducing drugs should use progestogen injection or an IUD.

Table 21.1 Risks of VTE associated with oestrogen containing contraception (cases per 100 000 women per year)

Healthy, non-pregnant, not using oestrogen-containing contraception[1]	2
Using COC containing levonorgestrel,[1] norgestimate, or norethisterone	5–7
Using COC containing gestodene, desogestrel, or drospirenone[1]	9–12
Pregnant women	60

There is no evidence to support the theory that by reducing the bowel flora responsible for recycling ethinylestradiol from the large bowel, broad-spectrum antibacterials reduce the effectiveness of hormonal contraceptives. Women taking broad-spectrum antibacterials that are not enzyme inducers do not need to use alternative forms of contraception.

Counselling points

If a woman is using hormonal contraception for the first time or is switching from one form to another it is important that the pharmacist ensures that she is aware of the following points:

• Confirm that the risk of VTE has been explained when deciding on form of hormonal contraception—if not, refer back to prescriber.
• When to take the first dose with respect to menstrual cycle and for how long alternative contraception should be continued after starting. This varies with the type of contraception—check SPC or *BNF*.
• What to do if a pill is missed, a patch is delayed or detached, or a vaginal ring is delayed, expelled, or broken.
• What to do if she vomits within 2h of taking pill.
• What to do if vomiting or diarrhoea last for >24h.
• Potential drug interactions (or lack of interaction), especially with respect to enzyme-inducing antibacterials and broad-spectrum antibacterials.
• ↑ risk of VTE with long-haul travel if on oral contraception, patch, or vaginal ring.

Emergency hormonal contraception (EHC)

Two types of EHC are available in the UK:

• Levonorgestrel 1.5mg—single dose taken as soon as possible after unprotected intercourse and ideally within 72h. If a woman is on an enzyme-inducing drug, she should take two tablets (unlicensed dose).
• Ulipristal 30mg, a progesterone receptor modulator—single dose taken within 120h of unprotected intercourse. It is probable that enzyme inducers reduce the efficacy of ulipristal but there is no information at present on adjusting doses to compensate.
• In the UK, levonorgestrel 1.5mg tablets (Levonelle One Step®) can be sold as a P medicine to women aged >16. Pharmacists can supply EHC to women aged <16yrs on prescription or via a PGD.

Further reading

Biswas J, Manna M, Webberle H (2008). Oral contraception. *Obstet Gynaecol Reprod Med* 18: 317–23.
Faculty of Sexual & Reproductive Healthcare (2012). 'Emergency Contraception', ℘ www.fsrh.org/pdfs/CEUguidanceEmergencyContraception11.pdf
Guillebaud J (2016). *Contraception Today: A Pocketbook for Primary Care Practitioners* (8th ed). Boca Raton, FL: CRC Press.

Reference

1. Faculty of Sexual & Reproductive Healthcare (2014). 'Venous Thromboembolism (VTE) and Hormonal Contraception', ℘ www.fsrh.org/standards-and-guidance/documents/fsrhstatementvteandhormonalcontraception-november/

Pre-eclampsia

Pre-eclampsia is a leading cause of maternal death in the UK. Rates of premature births and stillborn infants are also ↑ as a result of this condition. It is thought that hypertension in pregnancy is responsible for 8–10% of premature births. Hypertension in pregnancy can be classed as mild, moderate, or severe (see Table 21.2). 'Pre-eclampsia' is defined by NICE as hypertension that newly presents itself after 20wks of gestation with the presence of significant proteinuria (urinary protein:creatinine ratio of >30mg/mmol). Symptoms can include severe headache, visual disturbances, epigastric pain, vomiting, and severe swelling of the hands, legs, feet, or face. Eclampsia refers to the development of seizures in women with pre-eclampsia.

The risk of pre-eclampsia is ↑ in women with:
- chronic kidney disease
- autoimmune diseases
- type 1 or 2 diabetes
- pre-existing chronic hypertension
- history of hypertensive disorders in previous pregnancies.

Women who have suffered from pre-eclampsia in a previous pregnancy are at a higher risk of developing gestational hypertension or pre-eclampsia in future pregnancies.

Treatment

The only cure for pre-eclampsia is to deliver the baby. Often, pre-eclampsia will resolve itself within 6wks of delivery. However, raised BP may persist for up to 3 months in some women.

Pregnant women considered to be at high risk of pre-eclampsia should be given aspirin 75mg once daily from 12wks of gestation until the baby is delivered.

Women at moderate risk of pre-eclampsia should also receive aspirin 75mg once daily from 12wks of gestation until birth. Moderate risk factors include:
- first pregnancy
- age ≥40yrs
- interval between pregnancies >10yrs
- BMI >35 at first check-up
- family history of pre-eclampsia
- multiple pregnancies.

Table 21.2 Hypertension in pregnancy can be classed as mild, moderate, or severe.

Mild	140/90 to 149/99mmHg
Moderate	150/100 to 159/109mmHg
Severe	160/110mmHg and higher

Table 21.3 Labetalol doses

Oral	100mg twice daily (up to 2.4g/day in divided doses)
IV infusion	20mg/h, dose can be doubled every 30min up to a maximum of 160mg/h

Table 21.4 Alternative oral antihypertensives

Methyldopa	250mg twice a day up to a maximum of 3g/day in divided doses.
Nifedipine (modified release)	10mg–40mg twice a day
Hydralazine	25mg three times a day–75mg four times a day

Moderate and severe hypertension in pre-eclampsia should be treated first line with labetalol (see Table 21.3). The target BP is a diastolic BP of 80–100mmHg and a systolic BP of <150mmHg.

Alternative antihypertensive drugs should only be used after careful consideration of the side effects on mother and baby (see Table 21.4).

Caution

- Methyldopa should be stopped within 2 days of childbirth and replaced with an alternative. This is due to the ↑ risk of postnatal depression which can be caused as a side effect of therapy.
- Nifedipine is a tocolytic drug (unlicensed indication); it can be used to inhibit premature labour in addition to its effect on BP.
- Nifedipine modified release is preferred over immediate release as it is less likely to cause associated side effects, such as headache and flushing.
- Diuretics should be avoided in pre-eclampsia, hypertension, and oedema in pregnancy. This is because diuretics can contribute to a further reduction in the overall plasma volume of the woman, causing poor placental perfusion.
- ACE inhibitors and angiotensin II receptor blockers can ↑ the risk of congenital abnormalities if they are taken during pregnancy. Ideally, women should be advised to avoid these during pregnancy and switch to one of the preferred antihypertensive agents in pregnancy.

Further reading

National Institute for Clinical Excellence (2010). 'Hypertension in pregnancy: diagnosis and management (CG107)', ℘ www.nice.org.uk/guidance/cg107
Nelson-Piercy C (2015). *Handbook of Obstetric Medicine* (5th ed). Boca Raton, FL: CRC Press.
McKay G, Fisher M (2012). Nifedipine in pregnancy. *Practical Diabetes* 29(7): 295–6.

Hyperemesis gravidarum

Nausea and vomiting is a common problem which can affect between 50% and 90% of pregnancies. Women are usually affected during their first trimester of pregnancy, at around 6–8wks of gestation. Nausea and vomiting tends to subside after week 12 and rarely extends into the second trimester. Only 1% of pregnant women will go on to develop symptoms severe enough to warrant a diagnosis of hyperemesis gravidarum. These women need to be treated in hospital.

Key features of hyperemesis gravidarum can include:
- persistent vomiting
- weight loss of >5% of the pre-pregnancy weight
- dehydration
- deranged electrolytes
- raised levels of ketones in the blood.

A serious complication of hyperemesis gravidarum can be Wernicke's encephalopathy, caused by a thiamine deficiency as a result of excessive vomiting. Treatment, therefore, often requires fluid and vitamin replacement, in addition to antiemetic therapy.

Lifestyle advice
- Avoid triggers likely to exacerbate nausea and vomiting, these may include certain foods or smells.
- Small, frequent meals should be eaten. Plain, dry foods are recommended. Patients should keep well hydrated.
- Fatty foods and diets high in carbohydrates are thought to ↑ the risk of hyperemesis gravidarum. It is believed that diets low in carbohydrates and high in protein may be associated with a lower risk of nausea and vomiting.
- Folic acid 400 micrograms once daily is recommended for all pregnant women before 12wks of gestation.

Antiemetic therapy
Antiemetic drugs are key to successfully treating hyperemesis gravidarum. Studies show many to be highly effective in comparison to placebo. Although studies of safety and efficacy are lacking, there is sufficient experience of their use in pregnancy to confidently use these agents. There is little evidence to support one antiemetic over another; however, there are varying side effects between these drugs which should be considered before choosing an agent.

The following drugs can be used in pregnancy at the standard doses for the treatment of nausea and vomiting:
- H_1 receptor antagonists—cyclizine and promethazine.
- Phenothiazines—prochlorperazine and chlorpromazine.
- Dopamine antagonists—metoclopramide and domperidone.
- 5-HT_3 receptor antagonist—ondansetron.

Intravenous fluid therapy

- Appropriate choices for fluid replacement include sodium chloride 0.9% and Hartmann's solution for injection (sodium lactate IV infusion, compound).
- Fluids containing glucose should be avoided as IV glucose can precipitate Wernicke's encephalopathy in patients with a thiamine deficiency.
- Hyponatraemia as a result of persistent vomiting should be corrected. This should be done gradually. If the sodium is corrected too rapidly, the patient is at risk of neurological disorders.
- Hypokalaemia should also be corrected, using 40mmol of potassium (K^+) per litre of compatible fluid.
- Fluid and electrolyte balances should be assessed frequently and corrected as appropriate.

Thiamine (vitamin B_1)

Wernicke's encephalopathy can be prevented and treated by replacing thiamine. Thiamine is available as oral and IV preparations. Thiamine should be given to all women who have suffered from persistent vomiting:

- Oral thiamine is poorly absorbed and therefore doses should be split in order to improve absorption.
- Oral thiamine dose = 25–50mg two to three times a day.
- If the patient cannot tolerate oral thiamine, an IV vitamin B preparation should be used, e.g. Pabrinex®.

Corticosteroids

The evidence base for the use of corticosteroids is controversial. The trial data is often from very small populations of women with intractable vomiting. Outcomes range from dramatic improvement of symptoms, to no significant difference when compared with standard antiemetic and fluid therapy. Systemic steroid therapy has been linked with an ↑ risk of cleft palate formation in some studies. However, there is no conclusive evidence of an ↑ in the incidence of cleft palate in infants exposed to steroids *in utero*. As a result, the general consensus is that corticosteroid treatment should be initiated by a specialist as a last-line treatment option when standard therapies have failed. Corticosteroid therapy should be discontinued after 3 days if no clinical improvement is seen. Furthermore, if treatment with corticosteroids is successful, therapy should continue at the lowest dose to provide symptom control and for the shortest possible duration. A typical dosing regimen for this indication is hydrocortisone IV 100mg twice daily followed by prednisolone PO 40–50mg once daily when symptoms show improvement, the oral dose should then be tapered down, gradually.

Pyridoxine (vitamin B_6)

There is little evidence to suggest that pyridoxine is beneficial to women suffering from nausea and vomiting in pregnancy or hyperemesis gravidarum.

Ginger

- Ginger has been used for many years as an agent for the treatment of pregnancy-induced nausea and vomiting. However, the evidence for the use of ginger has always been limited.
- In recent years, systematic reviews have been carried out to assess the data.
- Ginger has been found to be significantly better at reducing the frequency of nausea and vomiting than placebo.
- The majority of trials used a maximum of 1g of ginger daily (often as a divided dose of 250mg four times a day). This is deemed to be a safe and effective dose.
- Ginger biscuits were also found to reduce nausea in pregnant women when compared with placebo.
- As with all herbal medications, the associated drug interactions should be taken into account on a patient-by-patient basis and therefore this treatment may not be suitable for all women.

Non-pharmacological treatments of hyperemesis

The following complementary therapies have been shown in a small number of trials to produce positive outcomes such as reducing the duration of nausea and vomiting and the need for antiemetic drugs:

- Acupuncture
- Acupressure
- Hypnosis
- Progressive muscle relaxation (in combination with antiemetic therapy).

Further reading

Drug and Therapeutics Bulletin (2013). Management of hyperemesis gravidarum. *Drug Ther Bull* 51(11): 126–9.

Jarvis S, Nelson-Percy C (2011). Management of nausea and vomiting in pregnancy. *BMJ* 342: d3606.

Ding M, Leach M, Bradley H (2012). The effectiveness and safety of ginger for pregnancy – induced nausea and vomiting: a systematic review. *Women Birth* 26: 26–30.

Therapy-related issues: malignant diseases and immunosuppression

Policy for the administration and handling of cytotoxic drugs

The term cytotoxic drug or systemic anticancer treatment (SACT) is used to refer to all drugs with direct anti-tumour activity including conventional anticancer drugs, monoclonal antibodies (e.g. rituximab, alemtuzumab), targeted treatments (e.g. erlotinib, imatinib), and drugs such as thalidomide.

Cytotoxic drugs are used in the treatment of cancers and certain other disorders. They act by killing dividing cells, by preventing their division. In addition to malignant cells, they also act on normal cells. Therefore their use poses certain risks to those who handle and receive them. It is important to ensure the safety of staff and patients who come in contact with these drugs.

- Cytotoxic drugs may only be reconstituted in facilities specifically approved for the purpose.
- Staff who prescribe, clinically screen, reconstitute, label, administer, and dispose of cytotoxic drugs must be appropriately trained and assessed as competent and must follow the local approved procedures.
- In areas where cytotoxic drug use is infrequent, a risk assessment must be carried out before a cytotoxic drug is requested. This should assess the availability of appropriate equipment and evidence of training, and demonstrate competence in safe administration of the drugs.
- Oral anticancer medicines must be prescribed, dispensed, administered, and monitored using the same standards as for injectable chemotherapy.
- Wherever possible, all cytotoxic medications should be initiated, and as much as feasible, administered within normal working hours.
- In circumstances where cytotoxic medications are to be prepared out of hours, be aware of local policies on how to proceed.

Cytotoxic drug procedures

- Any area in the hospital (including the wards, out-patient or day-case areas, and pharmacy) using cytotoxic drugs should have available current information on the type of agents used. This information should include relevant health and safety information (Control of Substances Hazardous to Health (COSHH) Regulations 2002, as amended).
- Cytotoxic drugs are occasionally used to treat clinical disorders other than cancer. In such instances, the patient should be referred to a clinical area where cytotoxic drugs are used routinely. Alternatively, a competent practitioner from such an area can administer the drug in the patient's own ward. A trained member of staff must undertake a risk assessment to determine by whom and in what circumstances the drug can be administered.

Prescription, preparation, and reconstitution of cytotoxic drugs

Ideally, all chemotherapy prescriptions are prescribed on an electronic chemotherapy prescribing system. In non-cancer areas, prescriptions may be handwritten on standard prescription charts, and they must be written legibly and signed in indelible black ink. In some cases, prescriptions might be computer generated, either on an approved chemotherapy chart or on a standard prescription chart. Cytotoxic drugs may only be prescribed by consultant haemato-oncologist or solid tumour oncologist medical staff. Specialist registrars, specialist non-career grades, and non-medical prescribers can prescribe chemotherapy when appropriately trained. The chief pharmacist is responsible for ensuring that cytotoxic drug reconstitution services are provided in appropriate facilities. In exceptional circumstances, they can designate other areas for reconstitution.

Dispensing, labelling, and transportation of cytotoxic drugs

- Syringes, infusion devices, and infusion fluids containing cytotoxic drugs must be clearly labelled, to identify the potential cytotoxic hazard, and placed inside a sealed plastic bag.
- Cytotoxic drugs must be packaged and transported in designated transport bags or boxes. These should be sturdy, secure, and leak-proof and should be clearly labelled: CYTOTOXIC DRUG—HANDLE WITH CARE. Additional precautionary labels should be added to the containers and the transport bags or boxes as appropriate, e.g. room temperature or refrigerate storage required.
- All staff involved in transportation of cytotoxic drugs must be trained to follow the 'cytotoxic spillage' procedure.
- The designated cytotoxic drugs reconstitution services must be notified at once if the integrity of a container received is suspect.
- *Oral cytotoxic drugs* should be transported in the same way as non-cytotoxic medication. In-patient supplies should be labelled as 'cytotoxic' on the normal prescription label.
- Reference should also be made to the dispensing and labelling oral chemotherapy NPSA rapid response report.[1] The report included:
  - Staff verifying or dispensing prescriptions must have access to the protocol and treatment plan from the hospital that initiated treatment and to advice of an oncology specialist pharmacist in that hospital—such that they can confirm that the prescribed dose is appropriate for the patient and that the patient is aware of the required monitoring arrangements.
  - Dispensary staff should work to detailed standard operating procedures.
  - Label details should comply with the local prescribing label guidelines.
  - All dispensed containers should be labelled with a 'Cytotoxic' warning label.
  - Automated dispensing systems should only include oral anticancer medicines that are available as unit doses (e.g. temozolomide and idarubicin). A local risk assessment should be carried out prior to inclusion.
  - Tablets or capsules should not be handled directly. All staff should use a 'no touch' technique or wear gloves to minimize risks of exposure.
  - Counting triangles designated only for use for cytotoxic drugs should be used. These should be cleaned after use with industrial methylated spirit 70%, or an alternative locally approved agent, and a wipe. Wipes should be disposed of as cytotoxic waste.

- Automated counting machines should *never* be used for oral anticancer medicines.
- During normal working hours, all quantities of oral anticancer medicines should have a physical double-check (count) prior to release to patient.
- Ideally, tablets should never be crushed or halved and capsules should never be opened. Where a commercial liquid preparation is not available and the pharmacy is able to extemporaneously prepare a formulation, this must be done in an isolator.
- Oral anticancer medicines should not be dispensed in compliance aids or monitored dose systems.
- When dispensing tablets or capsules, a sufficient quantity for the complete cycle of treatment should be supplied.
- When dispensing short courses of oral anticancer drugs in liquid formulations, the exact quantity required (plus an overage of ~10mL) should be supplied. Work over a leak-proof tray to contain any spillage. For patients on maintenance treatment (e.g. mercaptopurine for paediatric leukaemic patients), it is more appropriate to dispense a complete original container.
- All patients must receive appropriate written information. This should either be in the form of manufacturer's patient information leaflet or a locally approved information leaflet.
- Oral anticancer medicines should not be supplied to a patient unless he/she has received education relating specifically to the medicines, the intended treatment plan, and likely side effects. It is important that the patient accepts their roles and responsibilities relating to their treatment.

Administration of cytotoxic drugs

- Cytotoxic drugs should be administered in a dedicated therapeutic environment with appropriate facilities for safe administration and within safe working staffing levels.
- The area should also have an annual risk assessment undertaken to ensure fitness for purpose, in line with the recommendations of the NPSA alert promoting the use of injectable medicines.[2] This assessment should encompass 'Equality Impact Assessments'.
- Checks of medical equipment used within the area must be undertaken on an annual basis.
- Areas designated for the administration of cytotoxic drugs should have all relevant policy and protocol documents available.
- Facilities should include easy access to expert help and all the equipment necessary for the management of emergencies.
- Relevant clinical laboratory results, as defined by chemotherapy protocols, must be reviewed before administration, and appropriate action taken.
- The following checks are advised to be made by two qualified staff members, one of whom must be registered as competent in cytotoxic drug administration, depending on local policy:
  - Visual check of the product (to include signs of leakage, contamination, or breakdown products).

- The drug has been appropriately stored and is within its expiry date.
- Patients must be identified positively using three patient identifiers, as defined in the locally approved policy.
- The following prescription details must be checked:
  —Protocol
  —Dose
  —Diluent (if relevant)
  —Route of administration (chemotherapy can be given via various routes including PO, IV, SC, IM, intrathecal, intrareservoir, and topically)
  —Frequency.
- Staff should use personal protective equipment and clothing if handling and administering cytotoxic drugs. This includes gloves, an apron, and in some cases protection for the face (either goggles or a mask).

Accidental spillage

- All areas in which cytotoxic agents are stored, prepared, and administered should have a spill kit available for use at all times. These kits are usually obtained from the pharmacy department. The kit includes instructions on how to proceed safely. Staff should be familiar with the instructions before dealing with a spill.
- A trained healthcare professional should deal with the spill immediately. After use, the spillage kit should be replaced.
- Be familiar with your local policy and location of spillage kits in areas using cytotoxic drugs.

Disposal of product waste

- Cytotoxic waste should be disposed of separately to normal clinical waste and marked as being cytotoxic, according to local policy. The incorrect disposal of cytotoxic waste can result in prosecution under the Special Waste Regulations 1996.
- Cytotoxic waste includes vials that have contained cytotoxic drugs, syringes, needles, IV bags, infusion sets used to administer cytotoxic drugs, gowns and gloves, and urinary catheters and drainage bags from patients undergoing cytotoxic therapy.
- Cytotoxic waste should be disposed of according to local policy and clearly marked with cytotoxic residue tape.
- Hospitals have specific policies on the storage and collection of cytotoxic waste to ensure that it does not enter the normal clinical waste stream.

Disposal of excreta and blood

- Precautions should be taken to prevent occupational skin contact.
- Because cytotoxic drugs have varying half-lives, specific information about them will be found on safety datasheets. If the information is not specified, it is deemed GCP to apply universal precautions for 48h after administration.
- Patients and relatives (particularly pregnant mothers) who handle body fluids at home should be given appropriate advice.

- Gloves must be worn when handling all body fluids (e.g. blood, urine, faeces, colostomy and urostomy bags, nappies) during and after the administration of cytotoxic drugs.
- Linen contaminated with body fluids and cytotoxic drugs must be handled according to the local policy for handling cytotoxic contaminated waste.
- If contamination of the skin, eyes, or mucous membranes is suspected, the area should be rinsed thoroughly with large amounts of water and then washed with soap and water.

Incidents arising from handling and administration of cytotoxic drugs

- Any incident involving prescribing, administration, and disposal of cytotoxic drugs must be reported according to the local incident reporting system.
- The most probable incident for staff is accidental exposure to the drug during the set-up and administration of the drug. This might result from a bag leaking or bursting, or problems with the line *in situ*.
- If there is eye and skin contamination, rinse the affected area with copious amounts of tap water and seek further treatment, if needed. The occupational health department should be notified of all cases of staff exposure to organize risk assessment and follow-up care plans.
- For patients, the most probable incidents arising are extravasation during treatment (see ➜ 'Principles of extravasation', pp. 545–6).

Handling cytotoxics during pregnancy

There should be no significant exposure to cytotoxic drugs if good handling practices are strictly adhered to.

Managers must ensure that a COSHH assessment is carried out in all areas where cytotoxic drugs are handled in order to assess the level of risk and adequacy of control measures in place. Directions on how risk assessment can be completed can be found at the HSE website.[3] The risk assessment should assume that there may be an expectant mother working in the environment in the following 12 months.

Employees should notify their managers as soon as possible if they are pregnant. This is particularly important as the greatest risk is during the first 3 months of pregnancy, when rapid cell division and differentiation occurs. This is also to comply with HSE guidance where all pregnant staff should be removed from duties involving the preparation of cytotoxic drugs. Pregnant staff should refer to their local policy with regard to handling cytotoxic drugs, because this group of drugs is potentially mutagenic, teratogenic, and carcinogenic.

See ➜ 'Drugs in pregnancy', pp. 188–91, for recommendations on handling potentially teratogenic drugs in pregnancy.

Intrathecal chemotherapy

See ➜ 'Intrathecal administration of chemotherapy', pp. 541–3.

Further reading

Allwood M, Stanley A, Wright P (2002). *The Cytotoxics Handbook* (4th ed). Abingdon: Radcliffe Medical Press.

Hyde L, Dougherty L (2008). Safe handling of cytotoxic drugs. In: Dougherty L, Lister S (eds), *The Royal Marsden Hospital Manual of Clinical Procedures* (7th ed). Oxford: Blackwell.

References

1. NPSA (2008). 'Oral anti-cancer medicines: risks of incorrect dosing (NPSA/2008/RRR001)', ◌ www.nrls.npsa.nhs.uk/resources/?entryid45=59880

2. NPSA (2008). 'Promoting safer use of injectable medicines (NPSA/2007/20)', ◌ www.nrls.npsa.nhs.uk/resources/?entryid45=59812

3. HSE. 'Risk management', ◌ www.hse.gov.uk/risk/index.htm

Clinical screening of chemotherapy prescriptions

All chemotherapy prescriptions must be checked and authorized by an oncology pharmacist who has undertaken the appropriate specialist training and local accreditation. Where possible, chemotherapy should be prescribed using an electronic chemotherapy prescribing system.

Validating prescription details

- Check that doses have been correctly calculated and prescribed.
- Ensure that generic drug names have been used and the dosage form is specified.
- Check maximum doses according to the protocol.
- Check patient weight, height, and body surface area (BSA). Ensure that weight has been taken within time frames specified in local protocols—e.g. if it is >2 months since a patient has been weighed and no new weight is recorded, ask for the patient to be weighed.
- BSAs are often rounded. Do not query a discrepancy unless it is >0.1m^2 for adults.
- Oncology patients might have their BSA capped at 2m^2 or 2.2m^2, or calculated using ideal body weight, but this does not happen routinely. Check the local policy. For example, obese patients—confirm with the prescriber that BSA has not been capped if >2m^2 or >2.2m^2. There is no evidence for capping doses in obese patients.[4]
- Haematology patients may not have their BSA capped—check the local policy.
- Drug dosages should be expressed in metric notation. The word *units* should never be abbreviated.
- For rounding doses, be aware that the exact dose might have to be rounded to account for tablet or vial size, or dose banded according to local policy.
- Check cumulative doses—e.g. anthracyclines (doxorubicin has a maximum cumulative dose of 450mg/m^2) and bleomycin (maximum cumulative dose of 400 000IU).
- Check local policy for variation in the dispensed dose compared with the prescribed dose that has been agreed (often 5% variation is agreed).
- Administration rate and route should be specified.
- Administration schedule and duration of treatment should be included.
- For oral anticancer agents, calculate the exact number of tablets or capsules to be supplied and annotate the prescription accordingly.
- Ensure prescriber is authorized to prescribed chemotherapy and their signature is recognized. (According to the NHS Cancer Measures, only Consultants and Specialists in Oncology and Haematology and Staff and Associate Specialists in Oncology/Haematology are allowed to initiate a course of chemotherapy. Staff Grades and Non-Medical Prescribers with adequate training and experience in Oncology/Haematology are allowed to prescribe chemotherapy on subsequent courses.)
- Ensure that the infusion fluid and volume are stated and appropriate.
- For routes other than IV, ensure that the route is prescribed in full (e.g. intrathecal, not IT).

Verification of cycle 1 prescriptions

- Check prescriber's details and signature (including electronic signature) are present and confirm prescriber is authorized to prescribe chemotherapy.
- Ensure regimen prescribed has been through local approval process, e.g. clinical governance and financial approval (e.g. Cancer Drug Fund (CDF), private patient (insurance), national list, national algorithm, one-off approval) and/or is included on a list of locally approved regimens.
- Ensure regimen prescribed is appropriate and is the intended treatment for patient's diagnosis, medical history, performance status and chemotherapy history (using treatment plan), clinical notes or electronic records.
- Check patient's name, date of birth, and hospital/NHS number.
- Check the date the order was generated, and time and date treatments are to be administered.
- Check that the BSA has been calculated correctly:

$$Surface\,area = \sqrt{(Height[cm] \times weight[kg])\,/\,3600}$$

- BSA is often capped at $2m^2$ or $2.2m^2$. Check your local policy!

(The American Society of Clinical Oncology (ASCO)[4] recommends that actual body weight be used when selecting cytotoxic chemotherapy doses regardless of obesity status as there is no evidence that short- or long-term toxicity is ↑ among obese patients receiving full weight–based chemotherapy doses. Most data indicate that myelosuppression is the same or less pronounced among the obese than the non-obese when administered full weight-based doses.)

- Check the patient's treatment against the established protocol.
- Check the frequency of intended cycles and appropriate interval since any previous chemotherapy.
- Check the patient's age, because some doses/protocols are age related.
- Check for verification of dose modification or variance from the protocol and identification of the factors on which treatment modifications are based.
- Confirm the dose per day versus the dose per cycle with the protocol.
- Interpret critical laboratory values to see if a dose modification is required—e.g. impaired renal function, clotting disorders, and LFTs (if appropriate for drug).
- Check that the correct drugs have been prescribed and that all calculations have been performed correctly.
- Check if there are any drug interactions between the chemotherapy and the patient's regular medication/food.
- Check the patient's allergies and medication sensitivities.
- Check if there are any drugs contraindicated with the chemotherapy.
- Check that the appropriate supportive care for the patient is prescribed.

Second and subsequent cycles
- Check that the chemotherapy cycle is correct for the protocol.
- Check that the correct cycle was ordered.
- Check that the drugs were prescribed on the correct days and start dates.
- Check that there has been no significant change in the patient's weight that might significantly change the calculated BSA.
- Check response to previous treatment:
  - Blood indices—haematology/biochemical
  - Tolerability and adverse reactions.
- Check to see if any appropriate modifications have been made in relation to a previous response or critical laboratory values (normally in the protocol).

Clinical check
- What type of malignancy does the patient have? Is the chemotherapy appropriate for the malignancy?
- What is the patient's renal and hepatic function? Do any of the doses need adjusting to take this into account?
- Has the patient had any chemotherapy before? Do any of the drugs have a maximum cumulative lifetime dose (e.g. anthracyclines)?
- Other checks include allergies/reactions to previous chemotherapy and the extent of disease (need for prehydration or allopurinol).
- Check critical laboratory values—if white cell count (WCC), neutrophils, or haemoglobin are above or below a predefined limit, refer to individual protocols.
- Use the latest blood results available—check local protocols as to what is acceptable data limit.
- Check to see if any appropriate modifications have been made in relation to previous response or critical tests (normally in protocol, e.g. echo results for trastuzumab).
- Check if any supportive care has been prescribed—e.g. antiemetics.

Endorsing prescriptions
- Amend any abbreviations.
- Annotate generic names.
- Ensure infusion fluid, volume, and rate of administration are stated and appropriate.
- Check that the appropriate route is prescribed.
- For routes other than IV, ensure that the route is prescribed in full— e.g. intrathecal, not IT.
- For oral chemotherapy, ensure directions on the prescription are clear and unambiguous and include, where relevant, the intended period of treatment, including start and stop dates.
- Check that oral doses are rounded up or down to account for tablet size.
- Ensure the strength and number of oral tablets to be dispensed is clearly annotated.
- Pharmacist must ensure that a patient receiving oral chemotherapy understands how and when to take the medicines.

Annotations

- Sign and date the prescription to confirm that it is correct, safe, and appropriate.
- The following annotations should be made in the medical record:
  - Date.
  - 'Chemo ordered'—'confirmed' or 'awaiting confirmation (TBC)'.
  - Cycle number and date the cycle is due.
  - Any dose reductions.
  - Other relevant notes:
    —With the first cycle, annotate the drugs, doses, and frequency in the medical record, including reasons for alterations, so that it is clear exactly what the patient has received. Include the BSA, height, and weight that were used to calculate the doses and relevant biochemistry.
    —On the last cycle, record the cumulative dose of anthracyclines or bleomycin received.
  - Clinical pharmacist's signature and contact details.

Further reading

Allwood M, Stanley A, Wright P (2002). *The Cytotoxics Handbook* (4th edn). Abingdon: Radcliffe Medical Press.

British Oncology Pharmacy Association (BOPA) (2010). 'Competencies to Support Verification of Prescriptions for SACT', ℘ www.bopawebsite.org

British Oncology Pharmacy Association (BOPA) (2010). 'Guidance to Support BOPA Standards for Clinical Pharmacy Verification of Prescriptions for Cancer Medicines', ℘ www.bopawebsite.org

British Oncology Pharmacy Association (BOPA) (2013). 'Standards for Clinical Pharmacy Verification of Prescriptions for Cancer Medicines', ℘ www.bopawebsite.org

Royal College of Radiologists' Clinical Oncology Information Network (COIN) (2001). Guidelines for cytotoxic chemotherapy in adults. A document for local expert groups in the United Kingdom preparing chemotherapy policy documents. *Clin Oncol* 13: s209–48.

Reference

4. Griggs JJ, Mangu PB, Anderson H, *et al.* (2012). Appropriate chemotherapy dosing for obese adult patients with cancer: American Society of Clinical Oncology Clinical Practice Guideline. *J Clin Oncol* 30: 1553–61.

Chemotherapy dosing

Cancer chemotherapy drugs often have a narrow therapeutic window between the dose that is effective and the dose that can be toxic. Inappropriate dose reduction reduces chemotherapy efficacy. However, if doses are not ↓ in patients with organ dysfunction, this can lead to serious or life-threatening toxicity. It is essential that cytotoxic drugs are dosed correctly and adapted to individual patients to enable the maximum probability of a desired therapeutic outcome, with minimum toxicity.

Before administration of chemotherapy, each patient should be assessed for performance status, renal function, liver biochemistry tests, serum albumin level, and prognosis. Myelosuppression is the most common and dangerous toxicity of cytotoxics, so all patients must have a blood count before each cycle of chemotherapy. Patients should only be administered chemotherapy if their white blood cell count is >3.0 × 10⁹/L (or neutrophil count is >1.5 × 10⁹/L) and platelet count is >100–150 × 10⁹/L. There can be exceptions to this in some local policies or for patients with haematological malignancies and those undergoing intensive treatment with specialized support.

Doses of cytotoxics are usually calculated on the basis of BSA, which is measured in square metres (m²). The dose is quoted as units (e.g. milligrams, grams, or international units) per square metre. The patient's BSA is calculated using a nomogram from patient height and weight measurements or using the following calculation:

$$Surface\ area = \sqrt{(Height[cm]) \times weight[kg\ /\ 3600]}$$

This practice is derived from the relationship between body size and physiological parameters (e.g. renal function). The performance status of the patient and their renal and liver functions are also taken into account. Prior to each cycle of treatment, toxicities must be recorded using common toxicity criteria. Doses are modified if the patient experiences toxicity to treatment or changes in body weight occur. The size of the reduction depends on the nature and severity of the toxicity, taking into account whether the chemotherapy is palliative or curative in intent.

ASCO[5] recommends that actual body weight be used when selecting cytotoxic chemotherapy doses regardless of obesity status as there is no evidence that short- or long-term toxicity is ↑ among obese patients receiving full weight-based chemotherapy doses. Most data indicate that myelosuppression is the same or less pronounced among the obese than the non-obese when administered full weight-based doses.

Although it is conventional to prescribe chemotherapy according to BSA, it is acceptable to use pre-prepared standard doses for commonly used drugs to facilitate bulk preparation and rapid dispensing. This is known as 'dose banding'. The rounded dose must be within agreed limits—e.g. within 5% of the calculated dose.

However, there are some exceptions to calculation of doses on the basis of BSA. Drugs whose doses can be calculated using other parameters include the following:

- Asparaginase—the dosage is IU/kg body weight or IU/BSA.
- Bleomycin—IU, either per patient surface area or as a fixed dose.
- Carboplatin—the Calvert equation[6] can be used to calculate the dose of carboplatin in patients with or without renal impairment:

$$Dose\,(mg) = AUC \times (GFR + 25)$$

where AUC is the target area under the plasma concentration curve (AUC is usually in the range 4–7) and GFR is the glomerular filtration rate. For example, the dose of carboplatin for a patient with a GFR of 75mL/min, using an AUC of 5, would be:

$$5 \times (75 + 25) = 500mg\ carboplatin.$$

- Cytarabine—dosage in mg/kg for certain indications.
- Floxuridine—dosage in mg/kg.
- Mitomycin—dosage in mg/kg for certain indications.
- Trastuzumab IV—dosage in mg/kg.
- Bevacizumab—dosage in mg/kg.
- Abiraterone—fixed dose (1000mg daily for prostate cancer).
- Sunitinib—fixed dose (50mg daily for renal cell carcinoma).
- Pazopanib—fixed dose (800mg daily for renal cell carcinoma).

Some chemotherapy drugs (e.g. anthracyclines) have a maximum recommended cumulative lifetime dose. For example, doxorubicin has a maximum cumulative lifetime dose of 450mg/m² and bleomycin has a maximum cumulative lifetime dose of 400 000IU. If patients receive more than the maximum cumulative lifetime dose, they are at ↑ risk of potentially life-threatening toxicity.

Frequency of chemotherapy administration

Chemotherapy is administered in various treatment cycles ranging from 1 to 6wks. Cycle frequency is based on cancer type and treatment choice. Frequency and duration of treatment cycles continue to evolve and are not absolute. It is important to always verify treatment selection, frequency, and duration with established protocols. For example, a lot of chemotherapy is administered at 3wk intervals, with up to 8–12 cycles of treatment being administered.

Some examples of exceptions to 3wk administration intervals are as follows:

- Carboplatin—can be administered every 3 or 4wks.
- Irinotecan—administered every 2wks.
- Fluorouracil—can be administered once weekly every 2, 3, or 4wks, depending on dosage schedule.
- Mitomycin—administered every 6wks.
- Paclitaxel—can be administered once weekly (unlicensed).
- Docetaxel—can be administered once weekly (unlicensed).
- Abiraterone—daily administration until progression.
- Pazopanib—daily until progression.

Critical tests for chemotherapy to proceed on time

Chemotherapy should only be administered at the full protocol dose if the haematological and biochemical parameters are within the normal range. Biochemical parameters depend on the excreted route of the drug. Creatinine clearance should be monitored for renally cleared drugs and LFTs should be monitored for those drugs metabolized hepatically. Haematological parameters include the WCC, absolute neutrophil count (>1–1.5), and platelet count (>100).

If the biochemical or haematological parameters are not within the normal range, dose reduction or delaying subsequent doses must be considered. Doses are usually reduced by 20–25% initially. Chemotherapy is usually delayed by a week at a time.

Treatment guidelines

Oncology is an evolving field of practice. Treatments are becoming more individualized and targeted on the basis of genetics, tumour markers, and staging of disease. Check your local protocols for information on cancer treatments locally.

For more detailed information on the management of oncological disorders, refer to the *Oxford Handbook of Oncology*.[7]

Further reading

Allwood M, Stanley A, Wright P (2002). *The Cytotoxics Handbook* (4th ed). Abingdon: Radcliffe Medical Press.

Brighton D, Wood M (eds) (2005). *The Royal Marsden Hospital Handbook of Cancer Chemotherapy: A Guide for the Multidisciplinary Team*. Edinburgh: Churchill Livingstone.

Centre for Pharmacy Postgraduate Education (CPPE) (2015). 'Cancer: In Relation to Pharmacy Practice (CPPE Open Learning pack)', ℗ www.cppe.ac.uk/programmes/l/cancer-a-06

Hoskin P, Neal A (2009). *Clinical Oncology: Basic Principles and Practice* (4th ed). London: Hodder Arnold.

Murff S (2012). *Safety and Health Handbook for Cytotoxic Drugs*. Lanham, MD: Government Institutes.

National Chemotherapy Advisory Group (2009). 'Chemotherapy Services in England: Ensuring Quality and Safety', ℗ www.nelm.nhs.uk

National Confidential Enquiry into Patient Outcomes and Death (NCEPOD) (2008). 'NCEPOD Report, November 2008', ℗ www.ncepod.org.uk

NICE. 'Cancer Service Guidance', ℗ www.nice.org.uk/guidance/published?type=csg

NPSA (2008). 'Oral anti-cancer medicines: risks of incorrect dosing (NPSA/2008/RRR001)', ℗ www.nrls.npsa.nhs.uk/resources/?entryid45=59880

Summerhayes M, Daniels S (2003). *Practical Chemotherapy: A Multidisciplinary Guide*. Abingdon: Radcliffe Medical Press.

Williamson S, Polwart C (2008). *The Oral Anticancer Medicines Handbook* (3rd ed). Gateshead: North of England Cancer Network.

References

5. Griggs JJ, Mangu PB, Anderson H, *et al.* (2012). Appropriate chemotherapy dosing for obese adult patients with cancer: American Society of Clinical Oncology Clinical Practice Guideline. *J Clin Oncol* 30: 1553–61.

6. Calvert AH, Newell DR, Gumbrell LA, *et al.* (1989). Carboplatin dosage: prospective evaluation of a simple formula based on renal function. *J Clin Oncol* 7: 1748–56.

7. Cassidy J, Bissett D, Spence RAJ, *et al.* (eds) (2015). *Oxford Handbook of Oncology* (4th ed). Oxford: Oxford University Press.

Antiemetics for the prophylaxis of chemotherapy-induced nausea and vomiting

- Nausea and vomiting remain two of the most feared side effects of chemotherapy in cancer patients.
- Chemotherapy-induced nausea and vomiting can significantly affect a patient's quality of life, leading to poor compliance and even withdrawal from potentially useful or curative treatment.
- The goal of antiemetic therapy is to prevent nausea and vomiting completely.
- Antiemetics should be given regularly and prophylactically.
- Combinations of antiemetics are significantly more effective than single agents.
- Clinical practice guidelines ensure appropriate and cost-effective antiemetic use.
- Factors that need to be considered when choosing an antiemetic regimen include the following:
  - The chemotherapy emetic risk (Tables 22.1), dose, and schedule.
  - The type of nausea and vomiting being treated—acute, delayed, anticipatory, breakthrough, or refractory (Table 22.2).
  - The patient's risk of nausea and vomiting (Box 22.1).
  - Other underlying causes of nausea and vomiting (Box 22.2).
  - The mechanism of action and routes of administration of the antiemetic (Tables 22.3 and Boxes 22.3–22.8).
  - The adverse effects of the drugs.
  - The cost-effectiveness of the drugs.
  - Whether patients can self-administer the antiemetic.

Chemotherapy drug combinations have an additive emetic effect. If chemotherapy drugs from the same category are combined, the regimen is classified as a higher emetic risk. If drugs are from different categories, the emetic risk is determined according to the most emetic drug in the combination.

Table 22.1 Emetic risk of chemotherapy

High emetic risk (>90% frequency of emesis)	Moderate emetic risk (30–90% frequency of emesis)	Low emetic risk (10–30% frequency of emesis)	Minimal emetic risk (<10% frequency of emesis)
Busulfan high doses	Actinomycin-D	Arsenic trioxide	Alemtuzumab
Carmustine >250mg/m^2	Altretamine	Bendamustine	Amifostine <300mg/m2
Cisplatin ≥60mg/m^2	Amsacrine	Bexarotene	Asparaginase
Cyclophosphamide >1500mg/m^2	Azacitidine	Carmustine <100 mg/m^2	Axitinib
Dacarbazine	Carboplatin	Cyclophosphamide <750 mg/m^2	Bevacizumab
Doxorubicin >60 mg/m^2	Carmustine >100 mg/m^2 ≤250mg/m^2	Cytarabine <900 mg/m^2	Bleomycin
Doxorubicin/ epirubicin + cyclophosphamide combination	Cisplatin <60mg/m^2	Daunorubicin <50 mg/m^2	Bortezomib
Epirubicin >90 mg/m^2	Clofarabine	Doxorubicin <60mg/m^2	Bosutinib
Ifosfamide >2g/m^2	Cyclophosphamide >750 mg/m^2 and ≤1500mg/m^2	Doxorubicin (liposomal)	Brentuximab vedotin
Mustine	Cytarabine >900mg/m^2	Etoposide >120 mg/m^2	Busulfan <10mg
Streptozocin	Daunorubicin >50 mg/m^2	Gemcitabine	Capecitabine
	Doxorubicin <60 mg/m^2	Ixabepilone	Carbaxitaxel
	Epirubicin <90 mg/m^2	Methotrexate >250 <1000mg/m^2	Carfilzomib
	Estramustine	Mitoxantrone	Catumaxumab
	Idarubicin	Paclitaxel	Cetuximab
	Ifosfamide <2 mg/m^2	Procarbazine	Chlorambucil
	Irinotecan	Raltitrexed	Cladribine
	Lomustine	Tegafur uracil	Cladribine
	Melphalan >100mg/m^2	Teniposide	Cytarabine 100–200 mg/m^2
	Methotrexate >1000–mg/m^2	Topotecan	Dasatinib
	Mifamurtide	Trabectedin	Daunorubicin (liposomal)
	Oxaliplatin	Treosulphan	Decitabine
	Temozolomide (oral)	Vorinostat	Denileukin
	Vinorelbine (oral)		Dexrazoxane
			Docetaxel
			Doxorubicin (liposomal)
			Eribulin
			Erlotinib
			Etoposide >120 mg/m^2
			Everolimus
			Fludarabine
			Fluorouracil
			Gefitinib
			Gemtuzumab
			Hydroxycarbamide
			Imatinib

Table 22.1 (Contd.)

High emetic risk (>90% frequency of emesis)	Moderate emetic risk (30–90% frequency of emesis)	Low emetic risk (10–30% frequency of emesis)	Minimal emetic risk (<10% frequency of emesis)
			Ipilimumab
			Ixabepilone
			Lapatinib
			Lenalidomide
			Melphalan (oral)
			Mercaptopurine
			Methotrexate ≤250mg/m^2
			Mitomycin
			Mitoxantrone
			Omacetaxine
			Paclitaxel-albumin
			Nelarabine
			Nilotinib
			Ofatumumab
			Panitumumab
			Pazopanib
			Pegaspargase
			Pemetrexed
			Pentostatin
			Pertuzumab
			Pralatrexate
			Rituximab
			Romidepsin
			Sorafenib
			Sunitinib
			Temsirolimus
			Thalidomide
			Thiotepa
			Thioguanine
			Topotecan
			Trastuzumab
			Trastuzumab emantasine
			Valrubicin
			Vinblastine
			Vincristine
			Vindesine
			Vinorelbine

Table 22.2 Definitions of chemotherapy-induced nausea and vomiting

Acute	Nausea and vomiting experienced during the first 24h following chemotherapy administration
Delayed	Nausea and vomiting that occurs that occurs >24h after chemotherapy and may continue for up to 6 or 7 days after chemotherapy
Anticipatory	Nausea and vomiting that occurs prior to beginning of a new cycle of chemotherapy. Most common after previous chemotherapy cycles in which badly controlled nausea and vomiting was experienced. Can be exacerbated by anxiety
Breakthrough	Development of nausea and vomiting symptoms despite standard antiemetic therapy, which require treatment with an additional pharmacological agent
Refractory	Patients who have failed on both standard and rescue medication

Chambers, P. and Daniels, S. *Antiemetic Guidelines for Adult Patients Receiving Chemotherapy and Radiotherapy*. London Cancer New Drugs Group. November 2013 version 2.

Box 22.1 Patient risk factors which predict poor antiemetic control

Patients with more than three or four risk factors should be considered to receive additional antiemetics at the outset:
- ♀
- <30yrs old
- History of sickness—in pregnancy/travel sickness/with surgery
- Poor control with prior chemotherapy
- Underlying nausea and vomiting
- Anxiety.

Note: high alcohol intake can have a protective effect and ↓ risk of emesis.

Box 22.2 Other causes of nausea and vomiting to be considered

- Radiotherapy
- Radiosensitizers
- Infection
- Metabolic disorders
- Electrolyte disturbances (hypercalcaemia, hyperglycaemia, hyponatraemia)
- Uraemia
- Constipation
- GI obstruction
- Gastroparesis—tumour or chemotherapy induced (e.g. vincristine)
- Cachexia syndrome
- Metastases (brain, liver, or bone)
- Paraneoplasia
- Emetic medication (e.g. opioids, antibiotics, antifungals, or amifostine)
- Psychological factors (anxiety, anticipatory nausea and vomiting, vestibular dysfunction).

Box 22.3 Notes on appropriate antiemetic prescribing with chemotherapy

- Antiemetics should always be commenced before chemotherapy.
- Antiemetics should be administered regularly, prophylactically, and orally for at least 4 days for highly and moderately emetic chemotherapy.
- Oral and IV formulations of antiemetics are equally effective.
- Oral doses of antiemetics should be given at least 30min prior to chemotherapy.
- Optimal emetic control in the acute phase is essential to prevent nausea and vomiting in the delayed phase and to prevent anticipatory nausea and vomiting. The toxicity of the specific antiemetic(s) should be considered.
- 5-HT$_3$ receptor antagonists are equally efficacious and should be administered orally, and only for acute nausea and vomiting.
- 5-HT$_3$ receptor antagonists can be administered IV instead of orally if necessary.
- There is only evidence for the use of 5-HT$_3$ receptor antagonists for an additional day in the delayed phase for cyclophosphamide and carboplatin.
- Ondansetron (5-HT$_3$ receptor antagonist) may ↑ the risk of QT prolongation, leading to an abnormal and potentially fatal heart rhythm. Patients at particular risk include those with an underlying heart condition, those predisposed to low serum potassium and magnesium levels, and those taking other medications that lead to QT prolongation. Ondansetron should be avoided in patient with congenital long QT syndrome. ECG monitoring is recommended in patients with electrolyte abnormalities, congestive heart failure, bradyarrhythmias, or patients taking concomitant medications that prolong the QT interval. Refer to SPC for further information available at ℘ www.medicines.org.uk.
- Neurokinin receptor antagonists (e.g. aprepitant) can be considered as an adjunct to dexamethasone and a 5-HT$_3$ receptor antagonist to prevent acute and delayed nausea and vomiting with cisplatin-based chemotherapy.
- Fosaprepitant (an IV preparation of aprepitant) can be substituted for aprepitant in patients unable to tolerate oral medication.
- Optimal emetic control in the acute phase is essential to prevent nausea and vomiting in the delayed phase.
- Dexamethasone is not required when steroids are included in the chemotherapy regimen and for some haematology regimens.
- Dexamethasone should be given prophylactically where indicated. It is one of the most effective agents as a treatment for delayed emesis.
- Dexamethasone should be given no later than 2pm to minimize wakefulness in the night.
- If lorazepam is prescribed, ensure patients do not drive or drink alcohol due to the high risk of drowsiness.

(Continued)

Box 22.3 (*Contd.*)

- Consider administering antiemetics by IV infusion, SC, rectally, or sublingually (if available in those formulations) if the patient is unable to take oral antiemetics.
- Metoclopramide can be replaced with domperidone if the patient has extrapyramidal side effects.
- Metoclopramide should be prescribed at the lowest effective dose. Doses above 10mg three times daily ↑ the risk of extrapyramidal side effects and should be used with caution in line with MHRA guidance.
- Domperidone may be associated with an ↑ risk of serious ventricular arrhythmias or sudden cardiac death. The risk may be higher in patients >60yrs and at daily doses of >30mg. Domperidone should therefore be used at a maximum dose of 10mg three times daily and for the shortest time necessary as per MHRA guidance. Domperidone should be avoided in patients taking concomitant medication known to cause QT prolongation. Refer to SPC for further information (available at ℬ www.medicines.org.uk).
- If a patient is already taking antiemetics (e.g. cyclizine or prochlorperazine) for underlying nausea and vomiting before starting on chemotherapy, these drugs could be continued as a substitute for metoclopramide.

Table 22.3 Combinations of oral antiemetics to prevent chemotherapy-induced nausea and vomiting

High emetic risk	
Acutely	(Start antiemetics before chemotherapy (1h before orally))
	5-HT$_3$ receptor antagonist (Box 22.4) PO or IV on days of highly emetic chemotherapy
	+ Dexamethasone 6mg PO or IV twice daily on days of highly emetic chemotherapy, then 4mg PO twice daily for 1 day, then 4mg PO once daily for 1 day, then 2mg PO twice daily for 2 days
	+ Aprepitant 125mg PO once daily day 1, 80mg PO once daily days 2 and 3 *or* fosaprepitant 150mg IV over 20–30min day 1 only
	± Lorazepam 0.5–2mg PO/IV/sublingual every 4–6h days of highly emetic chemotherapy, and for 3 days after chemotherapy
	Consider prescribing prophylactic laxatives (e.g. senna) with 5-HT$_3$ receptor antagonists.
Delayed phase	Dexamethasone 4mg PO twice daily for 3–4 days, which can be reduced to 4mg daily for 1–2 additional days
	Neurokinin receptor antagonist (e.g. aprepitant 80mg daily for 2 days) given in addition to dexamethasone
	Metoclopramide 10mg PO three times a day for 3–4 days regularly, then if required

Table 22.3 (*Contd.*)

Moderate emetic risk	
Acutely	5-HT$_3$ receptor antagonist PO on days of moderately emetic chemotherapy
	Start 1h before chemotherapy
	+ Dexamethasone 6mg PO twice daily on days of moderately emetic chemotherapy, then 4mg PO twice daily for 1 day, then 4mg PO once daily for 1 day, then 2mg once daily for 2 days
	± Lorazepam 0.5–2mg PO/IV/sublingual every 4–6h on days of highly emetic chemotherapy, and for 3 days after chemotherapy
	Consider prescribing prophylactic laxatives (e.g. senna) with 5-HT$_3$ receptor antagonists
Delayed phase	Dexamethasone 4mg twice daily PO for 3 days
	Metoclopramide 10mg PO three times a day for 3–4 days, if required

Low emetic risk	
Acutely	Metoclopramide 10mg PO three times daily *or*
	Prochlorperazine 5–10mg PO four times daily *or*
	Dexamethasone 6mg PO twice daily for days of low emetic risk of chemotherapy
	± Lorazepam 0.5–2mg PO/IV/sublingual every 4–6h on days of highly emetic chemotherapy, and for 3 days after chemotherapy

Minimal emetic risk
No routine prophylaxis required
Metoclopramide, domperidone, prochlorperazine, or cyclizine can be prescribed if required

Note: for patients <30yrs old, consider domperidone instead of metoclopramide if the patient experiences extrapyramidal side effects.

Note: neurokinin receptor antagonists are moderate inhibitors of CYP3A4 and hence have the potential for drug interactions. Dexamethasone dose reduction is recommended when used in combination with neurokinin receptor antagonists.

Box 22.4 Recommended oral daily doses of serotonin 5-HT$_3$ receptor antagonists to be administered 1h before chemotherapy

- Granisetron 2mg daily
- Ondansetron 8mg twice daily
- Palonosetron 500 micrograms daily
- Orodispersible film ondansetron 8mg twice daily.

Box 22.5 Recommended IV doses of 5-HT₃ receptor antagonists to be administered if patients are unable to tolerate medicines by the oral route

- Granisetron 1mg daily
- Ondansetron 8mg daily
- Palonosetron 250 micrograms as a single dose 30min before treatment.

Box 22.6 Antiemetics for failure of control

- Aprepitant and dexamethasone are the most useful agents for delayed nausea and vomiting.
- To ensure absorption of antiemetics administered, consider SC, IV, topical (granisetron transdermal patch) or rectal administration if available (e.g. prochlorperazine 25mg rectally two to four times daily, or domperidone 30mg rectally—three times daily).
- Ensure antiemetics cover full period of nausea and vomiting.

Box 22.7 Suggested antiemetics for patients refractory to first-line antiemetics

Acutely

- Use antiemetics recommended for more emetic chemotherapy (for low or moderate emetic risk regimens).
- If highly emetic chemotherapy, consider *one* of the following options:
  - Add lorazepam 1mg PO/sublingual/IV every 8h if anxious (sedative and amnesic).
  - Consider levomepromazine 6.25–12.5mg PO as a single daily dose instead of metoclopramide.
  - Replace lorazepam and metoclopramide with levomepromazine 6.25–12.5mg PO or SC (in the evening) as a single daily dose (note: 12.5mg PO = 6.25mg SC).
  - Prescribe regular lorazepam 0.5–1mg with prochlorperazine 10mg oral four times daily instead of metoclopramide.
- Consider adding a neurokinin receptor antagonist to dexamethasone and a 5-HT₃ receptor antagonist on subsequent cycles of chemotherapy (e.g. aprepitant 125mg 1h before chemotherapy, then 80mg daily for 2 days).

Delayed

- *Dexamethasone 4mg twice daily* for up to 1wk after chemotherapy.
- Consider levomepromazine 6.25–12.5mg oral as a single daily dose instead of metoclopramide.

Anticipatory

Consider *lorazepam* 1mg oral at night (or dose up to 1mg three times daily) orally if anxious or anticipatory nausea and vomiting.

Box 22.8 Suggested non-drug/lifestyle measures that may help alleviate nausea and vomiting

- Avoid factors that precipitate nausea (sight/smell of food)
- Diet
- Small frequent meals
- Choosing healthy food
- Controlling amount of food consumed
- Eating food at room temperature
- Ginger
- Tonic water
- Sea-bands
- Acupuncture techniques.

Further reading

Basch E, Prestrud AA, Hesketh PJ, et al. (2011). Antiemetics: American Society of Clinical Oncology clinical practice guideline update. *J Clin Oncol* 29: 4189–98.

Chambers P, Daniels S (2013). *Antiemetic Guidelines for Adult Patients Receiving Chemotherapy and Radiotherapy, Version 2*. London: Cancer New Drugs Group.

Fauser AA, Fellhauer M, Hoffmann M, et al. (1999). Guidelines for antiemetic therapy: acute emesis. *Eur J Cancer* 35: 361–70.

Gralla RJ, Osoba D, Kris MG, et al. (1999). Recommendations for the use of antiemetics: evidence-based, clinical practice guidelines. *J Clin Oncol* 17: 2971–94.

MHRA (2012). Ondansetron: risk of QTc prolongation—important new intravenous dose restriction. *Drug Safety Update* 6(1).

MHRA (2013). Metoclopramide: risk of neurological adverse effects. *Drug Safety Update* 7(1): S2. ℘ www.mhra.gov.uk/home/groups/dsu/documents/publication/con300408.pdf

MHRA (2013). Ondansetron for intravenous use: dose-dependent QT interval prolongation—new posology. *Drug Safety Update* 6(12). ℘ www.mhra.gov.uk/Safetyinformation/DrugSafetyUpdate/CON296402

MHRA (2014, 25 April) 'New advice for domperidone'[Press release], ℘ www.mhra.gov.uk/home/groups/comms-po/documents/news/con409260.pdf

National Comprehensive Cancer Network (NCCN) (2014). 'NCCN Clinical Practice Guidelines in Oncology (NCNN Guidelines) Antiemesis v.2.2014', ℘ www.nccn.org

Roila F, Herrstedt J, Aapro M, et al. (2010). Guideline update for MASCC and ESMO in the prevention of chemotherapy and radiotherapy-induced nausea and vomiting results of the Perugia consensus conference. *Ann Oncol* 21(Suppl 5): v232–v243.

Stoner NS (2004). Evidence for selection and use of antiemetic agents and regimens: therapy-induced nausea and vomiting. In: Hoy A, Finlay I, Miles A (eds) *The Effective Prevention and Control of Symptoms in Cancer*, pp.145–54. Cardiff: Clyvedon Press.

Stoner NS (2004). Therapy-induced nausea and vomiting: assessment of severity and indications for treatment. In: Hoy A, Finlay I, Miles A (eds) *The Effective Prevention and Control of Symptoms in Cancer*, pp.139–44. Cardiff: Clyvedon Press.

Common Terminology Criteria for Adverse Events (CTCAE)

The CTCAE system is a standardized classification developed by the National Cancer Institute (NCI) used for the side effects of chemotherapy drugs. The adverse events are graded from 0 (none) to 5 (death) for all possible side effects. The CTCAE are used in cancer clinical trials, adverse drug reporting, and publications to ensure uniform capture of toxicity data. The full CTCAE table is available from the website ℘ http://evs.nci.nih.gov/ftp1/CTCAE/CTCAE_4.03_2010-06-14_QuickReference_5x7.pdf

Intrathecal administration of chemotherapy

Background

- Intrathecal chemotherapy is mainly used to treat CNS complications of haematological malignancy.
- The only drugs that can routinely be given by the intrathecal route are methotrexate, cytarabine, and liposomal cytarabine.
- However, other non-cytotoxic drugs can be administered by this route and include bupivacaine, opioids, baclofen, clonidine, gentamicin, hydrocortisone, and vancomycin.

Safe practice

- In the UK, there is a national policy that encompasses a range of standards that hospitals must comply with to enable staff to administer intrathecal chemotherapy.[8]
- To prevent inadvertent mix-up with other drugs, intrathecal chemo-therapy is segregated from IV chemotherapy. The separate delivery and locations for these drugs help to ensure that IV drugs are never present in the same location as intrathecal medications.
- To facilitate this, intrathecal medications should only be administered in a designated location, such as an anaesthetic room, at a standard time by competent registered staff. In this way, the pharmacy can release intrathecal medications to the doctor immediately before they are needed.
- Furthermore an NHS Patient Safety Alert in February 2014 instructed all hospitals to only use syringes and needles, and other devices with non-Luer connectors when delivering intrathecal chemotherapy, as they cannot connect with IV devices.[9]
- Also, at least two health professionals should independently verify the accuracy of all intrathecal doses before administration.

Frequently asked questions

Can you please explain the intrathecal route of administration?
Chemotherapy is injected into the area of the lower spine into the CSF. This injection is also termed 'spinal' or subarachnoid. It is mainly indicated when patients show clinical signs that their disease has spread into the CNS. Drugs can also be administered through an Ommaya reservoir, discussed later in this section.

Why have people been given the wrong drug intrathecally?
The main problem occurs as a result of inexperienced health professionals becoming involved in the process with the result that the drug vincristine (intended solely for the IV route) is administered in error using the intrathe-cal route. This results in immediate neural damage that normally results in death.

How are intrathecal products labelled?

The label on the product states that the drug is intended for intrathecal use only. The product is packaged and transported in a separate container from other IV chemotherapy products and collected by the person who is going to give the drug.

What range of volumes is administered intrathecally?

Generally, the volume administered varies with the dose, but the typical volume tends to be 5mL.

Who is allowed to prescribe and administer intrathecal products?

Since 2008, only haematology/oncology consultants or ST3 grades and above who were registered on the Trust Intrathecal Register of authorized personnel are allowed to carry out prescribing and/or administration of intrathecal chemotherapy. However, staff must be appropriately trained, deemed competent by a designated lead trainer, and registered for the administration task. Obviously, anaesthetists also administer intrathecal products, but are not allowed to administer cytotoxic chemotherapy intrathecally unless they are deemed competent and are authorized on the trust's register. Senior hospital officers can only be involved in administration if a risk assessment has been undertaken and a waiver that endorses their involvement has been signed by the chief executive.

What is an Ommaya reservoir?

It is a small, plastic, dome-like device with a small tube. The reservoir is placed under the scalp and the tube is placed into the ventricles so that it connects with the CSF. The Ommaya reservoir is permanent, unless there are complications. This device allows certain drugs to be administered into the CSF and allows CSF sampling without repeated need for lumbar puncture.

How are intrathecal products administered?

A spinal needle is inserted past the epidural space until the dura is pierced and the needle enters the CSF, which should flow from the needle. When CSF appears, care is needed not to alter the position of the spinal needle while the syringe for chemotherapy is being attached. The syringe is attached firmly to the hub of the needle and then injected slowly. When the injection is complete, the needle is removed.

Collecting

The staff member who is to administer the intrathecal chemotherapy should collect the drug in person by presenting the intrathecal prescription and any other chemotherapy prescriptions for that patient. The person must check the drug against the prescription before accepting the drug. It must be released only by a pharmacist authorized to do so. The drug should be carried to the patient from pharmacy in a dedicated container.

Administering

Frequently asked questions about administering include the following:

Where can intrathecal chemotherapy be administered?

This must be done only in designated areas.

When can intrathecal chemotherapy be administered?
This can only be done at designated times that have been approved locally, and must be undertaken within normal working hours.

Who checks the intrathecal chemotherapy at the bedside?
This should be done by a staff nurse authorized to perform this task. A final check must always be done by the administering doctor just before injection.

How should intrathecal chemotherapy be administered?
Access to the CSF should be obtained by a standard lumbar puncture procedure to obtain free flow of CSF. Injection of the chemotherapy must only be performed when the physician is confident that the spinal needle is in the intrathecal space. If assistance from an anaesthetist is required to perform the lumbar puncture, the chemotherapy must only be injected intrathecally by an authorized doctor, as outlined.

Pertinent points for nursing staff

For nurses to be able to check intrathecal drugs, they have to have received specific training related to these drugs and must be registered locally after competency assessment.

Pertinent points for pharmacists

Clinically screening prescriptions

Pharmacists must have been assessed as competent and registered to screen intrathecal chemotherapy. Follow the chemotherapy screening protocol.

Releasing the product to medical staff

Only pharmacists who have been authorized and registered are involved in this process. The staff member who is due to administer the intrathecal product presents the correct prescriptions to an authorized pharmacist who releases the product provided that there is documented evidence that any IV chemotherapy intended on the same day has already been administered.

References

8. Department of Health (2008). 'National guidance on the safe administration of intrathecal chemotherapy', ℘ http://www.dh.gov.uk
9. NHS England (2014). 'Patient safety alert on non-Luer spinal (intrathecal) devices for chemotherapy', ℘ www.england.nhs.uk/2014/02/20/psa-spinal-chemo/

Vinca alkaloids

Which drugs are contraindicated for use through the intrathecal route?

Vinca alkaloids (e.g. vincristine, vinblastine, vinorelbine, and vindesine) must never be given by this route. Vincristine is the most commonly used drug of this group. Wrong route administration of chemotherapy is in the 'The never events' list for NHS England 2013/14 update.

Neurotoxicity of vincristine

Vincristine and the other vinca alkaloids do not pass through the blood–brain barrier. They are always used intravenously. Peripheral neurotoxicity is one of the main side effects, which ↑ in a cumulative fashion with the total dose of treatment. Hence, when vinca alkaloids are inadvertently injected into the CSF the outcome is normally fatal. Since 1975, 14 people have died in the UK because vincristine was mistakenly given intrathecally—i.e. as a spinal injection.

How should vincristine to be labelled?

The label will state 'For IV use only—fatal if given by other routes'. The dose is be diluted to a fixed volume of 50mL for all adults and to a fixed concentration of 0.1mL/mL for paediatric patients.

Principles of extravasation

- Extravasation is defined as the accidental leakage of a liquid from its intended compartment into the subdermal or SC tissue surrounding the administration site.
- Extravasation is the inadvertent administration of IV administered vesicants into tissue instead of into the intended IV compartment. This can be caused by incorrect line insertion or breakdown of vasculature by vesicants. A number of agents used in cancer chemotherapy are extremely damaging if they extravasate or infiltrate into the tissues rather than remaining within the vasculature.
- If left undiagnosed or inappropriately treated, extravasation of chemotherapy can cause necrosis and functional loss of the tissue and limb concerned.
- Extravasation can occur with any IV injection. However, it is only considered to be a problem with compounds that are known to be vesicant or irritant.
- Appropriate treatment of extravasation within 24h should ensure that the patient has no further problems.

Signs and symptoms

Pain, burning, swelling, erythema, loss of blood return from the cannula, skin necrosis, inflammation, and discomfort. Other signs include a drip flow rate reduction or cessation of infusion.

Risk factors

Risk factors associated with extravasation include the following:
- Administration technique—↑ risk if staff are inadequately trained.
- Administration device—use of unsuitable cannulae (e.g. cannulae 24h old), large-gauge catheters, unsecured IV devices.
- Location of cannulation site—the forearm is the favoured site, avoid small, fragile, or hard sclerosed veins.
- Distractions during IV infusion.
- Patient factors:
  - Underlying conditions, such as lymphoedema, diabetes, and peripheral circulatory diseases.
  - Patient's age—additional precaution required for paediatric and elderly patients.
- Concurrent medication—e.g. steroids and anticoagulants.
- Physical properties of the administered drug–e.g. high vesicant potential of medication infused.

Prevention

- Extravasation is best prevented using one or more of the following techniques:
  - Avoid areas of joint flexion for IV sites.
  - Use the most appropriate sized catheter for the size of the vein and flow rate, usually the smallest gauge catheter possible.
  - Use of central line for slow infusions of high-risk drugs.
  - Administer cytotoxic drugs through a recently sited cannula.

- Ensure cannula cannot be dislodged during drug administration.
- Ensure that the cannula is patent before administration by confirming positive blood return through the catheter.
- If there has been a failed attempt to cannulate, avoid re-cannulation in the same vein further away from the heart.
- Administer vesicants by slow IV push into the side arm of a fast-running IV infusion of a compatible solution.
- Administer the most vesicant drug first.
- Assess the site continuously for any signs of redness or swelling.
- Ensure that the patient is aware of extravasation risks and reports any burning or pain on administration of the drug.
- Take your time—do not rush.
- Stop the infusion or injection immediately if an extravasation is thought to have occurred and follow the local extravasation policy.
- An extravasation policy and kit must be available in all areas where chemotherapy is administered.
- Check your local extravasation policy, and be aware of the location of extravasation kits.

Further reading

Allwood M, Stanley A, Wright P (2002). *The Cytotoxics Handbook* (4th edn). Abingdon: Radcliffe Medical Press.
European Oncology Nursing Society, European Society of Medical Oncology (2012). 'Extravasation Guidelines', http://www.cancernurse.eu/education/guidelines.html
'National Extravasation Information Service' website, http://www.extravasation.org.uk
Schulmeister L (2011). Vesicant chemotherapy extravasation management. *Br J Nurs* 20(19): S6–S12.
United Kingdom Oncology Nursing Society (UKONS) (2008). *Anthracycline Extravasation Management Guidelines*. London: UKONS.

Extravasation of chemotherapy in adult patients

A number of agents used in cancer chemotherapy are extremely damaging if they extravasate or infiltrate into the tissues, rather than remaining within the vasculature (Table 22.4). Extravasation with cancer drugs can be classified into five categories, according to the reaction that is caused by the substance passing into the surrounding tissue:

Definitions of cytotoxic drug classification

- *Vesicant*: an agent that has the potential to cause pain, inflammation, blistering, and irreversible tissue damage, including necrosis and loss of limb function and mobility.
- *Exfoliants*: an agent that is capable of causing inflammation and skin shedding, but less likely to cause tissue damage.
- *Irritant*: an agent that causes pain and inflammation at the administration site and/or along the vein, but rarely results in irreversible tissue damage.
- *Inflammatory agents*: an agent capable of causing mild to moderate inflammation.
- *Neutral*: an inert or neutral agent that does not cause inflammation or damage.

Extravasation might have occurred if there is evidence of the following:
- Pain, stinging, or burning on administration, either at the cannulation site or in the surrounding area.
- Swelling, inflammation, redness, or erythema around or above the cannulation site.
- Redness or heat at or around the area/site of administration.
- Reduced IV flow rate and/or resistance; lack of return of blood from cannula.

If the patient makes a complaint, stop the administration and check the site. If extravasation is suspected, the nursing/medical staff should follow the following directions:
- The administration of the infusion/injection must be stopped and the cannula left in place.
- The healthcare professional administering the treatment should remain with the patient and ask a colleague to collect the extravasation kit and summon a doctor to examine and prescribe the appropriate treatment, according to the local extravasation policy.
- If a vesicant or exfoliant drug (Table 22.4) has been extravasated, the plastic surgical specialist registrar on-call 24h should be contacted according to the local policy. An emergency intervention/antidote might be required, according to the local policy.
- Disconnect the infusion and aspirate as much of the fluid from the extravasation site, through the cannula if possible, with a 10mL syringe.
- Mark the affected area. If possible take digital images of the site.
- The cannula can then be removed.

Table 22.4 Extravasation classification of anticancer drugs

Vesicants	Exfoliants	Irritants	Inflammatory agents	Neutrals
Amsacrine	Aclarubicin	Bortezomib	Etoposide phosphate	Arsenic trioxide
Bendamustine*		Cabazitaxel	Eribulin	Asparaginase
Carmustine	Cisplatin	Carboplatin	Fluorouracil	Bevacizumab
Dacarbazine	Daunorubicin (liposomal)	Etoposide	Methotrexate	Bleomycin
Dactinomycin	Docetaxel	Irinotecan	Pemetrexed	Cetuximab
Daunorubicin	Liposomal doxorubicin (Caelyx®)	Ixabepilone	Raltitrexed	Cladribine
Doxorubicin	Floxuridine	Teniposide	Temsirolimus	Cyclophosphamide
Epirubicin	Oxaliplatin			Cytarabine
Idarubicin	Topotecan			Fludarabine
Mechlorethamine				Gemcitabine
Mitomycin				Ifosfamide
Mitoxantrone				Interferons
Mustine				Interleukin 2
Paclitaxel*				Ipilimumab
Streptozocin				Melphalan
Trabectedin				Monoclonal antibodies
Treosulfan				Pentostatin
Vinblastine				Rituximab
Vincristine				Thiotepa
Vindesine				Trastuzumab
Vinflunine				
Vinorelbine				

* Some texts class these as irritants/vesicants.

Note: as new drugs are being licensed regularly, confirm vesicant nature of any new drugs, prior to drug administration.

- The extravasated area should be covered with a sterile gauze dressing. Depending on the extravasated drug and the local policy, heat can be applied to disperse the extravasated drug or the area can be cooled to localize the extravasation. Check the local policy to see whether a heat or cold pack should be used for the extravasated drug. For example:
  - Vinca alkaloids—warm pack
  - Oxaliplatin—heat pack
  - Other vesicant drugs—cold pack
  - Other non-vesicant drugs—cold pack.
- The site should be elevated while swelling persists.
- Analgesia should be provided, if required.
- For the management of each individual drug, refer to the management plans in the local policy.
- The following documents should be completed, according to local policy:
  - Standard local documentation for extravasation—file in patient's notes.
  - Record in patient's notes.
  - Local incident form.
- The patient's consultant should be informed within 24h (at the discretion of the specialist registrar on-call).

Follow-up care

- If IV chemotherapy is to be continued on the same day as an extravasation incident, if possible avoid using the limb where the extravasation has occurred.
- Review the extravasation site (suggested at ~24h and at 7 days). If not ulcerated, advise gradual return to normal use. For subsequent cycles of chemotherapy, consider surgical opinion if persistent pain, swelling, or delayed ulceration occurs.
- Inform risk management of the outcome.

Extravasation risk for chemotherapy products

There is no standard test to determine a drug's extravasation risk. The absolute risk is determined by extravasation reports originating from clinical practice and therefore controversy will exist for certain drugs.

Guidelines for the use of hyaluronidase for an extravasated vinca alkaloid

Hyaluronidase may be indicated for a suspected or known extravasation of vinca alkaloids. It should be administered within 1h of the extravasation, before applying hydrocortisone cream. 1500IU of hyaluronidase is diluted in 1mL of water for injection. A 25G or 27G needle is used to administer the dose intradermally or SC around the peripheral extravasation at approximately five separate sites. Clean the skin and change the needle after each injection. Consider infusing 0.4mL of the dose directly through the affected IV catheter if there is no blood return, prior to removing the catheter.

Guidelines for the use of dexrazoxane for an extravasated anthracycline

Dexrazoxane is a DNA topoisomerase II inhibitor licensed for administration after an anthracycline (doxorubicin, epirubicin, daunorubicin, idarubicin) extravasation of ≥3mL. The dose should be administered in the opposite limb over 1–2h within 6h of the extravasation:

- Day 1: 1000mg/m^2
- Day 2: 1000mg/m^2
- Day 3: 500mg/m^2

The dose should be capped at a BSA of 2m^2, with a single dose not exceeding 2000mg.

Suggested contents of an extravasation kit

- Cold/hot packs × 2 (one to be stored in the freezer and one to be microwaved for a hot pack)
- Hyaluronidase 1500IU injection
- 10mL water for injection × 2
- 2mL syringes
- 10mL syringes
- 25G needles
- Copy of local extravasation policy
- Extravasation incident forms
- Patient extravasation information leaflet
- Consent form for photographs
- Gloves and apron
- Gauze swab and tape
- Alcohol swabs
- Drug chart and pen.

Further reading

Allwood M, Stanley A, Wright P (2002). *The Cytotoxics Handbook* (4th edn). Abingdon: Radcliffe Medical Press.

European Oncology Nursing Society, European Society of Medical Oncology (2012). 'Extravasation Guidelines'. ⅆ http://www.cancernurse.eu/education/guidelines.html

'National Extravasation Information Service' website, ⅆ http://www.extravasation.org.uk

Schulmeister L (2011). Vesicant chemotherapy extravasation management. *Br J Nurs* 20(19): S6–S12.

United Kingdom Oncology Nursing Society (UKONS) (2008). *Anthracycline Extravasation Management Guidelines*. London: UKONS.

Extravasation of chemotherapy in paediatric patients

Central venous catheters

- The majority of chemotherapy administered to children is given through indwelling central venous catheters.
- It is very unusual for administration of chemotherapy through indwelling central venous catheters to result in any problems with extravasation.
- The very occasional problems that occur with leakage or rupture of indwelling lines must be dealt with on their individual merits, taking account of such factors as site of the leak, type of drug being administered, and volume of drug thought to have been extravasated.

Peripheral catheters

- The same principles regarding extravasation apply to paediatric patients as for adult patients. However, treatment will differ and should be according to a local policy.
- The cannula should be sited on the dorsum of the hand or foot, and *never* sited at the antecubital fossa or any other deep vein that cannot be carefully monitored.
- During the administration of bolus chemotherapy, very careful attention must be paid to ensure that there is no evidence of extravasation at the time of the injection, with intermittent careful aspiration throughout to demonstrate patency and correct positioning.
- Administration must be stopped immediately if there is swelling around the site of the cannula. Some patients can experience discomfort during IV injection and therefore pain is a less reliable sign of extravasation. Some drugs can induce marked amounts of flare, even when being delivered safely into the vein, and therefore the presence of flare is not an indication that extravasation is occurring.
- Infusion chemotherapy should be administered using a pressure-monitoring pump, with the pressure limit set as low as possible.
- Antidotes are usually avoided in paediatric extravasations because some antidotes can cause more damage than the extravasation itself.
- Suggested contents for a paediatric extravasation kit:
  - Hot pack
  - Cold pack
  - Copy of local extravasation policy
  - Extravasation documentation forms.

- Problems of extravasation are most likely to occur with the administration of vincristine or vinblastine. Extravasations with vincristine or vinblastine should be regarded as an emergency. If there is an extravasation of either of these two drugs, it is appropriate to call the plastic surgeons so that the site of the extravasation can be extensively irrigated. Arrangements should be made quickly for the patient to be taken to theatre and anaesthetized and the area irrigated.
- The lead consultant for the patient or the haematology/oncology consultant in charge at the time should be notified of the event immediately.

Further reading

Allwood M, Stanley A, Wright P (2002). *The Cytotoxics Handbook* (4th edn). Abingdon: Radcliffe Medical Press.

Therapy-related issues: nutrition and blood

Administration sets

A standard administration set, which does not have a filter chamber, is suitable for most IV infusions except the following:

- Blood and blood products—a blood administration set has an integral filter chamber.
- Platelets—a special administration set is usually supplied with platelets.
- Neonates and paediatrics—a burette should be used.

Rates

These sets deliver different number of drops/mL:

- Standard administration set—20 drops/mL.
- Blood administration set—15 drops/mL.
- Burette—60 drops/mL.

Note: an amiodarone infusion alters the surface tension of the infusion, resulting in a different number of drops/mL.

Changing administration sets

Administration sets should normally be changed every 24h as a precaution on microbiological grounds, although a number of studies have shown that, during administration of crystalloid infusions, there is not an ↑ in infection rates if administration sets are left unchanged for up to 72h. Contamination of infusion fluid during manufacture is extremely rare. However, if drugs are added to infusion fluids at ward level, the risk of microbial contamination is high and sets must be changed every 24h.

Administration sets should be changed every 24h for:

- parenteral nutrition
- blood and blood products
- infusions to which drugs have been added.

Calculating flow rates

If an infusion depends on gravity for its flow, there will be a limitation to its rate and accuracy of delivery. The rate of administration also needs to be calculated, using the following formula:

$$\text{no of drops/min} = \frac{\text{quantity to be infused(mL)} \times \text{no of drops/mL}}{\text{no of hours over which infusion is to be delivered} \times 60\text{min}}$$

The number of drops/mL depends on the administration set and the viscosity of the fluid. If greater safety is required, a burette administration set can be used, particularly if large bolus volumes could be harmful (e.g. in children or in patients with cardiac failure).

The burette set has a discreet 150–200mL chamber that can be filled from the infusion bag, as necessary, depending on the flow rate. This enables the nurse to ensure that the patient receives no more than the prescribed hourly rate.

Peripheral venous access devices

- Provides a relatively easy method for obtaining immediate IV access.
- Used for short-term drug and/or fluid administration and blood transfusion. Principal problems associated with peripheral cannulae are infection, occlusion, phlebitis, and extravasation.

For central venous access see ➜ 'IV therapy at home', pp. 592–6.

Size of cannula

The size of cannula is relevant to the potential trauma it may cause to the vein in which it rests. Cannula size relates to the diameter and is stated in gauge size, where the ↑ in gauge number is inversely proportional to the diameter of the cannula (Table 23.1).

The cannula should be considered as a wound with direct entry to the vascular system and must be treated as any other wound using an aseptic technique.

Dressings should be changed only if they are bloodstained or have become wet or stained, or when fluid has collected at the insertion point. If they are dry and intact it is preferable to leave them alone to minimize exogenous infection or dislodgement of the cannula at the site.

If there are any signs of inflammation or pain, the cannula should be removed. If it is not in regular use, removal should also be considered. Most institutions recommend that peripheral cannulae should not remain in place for longer than a specified period (e.g. 48h).

Table 23.1 Cannula sizes

Size (gauge)/actual diameter (mm)	Colour	Use	Flow rate (mL/min)
22G/0.8mm	Blue	For small fragile veins	35
20G/1mm	Pink	For IV drug and fluid administration in patients who have fragile veins	60
18G/1.2mm	Green	Standard size for IV drug and fluid administration	100
16G/1.7mm	Grey	For patients requiring rapid IV fluid replacement	200
14G/2mm	Brown	Used in theatre for rapid transfusion	350

Intravenous (IV) administration pumps and other devices

Classification

The Medical Devices Agency (MDA) has developed a classification for pumps according to the perceived risk and suitability of a device for a specific clinical purpose:

- Neonatal—the highest risk category.
- High-risk infusions—infusion of fluids in children, where fluid balance is critical, or the infusion of drugs (e.g. cardiac inotropes) or cytotoxic drugs where consistency of flow and accuracy are important.
- Lower-risk infusions—delivery of simple electrolytes, parenteral nutrition, and infusional antibiotics.

Neonatal

The required characteristics of neonatal devices are as follows:

- High accuracy.
- Consistency of flow delivery, with very low flow rates.
- Flow rate increments in mL/h.
- Very short occlusion and low-pressure alarm times.
- Very low bolus volume on release of occlusion.

High-risk infusion pumps

The required characteristics of high-risk infusion pumps are as follows:

- High accuracy.
- Consistency of flow delivery.
- Short occlusion and low-pressure alarm times.
- Low bolus volume on release of occlusion.

Lower-risk infusion pumps

The characteristics of lower-risk infusion pumps are as follows:

- Lower accuracy over the long and short terms.
- Less consistent flow.
- Rudimentary alarm and safety features.
- Higher occlusion alarm pressure.
- Poorer overall occlusion alarm response.

IV pumps and syringe drivers are increasingly being used to control infusions in general wards, in addition to specialist clinical areas. Operators have a responsibility to ensure that they are fully conversant with any device being used. Training is provided initially by company representatives, although long-term, local, on-the-job competency training is the usual method employed.

There is a continuously expanding range of infusion devices, which vary slightly in design. However, there are normally a number of common features that operators need to be familiar with to understand the appropriate clinical use of each device.

Most devices require a specific administration set, cassette, or syringe. The use of the incorrect type can have a detrimental effect on patient care.

If a pump is designed to use a variety of sets or syringes, it normally must be programmed with information regarding the type and size being used.

Devices can be grouped into four main types:

- Infusion devices using a syringe:
  - Syringe infusion pumps
  - Syringe drivers
  - Anaesthetic pumps
  - Patient-controlled analgesia pumps.
- Infusion devices using gravity controllers:
  - Drip-rate controllers
  - Volumetric controllers.
- Infusion pumps:
  - Drip-rate pumps
  - Volumetric pumps
  - Patient-controlled analgesia pumps.
- Ambulatory pumps:
  - Continuous infusion
  - Multimodality pumps
  - Patient-controlled analgesia pumps.

Syringe infusion pumps

These are devices in which a syringe containing fluid or a drug in solution is fitted into the pump and the plunger of the syringe is driven forwards at a predetermined rate. These pumps are usually set to run at mL/h.

Application

Designed for the accurate delivery of fluids at low flow rates. Therefore syringe pumps are ideally selected for the safe infusion of fluids and drugs to neonates or children and drugs to adults. Often used in anaesthesia and critical care areas. Commonly used for the administration of patient-controlled analgesia.

Gravity controllers

Electronic devices that achieve the desired infusion rate on the principle of restricting flow through the administration set by an infusion force that depends on gravity (drip-rate control) or via a dedicated rate-controlling administration set.

Application

Suitable for most low-risk infusions such as IV fluids (e.g. sodium chloride or glucose 5% solutions). Not recommended for total parenteral nutrition (TPN).

Volumetric pumps

Application

Preferred for larger flow rates. They usually weigh between 3 and 5kg, and are designed to be 'stationary'. Volumetric pumps have the facility to work off mains power or a battery. The infusion rate is set using mL/h and most devices can be programmed to between 1 and 1000mL/h, although if used at rates <5mL/h, accuracy might ↓. Most pumps use a linear peristaltic pumping action.

The pump can often be programmed to stop infusing after a set volume, which useful if it is necessary to give a proportion of an infusion bottle or bag.

Ambulatory pumps
Small portable devices
They can use a small syringe but most use a reservoir bag of volume 100–250mL. Pumps are preprogrammable.

Implanted pumps
Implanted pumps have been developed for those ambulatory patients who need long-term low-volume therapy. These pumps are small and are implanted subcutaneously. The drug is then infused through an internal catheter into a vein, an artery, or an area of dedicated tissue.

Disposable pumps
These are non-electronic devices, which are generally very lightweight and small. Usually very 'user-friendly', requiring the minimum of input from the patient. They do not require a battery.

Disposable pumps work on a variety of principles:
- An elastomeric balloon, which is situated inside a plastic cylinder. When the balloon is filled with the infusion fluid, the resulting hydrostatic pressure inside the balloon is enough to power the infusion. The drug is infused through a small-bore administration set, which usually has a rate restrictor at the patient end.
- SideKick® exerts mechanical pressure from a spring-loaded device.
- SmartDose® works by generation of CO_2 in the space between a rigid plastic outer cylinder and the infusion bag.

Management of flow control devices
Any technical equipment will only function optimally if maintained appropriately and standardized, because devices are often moved with patients through various wards and departments. Care should be taken to comply with the manufacturer's instructions regarding storage of their product.

Management of magnesium imbalance

The normal range of magnesium is 0.7–1.0mmol/L.

Hypomagnesaemia

Causes of hypomagnesaemia
- Malnutrition
- Burns
- Trauma
- Alcoholism
- Medications—e.g. amphotericin, cisplatin, ciclosporin, loop diuretics.

Complications of hypomagnesaemia
- Hypokalaemia
- Hypocalcaemia
- Tetany
- Seizure
- Arrhythmias
- Cardiac arrest.

Preparations for replacement
- Magnesium glycerophosphate tablets (4mmol)
- Magnesium aspartate sachets (10mmol/sachet)
- Magnesium sulfate 50% solution 5g in 10mL (20mmol/10mL).

Mild hypomagnesaemia (0.5–0.7mmol/L) or asymptomatic patients
- Magnesium glycerophosphate tablets (4mmol): one or two tablets three to four times daily. Tablets can be dispersed in water and a 1mmol/mL liquid preparation is also available. Both preparations are unlicensed.
- Magnesium aspartate sachets (10mmol/sachet): one or two sachets daily. Sachets should be dissolved in 10mL of water. This preparation may be particularly useful in patients with short bowel syndrome.

Moderate to severe hypomagnesaemia (<0.5mmol/L) or symptomatic patients
- Magnesium sulfate injection of 10–20mmol (2.5–5g) in 1L infusion fluid over 12h daily until serum magnesium is within the normal range.
- The volume of fluid is not critical but consider the following:
  - The maximum peripheral concentration is 20% (20mmol in 25mL) because the injection has a very high osmolality.
  - The maximum rate is 150mg/min (20mmol over a period of 40min).
- Magnesium sulfate is compatible with sodium chloride 0.9% solution, glucose 5% solution, and sodium chloride/glucose solution.

Monitoring
Magnesium levels for symptomatic patients should be checked daily until corrected. Note that plasma levels might be artificially high while magnesium equilibrates with the intracellular compartment. However, if toxicity is suspected, treatment should be discontinued.

Hypermagnesaemia

Causes of hypermagnesaemia
- Renal insufficiency
- Hypothyroidism
- Medications (lithium).

Complications of hypermagnesaemia
- Hypotension
- Bradycardia
- Confusion
- Respiratory depression
- Coma.

Non-pharmacological treatment
- Treat underlying disorder
- External cardiac pacing (symptomatic)
- Mechanical ventilation (symptomatic)
- Dialysis (use only in emergency situations unless patient is already on dialysis).

Pharmacological treatment
- 1000mg calcium gluconate: slow IV push over 10min.
- Hydration with sodium chloride 0.9% solution (200mL/h).
- Add calcium gluconate 1000mg to each litre of fluid.
- Loop diuretics (e.g. furosemide 40mg IV push) to maintain urine output.

Monitoring
Serum magnesium every 2h until normalized and patient is asymptomatic.

Management of phosphate imbalance

The normal range of phosphate is 0.7–1.45mmol/L.

Hypophosphataemia

Causes of hypophosphataemia
- Malnutrition
- ↑ urine excretion of phosphorus
- Hyperparathyroidism
- Refeeding syndrome
- Medications.

Complications of hypophosphataemia
- Myalgias
- Peripheral neuropathy
- Paralysis
- Rhabdomyolysis
- Seizures
- Acute respiratory failure.

Treatment of hypophosphataemia
See Table 23.2.
- Mild hypophosphataemia: 0.61–0.69mmol/L.
- Moderate hypophosphataemia: 0.41–0.60mmol/L.
- Severe hypophosphataemia: <0.40mmol/L.
- Oral supplementation should be considered as first line in all patients who can tolerate oral therapy and who do not have a sodium restriction.
- Check plasma calcium. If high, seek specialist advice prior to supplementation.
- Half the dose in renal impairment and in patients <40kg.

Table 23.2 Treatment of hypophosphataemia

	Moderate (0.4–0.6mmol/L) Asymptomatic	Moderate (0.4–0.6mmol/L) Symptomatic	Severe (<0.4mmol/L)
Patient able to tolerate oral or enteral therapy	Phosphate-Sandoz® effervescent tablets: 2 tabs twice daily (16mmol phosphate/tab)	Oral therapy not appropriate	
Patient on IV therapy only	20mmol phosphate as sodium glycerophosphate in 0.9% sodium chloride or 5% glucose over 12h. Dilution volume ≤50mL must be administered via central access	20mmol phosphate as sodium glycerophosphate in 0.9% sodium chloride or 5% glucose over 6h. Dilution volume ≤50mL must be administered via central access	

Monitoring
Serum levels need to be checked 6h after the end of the infusion to enable time for distribution.

Hyperphosphataemia

Causes of hyperphosphataemia
- Renal insufficiency
- Acidosis
- Hypoparathyroidism
- Tumour lysis syndrome
- Medications—e.g. phosphate supplements, bisphosphonates.

Complications of hyperphosphataemia
- Calcium–phosphate complex formation and deposit in muscle
- Tetany
- Mortality.

Non-pharmacological treatment
- Treat underlying condition.
- Dialysis—use only in emergency situations, unless patient is already on dialysis.

Pharmacological treatment
- Phosphate binders:
  - Calcium carbonate 1250mg oral three times daily with each meal.
  - Calcium acetate 1000mg oral three times daily with each meal (adjusted to requirements).
  - Sevelamer 800–1600mg oral three times daily with each meal.
  - Lanthanum carbonate 750–1000mg three times daily with each meal.
  - Aluminium-based products are not usually recommended because of aluminium toxicity.
- Seek specialist information for dosing schedule.

Monitoring
- Serum phosphorus levels until normal.
- Serum calcium levels.

Management of hypokalaemia

Causes of hypokalaemia

- Excessive loss through GI tract or kidney
- Hypomagnesaemia
- Intracellular shift
- Medications—e.g. diuretics.

Complications of hypokalaemia

- Nausea/vomiting
- Weakness/fatigue
- Constipation
- Paralysis
- Respiratory failure
- Arrhythmias
- Sudden death.

Treatment of hypokalaemia

Treatment is summarized in Table 23.3.

Table 23.3 Treatment and monitoring of hypokalaemia

Serum potassium level (mmol/L)	Degree of hypokalaemia	Treatment
3.0–3.4	Mild or asymptomatic hypokalaemia	Oral potassium replacement is preferred for patients who are asymptomatic. IV replacement: 40mmol in 1L of sodium chloride 0.9% solution or glucose 5% solution administered peripherally (or centrally) over at least 6h
<3.0	Severe or symptomatic hypokalaemia	IV replacement with 40mmol in 500mL sodium chloride 0.9% solution or glucose 5% solution administered peripherally (or centrally) over at least 4h or over at least 2h through a central line with continuous ECG monitoring of heart rate and rhythm; repeat according to serum potassium levels
Monitoring	Serum potassium level every 1–6h if severe or symptomatic or if IV treatment ongoing	Testing serum magnesium may be indicated if hypokalaemia is resistant to treatment, and magnesium correction warranted if low

Risks associated with IV potassium

- Rapid administration of IV potassium or administration of concentrated IV potassium can result in hyperkalaemia paralysis, respiratory failure, arrhythmias, and asystole.
- Potassium should *not* be administered undiluted or by IV push.
- Peripheral administration of potassium may lead to burning, phlebitis, and necrosis, less concentrated solutions should be used peripherally.

Safety measures for IV potassium

- In July 2002, the National Patient Safety Agency (NPSA) in the UK issued a patient safety alert to prevent further fatalities following accidental overdose with IV potassium chloride concentrate that had been misidentified for sodium chloride 0.9% solution and water for injections.
- The risks associated with IV potassium chloride are well known. Potassium chloride, if injected too rapidly or in too high a dose, can cause cardiac arrest within minutes. The effect of hyperkalaemia on the heart is complex—virtually any arrhythmia could be observed.
- The true incidence of potassium-related fatalities and incidents is unknown.
- The alert identified safe medication practice recommendations concerning the prescribing, distribution, storage, and preparation of potassium chloride solutions in hospitals.
- The NPSA recommended withdrawal of concentrated potassium solutions from ward stock to be replaced by ready-to-use infusion products.
- The NPSA recommended that new control arrangements be introduced in critical care areas continuing to use potassium chloride concentrate ampoules and development of the use of pre-filled potassium syringes.
- Although recommendations have ↓ the risk to patients, staff still need to be vigilant to minimize and prevent harm to patients from incompetent/dangerous practice.

Minimizing risk: points pharmacists should encourage

- Labelling—the labelling format used differs between different manufacturers. The font size of K^+ details should be ↑ to improve identification. Historically, there has been a reliance on specifying the K^+ concentration as a percentage rather than mmol/volume on products as the primary focus. The latter should become main emphasis in future.
- Storage—decanting from boxes should be discouraged. Although most ward areas have limited storage space, it is GCP to segregate K^+-containing bags from other infusion fluids.
- Develop and publish a local range of infusions (e.g. Table 23.4).
- Staff competency needs to be established for IV fluid administration.

Concentrated K^+-containing products

Critical areas, high-dependency areas, and cardiac theatres that are allowed to store ampoules of potassium chloride locally should have a risk assessment performed periodically to overview the prescribing, ordering, storage, and administration processes. Other areas, such as general theatres, should not have access to concentrated ampoules of K^+.

Training development

The process from prescribing through to administration needs to be mapped and used as a backbone to develop multidisciplinary training.

Table 23.4 Suggested example of formulary for K+-containing IV fluids

Approved name	Manufacturer	Bag price*	Notes
Potassium chloride 20mmol in 50mL, sodium chloride 0.9% in pre-filled syringe	NHS manufacturer	£6	20mmol in 50mL (critical care only)
Potassium chloride 0.15%, glucose 10% (500mL)	Baxter	£6	10mmol in 500mL
Potassium chloride 0.15%, glucose 10%, sodium chloride 0.18% (500mL)	IVEX	£5	10mmol in 500mL
Potassium chloride 0.15%, glucose 2.5%, sodium chloride 0.45% (1000mL)	Fresenius Kabi	£5	20mmol in 1L
Potassium chloride 0.15%, glucose 4%, sodium chloride 0.18% (1000mL)	Fresenius Kabi	£1	20mmol in 1L
Potassium chloride 0.15%, glucose 5% (1000mL)	Fresenius Kabi	£1	20mmol in 1L
Potassium chloride 0.15%, sodium chloride 0.9% (1000mL)	TPS	£1	20mmol in 1L
Potassium chloride 0.15%, sodium chloride 0.9% (500mL)	TPS	£1	10mmol in 500mL
Potassium chloride 0.3%, glucose 4%, sodium chloride 0.18% (1000mL)	Fresenius Kabi	£1	40mmol in 1L
Potassium chloride 0.3%, glucose 5%, sodium chloride 0.18% (500mL)	Fresenius Kabi	£1	20mmol in 500mL
Potassium chloride 0.3%, glucose 5% (1000mL)	Fresenius Kabi	£1	40mmol in 1L
Potassium chloride 0.3%, sodium chloride 0.9% (1000mL)	Fresenius Kabi	£1	40mmol in 1L
Potassium chloride 0.3%, sodium chloride 0.9% (500mL)	Fresenius Kabi	£1	20mmol in 500mL
Potassium chloride 0.6% sodium chloride 0.9% (500mL)	Baxter	£5	40mmol in 500mL
Potassium chloride 0.6%, sodium chloride 0.9% (1000mL)	Baxter	£5	80mmol in 1L
Potassium chloride 3%, sodium chloride 0.9% (100mL)	Baxter	£4	40mmol in 100mL

*Prices listed as guide only. Cost will vary locally.

Guidelines for the treatment of hypocalcaemia

- The normal range of total calcium is 2.15–2.60mmol/L.
- The normal range of ionized calcium is 1.1–1.4mmol/L.

Causes of hypocalcaemia

- Malabsorption, inadequate intake, vitamin D deficiency
- Hypoalbuminaemia
- Hyperphosphataemia
- Hypomagnesaemia
- Pancreatitis
- Hypoparathyroidism.

Complications of hypocalcaemia

- Dysrhythmias
- Muscle cramping
- Paraesthesiae
- Seizures
- Stridor
- Tetany.

Non-pharmacological treatment

Treat the underlying disorder. The most common cause of low total serum calcium is hypo-albuminaemia. Therefore it is important to measure ionized calcium or correct the total serum calcium using the formula:

$$Ca_{corrected} = [(40 - Alb_{measured}) \times (0.02)] + Ca_{measured}$$

Preparations for replacement

- Calcium gluconate 10% (0.1g/mL)—injection contains 0.22mmol/mL of calcium.
- Calcium chloride 14.7% (0.147g/mL)—injection contains 1mmol/mL of calcium.
- Calcium solutions (especially calcium chloride) are irritants and care should be taken to prevent extravasation.

Dilution

- A calcium gluconate 10% injection can be given undiluted, or diluted in glucose 5% solution or sodium chloride 0.9% solution.
- A calcium chloride 14.7% solution should ideally be diluted in at least twice its volume of glucose 5% solution or sodium chloride 0.9% solution for peripheral administration. Calcium chloride can be given un-diluted by central line administration only.

Emergency elevation of serum calcium in symptomatic patients

- Give 2.25mmol IV stat over 10min.
- This is equal to either of the following:
  - 10mL of calcium gluconate 10% solution.
  - 2.25mL of calcium chloride 14.7% solution.

Hyperkalaemia and disturbance of ECG function

- 2.25–4.5mmol of calcium over 10–20min, depending on dose (up to a maximum rate of 0.2mmol/min).
- This is equal to either of the following:
  - 2–4mL of calcium chloride 14.7% injection.
  - 10–20mL of calcium gluconate 10% injection.
  - Titrate dose according to ECG.

Monitoring

For symptomatic patients calcium and albumin levels should be checked every 4h until corrected. Serum phosphate and magnesium levels should be monitored periodically.

Suggested dosing in asymptomatic hypocalcaemic patients

IV infusion to give 9mmol daily, which might need to be repeated at intervals of 1–3 days, as follows:

- 40mL of calcium gluconate 10% injection over 4h can be given neat or diluted in glucose 5% solution or sodium chloride 0.9% solution.
- 9mL of calcium chloride 14.7% injection over 4h diluted in 100mL of glucose 5% solution or sodium chloride 0.9% solution.

If the patient is absorbing oral medication, consider the use of soluble calcium tablets in divided doses.

Prescribing IV fluids

Fluid therapy is a fundamental part of patient care. IV fluid therapy should be reserved for patients who cannot meet their requirements via the oral or enteral route. It should be reviewed daily and stopped as soon as possible.

When prescribing IV fluids the 'five Rs' should be remembered: Resuscitation, Routine maintenance, Replacement, Redistribution, and Reassessment.

Patients should have an IV fluid management plan, which should include details of the IV fluid and electrolyte prescription over the next 24h as well as an assessment and monitoring plan.

Routine maintenance

- A patient who is unable to take fluid by mouth needs a basic IV regimen. In temperate climates, this should be restricted to 25–30mL/kg/day of water *and*
- Basic electrolyte requirements of ~1mmol/kg/day of sodium, potassium, and chloride *and*
- ~50–100g/day of glucose (equivalent to 1000–2000mL of glucose 5%). Note: this will not address patients' nutritional needs and care should be taken if patients are at risk of developing refeeding syndrome or are already receiving IV nutrition.
- Use of 25–30ml/kg/day sodium chloride 0.18% in 4% glucose with 27mmol/L on day 1 should be considered when prescribing for routine maintenance alone.
- Prescribing >2.5L per day ↑ the risk of hyponatraemia.
- Obese patients will need to have their IV fluid prescription adjusted to their ideal body weight. Patients rarely need more than 3L of fluid a day. Expert advice should be sought for patients with a BMI >40kg/m^2.

Assessment and monitoring

- Patients' likely fluid and electrolyte requirements can be assessed from their history, clinical examination, current medications, clinical monitoring, and laboratory testing.
- Check fluid charts, and note any losses from drains or catheters as well as NGT output, stoma output, and vomiting and/or diarrhoea.
- Most body fluids contain salt (Table 23.5), but at lower levels than plasma. Thus replacement requires a mixture of sodium chloride and glucose.
- Clinical history and examination should include any previous limited intake, thirst, the quantity and composition of abnormal losses, and any co-morbidities. This can be assisted by the measurement of changes in electrolytes, packed cell volume (PCV), and plasma proteins.
- Pulse, BP, capillary refill, JVP, the presence of pulmonary or peripheral oedema, and weight should also be monitored.
- Patients with heart failure are at greater risk of pulmonary oedema if over-hydrated. They also are unable to tolerate ↑ salt load because sodium retention accompanies heart failure.
- Patients with liver failure, despite being oedematous and often hypo-natraemic, have ↑ total body sodium. Therefore sodium chloride is best avoided in fluid regimens.

Table 23.5 Composition of commonly used crystalloids

	Na+ (mmol/L)	K+ (mmol/L)	Cl- (mmol/L)	Glucose (mmol/L)	Ca2+ (mmol/L)	Bicarbonate (mmol/L)
Sodium chloride 0.9%	154	0	154	0	0	0
Sodium chloride 0.18%/4% glucose	31	0	31	222 (40g)	0	0
Sodium chloride 0.45%/4% glucose	77	0	77	222 (40g)	0	0
5% glucose	0	0	0	278 (50g)	0	0
Hartmann's	131	5	111	0	2	29 (lactate)

Resuscitation

- Crystalloids containing sodium in the range 130–154mmol/L should be used, with a bolus of 500mL over <15min.
- Fluids using tetrastarch should not be used for resuscitation.
- Human albumin solution 4–5% can be considered only for patients with severe sepsis.

Abnormal losses: fluid management of the surgical patient

Planning an IV fluid therapy regimen

- Ensure adequate preoperative hydration.
- Minimize insensible losses during surgery:
  - Humidify inspired gases, minimize sweating by ensuring adequate anaesthesia, and, where possible, cover the patient to ensure adequate ambient temperature.
- Replace losses, such as blood loss.

Preoperative considerations

For routine elective surgery, the patient is kept NBM for 6–12h and takes little oral fluid for 6h postoperatively. A fluid deficit of 1000–1500mL arises, but this will be quickly corrected when the patient is drinking normally. IV fluid therapy is not required for many routine operations in adults, provided that the patient is not dehydrated. IV therapy is indicated preoperatively if the patient is likely to be NBM for >8h. Anaesthetists might set up an IV infusion of Hartmann's solution just before induction. On return to the surgical ward, this should be switched to sodium chloride or glucose as required, because there is no evidence that further treatment with Hartmann's solution has a clinical benefit compared with other crystalloids.

Perioperative considerations and blood loss

Operative blood loss of up to 500mL can be replaced with crystalloid solution (remembering that four times as much crystalloid solution will be needed). Use the following replacement fluids for blood loss:

- <500mL—use crystalloid solution.
- 500–1000mL—use colloid solution.
- >1000mL or Hb <10gdL—use whole blood.

Other replacement fluid is more appropriate if there is excess fluid loss from a specific compartment.

Hartmann's solution causes the least disturbance to plasma electrolyte concentrations and avoids postoperative fluid depletion. An allowance of 1mL/kg body weight/h should be begun at the start of anaesthesia to replace essential losses intraoperatively.

Postoperative considerations

- Normal fluid requirement is 2–3L/24h.
- Electrolyte requirements: Na^+, 2mmol/kg body weight; K^+, 1mmol/kg body weight.
- Low urine output (night after surgery) almost always results from inadequate fluid replacement, but might be a consequence of the anaesthetic technique. (K^+ is not normally administered during the first 24h in such patients.) Check JVP/CVP for signs of cardiac failure and consider fluid challenge, if appropriate.
- Check operation notes for extent of bleeding in theatre.
- Losses from gut—replace NGT; aspirate volume with sodium chloride 0.9% solution.
- Additional monitoring of urinary sodium can be useful in patients with high GI losses:
  - Reduced urinary sodium (<30mmol/L) may indicate total body depletion, even if plasma sodium levels are normal.
  - It can also be used to guide negative sodium balance in patients with oedema.
  - Note that urinary sodium values may be misleading in patients with impaired renal function or those on diuretic therapy.

Table 23.6 Composition of gastrointestinal body fluid

	Volume (L/24h)	Na^+ (mmol/L)	K^+ (mmol/L)	Cl^- (mmol/L)	HCO_3^- (mmol/L)	pH
Saliva	0.5–1.5	20–80	10–20	20–40	20–60	7–8
Gastric juice	1.0–2.0	20–100	5–10	120–160	0	1–7
Bile	0.5–1.0	150–250	5–10	40–120	20–40	7–8
Pancreatic juice	1.0–2.0	120–250	5–10	10–60	80–120	7–8

- Losses from surgical drains (see Table 23.6 for body fluid composition)—
  replace significant losses. However, calculate total fluid loss (24h) as follows:
  - Estimate skin and lung loss = (10 × body weight)mL.
  - Estimation of stool losses = 50mL.
  - Estimation of urine losses, normally measured directly.
  - Drain loss/NGT loss.

Design a fluid regimen
- Calculate fluid losses and replace them (as outlined).
- Calculate Na^+ and K^+ requirements.
- Measure plasma U&Es if patient is ill.
- Start oral fluids as soon as possible.

For example, a fluid regimen for a 60kg patient would be calculated as follows:
- Fluid losses:
  - Patient urine output 1500Ml.
  - Fluid losses = (10 × 60) + 1500 + 50mL = 2150mL.
  - NGT loss = 1000mL.
- Na^+ requirement = 2 × 60 = 120mmol.
- K^+ requirement = 1 × 60 = 60mmol.
- Volume of sodium chloride 0.9% solution that will provide sodium requirement = 1000mL (154mmol Na^+).
- Amount of K^+ required = 60mmoL.
- Remember that glucose 5% solution can be considered as isotonic water and will be used to make up the difference for the patient's fluid requirement.
- NGT replacement = 1000mL sodium chloride 0.9% solution.

Hence, a suitable 24h regimen for a 60kg patient with 1.5L urinary output and 1L NGT losses would be as follows:
- 2 × 1000mL sodium chloride 0.9% solution + 20mmol potassium chloride.
- 1000mL glucose 5% solution + 20mmoL potassium chloride.
- Each bag runs for a period of 8h.
- Start oral fluids as soon as reasonable, depending on the patient's condition/indication for surgery.

Special conditions that need more specialist fluid knowledge
- Haemorrhagic/hypovolaemic shock
- Septic shock
- Heart or liver impairment
- Excessive vomiting

Fluid balance
During a lifetime, the water content and fluid compartments within the body alter. In infants, fluid content is 70–80% of body weight. This progressively ↓, reaching 60% of body weight at age 2yrs. In adults, the fluid content accounts for 60% of body weight in ♂ and 55% in ♀, and the ratio of extracellular fluid (ECF) to intracellular fluid (ICF) is 1:3.

For example, the fluid content of a 70kg ♂ is as follows:
- Total fluid = 42L.
- ICF – 67% of body water = 28L.
- ECF – 33% of body water = 14 (25% of intravascular space = 3.5L; 75% of interstitium = 10.5L).

Compartment barriers

- The fluid compartments are separated from one another by semi-permeable membranes through which water and solutes can pass. The composition of each fluid compartment is maintained by the selectivity of its membrane.
- The barrier between plasma and the interstitium is the capillary endothelium, which allows free passage of water and electrolytes but not large molecules such as proteins.
- The barrier between the ECF and the ICF is the cell membrane.

Transport mechanisms

- Simple diffusion—movement of solutes down concentration gradients.
- Facilitated diffusion—again depends on concentration gradient differences, but also relies on the availability of carrier substances.
- Osmosis—movement of solvent through semipermeable membranes.
- Active transport—e.g. Na^+/K^+ exchange pump.

Osmolality

- Osmotic pressure is generated by colloids impermeable to the membrane.
- Water distributes across in either direction if there is a difference in osmolality across the membrane.
- Osmolarity is the number of osmoles per litre of solution.
- Osmolality is the number of osmoles per kilogram of solvent or solution.
- The osmolality of blood is 285–295mOsm/L.

Tonicity

Molecules that affect the movement of water (e.g. sodium and glucose) are called 'effective osmoles' and contribute to compartment osmolality (sometimes termed 'tonicity'). The normal range of serum osmolality is 285–295mOsm/L. The measured osmolality should not exceed the predicted value by >10mOsm/L. A difference of >10mOsm/L is considered an osmolal gap. Causes of a serum osmolal gap include the presence of mannitol, ethanol, methanol, ethylene glycol, or other toxins (usually small molecules) in very high concentrations. (The propylene glycol in lorazepam can cause hyperosmolarity and hyperosmolar coma in some patients, particularly when lorazepam is used as a continuous infusion.)

Serum osmolality is calculated as follows:
- Serum osmolality = $[2 \times (Na^+ + K^+)] + (glucose/18) + (BUN/2.8)$
- Where BUN is blood urea nitrogen. Na^+ and K^+ are in mmol/L, and glucose and BUN are in mg/dL. To convert glucose from mmol, divide by a factor of 0.05551. To convert BUN from mmol, divide by a factor of 0.3569.

Table 23.7 Fluid balance—average daily water balance

Input (mL of water)	Output (mL of water)
Drink: 1500	Urine: 1500
In food: 800	Insensible losses (lungs and skin): 800
Metabolism of food: 200	Stool: 200
Total: 2500	Total: 2500

Knowledge of fluid distribution

- Glucose 5% solution distributes through the ECF with a resultant fall in ECF osmolality, water distributes into the cells, and thus glucose 5% solution distributes throughout the body water.
- Conversely, a person marooned on a life raft with no water loses water from all compartments.
- Sodium chloride 0.9% solution contains 154mmol/L of sodium with an osmolality of 300mOmol/L. When infused, most of the solution stays in the ECF, which is of a similar osmolality.
- Conversely, if water and electrolytes are lost together (e.g. severe diarrhoea), fluid is mainly lost from the ECF.
- With ECF losses, sodium and water are lost together, so the sodium concentration in the remaining ECF does not change.
- However, protein and red cells are not lost so their concentration rises.
- If plasma alone is lost, only the PCV rises.
- Extra fluid for continuing losses should resemble as closely as possible the fluid that has been lost.

The body is normally in positive water balance (Table 23.7), with the kidney adjusting for varying intakes and losses by altering water clearance. The kidney requires 500mL of water to excrete the average daily load of osmotically active waste products at maximal urinary concentration.

Nutritional support in adults

Parenteral support

Poor nutritional status is a major determinant of a patient's morbidity (as a consequence of depressed cell-mediated immunity and wound healing) and mortality.

The decision to provide nutritional support must be as a result of a thorough clinical assessment of the patient's condition ideally by a nutrition support team. Parenteral nutritional support should be for patients who are malnourished or likely to become so, and in whom the GI tract is not sufficiently functional to meet nutritional needs or is inaccessible.

Appropriate indications for parenteral nutrition

- Short bowel syndrome.
- GI fistulae.
- Prolonged paralytic ileus.
- Acute pancreatitis if jejunal feeding is contraindicated.
- Conditions severely affecting the GI tract, such as severe mucositis following systemic chemotherapy.

Guide to calculating parenteral nutritional requirements in adults

Nutritional assessment

Assessment is essential for the correct provision of nutritional support. A variety of techniques are available to assess nutritional status. Some of the common criteria used to define malnutrition are recent weight loss (BMI) (see Table 23.8).

Identifying high-risk patients

- Unintentional weight loss—5–10% is clinically significant.
- ↓ oral intake—can result from vomiting, anorexia, or NBM.
- Weight loss—take oedema, ascites, or dehydration into consideration.

BMI is useful for identifying malnourished underweight patients, but a normal BMI does not rule out malnutrition, especially in an increasingly obese population.

Table 23.8 Body mass index

$BMI = \dfrac{Weight(kg)}{Height^2(m)}$	Normal: ♀ 20–25 ♂ 22–27

Normal nutritional requirements

The Schofield equation is used typically in the UK; the Harris–Benedict and Ireton–Jones equations are commonly referred to in US texts.

It is always best to be cautious and start low and titrate up, depending on tolerance and clinical response. Use actual bodyweight if BMI >30kg/m². A useful starting point in obese patients is to use 75% of body weight or alternatively feed to basal metabolic rate (BMR), without stress or activity factors added.

Macronutrients

- Calories
- Schofield equation
- Calculate BMR (W = weight in kilograms) (Table 23.9).

Add activity factor and stress factor as follows:
- Activity:
  - Bedbound/immobile: +10%
  - Bedbound mobile/sitting: +15–20%
  - Mobile: +25% upwards.
- Stress: percentage added for stress varies widely depending on the clinical condition, but it is typically in the range 0–30%.

Harris–Benedict equation

♂: $BMR = 66.473 + (13.751 \times BW) + (5.0033 \times HT) - (6.755 \times age)$

♀: $BMR = 655.0955 + (9.463 \times BW) + (1.8496 \times HT) - (4.6756 \times age)$

where BW is body weight in kilograms, HT is height in centimetres, and age is in years.

Total caloric requirement is obtained by multiplying the BMR by the sum of the stress and activity factors. Stress conditions and activity factors need to be factored to calculate specific requirements.

Composition of parenteral nutrition regimens

- If possible, a balance of glucose and lipids should be used to provide total amount calories calculated.
- Glucose provision should be within the glucose oxidation rate (GOR) if possible.
- Normal GOR is 4–7mg/kg body weight/min.

Table 23.9 Calculation of BMR

♀ (kcal/day)		♂ (kcal/day)	
18–29yrs	(14.8W) + 692	18–29yrs	(15.1W) + 692
30–59yrs	(8.3W) + 846	30–59yrs	(11.5W) + 873
60–74yrs	(9.2W) + 687	60–74yrs	(11.9W) + 700
>75yrs	(9.8W) + 624	>75yrs	(8.3W) + 820

Nitrogen
- Normal nitrogen requirements are 0.14–0.2g/kg body weight.
- Requirements in catabolic patients can be in the range of 0.2–0.3g/kg body weight.
- Non-renal nitrogen losses should be taken into consideration—e.g. wound, fistula, and burn losses.

Electrolytes
- Sodium (normal range 0.5–1.5mmol/kg body weight):
  - Sensitive to haemodilutional effects. Actual low sodium level is usually only as a result of excessive losses, and a moderately low level is unlikely to be clinically significant.
  - Renal excretion can be a useful indicator. Aim to keep urine sodium >20mmol/L.
- Potassium (normal range 0.3–1.0mmol/kg body weight):
  - Affected by renal function, drugs, or excessive losses.
- Calcium (normal range 0.1–0.15mmol/kg body weight):
  - Sensitive to haemoconcentration and haemodilution. Minimal supplementation generally adequate in short-term parenteral nutrition.
- Magnesium (normal range 0.1–0.2mmol/kg body weight):
  - Renally conserved. Minimal amounts generally suffice unless patient has excessive losses.
- Phosphate (normal range 0.5–1.0mmol/kg body weight):
  - Influenced by renal function, re-feeding syndrome, and onset of sepsis.

Trace elements and vitamins
Commercial multivitamin and mineral preparations (e.g. Solivito N®, Decan®, Additrace®, and Cernevit®) are suitable for most patients in the short to medium term. Requirements for long-term patients are dictated by monitoring.

How specific clinical conditions can affect parenteral nutrition requirements and provision

Re-feeding syndrome
- Start with low calories/day (max. 20kcal/kg body weight/day).
- Monitor and supplement potassium, magnesium, and phosphate as required.
- Ensure adequate vitamin supply, especially thiamine.

Acute kidney injury
- Consider fluid, potassium, and phosphate restriction.
- Sodium restriction can also help to ↓ fluid retention.

Chronic renal failure
- Influenced by dialysis status.
- Consider need for nitrogen, potassium, and phosphate restriction.

Acute liver failure
- Use dry body weight to calculate requirements (especially if ascites is present).
- Patients might require sodium and fluid restriction. Protein restriction is not necessary.
- Provision of nutrition usually outweighs risks of abnormal LFTs.

Congestive cardiac failure
- Consider need for sodium and fluid restriction.

Practical issues concerning parenteral nutrition

The identification and selection of patients who require parenteral nutrition, and the subsequent provision and monitoring of this treatment, consist of a number of overlapping phases.

If there is concern with regard to a patient's nutrition they should be referred to the ward dietician for a full assessment.

Initiation of parenteral nutrition

Once referred to the nutrition support team, the patient will be formally assessed and, if it is felt appropriate, line access will be planned. For short-term parenteral nutrition (7–10 days), this will usually be a peripherally inserted venous catheter (PICC). A tunnelled central line will be used if the anticipated duration of parenteral nutrition is longer or peripheral access is limited.

Before initiating parenteral nutrition, baseline biochemistry should be checked (Table 23.10) and fluid and electrolyte abnormalities corrected. In those at risk of developing re-feeding syndrome, additional IV vitamins might be required.

Early monitoring phase

During the first week of parenteral nutrition (and subsequently if the patient is 'unstable' with respect to fluid and electrolyte or metabolic issues) the patient is monitored intensively. This consists of a minimum set of mandatory ward observations, and appropriate blood and other laboratory tests. The aim is to optimize nutritional support, while remaining aware of the other therapeutic strategies in the patient's overall care plan.

It might be necessary to modify either nutritional support or the overall patient care plan to obtain the best patient outcomes.

Stable patient phase

After the patient is stabilized on parenteral nutrition, a less intensive monitoring process is required.

Re-introduction of diet

At a certain point, diet or enteral feed is usually introduced in a transitional manner. Liaison with the ward dietician is essential and, if appropriate, reduction or cessation of parenteral nutrition is recommended.

Cessation of parenteral nutrition

Parenteral nutrition is usually stopped when oral nutritional intake is deemed adequate for the individual patient. As a general rule, cessation of parenteral nutrition is determined by a variety of factors and is a multidisciplinary decision.

IV access

Peripheral cannulae (Venflons®) should not be used routinely for the administration of parenteral nutrition. They should only be used in the short term for the administration of 'peripheral formulated' parenteral nutrition.

Table 23.10 Suggested monitoring guide (please refer to local guidelines)

	Baseline	New patient or unstable	Stable patient
Blood biochemistry			
Urea and creatinine	Yes	Daily	Three times weekly
Sodium	Yes	Daily	Three times weekly
Potassium	Yes	Daily	Three times weekly
Bicarbonate	Yes	Daily	Three times weekly
Chloride	Yes	Daily	Three times weekly
LFTs: bilirubin	Yes	Daily	Three times weekly
ALP	Yes	Daily	Three times weekly
AST or ALT	Yes	Daily	Three times weekly
Albumin	Yes	Daily	Three times weekly
Calcium	Yes	Daily	Three times weekly
Magnesium	Yes	Daily	Three times weekly
Phosphate	Yes	Daily	Three times weekly
Zinc	Yes	Weekly	Every 2 weeks
Copper	Yes	Monthly	Every 3 months
CRP	Yes	Three times weekly	Three times weekly
Full blood count	Yes	Three times weekly	Weekly
Coagulation			
APTT	Yes	Weekly	Weekly
INR	Yes	Weekly	Weekly
Lipids			
Cholesterol	Yes	Weekly	Weekly
Triglycerides	Yes	Weekly	Weekly

LFT, liver function test; ALP, alkaline phosphatase; AST, aspartate amino-transferase; ALT, alanine aminotransferase; CRP, C-reactive protein; APTT, activated partial thromboplastin time.

PICC lines are usually used for medium- to long-term venous access (2–6 months).

Tunnelled cuffed central venous catheters (CVs) are inserted via the subclavian (or jugular) vein for long-term feeding.

A dedicated single-lumen line is the safest route for parenteral nutrition administration. There is a greater risk of infection the more times a line is manipulated. Aseptic technique should be used. Nothing else should be given through this lumen, nor should blood be sampled from the line under normal circumstances (it might be appropriate for blood sampling in patients receiving parenteral nutrition at home).

If a multilumen line must be used for clinical reasons, one lumen should be dedicated for parenteral nutrition use only. Again, ideally, nothing else should be given through this lumen, nor should blood be sampled from it.

Prescribing parenteral nutrition

Patients' nutritional requirements are based on standard dietetic equations. A regimen close to a patient's requirements should be provided in a formulation prepared to minimize risk.

Nitrogen

Protein in parenteral nutrition is provided in the form of amino acids. Individual nitrogen requirements are calculated.

Carbohydrate and lipid

The energy in parenteral nutrition is generally described as non-protein calories (i.e. the figure excludes the energy provided from amino acids).

Total energy intake is best given as a mixture of glucose and lipid, usually in a ratio of 60:40. This might be varied if clinically important glucose intolerance develops or if there is a requirement for a lipid-free parenteral nutrition bag.

Volume

The overall aim is to provide all fluid volume requirements, including losses from wounds, drains, stomas, fistulae, etc., through parenteral nutrition. However, if these losses are large or highly variable, they should be managed separately.

Electrolytes

These are modified according to clinical requirements, with particular regard to extra-renal losses. Electrolytes should be reviewed daily initially and modified as necessary. Monitoring of urinary electrolyte losses is useful.

Vitamins, minerals, and trace elements

These are added routinely on a daily basis. Extra zinc or selenium might be required in patients with large GI losses. Patients on long-term parenteral nutrition will have routine micronutrient screening (Table 23.11).

Other medications

No drug additions should be made to parenteral nutrition on grounds of stability, unless stability work is undertaken. Additions of certain drugs (e.g. heparin) are known to lead to incompatibility.

Recommended monitoring/care (early monitoring phase)

- Daily weight (before starting parenteral nutrition and daily thereafter).
- Take temperature and BP reading every 4–6h. (Also observe for clinical evidence of infection and general well-being.)
- Accurate fluid-balance chart and summary (to maintain accurate fluid balance and homeostasis). Bag change should be undertaken at the same time of day.
- Capillary glucose monitoring (BMS) every 6h during the first 24h, and then twice or once daily until stable (generally, the glucose target should be 4–10mmol/L). Return to BMS every 6h when parenteral nutrition is being weaned off.
- Daily assessment for CVC/PICC site infection or leakage. Change dressing for CVCs at least every 72h and more frequently if loose, soiled, or wet. Change PICC dressings weekly.
- 24h urine collections for nitrogen balance and electrolytes should be undertaken according to local practice.

Storage of parenteral nutrition on ward

Bags not yet connected to the patient must be stored in a refrigerator (at 2–8°C). Bags stored in a drug refrigerator must be kept away from any freezer compartment to prevent ice crystal formation in the parenteral nutrition.

Bags that have been refrigerated should be removed at least 1–2h before being hung and infused, to enable the solution to reach room temperature. Bags connected to the patient should be protected from light using protective covers.

Children's parenteral nutrition regimens

Parenteral nutrition in children

Infants and children are particularly susceptible to the effects of starvation. The small preterm infant (1kg) contains only 1% fat and 8% protein, and has a non-protein caloric reserve of only 110kcal/kg body weight. With growth, the fat and protein content rises, so a 1yr-old child weighing 10kg will have a non-protein calorie reserve of 221kcal/kg body weight. All non-protein content and one-third of the protein content of the body is available for calorific needs at a rate of 50kcal/kg body weight/day in infants and children.

A small preterm baby (<1.5kg) has sufficient reserve to survive only 4 days of starvation, and a large preterm baby (>3kg) has enough for ~10–12 days. With ↑ calorific requirements associated with disease this might be reduced dramatically to <2 days for small preterm infants and perhaps 1wk for a large preterm baby.

Indications for parenteral nutrition

Some children require short-term parenteral nutrition in the following clinical situations:
• Major intestinal surgery
• Chemotherapy
• Severe acute pancreatitis
• Multiorgan failure in extensive trauma, burns, or prematurity.

Others will need long-term parenteral nutrition if there are prolonged episodes of intestinal failure—e.g. in the following clinical situations:
• Protracted diarrhoea of infancy
• Short bowel syndrome
• Gastroschisis
• Chronic intestinal pseudo-obstruction.

Nutritional requirements

See Table 23.11.

Fluid requirements also depend on the child's size, abnormal losses (e.g. diarrhoea, fever), surgical procedures, and disease state. The requirements for fluid to body weight are much greater in very small children than in older children and adults. Infants have a much larger body surface area relative to weight than older patients. Infants lose more fluid through evaporation and dissipate much more heat per kilogram. The use of radiant heaters and phototherapy further ↑ a neonate's fluid loss, resulting in ↑ fluid requirement. Children with high urinary outputs, ↑ ileostomy or gastrostomy tube outputs, diarrhoea, or vomiting should have replacement fluids for these excessive losses in addition to their maintenance fluid requirements.

The child's weight and assessment of intake and output can be used to estimate hydration status. It is important that children receiving parenteral nutrition are weighed regularly (initially daily, then twice or three times weekly with growth plotted when their condition stabilizes) and their fluid balance is monitored when parenteral nutrition is prescribed.

Table 23.11 Estimated average requirements for fluid, energy, protein, and nitrogen

Age (yrs)	Fluid (mL/kg/day)	Energy (kcal/kg /day)	Protein (g/kg/day)	Nitrogen (g/kg/day)
Preterm	150–200	130–150	3.0–4.0	0.5–0.65
0–1	110–150	110–130	2.0–3.0	0.34–0.46
1–6	80–100	70–100	1.5–2.5	0.22–0.38
6–12	75–80	50–70	1.5–2.0	0.2–0.33
12–18	50–75	40–50	1.0–1.3	0.16–0.2

Energy sources

The body of a child requires energy for physical growth and neurological development.

Carbohydrate

Glucose is the carbohydrate source of choice in parenteral nutrition. To prevent hyperosmolality and hyperinsulinaemia, glucose infusions are introduced in a stepwise manner. In infants, glucose is introduced at 5–7.5% glucose and ↑ by 2.5% each day to an upper limit on glucose infusion rate of 4–7mg/kg body weight/min. In older children parenteral nutrition is started at 10–15% and ↑ daily to 20%, as tolerated.

The amount of glucose depends on the type of feeding line inserted. The glucose concentration in parenteral nutrition infused peripherally is limited to 12.5%. If central access is available, up to 20% glucose can be infused. Infusion of parenteral nutrition with glucose concentrations >20% has been associated with cardiac arrhythmias.

The infant with very low birthweight has low glycogen reserves in the liver and a diminished capacity for gluconeogenesis. Hepatic glycogen is depleted within hours of birth, depriving the brain of metabolic fuel. Thus providing exogenous glucose through parenteral nutrition is a priority. Preterm infants, especially those with birthweights <1000g, are relatively glucose intolerant because of insulin resistance. Infusion of glucose >6mg/kg body weight/min may lead to hyperglycaemia and serum hyperosmolality, resulting in osmotic diuresis. Tolerance to glucose improves on subsequent days. It is generally recommended that the glucose infusion rate does not exceed 9mg/kg body weight/min for premature infants after the first day of life and that ↑ is implemented gradually as the infant develops.

Lipids
- Regimens require fat as a source of essential fatty acids. Fat is an important parenteral substrate because it is a concentrated source of calories in an isotonic medium, which makes it useful for peripheral administration.
- Fat is a useful substitute for carbohydrate if glucose calories are limited because of glucose intolerance. It is available as emulsions of soybean, soybean–safflower oil mixtures, or olive oil. The major differences are their fatty acid contents.

- Essential fatty acid deficiency can develop in the premature newborn during the first week of life on lipid-free regimens. There is a maximum lipid utilization rate of 3.3–3.6g/kg body weight/day. Above these values, there is ↑ risk of fat deposition secondary to the incomplete metabolic utilization of the infused lipid.
- IV fat should be commenced at a dose not exceeding 1g/kg body weight/day and ↑ gradually to a maximum of 3g/kg body weight/day, depending on age. Tolerance should be assessed by measuring serum triglyceride and free fatty acid concentrations.

Nitrogen

Nitrogen is needed for growth, the formation of new tissues (e.g. wound healing), and the synthesis of plasma proteins, enzymes, and blood cells.

Requirements vary according to age, nutritional status, and disease state. Infants and children experiencing periods of growth have higher nitrogen requirements than adults. Low-birthweight infants have relatively high total amino acid requirements to support maintenance, growth, and developmental needs.

Amino acid intakes of 2.0–2.5g/kg body weight/day result in nitrogen retention comparable to the healthy enteral-fed infant. Rates of up to 4g/kg body weight/day might be required. Because the amino acid profile varies between commercial brands, their nitrogen contents are not equivalent and protein requirements are calculated as grams of amino acids rather than grams of nitrogen in children.

Choice of amino acid solution

The proteins of the human body are manufactured from 20 different amino acids. There are eight essential amino acids. Premature infants and children are unable to synthesize/metabolize some of the amino acids that are 'non-essential' for adults. The use of amino acid solutions designed for adults have resulted in abnormal plasma amino acid profiles in infants. Infants fed with adult amino acid solutions have been shown to develop high concentrations of phenylalanine and tyrosine and low levels of taurine.

Paediatric amino acid solutions

Amino acid solutions specifically designed for neonates have been developed, as follows:
- Higher concentration of branch-chain amino acids (leucine, isoleucine and valine) and lower content of glycine, methionine and phenylalanine.
- Higher percentage of amino acids essential for preterm infants, with wider distribution of nonessential amino acids.
- Contain taurine.

The amino acid preparations available are based on either the amino acid profile of human milk (Vaminolact®) or placental cord blood (Primene®).

Electrolytes

Normal baseline electrolyte requirements are shown in Table 23.12.

Trace elements

Requirements for trace elements are shown in Table 23.13.

Vitamins

Requirements for vitamins are shown in Tables 23.14 and 23.15.

Table 23.12 Normal baseline electrolyte requirements

Electrolytes	Requirements according to age (mmol/kg body weight/day)	
	Infants	Children
Sodium	2.0–3.5	1.0–2.0
Potassium	2.0–3.0	1.0–2.0
Calcium	1.0–1.5	0.5–1.0
Magnesium	0.15–0.3	0.1–0.15
Phosphate	0.5–1.5	0.12–0.4
Chloride	1.8–1.5	1.2–2

Table 23.13 Requirements for trace elements

Element	Requirements according to age (micrograms/kg body weight/day)		
	Preterm	Infants	Children
Zinc	100–500	50–100	50–80
Copper	30–60	20–50	20
Selenium	N/a	2–5	2
Manganese	N/a	1	1
Iron	100–200	20–100	100

Table 23.14 Requirements for water-soluble vitamins

Vitamin	Requirements according to age		
	Preterm	Infants	Children
B_1 (mg)	0.1–05	0.4–1.5	1.0–3.0
B_2 (mg)	0.1–0.3	0.4–1.5	1.0–3.0
B_6 (mg)	008–0.4	0.1–1.0	1.0–2.0
B_{12} (micrograms)	0.3–0.6	0.3–30	20–40
C (mg)	20–40	20–40	20–40
Biotin (micrograms)	5–30	35–50	150–300
Folate (micrograms)	50–200	100–200	100–200
Niacin (mg)	2–5	5–10	5–20

Table 23.15 Requirements for fat-soluble vitamins

Vitamin	Preterm	Infant	Children
A (micrograms)	75–300	300–600	500–800
D (micrograms)	5–10	10–20	10–20
E (mg)	3–8	3–10	10–15
K (micrograms)	5–80	100–200	N/a

Administration of nutrition

- The aqueous phase runs over a period of 24h and the solution is filtered using a 0.2μm filter.
- Lipid normally runs over a period of 20–24h and is filtered using a 1.2μm filter, although some centres prefer not to use filters.
- The weight used for calculation is usually the actual weight of the child.

Complications

Catheter related
Complications could be due to catheter insertion (e.g. malposition, haemorrhage, pneumothorax, air embolism, or nerve injury) or might occur subsequently (e.g. infection, occlusion, or thromboembolism).

Metabolic related
In stable patients with no abnormal fluid losses or major organ failure, severe biochemical disturbances are unusual.

Parenteral nutrition-associated cholestasis
The aetiology seems to be multifactorial, including the absence of enteral feeding, overfeeding, prematurity, surgery, and sepsis. It might progress to cirrhosis. Excessive calories, particularly glucose overload, can lower serum glucagon concentrations, which ↓ bile flow. Early initiation of oral calorie intake is the single most important factor in preventing or reversing cholestasis. Small intestinal bacterial overgrowth, which often occurs in the presence of intestinal stasis, can impair bile flow, leading to cholestasis.

Monitoring children receiving parenteral nutrition in hospital

Requires clinical and laboratory monitoring, observations, and assessment of growth. Growth is conveniently assessed by accurate measurement of weight and height, and development assessment is plotted over time. Fluid balance, temperature, and basal metabolism need to be assessed daily.

Laboratory monitoring
- Initial assessment—daily for first 3–4 days, then twice weekly.
- Full blood count.
- Blood test: sodium, potassium, urea, glucose.
- Calcium, magnesium, phosphate, bilirubin, ALP, AST, ALT, blood glucose albumin, triglycerides, cholesterol.
- Copper, zinc, selenium, vitamins A and E: baseline measurement.
- Urine: sodium and potassium (baseline).
- Continued monitoring depends on the child's clinical condition.

Enteral feeding

Enteral feeding should be considered in patients with a functioning GI tract who are unable to meet requirements with ordinary diet, food fortification, and/or oral nutritional supplements.

Enteral nutrition is contraindicated in patients with intestinal obstruction, paralytic ileus, GI ischaemia, intractable diarrhoea, and diffuse peritonitis. Enteral access device selection is based on several patient-specific factors, including GI anatomy, gastric emptying, tube placement duration, and aspiration potential.

Post-pyloric feeding is indicated if there is gastric outflow obstruction or severe pancreatitis, or if the patient is at risk from aspiration with intragastric feeding.

Types of tube feeding

Intragastric feeding
- Nasogastric (NG)
- Percutaneous endoscopic gastroscopy (PEG).

Post-pyloric feeding
- Nasojejunal
- Nasoduodenal
- PEG
- Percutaneous endoscopic jejunostomy
- Surgically placed jejunostomy.

Feeding tube specific issues

Site of delivery
- Gastric tubes end in the stomach, whereas jejunal tubes end in the jejunum.
- Sterile water must be used for jejunal tubes because of gastric acid barrier bypass.

Number of differences between tubes apart from site of feed delivery
- Bore size—fine-bore tube is designed for administration of feeds, and wide-bore tube is designed for aspiration.
- Number of lumens.
- Rate of flow.
- Length.

Complications of tubes
- Removal by patient.
- Oesophageal ulceration or strictures.
- Incorrect positioning of tube.
- Blockage.

Categories of feed

Polymeric feeds
Contain whole protein, carbohydrate, and fat, and can be used as the sole source of nutrition for those patients without any special nutrient requirements. Standard concentration is 1kcal/mL with 40–50g/L protein, but they can vary in energy density (0.8–2kcal/mL) and can be supplemented with fibre, which can help improve bowel function if this is problematic.

Elemental feeds

Contain amino acid and glucose or maltodextrins; fat content is very low. Used in situations of malabsorption or pancreatic insufficiency. Because of their high osmolality, they should not be used in patients with short bowel syndrome.

Disease-specific feeds and modular supplements

Certain clinical conditions require adjustment in diets—e.g. high-energy, low-electrolyte feeds for patients requiring dialysis, and low-carbohydrate and high-fat diets for patients with CO_2 retention (for certain patients on ventilators) as carbohydrate leads to more CO_2 production compared with calorific equivalent amounts of protein or fat.

Modular supplements are used for a variety of conditions—e.g. mal-absorption and hypoprotein states. They are not nutritionally complete and hence are not suitable as the sole source of food. These feeds contain extra substrates that are claimed to alter the immune and inflammatory responses. These substrates include glutamine, arginine, RNA, omega-3 fatty acids, and antioxidants.

Administration of tube feeds

For intragastric feeds, diet can be delivered at a continuous rate over a period of 16–18h daily. Alternatively, intermittent boluses of 50–250mL can be administered by syringe over a period of 10–30min four to eight times a day, although complications such as aspiration and delayed gastric transit times have been reported more frequently with this approach.

Post-pyloric feeding is generally performed by continuous infusion because it is deemed more physiological.

Table 23.16 Checklist of information to be included in the discharge plan

Patient	Vascular access device	Treatment
Relevant past medical history	Type of device	Pathology and infecting organism
Problems/side effects experienced	When inserted or placed, and by whom	Details of antimicrobial regimen, drug, dose, etc.
Frequency and timing of clinic visits during treatment	If centrally placed, where is the tip?	Administration details
Blood monitoring and frequency	Possible complications—signs, symptoms, prevention, and management	Side effects
Length of time on treatment	Day-to-day care of the line	Monitoring requirements and action required if results are abnormal
Finish/review date for treatment	Who to contact if there are any difficulties with the device	
How to access help	Who will remove the device and how	

Complications from feeds

Diarrhoea

Diarrhoea is the most common complication associated with enteral nutrition, occurring in 21–72% of patients. Severe diarrhoea can cause life-threatening electrolyte changes and hypovolaemia. Management is by excluding other explanations (e.g. colitis, laxative use, antibiotics, and malabsorption).

Concomitant medications need to be rationalized. Antidiarrhoeal medications (codeine phosphate and/or loperamide) are often useful and fibre can help in some cases.

If diarrhoea persists after treatment, consider switching to the post-pyloric route.

Constipation

Usually a result of a combination of inadequate fluid, dehydration, immobility, and drugs. If functional pathology is excluded, management is by laxatives, suppositories, and fibre-containing feeds.

Vomiting, aspiration, or reflux

Both nasogastric and post-pyloric feeding can ↑ the risk of aspiration. Both can interfere with oesophageal sphincter function, and wide-bore tubes cause more problems than fine-bore tubes. Standard antiemetics and pro-kinetics are usually effective.

Metabolic complications

Re-feeding syndrome

Excess carbohydrate stimulates insulin release, which leads to intracellular shifts of phosphate, magnesium, and potassium that can lead to cardiac arrhythmias or neurological events. Emaciated patients must have their feed introduced gradually at a rate of 20kcal/kg body weight and electrolytes replaced in accordance with daily blood levels.

Vitamin/trace element deficiencies

Incidence is rare as commercially available feeds are nutritionally complete. Patients being fed over extended periods should be monitored appropriately.

Hyperglycaemia

Important in the critically ill. It is imperative that blood glucose is monitored and controlled because good glycaemic control reduces mortality rates in the critically ill.

Drug administration in patients with feeding tubes

The administration of medication to patients with feeding tubes can be challenging, and a number of issues need to be considered in parallel with the patient's medical problems. These issues include the following:

- The continued need for the patient's regular medicines and the consequences of medication withdrawal or administration delay, both medically and legally.
- The intention to tube feed and subsequent compliance of the patient to retain the tube.
- Institutional ability to site percutaneous tubes.
- Availability and appropriateness of different formulations of medication.

Formulation difficulties

Pharmacists will be involved in influencing the choice of medication formulation on the basis of their training and experience.

Is there a formulation available for use by a licensed route? Use alternative routes of administration, if appropriate (i.e. buccal, IM, IV, intraosseous, transdermal, topical, nebulized, rectal, SC, sublingual, etc.)

Pharmacists should also be able to calculate the cost implications of the different formulations and, importantly, should facilitate long-term choice, particularly if the parenteral route cannot be used in the long term.

- Is there a commercial oral solution, suspension, or soluble solid dose form?
- Oral liquid—dilute with 10–30mL sterile water or enteral formula if hyperosmolar.
- Oral immediate-release tablet—crush to fine powder and mix with 10–30mL water.
- Oral immediate-release capsule—open capsule and crush contents to fine powder. Mix with 10–30mL sterile water.
- Oral soft gelatin capsule (e.g. acetazolamide, nifedipine)—remove liquid contents with a needle and syringe. Then mix with 10–30mL of sterile water
- IV liquid preparation—draw dose into an amber oral syringe prior to administration
- Soluble tablets dissolved in 10mL of water are often the best option for tube-fed patients.
- Refer to specific manufacturer's advice for feed-tube administration.
- Remember to shake liquid preparations before administration.
- Viscous liquids might have to be diluted with water to ↓ tube blockage.
- Liquids with high osmolality or sorbitol content can lead to diarrhoea.
- Does the crushed tablet or capsule contents disperse fully or form a workable suspension that will not clog or block the feeding tube?
- Is the parenteral formulation of the product suitable for enteral use?
- Osmolality concerns for parenteral product.
- Additives in injections might make administration through a tube unsuitable.
- Is there a therapeutic substitute that can be administered via a tube?

Administration of medication through a tube

- Do not add medication directly to the feed.
- Only administer one medication at a time.
- Use an oral syringe if possible.
- Flush the tube with 50mL water immediately after stopping the feed.
- Add the volume of water used to fluid balance charts.
- Draw identified formulation into appropriate 50mL syringe.
- Attach the tube and apply gentle pressure.
- Flush with a minimum 15mL of water between different medicines.
- Flush with 50mL of water after the last medication.
- If drug is to be taken on an empty stomach, for gastric tubes, stop feed for 30min before the dose and resume feeding 30min afterwards. These measures are not relevant for jejunal tubes.
- Add the total volume of flushes and medicine to fluid balance chart.

Specific drug/tube feeding problems

Drug-specific issues

- Absorption could be unpredictable because the tube might be beyond the main site of absorption for the specific drug.
- Formulation issues of medication being administered through feeding tubes.
- Crushing destroys the formulation properties of tablets, altering peak and trough levels.
- Detrimental clinical effect for certain slow-release products (e.g. nifedipine LA), causing severe hypotension if inadvertently given crushed.

Adsorption onto feeding tubes

Examples are phenytoin, diazepam, and carbamazepine. Dilute with at least 50mL of water and flush the tube well.

Interactions causing blockage

Antacids and acidic formulations could cause precipitation because of an acid–base reaction.

Feed ↓ drug absorption

- Phenytoin—50–75% reduction in serum levels when given with enteral nutrition. Hold tube feeding for 2h before and after each dose as well as flushing the tube before and after each phenytoin dose.
- Fluoroquinolones (ciprofloxacin, levofloxacin, moxifloxacin)—give enterally via large-bore feeding tube. Crush tablets and mix with 20–30mL of water prior to administration. Hold tube feeding for 2h before and 4h after administration. Ciprofloxacin suspension should not be administered via the feeding tube. It has a thick consistency that may clog the tube, and since it is an oil-based suspension it does not mix well with water.
- Warfarin—reductions in absorption may occur because enteral feeding solutions may bind warfarin.

Drug–feed interactions
If vitamin K is in present in the feed it means that doses of warfarin might need to be amended (monitor INR).

Bioequivalence
Different formulations might necessitate adjustment of dose (e.g. phenytoin tablets and liquid).

Further reading

Beckwith MC, Feddema SS, Barton RG, *et al.* (2004). A guide to drug therapy in patients with enteral feeding tubes: dosage form selection and administration methods. *Hosp Pharm* 39: 225–37. ℘ http://www.bapen.org.uk

IV therapy at home

Patients who are medically stable but require prolonged courses of IV drugs (usually antimicrobials) can benefit from IV therapy at home. This is often referred to as Outpatient Parenteral Antimicrobial (or antibiotic) Therapy (OPAT), though the principles discussed in this section apply to any IV therapy given outside a secondary care setting. Suitable indications or therapies are as follows:

- Bone infections
- Endocarditis
- Cystic fibrosis
- Cytomegalovirus infection
- Total parenteral nutrition
- Immunoglobulins.

The advantages of treating these patients at home are as follows:

- Releases hospital beds for other patients.
- Reduces patient exposure to hospital-acquired infection.
- ↑ patient autonomy.
- Improved patient comfort and convenience.
- Some patients can to return to work or study while therapy continues.

Despite the potential benefits, IV therapy at home should not be undertaken lightly. All IV therapy is potentially hazardous and complications, such as line sepsis or blockage, are potentially more probable and risky in the community.

It is recommended that a multidisciplinary home IV team is set up to oversee the process and that guidelines are drawn up to ensure that home IV therapy is done safely and effectively.[1,2]

Home IV therapy team

The following people should be included in the team. They may not have hands-on involvement in every patient but should be available for advice and support:

- Clinician with an interest in home IV therapy (e.g. microbiologist, infectious diseases physician).
- Home IV therapy specialist nurse(s)/community liaison nurse(s).
- Antimicrobial/Infectious Diseases pharmacist.
- Community representative (GP or community nurse).
- For paediatric OPAT (p-OPAT) the doctor and nurse (at least) should have paediatric training.
- 24h access to key member(s) of the team (usually the specialist nurse and/or a clinician) is essential.
- For individual patients, the medical and nursing team responsible for the patient's care should liaise with the home IV team and be involved in assessment, discharge planning, and follow-up.

IV access

Venous access through short peripheral lines (Venflons®) is unsuitable for home delivery (unless for courses of only a few days) because it is designed for short-term use and should be replaced every 48–72h. Peripheral access

is also unsuitable for irritant or hyperosmolar infusions (e.g. TPN). Central venous access is preferred for the following reasons:
• It can remain in place for prolonged periods.
• It can be used for irritant or hyperosmolar infusions.
• It is easier for patients to self-administer through a central line.

Three types of central IV access are used for home IV therapy:
• *Central line* (e.g. Hickman® or Groshong®)—the line is inserted, usually through the subclavian vein, and is threaded through a sub-cutaneous tunnel to exit on the chest wall. The tip lies in the superior vena cava or just inside the right atrium. Central lines are inserted under general or local anaesthetic. In some hospitals specialist nurses insert central lines. Central lines might have one or more lumens, but for IV therapy at home a single lumen line is recommended to ↓ complications. These lines can remain in place for many months.
• *Port-A-Cath*®—a central venous access device, consisting of a small reservoir (the port) attached to a catheter. The port is implanted into the chest wall, with the catheter inserted into the subclavian or internal jugular vein. The reservoir is covered with a thick rubber septum, which is accessed through the skin using a special needle known as a Huber® needle. Port-A-Caths® are inserted under general anaesthetic. They can remain in place for years. Because of the cost and complexity of insertion, Port-A-Caths® are only suitable for patients who require prolonged or repeated IV therapy (e.g. cystic fibrosis patients).
• *Peripherally inserted central catheters (PICCs)*—these are fine flexible catheters inserted into the basilic or cephalic vein at the ante-cubital fossa, in a similar manner to peripheral venous access. Using a guidewire, the catheter is threaded up the axillary vein and into a central vein. PICC lines are inserted under local anaesthetic and are the least complex of the three types to insert. They can remain in place for several weeks or months. PICC lines are the least costly and complex and therefore are usually the preferred type of access.

To preserve the patency of central lines and avoid septic complications, guidelines should give advice on handling the line, including the following:
• Aseptic technique for drug administration.
• Flushing the line between doses.
• Use of heparinized saline to avoid clot formation within the line.
• Dressing and cleaning the insertion site.
• Care of the line when not in use.
• Procedure if the line is blocked or damaged.
• Procedure if there are signs of infection/cellulitis around the insertion site or signs/symptoms of sepsis.

Assessment and discharge planning

The home IV team should take responsibility for assessing whether the patient is suitable for IV therapy at home and for planning the discharge jointly with other nursing/medical staff caring for the patient. It is important that sufficient time is allowed to ensure that assessment, training, and general organization of the discharge are carried out adequately. Ideally patients should be referred to the OPAT team a minimum of 48h before discharge.

Patients should have the following characteristics:
- Medically stable.
- Not likely to misuse the line.
- Psychologically able to cope with IV therapy at home (patient and parents/carers).
- Willing to have IV therapy at home.
- Able to recognize problems and act accordingly.

The patient's home circumstances must also be taken into GP account:
- Is there another responsible adult who can support the patient and, if necessary, contact medical services themselves?
- Does the patient have a telephone?
- Are there reliable water and electricity supplies?
- Is there somewhere cool, dry, and safe to store drugs (out of reach of children)?
- Does the patient have a fridge, if needed, for drug storage (and do children have unsupervised access to this fridge)?
- Are there children or other people in the house who might be distressed by seeing drugs being administered IV?
- Does the patient have some means of transport to out-patient appointments?

Procedures for children receiving IV therapy at home are much the same as those for adults, but special attention must be paid to ensuring that home circumstances are suitable and that parents do not feel too pressured, especially if they are responsible for administering the drugs.

The OPAT management plan should be written in the patient's medical records (Table 23.16). A copy should be supplied to the GP, and patients should be provided with written information on the drugs, their administration, and their side effects, and given monitoring and emergency contact details.

Drug selection and administration

Drug selection primarily depends on the condition being treated. Ideally, drugs that are administered once daily should be used. In most UK schemes, IV infusions are avoided and wherever possible drugs are administered by slow IV push because this is a less complex and time-consuming method of drug administration. Where IV infusion cannot be avoided (e.g. vancomycin), the drug should be administered through a volumetric pump rather than a gravity drip. In some situations, it can be more appropriate to use an ambulatory infusion device such as an elastomeric pump (e.g. Homepump Eclipse®) or other system (e.g. Sidekick®), rather than a volumetric pump. Discussion of these devices is beyond the scope of this chapter.

Guidelines should give advice on drug administration. Issues that must be considered are as follows:
- Who will administer the drug—e.g. patient, parent/carer, community nurse?
- What training will they require?
- Who will do the training?

Many patients or their carers are capable of administering IV therapy provided that they receive suitable training and support. However, if therapy is only to continue for a week or less it is probably not worth the time taken to train a patient or carer. In some areas community nurses can administer the drugs, but they might also need additional training. Training is usually provided by a specialist nurse.

Training should include recognition of adverse effects and what action to take. This includes possible allergic or anaphylactic reactions.

It is recommended that the first dose of the drug is administered in a supervised setting so that the patient can be monitored for acute side effects. This can be in the patient's home if the drug is administered by a person competent and equipped to identify and manage anaphylaxis.

Guidelines should include procedures for disposal of clinical waste (e.g. used dressings), sharps, and empty vials. These should follow local practice—e.g. some areas might accept sharps boxes for disposal in the community, whereas others might require them to be returned to the hospital.

Community support

The patient's GP should be willing for the patient to go home with IV therapy. Even if they are not administering the drug, community nurses might be involved in other aspects of patient care and so should be kept informed. Good communication between the home IV therapy team and community healthcare workers is essential. Contact details for the hospital clinician and specialist home IV therapy nurse should be provided, including out-of-hours contact details.

Follow-up

Before discharge, follow-up arrangements should be planned. This should include the following:
- What to do if the patient has a significant ADR—who is responsible for managing this?
- Blood tests for monitoring ADR and TDM:
  - Who will take blood?
  - What tests are required?
  - Frequency.
  - How will the results be communicated and to whom?
  - Who will act on the results?
- The specialist home IV therapy nurse will usually be the main point of contact.
- The referring team should follow up the patient with respect to presenting indication, in addition to follow-up from the home IV therapy team.
- Duration of IV therapy is usually decided before discharge. It should be agreed which team is responsible for review of this and for provision of oral follow-on therapy.
- The home IV therapy team is usually responsible for line removal (as appropriate) at the end of the IV course.

The role of the pharmacist

The pharmacist is an important member of the home IV team. Their role includes the following responsibilities:

- Advice on drug stability and compatibility.
- Advice on drug administration, including infusion rates, and ambulatory infusion devices.
- Ensuring the supply of IV and ancillary drugs on discharge.
- Ensuring that follow-on oral therapy is prescribed.
- Provision of anaphylaxis kits if needed.
- Liaison with homecare companies.
- Supporting the training of patients, and community nurses.

The American Society of Health System Pharmacists has published guidelines on the pharmacist's role in home care which includes home IV therapy.[3] It should be borne in mind that these guidelines reflect the US system of healthcare and so some aspects might not be relevant to non-US pharmacists.

Drugs for home IV therapy at home fall into the 'hospital at home' category and, as such, all supplies should be supplied by the hospital either directly or through a homecare company. Thus community pharmacists are rarely involved in IV therapy at home. However, it is important that hospital pharmacists liaise with their community colleagues as appropriate—e.g. where oral follow-on therapy might be prescribed by the GP.

Homecare companies

A number of companies provide support services for home IV therapy. The service may range from supply of drugs and ancillaries direct to the patient's home to provision of the IV drug in an ambulatory infusion device to full nursing support. Pharmacists should ensure that they are familiar with the services being provided by the homecare companies used and that local procedures are complied with.

Outcome measures

It is good practice to record outcomes and to audit practice in OPAT. This might include THE FOLLOWING:

- Cure/partial cure rates.
- Treatment failure.
- Hospital admission/readmission due to medical deterioration or complications of OPAT.
- ADRs.
- OPAT complications such as line infection.
- Patient satisfaction questionnaires.

The British Society for Antimicrobial Chemotherapy (BSAC) has developed a toolkit for measuring outcomes and a national registry (⌂ www.e-OPAT.com).

References

1. Chapman A, Seaton RA, Cooper MA, et al. (2012). Good practice recommendations for outpatient antimicrobial therapy in adults in the UK: a consensus statement. J Antimicrob Chemother 67(5): 1053–62.
2. Patel S, Abrahamson E, Goldring S, et al. (2015). Good practice recommendations for paediatric outpatient parenteral antibiotic therapy (p-OPAT) in the UK: a consensus statement. J Antimicrob Chemother 70(2): 360–73.
3. American Society of Health System Pharmacists (2000). ASHP guidelines on the pharma-cist's role in home care. Am J Health Syst Pharm 57: 1252–7.

Therapy-related issues: musculoskeletal

Rheumatoid arthritis

Rheumatoid arthritis is an autoimmune disease which causes joints lined with synovium to become inflamed, swollen, stiff, and painful, leading to joint erosion. It is a multisystem disorder which can affect many organs including the eyes, lungs, heart, and blood vessels and is associated with significantly ↑ mortality. The aim of treatment is to ↓ pain and inflammation, prevent joint damage, and ultimately induce remission of disease.

Disease-modifying antirheumatic drugs (DMARDs) should be started early, ideally within 3 months of the start of persistent symptoms, to avoid joint damage. Symptomatic relief may be used until the DMARDs take effect, and as an adjunct. A multidisciplinary approach is essential.

Symptomatic relief

- Analgesics
- NSAIDs
- Corticosteroids—intra-articular (IA), intramuscular (IM), or oral
- Rest joints when they are actively inflamed
- Exercise to maintain muscle power
- Joint supports and aids provided by occupational therapists and physiotherapists

Disease-modifying antirheumatic drugs

See Table 24.1.
- Use a combination of at least two for significantly active disease, usually including methotrexate.
- If a single DMARD is used, ↑ the dose rapidly to a therapeutic level.
- When the disease is controlled, DMARDs can be cautiously reduced.
- May take up to 3 months for full therapeutic effect. Therefore short-term glucocorticoids may be required in this period (IA, IM, or oral).
- Monitoring is required (see Table 24.1).
- Live vaccines should be avoided but annual influenza and pneumococcus vaccines are recommended.
- Avoid exposure to chicken pox/shingles.

Biologic therapies

See Table 24.2.
The role of biologics in the treatment of rheumatoid arthritis is rapidly evolving. In England and Wales, NICE guidance advises that patients with persistent highly active RA (a Disease Activity Score-28 (DAS28)[1] score of >5.1) despite DMARD therapy are eligible to start biologics, and can continue if the DAS28 improves by ≥1.2.
- Biologics are associated with ↑ risk of serious infection and their use is contraindicated in patients with current sepsis.
- Screen patients for mycobacterial infections (e.g. CXR) before biologics are initiated—if necessary give TB prophylaxis.
- Can exacerbate heart failure—assess patients prior to initiation.

Table 24.1 Disease-modifying antirheumatic drugs (DMARDs)

DMARD	Dose	Other clinical information	Suggested monitoring regimen
Methotrexate	7.5–10mg weekly ↑ to 25mg weekly	Folic acid 5mg may be given 3–4 days after the methotrexate, ↑ as necessary, but avoiding the day of methotrexate. Patient information and shared care card should be given as per NPSA alert. NSAIDs may be continued with regular monitoring; however, over-the-counter NSAIDs should be avoided. May be changed to SC route for maximum bioavailability and improved tolerability The strength and form of methotrexate must be clearly stated	FBC, LFTs, U&Es, ESR, and CRP every 2wks for 3 months then monthly
Sulfasalazine	500mg daily ↑ by 500mg weekly to 1g twice a day. Maximum 3g daily	May colour urine orange and stain soft contact lenses yellow. May be used in pregnancy (up to 2g/day) and breastfeeding. Contraindicated in hypersensitivity to sulphonamides and aspirin. Enteric-coated tablets may improve tolerability	FBC, U&Es, LFTs, ESR, and CRP monthly for 3 months then 3-monthly
Hydroxychloroquine	200–400mg daily, maximum 6.5mg/kg	Patients should be advised to report any visual disturbances. May be continued in pregnancy	Regular blood monitoring is not required. Visual acuity should be monitored annually by an optometrist
Leflunomide	10–20mg daily, occasionally 30mg daily	Long elimination half-life. Teratogenic—♀ planning to have children should discontinue leflunomide for 2yrs or have colestyramine washout procedure. ♂ should stop leflunomide 3 months before trying to father a child	FBC, LFTs, U&Es, ESR, CRP, BP, and weight monthly for 6 months then 2-monthly
Azathioprine	1mg/kg/day for 4–6wks, ↑ to 2–3mg/kg/day	Thiopurine S-methyltransferase (TPMT) must be measured before starting azathioprine. If patient started on allopurinol reduce azathioprine dose to 25% of original dose	FBC, LFTs, U&Es, CRP, and ESR weekly for 6wks, fortnightly until stable then monthly

(Continued)

Table 24.1 (Contd.)

DMARD	Dose	Other clinical information	Suggested monitoring regimen
Ciclosporin	2.5mg/kg/day in 2 divided doses for 6wks. ↑ at 2–4wk intervals to maximum 4mg/kg/day	Bioavailability varies with formulation—prescribe by brand name. Reduce diclofenac dose by 50%, avoid colchicine, St John's wort and doses of simvastatin above 10mg	U&Es, FBC, ESR, CRP, BP, and urinalysis fortnightly for 3 months, then monthly. LFTs monthly. Lipids every 6 months
Mycophenolate	500mg daily ↑ by 500mg weekly to 1–2g daily. Maximum 3g daily	Used to treat systemic vasculitis and systemic lupus erythematosus. Antacids and magnesium supplements reduce mycophenolate absorption	FBC weekly for 6wks then monthly. LFTs, U&Es, ESR, and CRP monthly
Gold	10mg test dose. 50mg IM weekly until total of 1g then review	Given by deep IM injection. Patients should be observed for 30min after injection due to risk of anaphylaxis. Benefit not usually seen until cumulative dose of 500mg given. Stop if no response after 1g	FBC and urinalysis before each injection. CRP, ESR, and U&E at least 3-monthly
Penicillamine	125mg daily ↑ by 125mg every 4wks to 500mg daily in divided doses. Maximum 1g daily	Take on an empty stomach and avoid taking iron/zinc/indigestion remedies at the same time as penicillamine. Stop if no response after 3 months on the maximum dose	Urinalysis with blood tests every 2wks. FBC, U&Es, ESR, CRP, and LFT every 2wks until stable then monthly

Table 24.2 Biologic therapies

Biologic	Dose	Action	NICE approval
Infliximab	RA: 3mg/kg by IV infusion over 2h at 0, 2, and 6wks then every 8wks with methotrexate. Can ↑ in steps of 1.5mg/kg to 7.5mg/kg Use with methotrexate AS and PsA: 5mg/kg at 0, 2, and 6wks then every 6–8wks	TNF-α inhibitor	RA: for patients with inadequate response to 2 DMARDs including methotrexate Also for patients with severe active RA with inadequate response to or intolerance of other DMARDs including at least 1 anti-TNF and who have a contraindication to or intolerance of rituximab AS: not recommended PsA: when response to 2 DMARDs has been inadequate
Etanercept	RA: 25mg twice weekly or 50mg weekly SC in combination with methotrexate unless not tolerated or contraindicated AS and PA: 25mg twice weekly or 50mg weekly SC	TNF receptor fusion protein	RA: for patients with inadequate response to 2 DMARDs including methotrexate Also for patients with severe active RA with inadequate response to or intolerance of other DMARDs including at least 1 anti-TNF and who have a contraindication to or intolerance of rituximab or methotrexate AS: severe active AS when 2 NSAIDs have not been effective PsA: when response to 2 DMARDs has been inadequate
Adalimumab	RA: 40mg every 2wks SC with methotrexate unless not tolerated or contraindicated AS and PsA: 40mg every 2wks	TNF-α inhibitor	RA: for patients with inadequate response to 2 DMARDs including methotrexate Also for patients with severe active RA with inadequate response to or intolerance of other DMARDs including at least 1 anti-TNF and who have a contraindication to or intolerance of rituximab or methotrexate AS: severe active AS when 2 NSAIDs have not been effective PsA: when response to 2 DMARDs has been inadequate

(Continued)

Table 24.2 (Contd.)

Biologic	Dose	Action	NICE approval
Golimumab	RA and PsA: 50mg once a month with methotrexate AS: 50mg once a month	TNF-α inhibitor	RA: for patients with inadequate response to 2 DMARDs including methotrexate Also for patients with severe active RA with inadequate response to or intolerance of other DMARDs including at least 1 anti-TNF and who have a contraindication to or intolerance of rituximab AS: severe active AS when 2 NSAIDs have not been effective PsA: when response to 2 DMARDs has been inadequate
Rituximab	RA: 1g by IV infusion 30min after 100mg IV methylprednisolone. Followed by a further dose after 2wks. May be repeated after 6 months. In combination with methotrexate	Depletes B lymphocytes	Severe active RA and inadequate response or contraindication to other DMARDs including 1 or more tumour necrosis inhibitor
Certolizumab	RA and PsA: 400mg SC at 0, 2, and 4wks then 200mg every 2wks in combination with methotrexate unless not tolerated or contraindicated AS: 400mg SC at 0, 2, and 4wks then 200mg every 2wks	TNF-α inhibitor	RA: for patients with inadequate response to 2 DMARDs including methotrexate. The manufacturers provide the first 12wks treatment free of charge

Tocilizumab	RA: 8mg/kg (maximum 800mg) by IV infusion over 1h every 4wks Or 162mg SC weekly In combination with methotrexate unless not tolerated or contraindicated	Inhibits interleukin-6	RA: for patients with inadequate response to 2 DMARDs including methotrexate Also for patients with moderate or severe active RA that has responded inadequately to 1 or more anti-TNFs and whose RA has responded inadequately to rituximab or in whom rituximab is contraindicated or not tolerated
Abatacept	RA: <60kg 500mg; 60–100kg 750mg; >100kg 1000mg IV as a 30min infusion at 0, 2, and 4wks then every 4wks Or 125mg SC weekly In combination with methotrexate	Attenuates T-lymphocyte activation	RA: for patients with highly active disease who have tried methotrexate and another DMARD Also for patients with severe active RA with inadequate response to or intolerance of other DMARDs including at least 1 anti-TNF and who have a contraindication to or intolerance of rituximab or methotrexate
Anakinra	RA: 100mg daily SC	Inhibits interleukin-1	Not recommended

AS, ankylosing spondylitis; PsA, psoriatic arthritis; RA, rheumatoid arthritis.

- Caution is required in patients with demyelinating diseases as anti-TNF therapies have been associated with demyelinating syndromes in a few cases.
- Contact with chickenpox should be avoided.
- Before surgery, the benefit of stopping treatment to reduce the risk of infection, and improve would healing, should be balanced against the risk of a flare. If stopping, stop three to five times the half-life of the biologic before surgery, and restart once there is good wound healing and no evidence of infection.
- Patients starting biologics should be given an alert card and information leaflet, e.g. leaflets available at the Arthritis Research UK website.[2]

References

1. 'DAS-score' website, ℘ www.das-score.nl/das28/en
2. 'Arthritis Research UK' website, ℘ www.arthritisresearchuk.org

Ankylosing spondylitis

Ankylosing spondylitis is an inflammatory disease affecting the spine and causing back pain, stiffness, and joint fixation. The large peripheral joints can also be affected.

- Conventional treatment is with physiotherapy and NSAIDs including COX-2 inhibitors.
- Methotrexate and sulfasalazine are only used for peripheral joint disease.
- Adalimumab, etanercept, or golimumab are NICE approved for patients who have persistent active disease (Bath Ankylosing Spondylitis Disease Activity Index[3] ≥4 and/or spinal pain visual analogue scale ≥4) that has not responded to at least two NSAIDs (see ➔ Table 24.2, pp. 601–3).

Reference

3. 'Bath Ankylosing Spondylitis Disease Activity Index' website. ℞ www.basdai.com

Psoriatic arthritis

Psoriatic arthritis is a chronic inflammatory arthropathy of variable and unpredictable course associated with psoriasis of the skin or nails.

- NSAIDs and corticosteroid injections for symptomatic relief.
- Methotrexate, leflunomide, and sulfasalazine are the DMARDs of choice (only leflunomide is specifically licensed). Early introduction improves prognosis. The risks of hepatotoxicity are slightly greater than for the same drugs used in rheumatoid arthritis and monitoring is essential.
- Patients with poor response may be changed to alternative DMARDs (e.g. ciclosporin).
- Etanercept, adalimumab, golimumab, or infliximab may be used (in accordance with NICE guidelines) in patients with active and progressive psoriatic arthritis not responsive to adequate trials of at least two DMARDS either individually or in combination.
- Ointments, topical retinoids, UV light therapy for the psoriasis.

Further reading

'Arthritis Research UK' website. ℞ www.arthritisresearchuk.org
'National Institute for Health and Care Excellence' website. 'Musculoskeletal conditions' ℞ https://pathways.nice.org.uk/pathways/musculoskeletal-conditions

Osteoarthritis

Osteoarthritis is the most common form of joint disease in the UK, causing pain, stiffness, swelling, and crepitus.

Risk factors include:
- age—late 40s onwards
- gender—♀
- obesity
- previous joint injury
- occupation involving repetitive movements
- genetic factors.

Patients should receive information (oral and written) enabling them to be actively involved in designing a management plan including the following options:

Self-management

- Exercise, general aerobic and muscle strengthening, physiotherapists can advise
- Weight loss if obese
- Reducing strain on joints, e.g. joint supports, wearing low heeled shoes with shock-absorbing soles, using a walking stick, handrails, tap turners, pacing activities through the day
- Local heat or cold
- TENS.

Pharmacological management

- Paracetamol
- Topical NSAIDs
- Opioid analgesics if paracetamol and topical NSAIDs are insufficient
- Oral NSAIDs including COX-2 inhibitors if paracetamol and topical NSAIDs are insufficient. Consider patient risk factors and try to avoid if on aspirin. Add a PPI
- Capsaicin cream
- IA steroid injections for moderate to severe pain.

Joint replacement may also be discussed as a treatment option.

The following have not been shown to be effective and are not recommended by NICE:
- Glucosamine and chondroitin
- Rubefacients
- IA hyaluronic acid injections
- Acupuncture.

Further reading

'Arthritis Research UK' website, ℳ www.arthritisresearchuk.org
'NICE' website, ℳ www.nice.org.uk

Osteoporosis

Osteoporosis is a condition involving ↓ bone mass and weakening of the bone micro-architecture, leading to ↑ fragility and risk of fracture, most commonly of the spine, wrist, and hips.

Risk factors

- ↑ with age
- Gender—most common in postmenopausal ♀, especially when menopause was before age 45
- Previous fragility fracture as defined as a fall from standing height or less
- Treatment with oral corticosteroids
- History of falls
- Parental history of hip fracture
- BMI <19
- Excessive alcohol or smoking
- Lack of calcium or vitamin D
- Other conditions including rheumatoid arthritis, coeliac disease, hyperthyroidism, type 1 diabetes, chronic kidney disease, Crohn's disease
- Sedentary lifestyle.

In patients at risk of falls, efforts should be made to minimize risks.

Lifestyle factors

Encourage:
- a balanced diet, containing calcium and vitamin D
- BMI between 20 and 25
- regular weight-bearing exercise
- reduce alcohol intake to <3 units/day and stop smoking.

Treatments

Treatment algorithms (e.g. NICE Clinical Guideline 146, TA160/161), involve assessing risk factors and bone mineral density (BMD) and selecting treatment.

Calcium and vitamin D

Patients should have normal calcium and vitamin D levels before starting treatment for osteoporosis:
- 25-hydroxyvitamin D serum level:[3]
    - <30nmol/L is deficient
    - 30–50nmol/L is inadequate in some people
    - >50nmol/L is sufficient
- If rapid vitamin D level correction is necessary, the following regimens can be used:
    - Colecalciferol 50 000 units weekly for 6wks (unlicensed preparation)
    - Colecalciferol 20 000 units 2 weekly for 7wks (unlicensed preparation)
    - Colecalciferol 3200 units daily for 13wks.
    - Followed by a maintenance of 800–2000 units daily.

Dietary sources of calcium are preferred. The aim is 700–1200mg/day:
- Pint of milk = 700mg
- Small matchbox-size piece of cheese = 200mg
- Small pot of yoghurt = 200mg.

If dietary intake insufficient, supplements (e.g. Adcal®, Calceos®, Calcichew®) may be used. It should be noted that while studies have shown an association between calcium supplements and a small ↑ in cardiovascular disease, this remains controversial.

Bisphosphonates

Bisphosphonates are first-line treatment for osteoporosis, acting by inhibiting osteoclast bone resorption. Bisphosphonates should not be used in patients with impaired renal function (GFR <35mL/min).

Alendronic acid is usually first choice, and is licensed for the treatment of osteoporosis in postmenopausal ♀, osteoporosis in ♂ at risk of fragility fractures, and steroid-induced osteoporosis. Bisphosphonate counselling points:
- Swallow whole, do not chew or dissolve in the mouth due to risk of oesophageal ulceration
- Take with a full glass of water, at least 200mL on rising after an overnight fast
- Do not eat or take other medicines or drink (other than water) for 30min after taking
- Sit or stand upright for at least 30min after taking
- Ensure good oral hygiene to avoid osteonecrosis of the jaw
- There is a small risk of atypical fracture with long-term use, but this is outweighed by the benefits of fracture prevention. In patients on treatment for >12 months with a new-onset unexplained thigh pain, stop the treatment until an urgent X-ray of the entire femur is performed.

Risedronate may be better tolerated than alendronic acid and may be used second line. If oral bisphosphonates are not tolerated due to GI side effects, yearly zoledronic acid 5mg by IV infusion is an option for steroid-induced osteoporosis.

Oral bisphosphonates should be reviewed after 5yrs and zoledronic acid after 3yrs.

If gastric symptoms develop because of the oral bisphosphonate then switch and do not add in gastroprotection.

Strontium ranelate

Strontium is believed to rebalance bone turnover in favour of bone formation. It is restricted to patients with severe osteoporosis where other treatments are contraindicated or not tolerated, due to concern about cardiovascular side effects.[4] It should not be used in patients with:
- ischaemic heart disease
- peripheral arterial disease
- cerebrovascular disease
- uncontrolled hypertension

Risk factors for ischaemic heart disease should be reviewed annually.

Denosumab

Denosumab is a monoclonal antibody to receptor activator of nuclear factor κ-B (RANK) ligand. It is given as a 60mg SC injection twice a year. Under NICE guidance[5] denosumab may be used for primary prevention of osteoporotic fractures in postmenopausal ♀ who are unable to take bisphosphonates and have a defined combination of T-score (comparison of the patient's BMD to that of a healthy 30yr-old) and risk factors, and for secondary prevention in postmenopausal ♀ who cannot take oral bisphosphonates.

Raloxifene

Raloxifene is a selective oestrogen receptor modulator, given orally at 60mg daily. It may be used in ♀ at risk of spinal fractures who cannot take bisphosphonates.

Teriparatide

Teriparatide is the active fragment of endogenous parathyroid hormone. It is given as a 20-microgram SC injection daily for 2yrs. Due to its high cost, it is only recommended for secondary prevention of fragility fractures in postmenopausal ♀ when other treatments have been tried or are contraindicated and who have defined T-scores.

Further reading

Arthritis Research UK' website, ℘ www.arthritisresearchuk.org
'NICE' website, ℘ www.nice.org.uk

References

3. National Osteoporosis Society (2013). *Vitamin D and Bone Health: A Practical Clinical Guideline for Patient Management*. Bath: National Osteoporosis Society. ℘ https://nos.org.uk/for-health-professionals/tools-resources/
4. Medicines and Healthcare products Regulatory Agency (March 2014). Strontium ranelate: cardiovascular risk. *Drug Safety Update* 7(8). ℘ www.gov.uk/drug-safety-update/strontium-ranelate-cardiovascular-risk
5. NICE (2010). 'Denosumab for the prevention of osteoporotic fractures in postmenopausal women [TA 204]', ℘ www.nice.org.uk/guidance/ta204

Gout

Gout is a type of arthritis caused by uric acid crystal deposition in joints and soft tissues, resulting in intense pain of sudden onset, swelling, and inflammation. The base of the big toe is most commonly affected, but it can occur in any joint. Attacks typically last 3–10 days and are usually recurrent.

Treatment of an acute attack of gout

- NSAIDs at maximum dose for 1–2wks, unless contraindicated. For patients at ↑ risk of peptic ulceration gastroprotection can be added or a COX-2 inhibitor used (e.g. etoricoxib 120mg daily), provided there are no cardiovascular contraindications. Aspirin or salicylates at analgesic doses should not be used, due to reduced uric acid excretion, but low-dose aspirin may be continued.
- Colchicine may be used as an alternative or in addition to a NSAID. Give 500 micrograms (two–) three times a day until pain relief is achieved, a total dose of 6mg is reached, or side effects become limiting (commonly sickness and diarrhoea). Note interactions with ciclosporin and erythromycin.
- If NSAIDs are contraindicated or ineffective, or if gout is refractory, corticosteroids may be needed. IA corticosteroid injections may be useful. Systemic corticosteroids may be needed for polyarticular disease (e.g. prednisolone 10mg daily for 2wks or methylprednisolone acetate 80–120mg).
- Allopurinol and uricosurics should not be started during an acute attack or for 2–3wks after the attack has resolved; however, they should be continued in patients already taking them.
- Simple analgesics may be used in addition if necessary.
- Diuretics should be stopped if for hypertension. If an alternative antihypertensive is required, losartan should be considered as it has modest uricosuric effects. Diuretics for heart failure should be continued.

Lifestyle changes

- During an acute attack the joint should be rested. Ice packs and splinting may be of benefit.
- If obese, a weight reduction programme should be adopted, but high-protein, low-carbohydrate diets should be avoided. Once the acute attack has subsided, moderate exercise should be encouraged.
- Alcohol should be restricted to <14 units per week for ♂ and ♀, particularly avoiding beer and fortified wine.
- Foods with a high purine content such as red meat, offal, game, shellfish, and yeast extracts should be avoided.

Management of chronic or recurrent gout

- Allopurinol should be started at 50–100mg daily and ↑ by 100mg every 2–4wks until symptom control is achieved, serum urate of <360µmol/L, or a dose of 300–600mg daily in divided doses is reached, occasionally 900mg is necessary. Allopurinol lowers urate levels by inhibiting xanthine oxidase. It is metabolized principally to oxypurinol which has a half-life of 13–30h and can accumulate in renal impairment, therefore reduced dosing is required. Withdraw immediately if a rash develops. Note interactions with azathioprine, mercaptopurine, and coumarins.

- A uricosuric may be used in patients with normal renal function and no history of renal stones if allopurinol is not tolerated. Sulphinpyrazone 100–200mg daily may be used, ↑ over 2–3wks to 600mg daily. Probenecid 1–2g daily is available (in the UK) on a named-patient basis.

- Febuxostat is a selective inhibitor of xanthine oxidase which may be used in patients who are intolerant of allopurinol or for whom allopurinol is contraindicated. It is started at 80mg daily and may be ↑ to 120mg daily after 2–4wks if serum urate <360µmol/L.

- Colchicine 0.5mg twice a day or low-dose NSAIDs should be given at the same time as allopurinol to prevent an acute attack, and continued for 1 month after normal serum urate is achieved.

Further reading

'Arthritis Research UK' website, ✇ www.arthritisresearchuk.org

Jordan KM, Cameron JS, Snaith M, et al. (2007). British Society for Rheumatology and British Health Professionals in Rheumatology guidelines for the management of gout. *Rheumatology* 46(8): 1372–4. ✇ http://rheumatology.oxfordjournals.org/content/46/8/1372.full

'Summary of Product Characteristics', available for drugs at the European Medicines Agency website, ✇ www.ema.europa.eu/

Zhang W, Doherty M, Bardin T, et al. (2006). EULAR Evidence based recommendations for gout. Part II: Management. Report of a taskforce of the EULAR Standing Committee for International Clinical Studies Including Therapeutics (ESCISIT). *Ann Rheum Dis* 65(10): 1312–24.

Therapy-related issues: skin

Wound care

The skin is the largest organ of the body and has the primary function of protecting underlying tissues and organs. Breaching this barrier exposes the underlying tissues and organs to:

- mechanical damage
- dehydration
- microbial invasion
- temperature variations.

The ideal wound dressing replicates the skin's protective qualities, in addition to promoting wound healing.

Factors affecting the healing process

For a wound to heal the following factors are required:

- Moist environment, but not excessively wet
- Warmth
- Oxygen
- Nutrition
- (Relatively) Free from contamination with microbes or foreign bodies, including slough and necrotic tissue.

A wound dressing should provide all these factors.

Some patients experience delayed wound healing and can develop chronic wounds (e.g. leg ulcers) despite good wound care. This might be caused by patient-related factors which inhibit wound healing, and these must be addressed as far as possible (Box 25.1). When cleaning a wound it is important to note that sodium chloride 0.9% should be used in preference to antiseptic solutions.

Classification of wounds

Various wound classifications exist. For the purposes of wound care, the following descriptions are the most useful because they correspond to dressing choice. Note that some wounds may show more than one of the following features:

- Epithelializing or granulating—a clean red or pink wound, usually shallow with minimal exudates.
- Sloughy—yellow slough covers part or all of the wound. This might be a dry or wet wound. Note that visible bone or tendon appears yellow.
- Necrotic—dead tissue creates a black, dry, leathery eschar.
- Infected—yellow or greenish in colour, with possible surrounding cellulitis of unbroken skin. The wound might have an offensive smell.

Box 25.1 Patient factors that inhibit wound healing

- Poor perfusion (e.g. peripheral vascular disease)
- Older age (usually linked to poor nutrition or other disease)
- Concurrent disease (e.g. diabetes, cancer, or anaemia)
- Drugs (e.g. steroids, cytotoxics, or NSAIDs)
- Smoking
- Immobility.

- Exuding—all the features listed so far (except necrotic) might produce exudates to varying degrees. High levels of exudates can lead to maceration of surrounding skin.
- Cavity—the wound might form a deep or shallow cavity. Sinuses are narrow cavities which can extend to some depth, including tracking to bone or between two wounds.
- Malodorous—fungating tumours and infected and necrotic wounds can all have an offensive smell.

These classifications broadly represent the stages of wound healing. Thus, as the wound heals, the type of dressing appropriate to the wound can change. Slough and necrotic tissue are effectively foreign bodies that inhibit wound healing. After these have been removed, the underlying tissue should be granulating. Patients should be warned that as debridement occurs the wound might appear to become bigger before it starts to heal. Occasionally pain associated with the wound can ↑ as the wound heals, due to the healing of damaged nerve endings.

It is important to review wound care on a regular basis. Frequency of reviews (and dressing changes) depends on the severity and nature of the wound. An infected or highly exuding wound might require daily dressing changes, but a granulating wound might only require re-dressing every few days. It is important to avoid renewing a dressing unnecessarily because this can expose the wound to cooling, dehydration, or mechanical damage. It is good clinical practice to prepare a wound care chart (Table 25.1). This ensures that all staff are informed about the nature of the wound, which dressings are being used, and the frequency of dressing changes/review. Including photographs of the wound enables progress (or deterioration) to be monitored.

Selection of wound dressing

There is no universal wound dressing and different types of dressing suit different wounds. The ideal dressing satisfies all the requirements described in Box 25.2 according to the environment in which it is being used. Dressings are divided into the following two categories:

- Primary dressings—applied directly to the wound surface
- Secondary dressings—placed over the primary dressings to hold them in place and/or provide additional padding or protection.

It is less important for secondary dressings to satisfy the ideal requirements.

Table 25.1 Wound care plan

Patient's name: _____	Date: _____
Photograph/diagram (number each wound and use numbering scheme when describing wounds):	Description of wound(s)
Dressings (number, as above):	Frequency of dressing changes:
Other information (e.g. analgesia required with dressing changes):	
Review date: _____	
Signature: _____	

Box 25.2 Characteristics of the ideal wound dressing
- Maintain moist environment
- Manage excessive exudates
- Allow oxygenation
- Provide a barrier to micro-organisms
- Maintain a warm environment (~37°C)
- Not shed particles or fibres
- ↓ or eliminate odour
- Cost-effective
- Acceptable to the patient.

Each time a dressing is changed, it exposes the wound to contamination, dehydration, and cooling. Thus, ideally, the frequency of primary dressing changes should be kept to a minimum. Secondary dressings can be changed more frequently, without disturbing the primary dressing.

Wound care has advanced greatly since the introduction of 'interactive' dressings. These dressings provide active wound management, usually by interacting with the wound surface (e.g. alginates form a gel on contact with exudates) rather than simply acting as a barrier. Selection of the correct dressing is important both to ensure that the wound is healed as efficiently as possible and to ensure cost-effective use because interactive dressings are usually more expensive than non-interactive dressings (Table 25.2).

Use of topical antimicrobials

These agents are not usually recommended because of the risk of development of resistance and high incidence of local sensitivity reactions (which could ultimately lead to systemic allergic reactions). There is little evidence that topical antimicrobials work, and infection should be treated systemically.

The following preparations are recommended for particular situations:
- Povidone iodine preparations, as either impregnated dressings or solutions can be used on wounds infected with bacteria, fungi, or protozoa. These should be stopped as soon as the infection is under control as povidone iodine has been shown to inhibit wound healing.
- Silver, either as silver sulfadiazine cream or as silver-impregnated dressings, is active against Gram-negative infection (e.g. *Pseudomonas* infection in burns) and MRSA. These preparations are often used inappropriately for any 'infected' wound. Use should be restricted because they are expensive and excessive use of the cream can cause irreversible black skin staining (argyria) because of deposition of silver into the skin.
- Metronidazole gel is used to inhibit anaerobic bacteria which cause the malodour associated with fungating tumours or necrotic wounds. Liberal application of metronidazole suppresses bacterial growth and thus ↓ odour. The surrounding skin should be protected from the gel to avoid maceration. Excessive use could (theoretically) lead to the emergence of metronidazole resistance. Where metronidazole gel is unavailable (e.g. in developing countries), the tablets can be crushed to a fine powder and sprinkled over the wound or mixed with an aqueous gel (e.g. KY® jelly) before application.

Table 25.2 Matching the dressing to the wound

Dressing type	Examples	Suitable for	Comment
Alginate	ActivHeal® alginate Sorbsan® Sorbsan® Plus Kaltostat®	Exuding, sloughy Ribbon or rope—cavity or sinus	'Plus' versions have a highly absorbent backing, suitable for highly exuding wounds
Foams	ActivHeal® foam Lyofoam® Allevyn®	Exuding or highly exuding wounds	Avoid adhesive versions on fragile skin, Do not use for cushioning
Films and membranes	Opsite® Tegapore®	Shallow, granulating	
Hydrocolloid	ActivHeal® hydrocolloid Granuflex® Comfeel® Plus	Sloughy, light to medium exudates	Not suitable for infected wounds or if frequent dressing changes required Avoid on fragile skin
Hydrofibres	Aquacel®	Sloughy, medium to high exudates Ribbon—cavity or sinus	
Hydrogels	ActivHeal® hydrogel Intrasite® Granugel® Actiform Cool®	Dry, sloughy	Always requires secondary dressing Actiform Cool® is reported to reduce pain
Low-adherent	Atrauman® Melolin® Mepitel® NA® NA Ultra®	Dry, lightly exuding, granulating	Even 'non-adherent' versions can stick to wound, causing trauma on removal.
Odour-absorbing	Clinisorb® Carbopad® VC	Malodorous	Apply over primary dressings
Padding	Gamgee®	Highly exuding	Secondary dressing only
Paraffin gauze	Jelonet®	Granulating	

Other special wound care agents

Chlorinated desloughing agents

These agents are no longer recommended. Although effective for debriding sloughy wounds, they are potential irritants and can delay healing because of cell toxicity and ↓ capillary blood flow. With more modern desloughing dressings available, the disadvantages of these agents outweigh the benefits.

Sugar paste and honey dressings

These can be used on sloughy, infected, and/or malodorous wounds. The antibacterial effect of the sugar or honey ↓ odour. Bacterial growth is inhibited because of the ↑ osmotic pressure in the wound, and honey (especially manuka honey) has some inherent antimicrobial effect. These dressings debride sloughy wounds and can promote angiogenesis. Pharmaceutical quality honey should be used as it is prepared according to set standards and gamma irradiated to reduce the risk of bacterial contamination. Sugar pastes are made from preservative-free icing or caster sugar. Thin pastes can be used in wounds with small openings, using a syringe to dribble the paste into the wound, and thick pastes are used for larger cavity wounds. The disadvantage of these dressings is that they might require frequent changes—twice daily or more.

Vacuum-assisted closure (VAC)

VAC therapy is a form of wound care where negative pressure is applied to a special porous dressing which is placed in the wound cavity or over a flap or graft. VAC helps to remove excess exudates and mechanically draws the edges of the wound inwards, promoting healing. It is suitable for any chronic open wound or acute and traumatic surgical wounds, and is used in plastic surgery to promote healing of grafts and flaps. VAC therapy should not be used on infected wounds (including those involving osteomyelitis) unless these are being treated with systemic antimicrobials. VAC is unsuitable for fistulae, which connect with body cavities or organs, and malignant or necrotic wounds, and should be used with caution on bleeding wounds.

Larval (maggot) therapy

Larvae of the common greenbottle are used in the management of necrotic or sloughy wounds. To feed, the larvae produce proteolytic substances that degrade dead tissue but have no adverse effect on living tissue.

Larvae are supplied either in a gauze bag—various sizes contain different numbers of larvae—or loose. The former presentation is often more acceptable to patients (and HCPs) and can be used on cavity wounds, where it might be difficult to locate and retrieve free larvae.

Larvae should usually be used within 48h of receipt, otherwise they will die because of lack of nutrients, and will generally survive for 3–5 days feeding on the wound. During this time, they ↑ in size, and as long as they are still active and ↑ in size, they are still effective.

The gauze bag or individual larvae are applied directly to the wound and covered with a non-adherent dressing, which is soaked in saline to ensure that the larvae are kept moist (but not drowning!). A non-occlusive secondary dressing should be used to cover them to prevent them from drying out and to ensure that they have sufficient O_2 to survive. Most interactive dressings are unsuitable (and unnecessary) for use on a wound being treated with larvae, they may also be lethal to larvae by ↑ osmotic pressure or ↓ O_2 supply. During treatment, the amount of exudate can ↑ and appear greenish in colour, but this is normal. It might be necessary to protect surrounding healthy skin from maceration caused by ↑ exudates by applying a barrier film.

Further reading

'*World Wide Wounds*' website—a peer-reviewed online wound care journal, sponsored by industry but with a code of practice to limit bias, ℘ www.worldwidewounds.com

Eczema

Eczema is an inflammatory skin condition. It nearly always causes itching but its appearance can vary, depending on the site, cause, and severity, and whether it is acute or chronic. Signs can include dryness, scaling, erythema, oedema, weeping, crusting, papules, and vesicles. The terms eczema and dermatitis are interchangeable.

- There are a number of different types of eczema (Table 25.3), but the most common is atopic eczema which affects 15–20% of school children and 2–10% of adults.[1]
- Atopic eczema often affects the face and hands in infants, and the face, neck, wrist, and elbow and knee flexures in children.
- Discoid/nummular eczema affects the limbs with round coin-shaped lesions. This form can be intensely itchy and scratching may lead to secondary infections.
- Gravitational eczema affects the lower legs.
- Pompholyx eczema produces itchy blisters which can form on the fingers, palms, and soles.
- Seborrhoeic eczema often affects the scalp, face, back, presternal area, groin, and armpits. In babies this is commonly described as 'cradle cap'.
- Allergic contact dermatitis is usually caused by a delayed hyper-sensitivity reaction to an allergen, although it can be an immediate reaction. Nickel and latex are common causes, but it should be noted that some medicines and excipients can act as allergens (e.g. neomycin, benzocaine, chlorocresol).
- Irritant contact dermatitis is caused by substances that damage the skin—e.g. acids, alkalis, solvents, and detergents. Once the causative irritant or allergen has been identified, steps should be taken to try and avoid it, or if that is not possible to minimize the risk of exposure.
- Photodermatitis is caused by the interaction between light and chemicals absorbed by the skin. This reaction may be as a result of an allergy or it be due to toxic effects of a substance (e.g. tetracyclines, retinoids, chemotherapeutic agents, NSAIDs).

Table 25.3 Classification of eczema

Exogenous	Endogenous
Allergic contact dermatitis	Atopic
Irritant contact dermatitis	Discoid/nummular
Photodermatitis	Gravitational/stasis/venous
	Pompholyx
	Seborrhoeic

Emollients

- Emollients should be used to rehydrate the dry skin usually associated with eczema.
- Soap should be avoided as it dries the skin—use an emollient soap substitute instead. Emollient bath oils can be added to bath water to enhance rehydration and ensure that the whole skin is treated.
- Aqueous cream is suitable as a soap substitute, but not as an emollient.[2]
- Emollients are best applied when the skin is moist (i.e. after shower or bath).
- They should be applied liberally and as frequently as possible, ideally three to four times daily and more during relapses.
- They should be applied in the direction of hair growth by smoothing rather than rubbing in.
- Ointments are better for dry scaly skin, but are also more greasy and difficult to wash off.
- Creams are better for wet weeping eczema and can help with pruritus because of the cooling effect as the water evaporates.
- Ensure sufficient supplies of emollients—600g/wk for an adult and 250g/wk for a child. Don't underestimate the quantities that will be required! The BNF contains a useful guide of suitable quantities for prescribing.
- Numerous generic and proprietary brands are available. It is important to find one that the patient is happy with and confident using.
- Some emollients may contain sensitizers, such as lanolin, or preservatives which can cause allergies and further exacerbate the eczema.
- Use of emollients should be continued even after the eczema has cleared.

Corticosteroids

Topical corticosteroids are an effective treatment for eczema and are the first-line treatment for atopic eczema exacerbations.[3] If not used correctly, there is a significant risk that their use will be ineffective or will cause adverse effects. Poor adherence is a major cause of treatment failure in atopic eczema.[4] The risks can be minimized and adherence improved by the following:

- Tailoring potency to the severity of the eczema, using the least potent corticosteroid that effectively controls the disease.
- Explaining how and when to step treatment up or down, including the maximum period of time to treat a flare before potency should be stepped down or healthcare advice should be sought to review the eczema.
- Using weaker corticosteroids on the face, genitals, and flexures.
- Labelling topical corticosteroids with the potency class on the tubes when they are dispensed.[5]
- Treating secondary infections promptly. Oral treatment is often necessary. There is only limited evidence to support corticosteroid/anti-infective combination creams and ointments.
- Applying emollient first and then waiting for at least 30min until the emollient has been absorbed before applying the corticosteroid.
- Applying gently in the direction of hair growth.
- Counselling on using thinly, the fingertip unit, and how much to apply.
- Counselling on how long to apply, how often to apply (no more than twice daily), and where to apply.

- Counselling on adverse effects and what to do if they notice them, but also reassuring the patient or carer that adverse effects are rare when the treatment is used correctly.

The fingertip unit

- Some patients or their carers may be inclined to undertreat eczema because of fear of medication side effects. Others may overtreat to keep it away. In order to standardize the amount used, the fingertip unit has been devised. It is defined as the amount of cream or ointment that can be applied to the terminal phalanx of an adult index finger and is ~500mg. The fingertip unit should not be used for emollients, which should always be used liberally. Table 25.4 shows the number of fingertip units which should be used to cover various parts of an adult's body.[6] Table 25.5 shows the number of fingertip units which should be used to cover various parts of a child's body at different age ranges.[7]

Table 25.4 The fingertip unit and how to assess the quantity of topical agents needed to cover a given body surface area (BSA) in adults

Area to be treated	No. of fingertip units	Approximate BSA (%)
Scalp	3	6
Face and neck	2.5	5
One hand (front and back) including fingers	1	2
One entire arm including entire hand	4	8
Elbows (large plaque)	1	2
Both soles	1.5	3
One foot (dorsum and sole), including toes	1.5	3
One entire leg including entire foot	8	16
Buttocks	4	8
Knees (large plaque)	1	2
Trunk (anterior)	8	16
Trunk (posterior)	8	16
Genitalia	0.5	1

Table 25.5 The fingertip unit in children

Age	Face and neck	Arm and hand	Leg and foot	Trunk (front)	Trunk (back) including buttocks
3–6mo	1	1	1.5	1	1.5
1–2 yrs	1.5	1.5	2	2	3
3–5yrs	1.5	2	3	3	3.5
6–10yrs	2	2.5	4.5	3.5	5.5

Topical calcineurin inhibitors

Topical tacrolimus and pimecrolimus are licensed for treating atopic eczema only. Their use in the UK is restricted to second-line treatment after corticosteroids have failed or the risks of further adverse effects (e.g. irreversible skin atrophy) are unacceptable. They are not recommended for treating mild atopic eczema.[8] Patients or carers should be given the following advice:

- To use thinly, and how much to apply with reference to the fingertip unit.
- That it is common to get initial skin irritation at the site being treated (e.g. burning, itching, feeling of warmth), but this usually subsides.
- Emollients should not be used within 2h of applying tacrolimus.
- Excessive exposure to UV light should be avoided.
- The medication may cause intolerance to alcohol (flushing and skin irritation).

Other topical treatments

- Wet wraps are wet bandages applied to the areas affected by eczema. A dry bandage layer is put over the top. The eczema may have been pretreated with emollients and/or topical corticosteroids. Wet wraps cool the eczema, enhance the absorption of the corticosteroid, and act as a barrier to scratching.
- Bandages containing ichthammol (to reduce itching), zinc oxide, or coal tar are used to treat lichenification.
- Ketoconazole shampoo and coal tar shampoos are effective treatments for seborrhoeic eczema.
- Potassium permanganate 0.1% solution can be used to treat eczema when it is weeping and wet. Care must be taken because it stains skin, clothes, and baths. It is important to prevent over-drying of the skin, therefore stop treatment when the exudation stops and only use on weeping areas not on normal skin.

References

1. Primary Care Dermatology Society and British Association of Dermatologists (2009). Guidelines for the Management of Atopic Eczema. ℘ www.nice.org.uk/guidance/ta81/resources/primary-care-dermatology-society2
2. Tsang M, Guy RH (2010). Effect of aqueous cream on human stratum corneum in vivo. *Br J Dermatol* 163: 954–8.
3. NICE (2004). 'Frequency of application of topical corticosteroids for atopic eczema (TA81)'. ℘ www.nice.org.uk/guidance/ta81
4. Beattie PE, Lewis-Jones MS (2003). Parental knowledge of topical therapies in the treatment of childhood atopic dermatitis. *Clin Exp Dermatol* 28: 549–53.
5. NICE (2007). 'Atopic eczema in under 12s: diagnosis and management (CG57)'. ℘ www.nice.org.uk/guidance/cg57
6. MeReC (1999). Using topical corticosteroids in general practice. *MeReC Bull* 10: 21–4.
7. Menter A, Korman NJ, Elmets CA, et al. (2009). Guidelines of care for the management of psoriasis and psoriatic arthritis. Section 3: Guidelines of care for the management and treatment of psoriasis with topical therapies. *J Am Acad Dermatol* 60: 643–59.
8. NICE (2007). 'Tacrolimus and pimecrolimus for atopic eczema (TA82)'. ℘ www.nice.org.uk/guidance/ta82

Psoriasis

Psoriasis is a chronic inflammatory skin disease characterized by raised erythematous scaly plaques, patches, or papules. The vast majority of cases are managed in primary care or the dermatology out-patient setting. It is relatively common, with a prevalence of 1.3–2.2% in the UK population, most commonly in adults before the age of 35yrs. Plaque psoriasis is the most common type of psoriasis (~90% of cases)

It is not known why psoriasis develops but there is a strong genetic component. A number of factors are known to trigger or exacerbate it, including drugs, so it is essential to establish a full and accurate drug history. Drugs recognized to worsen psoriasis or precipitate a relapse include:
- lithium
- chloroquine/hydroxychloroquine
- β-blockers
- ACE inhibitors
- terbinafine
- mepacrine
- bupropion
- ethanol
- NSAIDs.

There is no known cure for psoriasis; treatments are aimed at suppressing symptoms and inducing remission. Some treatments may be relatively safe but unpleasant or inconvenient to use. Other treatments, although well tolerated, have risks of severe toxicity to the liver, bone marrow, kidney, or unborn fetus, and may even ↑ the risk of malignancy. Thus it is essential to tailor treatment to each individual patient based on their age, sex, occupation, personality, general health, and resources, and their perception and understanding of the disease. The success of treatment depends on patient concordance, and all patients need to be carefully counselled on their treatment to ensure adherence. A list of the treatment options available is shown in Table 25.6.

Table 25.6 Treatment options for psoriasis

Topical therapies	Systemic therapies
Emollients	Psoralen + UVA radiation
Coal tar	Acitretin
Salicylic acid	Methotrexate
Dithranol	Ciclosporin
Corticosteroids	Biological agents
Vitamin D analogues	
Tazarotene	
UVB radiation	

Assessment of severity

This is usually determined by severity of symptoms and the percentage BSA covered by erythema, induration, and scaling in four main areas (head, arms, trunk, and legs).

There are also two assessment tools which can be used:
- PASI—Psoriasis Area and Severity Index
- DLQI—Dermatology Life Quality Index.

These tools have been validated in adult patients and also take into account the psychological impact of the disease. Patients with psoriasis may have low self-esteem, not necessarily related to the extent of the skin involvement. They may be limited in what they are able to do due to plaques on their hands and feet. Optimization of therapy and emotional support will be required, in differing degrees, for all patients.

Lifestyle recommendations

The following may affect symptoms of psoriasis and support or counselling may be provided in the appropriate area:
- Smoking cessation
- Alcohol moderation
- Weight management (including reducing high lipid levels).

Patients with psoriasis have an ↑ risk of cardiovascular co-morbidities, therefore the listed recommendations will further ↓ the patient risks.

Emollients

- Emollients have a beneficial effect in psoriasis. They help to re-establish the lipid layer and enhance rehydration of the epidermis.
- They are particularly useful in inflammatory psoriasis and palmoplantar plaque psoriasis.
- Apply liberally and frequently to soften and reduce scaling.

See ➲ 'Emollients' in 'Eczema', p. 620, for counselling points.

Coal tar

- This has been an effective treatment for inducing remissions in psoriasis for many years.
- Smelly, messy, and stains skin and clothing.
- Difficult to apply, resulting in reduced adherence.
- It is available as creams, shampoos, and paste bandages. Tar-based shampoos are the first-line treatment for scalp psoriasis.
- There is no evidence that using strengths of coal tar >5% is any more effective There is no firm epidemiological evidence to confirm worries surrounding links of topical cold tar and cutaneous/internal cancers.
- Crude coal tar is the most effective but this usually requires hospital admission.
- Can be used in combination with:
  - UVB radiation
  - steroid use during day and coal tar at night.

Salicylic acid

- A topical keratolytic agent.
- Used for hyperkeratotic psoriasis of the palms, soles, and scalp where penetration of other topical agents will be prevented by significant scaling leading to treatment failure.

Dithranol

- A very effective treatment for chronic plaque psoriasis.
- Like coal tar, its use has declined in recent years because of the widespread availability of more cosmetically acceptable treatments.
- Burns normal skin and is oxidized to a dye which stains skin and anything else it comes into contact with (e.g. hair, clothes, bed linen, and bathroom fittings).
- Wear disposable gloves and wash hands with cold water and soap.

Topical corticosteroids

- Effective treatment for some forms of psoriasis.
- Non-irritant compared with coal tar and dithranol.
- Clean and easy to use.
- Limited by adverse effects which include causing rebound exacerbation of psoriasis on discontinuation and precipitating unstable forms of psoriasis.
- Long-term use can also cause tachyphylaxis.
- Rarely used for widespread chronic plaque psoriasis, but reserved for delicate areas, such as the face, genitals, and flexures, or more resistant areas such as the scalp, palms, and soles.
- Use on the face, genitals, and flexures should be limited to mild potency topical corticosteroids—e.g. hydrocortisone 1%.
- Potent topical corticosteroids can be used initially on the scalp, palms, and soles, with the strength adjusted according to clinical improvement.

The NICE guideline on psoriasis includes following recommendations concerning the use of topical corticosteroids in psoriasis:

- No more than 100g moderate or higher potency preparations should be applied per month.
- Patients should be counselled on the use of the fingertip unit to ensure that they know how much ointment or cream to apply (see ➲ 'The fingertip unit', p. 621).
- Attempts should be made to rotate topical corticosteroids with alternative non-corticosteroid preparations.
- Use of potent or very potent preparations should be under dermatological supervision.
- Very potent steroids should not be used regularly for >4wks, and potent steroid for no >8wks at a time on any one site.
- Consider 4wk breaks between courses of potent or very potent corticosteroids.

Systemic corticosteroids are generally only used for erythrodermic psoriasis.

Vitamin D and its analogues
- Calcipotriol, a vitamin D analogue, is the first-line treatment for plaque psoriasis.
- Easy to apply.
- Does not smell or stain.
- Lacks many of the adverse effects of topical corticosteroids.
- Calcipotriol can irritate the skin, particularly in sensitive areas such as the scalp, face, and flexures, but this rarely leads to withdrawal of treatment.
- Calcitriol and the topical vitamin D analogue tacalcitol are both less irritant than calcipotriol.
- Avoid vitamin D and its analogues in patients with calcium metabolism disorders.
- Do not exceed maximum doses cited in the *BNF*. If the patient uses over the recommended dose, systemic absorption may occur leading to hypercalcaemia.

Tazarotene
- A topical retinoid.
- Effective treatment for mild to moderate plaque psoriasis involving up to 10% BSA.
- Local irritation is common, necessitating careful application, avoidance of normal skin, and titration of gel strength.
- Often used in alternation with a topical corticosteroid.
- Patients need counselling on washing hands after use, avoiding contact with sensitive areas, avoiding excessive exposure to UV radiation, and not applying cosmetics or emollients within 1h of application.

Ultraviolet B radiation
- An effective treatment of guttate psoriasis or plaque psoriasis that is unresponsive to topical treatment.
- Broadband UVB is less effective than narrowband (311 ± 2nm) therapy.
- Treatment is usually three times weekly, and 10–30 doses are required to achieve clearance.
- Dosage can be based on the minimal erythema dose or skin type.
- Used alone or combined with other treatments (e.g. tar, dithranol, calcipotriol, and oral retinoids) to enhance their effect.
- ↑ risk of cutaneous malignancies.

Ultraviolet A radiation and psoralen
- Topical or systemic administration of a psoralen followed by exposure to ultraviolet A radiation (PUVA) is an effective treatment for most forms of psoriasis and is used in some centres.
- There is no licensed psoralen available in the UK.
- ↑ risk of cutaneous malignancies.
- It can be combined with acitretin (not routine) or calcipotriol.

Patients receiving UVB or PUVA treatment should not be prescribed photosensitizing agents such as:

- amiodarone
- chlorpromazine
- nalidixic acid
- ofloxacin
- tacrolimus
- tetracyclines
- voriconazole.

Acitretin

- An oral retinoid which normalizes the epidermal cell proliferation in psoriasis
- Least effective of the systemic therapies when used alone, but it also lacks many of their toxicities.
- Titrate dose up to a target of 25mg (minimize mucocutaneous side effects).
- Often used in combination with topical therapies or PUVA.
- The effects of acitretin are ↑ by UV lights, therefore patients should be counselled on the risk of excessive sunlight and sunlamp exposure.
- Commonly causes drying of the skin and lips, which can be countered with regular use of emollient and lip salve.
- Less frequently, it also dries the mucous membranes and conjunctiva.
- Stringent controls are in place when acitretin is used in ♀ patients of child-bearing age because of its teratogenicity which can continue for up to 2yrs after cessation of treatment.

Methotrexate

- An effective treatment for severe psoriasis which cannot be controlled with topical therapies alone.
- Most patients are managed adequately with 7.5–15mg methotrexate weekly. Maximum of 25mg a week.
- The PASI and DLQI scores can be used to assess response.
- Can cause haematological, renal, and liver toxicity, which necessitates careful counselling of the patient on adverse effects and frequent monitoring of blood tests.
- Contraindicated in pregnancy.
- ♂ should be advised to avoid fathering children during therapy and for 3 months afterwards.
- Pharmacists screening prescriptions for methotrexate should ensure that they comply with local or national guidelines.

Ciclosporin

- Licensed in the UK for severe psoriasis when conventional therapy is ineffective or inappropriate.
- Efficacy has been fully demonstrated.
- Dose used is 2.5–3mg/kg/day. Up to a maximum of 5mg/kg/day after 4wks.
- The PASI and DLQI scores can be used to assess response.
- BP and renal function should be monitored during treatment.

Cytokine modulators

- Biological agents must only be initiated and supervised by specialist doctors.
- Adalimumab, etanercept, infliximab, and ustekinumab are all licensed and approved in the UK by NICE for the treatment of severe plaque psoriasis which has failed to respond to standard systemic treatments.
- To determine whether the patient is eligible for biological therapy the PASI and DLQI scores are used to assess severity. These scores are used by NICE and the British Association of Dermatologists to assess response to treatment also.
- No biologic is recommended over another. Consideration should be made for:
  - age of patient
  - nature of disease, severity, and impact
  - conception plans
  - co-morbidities
  - patient views
  - presence of psoriatic arthritis
  - cost.
- If a patient does not respond to one biologic then another can be tried after a washout period (usually four half-lives). This wash out time can be difficult for patients.
- Pharmacists have an important role to play in all patients on systemic immunosuppressants by:
  - counselling
  - monitoring
  - identifying important drug interactions
  - preventing prescribing errors and inappropriate prescribing
  - ensuring treatment duplication does not occur, e.g. patient with co-morbidities receiving biologic agents from two sources.

Further reading

British Association of Dermatologists. 'Psoriasis' (includes PASI and DLQI tools), ℳ www.bad.org.uk/healthcare-professionals/psoriasis

NICE (2012). 'Psoriasis: assessment and management (CG153)', ℳ www.nice.org.uk/guidance/cg153

Therapy-related issues: palliative care

Anorexia and cachexia

The dictionary definition of anorexia is a lack of appetite (for food). Cachexia is involuntary weight loss which can progress to an emaciated state. The majority of palliative care patients experience cachexia at some stage, and this difficult condition requires determination of the cause, if possible, and development of careful management. A number of Cochrane reviews have been published which summarize a fairly large volume of literature. The following interventions may be considered:

• Megestrol—evidence for effectiveness in stimulating appetite at doses ranging from 160 to 1600mg daily
• Medroxyprogesterone acetate—evidence of greater weight gain and appetite than placebo at doses of 300—800mg daily
• Corticosteroids—some evidence for short-term improvement in appetite but not weight gain
• Eicosapentaenoic acid found in oily fish—somewhat heterogeneous literature with an unclear picture for benefit. Possibly worth trying if other treatments fail.

These interventions are not without their own risks which need to be considered.

Constipation

Constipation is a common symptom in palliative care patients. It is related to opioid analgesic use, reduced food intake, and reduced activity. A patient diary can be helpful in determining the severity of the condition.

There is a lack of good-quality evidence for the effectiveness of laxatives, so a pragmatic approach is required. In general, it is necessary to combine an ↑ in fibre and fluid which is often not possible in this patient group. A pharmacological approach is therefore necessary with a stool softener and probably a stimulant in order to maintain good bowel function. Choices can be based on local formularies. Rectal laxatives may be necessary for hard impacted faeces. This is not a pleasant option for either patient or care staff, but may be the only option for some cases.

Peripheral opioid receptor antagonists are licensed for use in the UK, e.g. methylnaltrexone administered by injection. The licence is for opioid constipation in palliative care patients where other laxatives have failed. Methylnaltrexone is added to other laxative treatment. Doses should be reduced in renal failure. It is an expensive option with a 50% success rate which has still to find its place in palliative medicine.

Other drugs such as alvimopan are under development and may prove useful. A Cochrane review of these agents suggested that there is currently insufficient evidence for the use of naloxone or nalbuphine.

Fatigue

- Fatigue is among the most common symptoms in palliative care patients. It is not easily defined, but is commonly described by words such as lethargy, muscle weakness, tiredness, and mood disturbance.
- A number of assessment tools exist and these are useful to monitor both decline and improvement.
- A number of Cochrane reviews and other systematic reviews show benefit from a range of interventions. These include cognitive behavioural therapy, erythropoietin and similar agents, and exercise.
- A systematic review has shown that Chinese herbal medicine is not effective.
- Patients who are able to undertake therapeutic exercise regimens may find these to be helpful.

Hypercalcaemia of malignancy

- This is a common complication, especially in breast and lung cancer and in myeloma, and often occurs with bone metastases.
- Mild hypercalcaemia—corrected serum calcium 2.7–3.0mmol/L.
- Moderate to severe hypercalcaemia—corrected calcium ≥3.0mmol/L.
- Corrected calcium = measured calcium + (0.022 × (40 − albumin g/L)).

Signs and symptoms

- Nausea
- Vomiting
- Thirst
- Polyuria
- Constipation
- Headache
- Impaired consciousness.

The patient may be severely dehydrated and in renal failure.

Management

- Mild, asymptomatic—rehydrate and observation. Recheck calcium after 24h.
- Symptomatic—ensure hydration. Treat with bisphosphonates.
- Moderate to severe—urgent rehydration up to 3–6L in 24h and bisphosphonates.
- Stop any drugs that ↑ calcium levels—e.g. thiazide diuretics, lithium, calcium, and vitamin D supplements.[1]

Bisphosphonates inhibit osteoclastic bone resorption. A significant ↓ in serum calcium is generally observed 24–48h after IV administration and normalization is usually achieved within 3–7 days. If the patient is not normocalcaemic within this time a further dose can be given. Pamidronate should be infused at a concentration ≤60mg/250mL and a rate ≤60mg/h. Renal failure is a relative contraindication to the use of bisphosphonates and the dose should be administered at ≤20mg/h. The patient may be maintained on 4-weekly infusions or to prevent further skeletal events in patients with bone metastases from Ca breast consider ibandronic acid 50mg PO once daily. Oral bisphosphonates need to be taken after an overnight fast and no food for a further 30min, with a full glass of plain tap water with the patient in an upright position to maximize absorption and minimize gastro-oesophageal side effects.

Resistant hypercalcaemia not responding to pamidronate or recurring frequently can be treated with zoledronic acid 4mg IV depending on renal function. With repeated use of bisphosphonates, be aware of the rare possibility of osteonecrosis of the jaw.

In severe hypercalcaemia or with severe symptoms, calcitonin rapidly lowers serum calcium within hours, but the effect only lasts for hours and wears off altogether after a few days. Calcitonin 4–8IU/kg SC or IM every 6–12h for 2 days can be given along with bisphosphonate.

Denosumab is a human monoclonal IgG2 antibody which is now licensed to prevent skeletal events in adults with bone metastases from solid tumours. Supplementation may be needed for calcium and vitamin D levels unless hypercalcaemia is present. Be aware of local guidelines for this product due to its high cost and specificity.

Reference

1. Twycross R (2011). *Palliative Care Formulary* (4th edn). Nottingham: Palliativedrugs.com Ltd. ↪ www.palliativedrugs.com

Mouth care

Patients find mouth problems very distressing, and careful attention should be paid to dental hygiene and risk factors for dry mouth. Encourage regular mouth care to moisten and keep the mouth clean, e.g. four times daily on drug chart.

Dry mouth

- Check for candidiasis.
- Ice-chips, fresh pineapple, sugar-free gum. Rinse with 0.9% saline.
- Artificial saliva and topical saliva stimulants, preferably with neutral pH.
- Review medicines as some (e.g. hyoscine and tricyclic antidepressants) exacerbate dry mouth.

Sore mouth

- Candidiasis—fluconazole 50mg orally once daily or nystatin 100 000IU four times daily for 7 days.
- Soak dentures overnight and ensure that they are thoroughly cleaned.
- A coated tongue can be cleaned by allowing a quarter of a 1g effervescent ascorbic acid tablet to dissolve on the tongue up to four times daily for a week.
- Mucositis—chlorhexidine or benzydamine mouthwashes.
- Stomatitis—choline salicylate gel or beclomethasone soluble 500-microgram tablets dissolved in 20mL water and used as a mouthwash four times daily.
- Systemic analgesia may be needed if severe. Morphine sulfate solution 10mg/5mL can cause stinging though due to its alcohol content. Paracetamol soluble tablets may be useful.

Noisy breathing

Noisy breathing (sometimes called death rattle) occurs in significant numbers of people who are dying. The cause of noisy breathing remains unproven, but it is presumed to be due to an accumulation of secretions in the airways. It is managed either physically (repositioning and clearing the upper airways of fluid with a mechanical sucker) or pharmacologically. There are a number of treatment options (mainly anticholinergic drugs with some trials of atropine, hyoscine butylbromide, hyoscine hydrobromide, and glycopyrronium) but studies have found no difference in efficacy between these. A Cochrane review was unable to demonstrate any real effectiveness, and these options remain time-honoured rather than evidence-based treatments. Often repositioning of the patient to encourage drainage and explanation to the relatives is preferable to pharmacological management.

Insomnia

Insomnia is a common problem in palliative care. Daytime sleepiness can lead to night-time wakefulness therefore so-called sleep hygiene is an important consideration. A sleep log may be useful to assess how much sleep is actually achieved. There are many contributing factors to insomnia including anxiety, pain, medications, or limb movements. Pharmacists can help by reviewing those medicines that can induce sleep during the day-time (e.g. tricyclic antidepressants for neuropathic pain) and shifting the dose to later in the day. Ensure adequate pain relief is provided at night and any other contributory factors such as depression or delirium have been addressed. Discourage the use of stimulants including caffeine in the evening. If a pharmacological approach is decided upon, then use a benzodiazepine or a hypnotic with a short half-life but beware of the ↑ risk of falls in some patients.

Spinal cord compression

This is a complication of advanced cancer with tumour mass or bone compressing the dural sac and contents. This is a poor prognostic sign, with average survival of 4–6 months. 90% of patients present with back pain and 50% also have some neurological deficit—usually leg weakness with possible bowel or bladder involvement. Investigate with MRI of the whole spine or CT. Speed is of the essence to preserve mobility if the patient is ambulant at diagnosis.

Management

- Don't wait for confirmation, dexamethasone 16mg stat, then 8mg twice daily to reduce pain and spinal oedema. First 48h are crucial for the majority of clinical benefit. Taper steroids as appropriate thereafter.
- Radiotherapy within 24h if possible.
- Surgery if single site and patient has good performance status.

Malignant bowel obstruction

This is a complex problem which occurs mainly in patients with advanced gynaecological and GI cancers. The condition can range from a partial to a complete obstruction. Symptoms can include nausea and vomiting as well as abdominal distension and pain. In complete obstruction no faeces or flatus are passed. Surgery is usually the first option, but many patients may not be fit for such an intervention and other interventions such as stents may be tried.

Drug therapy includes antiemetics, usually parenteral metoclopramide or cyclizine if colic presents, anticholinergics such as hyoscine butylbromide, or other drugs to reduce the persistent nausea that can accompany this condition.

Other interventions include the use of octreotide which may prevent damage to the intestine such as oedema or necrosis and may improve intestinal transit. The beneficial effects seem to be seen in the early stages of obstruction.

Laxatives if appropriate such as docusate or glycerin suppositories may be useful as might a venting gastrostomy, e.g. Ryles tube to drain the built-up secretions and relieve the pressure of a distended abdomen.

Syringe drivers and compatibility of medicines

The syringe driver is a simple and cost-effective method of delivering a continuous subcutaneous infusion (CSCI), which can be used to maintain symptom control in patients who are no longer able to take oral medication because of persistent nausea and vomiting, dysphagia, or bowel obstruction, or are in end-of-life care. Commonly used medicines in syringe drivers are opioid analgesics, antiemetics, antisecretories, and anxiolytics. In addition to the CSCI, each of the medicines should be prescribed PRN for breakthrough symptoms and used to calculate the doses for the next driver. The prescription should be reviewed every 24h. Literature sources for compatible combinations of medicines are limited and the following is a guide for combinations known to be compatible when made up to 21mL with water for injection over 24h.

Two-medicine combinations

Up to *50mg morphine sulfate* may be combined with *one* of the following medicines:
- Cyclizine up to a maximum dose of 150mg
- Haloperidol up to a maximum dose of 10mg
- Metoclopramide up to a maximum dose of 75mg
- Midazolam up to a maximum dose of 30mg
- Hyoscine butylbromide up to a maximum dose of 120mg.

Three-medicine combinations

Up to *30mg of morphine sulfate* may be combined with the following medicines:
- Cyclizine (up to150mg) and haloperidol (up to 2.5mg)
- Cyclizine (up to 150mg) and midazolam (up to 20mg)
- Midazolam (up to 30mg) and metoclopramide (up to 40mg)
- Midazolam (up to 30mg) and haloperidol (up to 5mg)
- Midazolam (up to 30mg) and hyoscine butylbromide (up to 80mg)
- Haloperidol (up to 5mg) and hyoscine butylbromide (up to 80mg).

Any other combinations or diluents should be confirmed against the references in the ➔ 'Further reading' listing in this section or referred for specialist advice.

Further reading

American Society of Health-System Pharmacists (2016). *Handbook on Injectable Drugs* (19th edn). Bethesda, MD: American Society of Health-System Pharmacists.

Dickman A, Schneider J (2016). *The Syringe Driver: Continuous Subcutaneous Infusions in Palliative Care* (4th edn). Oxford: Oxford University Press.

End-of-life care

'One Chance to Get it Right' has been produced by the Leadership Alliance for the Care of Dying People.[2] It determines core principles of good care to enable a high standard of care for dying patients and to meet the needs of their family/carers.

The five 'Priorities for Care' are:

- The possibility that a person may die within the coming days and hours is recognized and communicated clearly, decisions about care are made in accordance with the person's needs and wishes, and these are reviewed and revised regularly.
- Sensitive communication takes place between staff and the person who is dying and those important to them.
- The dying person, and those identified as important to them, are involved in decisions about treatment and care.
- The people important to the dying person are listened to and their needs are respected.
- Care is tailored to the individual and delivered with compassion—with an individual care plan in place.

Follow local guidance for prescribing in the dying patient to manage their symptoms. Often this will mean formulating the required medicines for delivery in a syringe driver via the SC route.

If the patient does not require regular medication at this stage then ensure a range of anticipatory injectable medicines via the SC route are prescribed. If the patient is dying at home then having a small supply of these medicines already in the home will save time and anxiety for the GP or district nurse to administer as the symptoms present.

Reference

2. Leadership Alliance for the Care of Dying People (2014). *One Chance to Get it Right*. London: NHS England. ℘ www.gov.uk/government/uploads/system/uploads/attachment_data/file/323188/One_chance_to_get_it_right.pdf

Anaemia

Anaemia is a ↓ in red blood cells (RBCs), haematocrit, or haemoglobin (Hb) because of:
- blood loss—e.g. GI bleed
- deficient RBC production (erythropoiesis)—e.g. iron deficiency, vitamin B_{12} deficiency
- excessive RBC destruction (haemolysis)—e.g. G6PD deficiency (see ➲ 'G6PD deficiency', pp. 198–9).

Anaemia is not a diagnosis in its own right but a manifestation of an under-lying disorder (e.g. NSAID-induced GI bleed), and so should be investi-gated to determine the cause. A low Hb is defined as <13.5g/dL in ♂ and <11.5g/dL in ♀ but symptoms are uncommon until Hb is <7g/dL, although they may occur at higher Hb concentrations if there is an acute ↓ or limited cardiopulmonary reserve.

Signs and symptoms
- Fatigue
- Dyspnoea
- Faintness
- Headache
- Pallor (including conjunctival pallor).

Haematological investigations
- Mean cell volume (MCV)—a measure of RBC size
- Mean corpuscular haemoglobin (MCH)—a measure of the amount of Hb in RBCs
- Mean corpuscular haemoglobin concentration (MCHC)—a measure of the concentration of Hb in RBCs
- Haematocrit—a measure of the percentage of blood that is RBCs.

These investigations can help to indicate the mechanism of anaemia and thus help determine the cause (Table 26.1):
- Microcytic anaemia (i.e. MCV is low) indicates altered haem or globin synthesis
- Macrocytic anaemia (i.e. MCV is high) indicates impaired DNA synthesis
- Normocytic anaemia results from insufficient or inadequate response to erythropoietin
- Hypochromic anaemia (i.e. MCH and MCHC are low).

Table 26.1 Some causes of anaemia based on the MCV

Microcytic/ hypochromic	↓ MCV, ↓ MCHC (e.g. Fe deficiency) Thalassaemia Anaemia of chronic disease
Macrocytic	↑ MCV Reticulocytis (polychromasia on blood film) Vitamin B_{12} or folate deficiency Chronic liver disease Hypothyroidism Alcohol Myelodysplasia
Normocytic/ normochromic	↔ MCV, MCHC Anaemia of chronic disease (e.g. chronic infection, inflammation) Inflammatory disease or malignancy Acute blood loss Renal failure Myeloma

Iron-deficiency anaemia

Iron is present in the body at ~50mg/kg of which ~60% is in RBCs, 30% in body stores (as ferritin and haemosiderin), 5% in muscle cell myoglobin, and 5% in various enzymes or bound to transferrin. Dietary intake is needed to replace normal losses:

- 0.5–1mg/day in faeces, urine, sweat
- 0.5–0.7mg/day (averaged over the month) in menstruating ♀.

Pregnant ♀ need an additional 1–2mg/day.

Dietary intake comes from haem iron (in meat and fish) and non-haem iron (in grains, fruit, and vegetables). Haem iron is better absorbed than non-haem iron but the absorption of the latter may be ↑ by ascorbic acid or citric acid. Iron is mostly absorbed in the duodenum and jejunum, and the excess is excreted in the faeces.

A low Hb does not necessarily mean low iron and a full blood count as well as iron studies should be conducted to determine whether it is iron-deficiency anaemia and so iron supplements are required (Table 26.2).

Treatment

Treatment includes finding and treating the underlying cause (e.g. GI bleed, menorrhagia) as well as correcting the deficiency. Hb should be ↑ by 1–2g/L every day and continued for 3 months after normalization of Hb to replenish iron stores. Different iron salts contain different amounts of elemental iron (Table 26.3), but the aim is to give 100–200mg elemental iron per day (e.g. as ferrous sulfate 200mg three times daily). Other salts are sometimes better tolerated but may be more expensive. Modified-release or enteric-coated preparations supposedly improve tolerability, but may not be released until after the duodenum where absorption is poor.

Parenteral iron (as iron dextran or iron sucrose complex) has no advantage over oral iron as it replenishes Hb, at the same rate although iron stores are replenished more quickly, and it has been associated with hypersensitivity reactions. It is used in specific situations:

- Haemodialysis patients
- Intolerance to oral iron
- Poor compliance
- Continuing blood loss
- Documented malabsorption (e.g. IBD).

Prophylaxis with oral or parenteral (if fits listed criteria) iron may be given if there are risk factors for iron deficiency—e.g. pregnancy, malabsorption conditions (e.g. gastrectomy), haemodialysis.

Blood transfusion is not usually necessary in most patients unless Hb <7g/dL. It is potentially hazardous with a risk of transfusion reactions (hypersensitivity-type symptoms), fluid overload potentially leading to heart failure, and haemolytic reactions due to blood group or rhesus factor incompatibility. Fevers and mild allergic reactions are also fairly common, although rarely serious. Therefore transfusion should only be carried out in the following situations:

- Acute situation (e.g. haemorrhage)
- Comorbidity (e.g. IHD, heart failure, COPD)
- Patient symptomatic.

Table 26.2 Interpreting plasma iron studies

	Iron	TIBC	Ferritin
Iron deficiency	↓	↑	↓
Anaemia of chronic disease	↓	↓	↑
Chronic haemolysis	↑	↓	↑
Haemochromatosis	↑	↓ (or ↔)	↑
Pregnancy	↑	↑	↔
Sideroblastic anaemia	↑	↔	↑

TIBC, total iron-binding capacity.

Table 26.3 Ferrous iron content of different iron tablets

Iron salt	Tablet strength (mg)	Ferrous iron content (mg)
Ferrous fumarate	200	65
Ferrous gluconate	300	35
Ferrous sulphate	300	60
Ferrous sulphate, dried	200	65

Vitamin B$_{12}$ deficiency/pernicious anaemia
Vitamin B$_{12}$ is found in meat and dairy products but not in plants. Signs and symptoms include the following:
- General symptoms of anaemia
- Glossitis
- Angular cheilosis
- Peripheral neuropathy.

Causes include dietary (e.g. vegans), malabsorption (e.g. gastrectomy, Crohn's disease), lack of intrinsic factor (necessary for absorption). ↑ Hb, ↑ MCV, and ↓ B$_{12}$. Treatment is with parenteral vitamin B$_{12}$ (hydroxo-cobalamin)—initially alternate-day injections for 2wks to replenish stores and then every 3 months. Pharmacists need to be aware of the need for continuing maintenance injections in long-stay patients. Oral maintenance with cyanocobalamin is an option only if the deficiency is due to diet alone.

Folate deficiency
Folate is found in most foods, especially green vegetables, but it can be destroyed by cooking. Causes of folate deficiency include the following:
- Dietary deficiency
- Malabsorption
- ↑ requirements (e.g. pregnancy)
- ↑ losses (e.g. malignancy)
- Other causes (e.g. prematurity, folate antagonist drugs).

Folate deficiency is relatively common in patients with grossly deficient diets as stores are only sufficient for 3–4 months. Clinical presentation is similar to vitamin B_{12} deficiency but:
- there is a more rapid onset of symptoms
- neuropsychiatric disorders are rare.

Treatment

Treatment is with folic acid 5mg daily and patients should be encouraged to ↑ dietary intake. Coexisting vitamin B_{12} deficiency should be corrected.

Folate deficiency in pregnancy can lead to neural tube defects. ♀ who are pregnant or planning a pregnancy should be advised to take folate supplements:
- 400 micrograms daily before conception and for the first 12wks of gestation
- 5mg daily in ♀ with diabetes or sickle cell disease, or on anticonvulsants.

Therapy-related issues: miscellaneous

Introduction to critical care

For the purposes of critical care in the UK, patients are grouped into one of four levels of care, an allocation that changes according to severity of illness and degree of actual or potential organ support required by the patient.

- Level 0 patients have needs that can be met by normal ward care.
- Level 1 patients have needs that can be met on an acute ward with additional advice and support from the critical care team. They are at risk of their condition deteriorating, or have recently been relocated from higher levels of care.
- Level 2 patients require more detailed observation or intervention, including support for a single failing organ system or postoperative care, and include patients stepping down from higher levels of care (formerly known as high dependency unit (HDU) patients).
- Level 3 patients require advanced respiratory support alone or basic respiratory support together with support of at least two organ systems. This level includes all complex patients requiring support for multi-organ failure (formerly known as intensive care unit (ICU) patients).

This classification has meant that critical care has come to define a type of therapy, rather than a specific place where such therapy is administered. Critical care teams work in ICUs, HDUs, specialist surgical units, recovery areas, and perioperative care, and on general wards with outreach teams. Therefore critical care encompasses a diverse area for pharmacists to work within, and pharmacists working on general wards are increasingly coming into contact with critically ill patients. For the pharmacist who commits to a career in critical care, the UK Clinical Pharmacy Association critical care group have a mechanism in place to recognize advanced practice in critical care.[1]

Tips, hints, and things you should bear in mind

Critical care can at first be a daunting area within which to work. Patients are on the extremes of the physiological spectra, often accompanied by a frightening array of equipment that bristles with buttons and gaudy displays, issuing all manner of warning squeaks, pips, and beeps. The patient is cared for by experienced, efficient nurses and calm, intelligent doctors, and can be surrounded by teams of personnel attending to various functions of care. An enormous variety and quantity of data are generated, with the patient's notes quickly expanding in size. All this activity is being watched by tense, tired, and often tearful relatives or carers, who are constantly looking for the slightest sign that their loved one's condition is getting either better or worse.

Put the patient first

In all your endeavours and work, you must put the patient first. If there are limited resources and you have several patient care responsibilities, then you must do the best you can for the patients who need you the most.

Not all patients are model citizens. They may have led very colourful lives, and this can complicate their medical management and their dealings with relatives, or affect your own personal feelings for them. You must put these aspects aside in order to do your best for them.

You will have to come to terms with the fact that a significant proportion of patients will die despite your best efforts. This of course reflects the severity of their illness, not your performance, and you will need to remind yourself of this from time to time.

Remember the relatives, carers, and friends

The patient is not always alone. Loved ones visit and stay by the bedside without restrictions on visiting hours. As a member of the team, you will be asked about various aspects of the patient's care. As a junior pharmacist, you should refer requests for information about progress or planning to a member of the medical team. This ensures that visitors receive consistent information. You may still need to talk to relatives to obtain information about medications, or possibly because you are asked to discuss a specific aspect of care with them by the medical team. When you do so, employ great sensitivity. Loved ones have a lot of time to think and dwell on the consequences of the illness that brings the patient to critical care, and as such can be extremely fragile. Remember that certain aspects of the patient may not be known to them and should not be divulged, sometimes at the specific request of the patient. This can give rise to some extraordinary circumstances, yet you must still employ strict patient confidentiality. Because of the situation they find themselves in, visitors may not take in everything you are saying. They may also make their own interpretation of any information you are giving them or asking of them. Be as clear and concise as you can. Note the key points of conversation in the patient's notes and, if possible, ensure that the patient's nurse is party to the conversation. As well as acting as a witness, they can dig you out of a hole.

Do not worry

You may not know the nuances and subtleties of various standard critical care interventions such as the use of vasopressors or sedation and analgesia. In fact you are unlikely to, unless you have committed to a career in critical care pharmacy. Fortunately, intensivists tend to know a fair bit about these agents and so you should be assured that, at more junior levels of practice, such in-depth knowledge is not necessary in order to contribute meaningfully to the team.

Nor will you be expected to know the function of every piece of kit available at the bedside, and no one will expect you to be able to interpret pressure waveforms or scan results. Your role is not the same as everyone else's. In time, you may understand the intricacies of the available monitoring and supporting equipment, but for now, concentrate on the area that you know best—basic clinical pharmacy.

Develop a methodical approach

Every critical care patient requires a high degree of pharmaceutical care/ medicines management. You must know the patient's medical history, drug history, allergy history, admitting complaint, progress, pharmacokinetic reserve, and prescription as a minimum dataset from which to work. Making professional notes is important in order to record all pertinent information and to aid in planning the patient care (including follow-up).

Do not become overloaded with the huge amount of information available. Always summarize trends and interpret where possible. It is usual to think in terms of individual body systems in order to avoid missing anything out, but of course these are interrelated and so you must always step back and consider the patient as a whole. Remember that medicines are only one of the tools that can be utilized in the care of a patient. Try to think beyond just drugs (e.g. there are mechanical methods for venous thrombus prophylaxis, as well as anticoagulants).

Draw on what you know …

Your broad generalist knowledge of medicine is a bonus. Critical care teams are highly specialist, and despite the broad case mix, many of the patients present to intensive care for the same sorts of reasons and require the same sorts of treatments. The fact that you know a bit about other medications found outside critical care is very useful to the team.

Despite the fact that the majority of critically ill patients have disturbances of organ function that necessitate adjustments of dose, route, or choice of agent, this area is often not consistently tackled by medical staff and is one area where you can make a major contribution. Examples include dose adjustment in renal dysfunction or changes in route of administration because of surgery.

Looking out for, or avoiding, adverse drug reactions/interactions is very important. This can sometimes be more about refuting that such a reaction has taken place rather than the more usual situation of avoiding problems that may arise.

… and say when you don't know

Knowing your limitations is something to be respected. Do not bluff your way through an issue—it is obvious when you do and nobody likes it. It can result in inappropriate interventions in the short term and appropriate advice or interventions being ignored or treated as suspect in the future.

Recognize others' expertise

Everyone has expertise: medics, surgeons, nurses, physiotherapists, dieticians, relatives, and loved ones—everyone. There will be overlaps as well as gaps in knowledge and differences in opinion. Learn to live with it and collaborate. Do not create conflict. This will not help the patient.

Be aware and utilize other resources

Liaise with pharmacists from the service that the patient came from. Critical care is a support service, treating the sickest patients from many other services. Obtaining valuable advice from pharmacists who routinely work in those services will greatly aid in the provision of appropriate care for the patient.

Critical care units do not work in isolation from each other. Each unit is part of a larger network or group of units that covers a distinct geographical location. This means that, within each network or group, there will be other critical care pharmacists whom you can talk to or draw support from. Find out who they are and introduce yourself to them (face to face, by telephone, or by email), before you need their advice in a crisis. Each network or group will have standards of practice and therapeutic protocols (often called care bundles). Obtain copies and be familiar with them.

Reference

1. Middleton H (2011). How to build your professional portfolio (and why you should). *Clin Pharm* January, ☞ http://www.pharmaceutical-journal.com/career/career-feature/how-to-build-your-professional-portfolio-and-why-you-should/11072302.article

Delirium/acute confusional state

Large numbers of patients become delirious in critical care. Some studies put the incidence as high as 80%, although it is probably nearer to 50% in a general ICU population in the UK. Delirium is important—it is associated with excess mortality, ↑ length of stay, new admissions to care homes after leaving hospital, and ↑ likelihood of a long-term cognitive dysfunction (i.e. dementia).

Historically, delirium has been poorly recognized and treated. In particular, agitated delirium has been treated with sedation, which masks the condition without treating it, whilst non-agitated delirium goes unrecognized.

Detection

Detection should be through the routine use of a screening tool such as the Confusion Assessment Method modified for critically ill patients (CAM-ICU). Other tools also exist, such as the Intensive Care Delirium Screening Checklist (ISDSC) which some find easier to use. Routine screening ↑ recognition.

Prevention

Preventative measures are simple interventions such as avoiding dehydration, ensuring good sleep patterns and good nutrition, and normalizing the environment as much as possible. Humane attention to detail such as use of glasses and hearing aids make a difference, as well as interacting with the patient as much as possible.

Many medications may cause delirium. Good pharmaceutical care (reducing doses in renal failure and hepatic failure) and avoidance of precipitants such as drugs with anticholinergic activity, daily sedation breaks, and good sedative management all help.

Treatment

Pharmacological treatment options are based on a small evidence base. Antipsychotics are used at the lowest effective dose and withdrawn as the delirium clears. Specialist advice should be sought if delirium fails to clear after a week of therapy to rule out a more permanent decline in cognitive function (dementia). The aim of therapy is not to sedate the patient, but to clear the cognitive deficit. A sedative may be required in addition to keep a severely disturbed patient safe.

Haloperidol

Haloperidol is flexible; it has a wide dosing range and can be administered via a variety of routes (PO, NG, IV, IM). Typical doses are 1–5mg, depending on the degree of illness and age of the patient, given regularly every 6–8h. Avoid in patients with prolonged QTc interval.

Olanzapine

Olanzapine can be administered NG and IM. Typical doses are 2.5–10mg/day. It may be more effective in certain types of delirium and has fewer side effects than haloperidol.

Stress ulcer prophylaxis

Over three-quarters of ICU patients have endoscopic evidence of mucosal damage within 1–2 days of admission to intensive care, although in most cases the damage is superficial and will heal quickly. Clinical evidence for gastric bleeding occurs in up to a quarter of patients ('coffee grounds', melaena), and up to 6% of patients suffer clinically important bleeding that results in haemodynamic instability or a requirement for blood transfusions. The incidence of stress ulceration appears to be falling, probably because of general advances in the management of critically ill patients as well as specific prophylactic measures for stress ulceration.

Pathophysiology

It is thought that mucosal damage is brought about by a number of factors, such as disturbances in mucosal blood flow due to cardiovascular instability and hypoperfusion leading to a relative mucosal ischaemia, the presence of reduced gastric luminal pH, and altered mucosal protective mechanisms. At pH <4, the proteolytic enzyme pepsin destroys clots forming on damaged gastric mucosa, ↑ the likelihood of bleeding and the extent of gastric damage.

Risk factors

A large number of risk factors have been identified for stress ulceration including:
- >48h of mechanical ventilation
- coagulopathy
- acute kidney injury
- acute liver failure
- sepsis
- hypotension
- severe head injury
- history of GI bleeding
- burns covering >35% of body surface
- major surgery.

The two factors that are thought to contribute to development of a stress ulcer are mechanical ventilation for >48h and coagulopathy.

Aim of therapy

An ↑ in the gastric pH to >4 is thought to be sufficient to prevent superficial stress ulceration progressing to a more serious pathological state which is much more difficult to treat. Therefore the aim of therapy is to prevent further attack on already injured mucosa by reducing acidity and/or preventing proteolytic enzymes from attacking unprotected gastric mucosa. This can be differentiated from the aim of therapy for non-variceal upper GI bleeding where a higher pH is required (pH >6).

Methods of stress ulcer prophylaxis

Several large randomized placebo-controlled studies have been conducted, with conflicting results arising from each. The therapy of choice has changed a number of times over the years.

- H_2-receptor antagonists are usually used first line. Ranitidine 50mg given by bolus injection three times daily is common.
- PPI use is ↑, although there is at present no defining study that places this agent at the heart of stress ulcer prophylaxis therapy. Once-daily injections of omeprazole or pantoprazole have been used, and some centres use an extemporaneously prepared enteral formulation of omeprazole (simplified omeprazole suspension). Oro-dispersible lansoprazole tablets dissolved in a small volume of water are also used by some centres.
- The use of sucralfate has almost disappeared, and antacids are no longer used.

It is common practice to cease stress ulcer prophylaxis when full NG feeding is established, although the limited evidence available suggests that feed is not an effective form of stress ulcer prophylaxis.

Some surgical procedures may result in a reduced acid secretory function through denervation of the stomach (e.g. oesophagectomy), but the effect this has on stress ulcer formation has not been studied.

Pharmacological stress ulcer prophylaxis is so routine in critical care that the prescribing of prophylaxis becomes an almost reflex response. Stopping acid suppression therapy in patients with a total gastrectomy can be a common pharmacist's intervention. Partial gastrectomy may still require stress ulcer prophylaxis if the acid secretory function remains intact (i.e. where the antrum of the stomach remains).

Unwanted effects of stress ulcer prophylaxis

- One large study found an ↑ incidence of nosocomial pneumonia in the ranitidine arm. This has largely been ignored since it was not found in subsequent studies, although an ↑ incidence of pneumonia in an ambulatory population taking acid suppressant therapy has also been reported.
- There is growing evidence that the use of acid suppressants ↑ *Clostridium difficile* acquisition rates. This effect may be greater with PPIs than with H_2 antagonists.
- The use of pH testing strips to confirm the correct placement of enteral tubes is unreliable where acid suppressant therapy is used.
- Ranitidine is associated with a number of side effects, including cardiac rhythm disturbance, but the evidence that it causes thrombocytopenia is very poor.

Motility stimulants

The provision of early enteral feed is an important goal in critically ill patients and has several advantages over parenteral feeding. Haemodynamic disturbance, pre-existing disease states, and drugs used in the critically ill patient (e.g. adrenergic agents, opiates) frequently result in failure to absorb enteral feed in the patient.

It is usual to use markers such as bowel sounds and gastric residue volume on aspiration to assess gut motility, although neither method is particularly reliable.

Metoclopramide

Metoclopramide is widely used to promote gut motility. However, the evidence base in the critically ill is very poor. This dopamine antagonist possibly works through blockade of dopaminergic neurons in the stomach and small bowel that would normally inhibit GI motility. It also ↑ lower oesophageal sphincter tone. A typical dose is 10mg three times daily.

Erythromycin

The evidence base for erythromycin is stronger than that for metoclopramide and comes from several small-scale studies, but it is often reserved for second-line therapy after metoclopramide because of concerns about promoting antimicrobial resistance. Erythromycin acts as a motilin receptor agonist. The addition of erythromycin to a metoclopramide regimen is not evidence based, although simultaneously targeting different motility pathways may prove beneficial.

Typical doses range from 250mg twice daily to 200mg three times daily IV. Doses as small as 70mg have been shown to have an effect in adults. It is believed that smaller doses are more effective than larger doses, and this is consistent with the well-known upper GI effects of antibiotic doses.

Neostigmine

Neostigmine infusions have been used to promote normal bowel function in the critically ill. Neostigmine directly stimulates acetylcholine release from nerve plexi within the gut wall. A continuous infusion of 0.4–0.8mg/h has found to be an effective prokinetic based on frequency of stool production.

Domperidone

There is no evidence to support or refute the usefulness of domperidone for gut motility. Activation of dopaminergic fibres found in the smooth muscle of the GI tract inhibit smooth muscle contraction and so blockade of these fibres by dopamine antagonists may encourage smooth muscle contraction. Therefore it is possible that a role for domperidone and other dopamine antagonists may be found in the future.

Mechanical ventilation

Mechanical respiratory support may be required in patients with a certain degree of respiratory failure. Typically such failure can be described in terms of a failure to oxygenate blood, such as during an acute asthma attack (type 1 respiratory failure), or a failure to ventilate the lungs resulting in carbon dioxide retention, such as in exacerbations of COPD (type 2 respiratory failure). Patients who do not protect their airway (e.g. through the consequences of acute head injury) may also require respiratory support.

Non-invasive ventilation

Selected patients may initially be managed using a form of tight-fitting face-mask which acts as the interface between patient and ventilator. These come in a variety of shapes and sizes. A NGT is usually *in situ* in order to decompress the stomach, which can frequently become inflated as a result of swallowing air.

Invasive ventilation

The more typical method for connecting a ventilator to a patient is through the insertion of a plastic pipe into the patient's trachea, placed either through the upper airways (nasal passages or mouth) or through a stoma in the patient's neck under the larynx. An inflatable cuff at the end of the tube secures it in the trachea. The ventilator is attached to the other end of the tube. The act of tube placement is known as intubation.

Drugs used to facilitate intubation

Feeding a large-diameter tube through the mouth or nose into the trachea generates all manner of physiological responses, none of which are described as 'pleasant'. Various agents are used to manage or attenuate such a noxious stimulus.

Rapid-sequence induction

This technique is used to secure the patient's airway rapidly whilst minimizing the risk of soiling the airways with stomach contents. A sedative agent such as thiopental 3–4mg/kg is used in combination with a muscle relaxant such as suxamethonium (succinylcholine) 1–1.5mg/kg to facilitate the technique. Other sedative agents used include propofol 2mg/kg, etomidate 0.1–0.4mg/kg, or occasionally ketamine 1–2mg/kg. Alternative muscle relaxants include rocuronium 1mg/kg or vecuronium 80–100 micrograms/kg.

Awake intubation

This is used to secure an airway where a difficult intubation is anticipated, e.g. due to previous history or airway obstruction, unstable cervical spine fracture, or when anaesthetic induction is dangerous for the patient. Comfort for the patient is provided using topical anaesthetics such as lidocaine 4%, possibly with light sedation with an agent such as midazolam 1–2mg. Atropine 400–600 micrograms or glycopyrronium bromide 200–400 micrograms is given to dry up secretions.

Ventilation modes

A bewildering array of ventilation modes are used. The following is intended to be a brief overview of those most commonly used.

Continuous mandatory ventilation (CMV)

The ventilator controls movement of gas through the patient's lungs according to set parameters and takes no account of any residual breathing effort the patient may make. Set parameters can be volume based, pressure based, or a mixture of both.

Assist-control ventilation (ACV)

The ventilator controls movement of gas through the patient's lungs according to set parameters either when the patient triggers a breath (assisted breaths) or at the set respiratory rate if the patient fails to trigger a breath (controlled breaths).

Intermittent mandatory ventilation (IMV)

The ventilator controls movement of gas through the patient's lungs according to the parameters set at a mandatory respiratory rate, but allows spontaneous breathing to occur between mandatory breaths.

Synchronous intermittent mandatory ventilation (SIMV)

The ventilator controls movement of gas through the patient's lungs according to the parameters set at a mandatory respiratory rate, but allows spontaneous breathing to occur between mandatory breaths. Assisted breaths are synchronized with spontaneous breaths when their timing is sufficiently close.

Pressure support ventilation (PSV)

The ventilator augments the flow of gas moving into the patient's lungs in order to maintain a preset pressure in the ventilator circuit during inspiration. When the flow rate falls below a set value, the expiration cycle begins. PSV may be combined with other modes of ventilation to support spontaneous breaths.

Continuous positive airway pressure (CPAP)

The ventilator maintains the ventilator circuit pressure at a constant value above ambient pressure during spontaneous breaths.

Positive end-expiratory pressure (PEEP)

The ventilator maintains the ventilator circuit pressure at a constant value above ambient pressure during ventilator-generated breaths.

Bilevel positive airway pressure (BiPAP)

The ventilator maintains the ventilator circuit pressure at one value above ambient pressure during inspiration and at a lower value (still above ambient pressure) during expiration.

Vasoactive agents

A variety of agents can be used to manipulate the cardiovascular system in critical care. These agents should only be used after the patient has been adequately fluid resuscitated. Terminology is often used incorrectly and interchangeably:

- Inotropes—affect the force of contraction of the heart
- Chronotropes—affect the heart rate
- Vasopressors—↑ BP.

Charts of receptor activity are widely available. However, they can be tricky to use as different activities predominate at different infusion rates.

Adrenaline (epinephrine) (α_1^{+++}, β_1^{+++}, β_2^{++}, D_1^0, D_2^0)

Dose range effects

- Low doses (<0.01 micrograms/kg/min)—predominant β_2 stimulation leads to dilation of skeletal vasculature resulting in a fall in BP.
- Medium doses (0.04–0.1 micrograms/kg/min)—predominant β_1 stimulation leads to an ↑ in heart rate, stroke volume, and cardiac output.
- Large doses (0.1–0.3 micrograms/kg/min)—α_1 stimulation predominates leading to vasoconstriction which ↑ systemic vascular resistance and therefore ↑ BP.
- Larger doses (>0.3 micrograms/kg/min)—↑ α_1 stimulation causes reduced renal blood flow and reduced splanchnic vascular bed perfusion. GI motility and pyloric tone are also reduced.

Uses

Anaphylactic shock, severe congestive cardiac failure, septic shock, status asthmaticus.

Other effects

Infusions of adrenaline can lead to arrhythmias, hyperglycaemia, and metabolic acidosis.

Noradrenaline (norepinephrine) (α_1^{+++}, β_1^+, β_2^0, D_1^0, D_2^0)

Dose range effects

- Low doses (<2 micrograms/min)—predominant β_1 stimulation leads to an ↑ in heart rate, stroke volume, and cardiac output.
- Higher doses (>4 micrograms/min)—predominant α_1 stimulation leads to vasoconstriction. Baroreceptor-mediated bradycardia is possible.

Uses

↑ the mean arterial pressure—e.g. in septic shock, in severe head injury.

Other effects

Infusions of noradrenaline can lead to arrhythmias, hyperglycaemia, and metabolic acidosis. Not useful for cardiogenic shock because of ↑ afterload.

Dopamine (α_1^{++}, β_1^{++}, β_2^{++}, D_1^{+++}, D_2^{+++})

Dose range effects
- Low doses (<2 micrograms/kg/min)—predominant D_1 stimulation leads to ↑ renal, mesenteric, and coronary perfusion.
- Medium doses (2–5 micrograms/kg/min)—predominant β_1 stimulation leads to an ↑ in heart rate, stroke volume, and cardiac output.
- Large doses (>6 micrograms/kg/min)—predominant α_1 stimulation leads to vasoconstriction which ↑ systemic vascular resistance and therefore ↑ BP.

Uses
Cardiogenic shock. Should not be used as a 'renoprotective' agent, except occasionally when used it is used as a vasopressor on general wards to support BP (and hence improves renal perfusion).

Other effects
Infusions of dopamine can lead to arrhythmias, hyperglycaemia, and metabolic acidosis.

Dobutamine (α_1^{+}, β_1^{++}, β_2^{+}, D_1^{0}, D_2^{0})

Dose range effects
- Usual dose (2.5–10 micrograms/kg/min)—predominant β_1 stimulation leads to ↑ cardiac output.

Uses
Cardiogenic shock.

Other effects
BP may fall in hypovolaemic patients.

Dopexamine (α_1^{0}, β_1^{+}, β_2^{+++}, D_1^{++}, D_2^{++})

Dose range effects
- Usual dose (0.5–6 micrograms/kg/min)—strong β_2 stimulation leads to vasodilation. D_1 leads to ↑ renal perfusion. Splanchnic perfusion may also be ↑.

Uses
May be useful to improve splanchnic perfusion.

Other effects
Heart rate ↑ in a dose-dependent manner.

Phosphodiesterase inhibitors (non-receptor-mediated effect)

Pharmacology
Inhibits phosphodiesterase, causing an intracellular excess of cAMP which causes a calcium ion influx. This causes ↑ myocardial contractility and smooth muscle relaxation.

Uses
Cardiac failure.

Other effects
Hypotension due to vasodilation.

Renal replacement therapy

Acute kidney injury is a common feature of critical illness. Renal function will recover in the majority of patients although a proportion will go on to require chronic renal support. During the period of time it takes for the kidneys to recover, renal replacement therapy will be required to undertake some of the functions that the healthy kidneys would perform.

Terminology

Confusion often arises over the various techniques used for renal replacement therapy. Abbreviations add to the confusion, but there are basically two main renal replacement modes (dialysis or filtration), with a hybrid of the two also being commonly employed (diafiltration). The process is usually continuous (C), but can be intermittent (I). Blood follows a pressure gradient that is generated either by taking blood from an artery and returning it to a vein (arteriovenous or AV) or by taking blood from a vein and using the machine to generate the pressure gradient required before returning the blood to a vein (venovenous or VV). Putting the various abbreviations together with the mode of renal replacement gives the appropriate abbreviation for the technique (e.g. CVVHDF = Continuous VenoVenous HaemoDiaFiltration).

Haemodialysis (HD)

Not normally used in critical care, but may be used in a stable or pre-existing chronic renal failure patient.

Blood is pushed through thousands of small tubes made of a semi-permeable membrane (Fig. 27.1) Clearance of small (<2000Da), water-soluble molecules occurs by diffusion through a semipermeable membrane into dialysis fluid that bathes the tubes. Water may also be drawn off by altering the concentration of glucose in the dialysis fluid.

Clean fluid can be infused back into the patient if required, although this is unusual for this form of renal replacement.

Haemofiltration (HF)

Blood passes through thousands of small tubes made of a membrane full of small holes (typically 20 000Da in diameter). A pressure gradient pushes the patient's plasma through the holes (filtration) and this eluent is discarded (Fig. 27.2).

Clean fluid is infused back into the patient.

Haemodiafiltration (HDF)

This is a hybrid form which adds a dialysis element to haemofiltration by allowing dialysis fluid to be added to the eluent generated from the filter, thus diluting it and causing an additional diffusion process to occur.

Buffer

Whichever technique is employed, vast quantities of fluid are required for the process to take place. One of the many small molecules that are cleared is bicarbonate. Bicarbonate is central to the acid–base balance of the human body, and its steady removal in renal replacement therapy without replacement would lead to ↑ acidosis and ultimately to the patient's death.

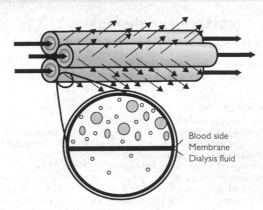

Fig. 27.1 Haemodialysis.

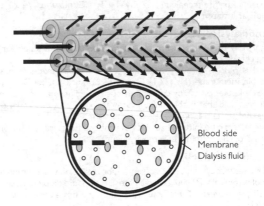

Fig. 27.2 Haemofiltration.

Initial stability difficulties precluded manufacturers from simply adding bicarbonate to the dialysis or replacement fluids (although this has now been overcome). Therefore a buffer was added to the fluids in the form of either lactate or acetate, both of which are converted to bicarbonate by the patient. This may become problematic if the patient cannot utilize the buffer.

Anticoagulation

The passage of blood through the extracorporeal circuit activates clotting pathways (Fig. 27.3). The resulting coagulation clogs the filter circuit, reducing its efficiency and ultimately destroying its patency.

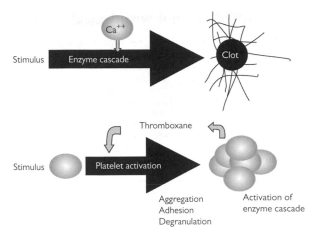

Fig. 27.3 Activation of the clotting cascade.

Anticoagulants are employed to maintain circuit patency, unless the patient is particularly coagulopathic.

Heparin
Heparin has long been used to maintain filter patency through its inhibitory effects on the enzyme cascade. It can be infused into the circuit or the patient to maintain an APTT of 1.5–2 times normal. Heparin is poorly cleared by renal replacement therapy. Attempts have been made to neutralize heparin with protamine before it is returned to the patient, but the technique is tricky and not widely used.

Epoprostenol
Prostaglandins produced by the endothelial lining of the vasculature inhibit the effect of thromboxane on platelet activation. This activity is lost in the artificial environment of an extracorporeal circuit. Epoprostenol can be infused into the circuit as a substitute at 1–5ng/kg/min, and occasionally at even higher doses. Hypotension is a problematic side effect. The combination of heparin and epoprostenol has been shown to be synergistic.

Citrate
Citrate has been used to bind up ionized calcium in the circuit, thus inhibiting several calcium-dependent steps in the clotting cascade and inhibiting calcium influx into platelets, preventing platelet activation. Large quantities of citrate are needed, and this results in a large solute load and metabolic alkalosis. Specialized fluids are required and sourcing citrate can be problematic. This technique, whilst promising, is not widely used.

Treatment of alcohol withdrawal

Early identification important to prevent progression

Alcohol withdrawal syndrome (AWS) occurs when an alcohol-dependent individual intentionally or unintentionally abruptly ceases drinking. Among hospitalized patients, as many as 1 in 5 patients are alcohol dependent and, due to abstinence in the hospital setting, 1 in 10 of such alcohol dependent patients will develop symptoms of AWS. Because the symptoms of AWS can be severe, including seizures and delirium tremens (DT), it is essential to establish the risk of developing AWS in all patients admitted to hospital. Early identification and treatment reduces their chances of progressing of severe AWS.

Alcohol withdrawal syndrome is characterized by a range of symptoms including tremor, paroxysmal sweats, nausea and vomiting, anxiety, agitation, headache, and perceptual disturbances. Seizures are occasionally observed. Half of patients who experience a seizure only suffer a single fit. Some patients with severe withdrawal will progress to delirium tremens. Symptoms usually appear within 6–24h of the last consumption of alcohol and typically persist for 72h, but can last for several weeks.

Many alcohol-dependent people require no medication when withdrawing from alcohol. Supportive care, including information on the withdrawal syndrome, monitoring, reassurance, and a low-stimulus environment, are effective in ↓ withdrawal severity. Many alcohol-dependent patients might not be obvious 'alcoholics'.

If medication is required, a benzodiazepine loading dose technique is usually employed. Benzodiazepines have been the drug class of choice for the prevention and treatment of AWS and its complications since the introduction of chlordiazepoxide 50yrs ago.

By modulating the inhibitory GABA neurotransmitter pathway, benzodiazepines replace the inhibitory effect of the ethanol that has been withdrawn

The patient is given repeated doses until symptoms have diminished to an acceptable level. Chlordiazepoxide or diazepam is effective in the prevention and treatment of acute alcohol withdrawal seizures. Because of the relatively large doses usually given, and the long half-lives, it might not be necessary to give any further medication for withdrawal relief. However, if symptoms reappear, further doses should be administered, titrated according to symptom severity.

Suggested withdrawal regimen

Therapy should be started as soon as the patient can tolerate oral medication. Patients should be sedated on admission with chlordiazepoxide 20mg four times daily for 1–2 days, followed by rapid tailing-off over the subsequent 3–4 days.
- Day 1—20mg four times daily + 10mg when required up to a maximum of 200mg daily.
- Day 2—20mg four times daily + 10mg when required up to a maximum of 200mg daily.
- Day 3—20mg three times daily.

- Day 4—20mg twice daily.
- Day 5—10mg twice daily.
- Day 6—STOP.

Review dose daily and titrate on individual patient basis

There is a clinical opinion that patients given the recommended maximum dose and still suffering symptoms of withdrawal should be given further doses every 2h until symptoms are controlled or they are obviously too drowsy to swallow any more!

Cautions

- Patients might experience seizures as the dose of benzodiazepine is tailed off.
- Patients who are sedated for too long might develop a chest infection.
- The dose should be adjusted to provide effective sedative and anticonvulsant endpoints while preventing oversedation, respiratory depression, and hypotension.
- Benzodiazepines can cause temporary cognitive slowing and may interfere with learning and planning. This, and the need to avoid benzodiazepine dependence, are reasons for keeping the length of treatment to a maximum of 5 days.
- Doses of benzodiazepine should be reduced in severe liver dysfunction. Alternatively, a shorter-acting benzodiazepine (e.g. lorazepam) can be used (seek specialist advice). Patients with chronic liver disease should have their dose assessed twice daily to avoid oversedation.
- A maximum 24h dose (10mg twice daily) should only be prescribed on discharge from hospital if necessary.
- Clomethiazole, although historically used for the treatment in alcohol withdrawal of in-patients, has the potential for life-threatening respiratory depression if the patient continues to drink alcohol, which precludes its use.

Thiamine and vitamin supplements

Poor nutrition is common in patients who drink for the following reasons:
- Inadequate intake of food
- Associated chronic liver disease
- Chronic pancreatitis
- Malabsorption (water-soluble and fat-soluble vitamins should be replaced and severely malnourished patients should be considered for enteral feeding).

Thiamine

Thiamine deficiency leads to polyneuritis with motor and sensory defects. Ophthalmoplegia (paralysis of the eye muscles), nystagmus, and ataxia are associated with Wernicke's encephalopathy, in which learning and memory are impaired; there is an ~10–20% mortality. Korsakoff's psychosis is characterized by confabulations (the patient invents material to fill memory blanks) and is less likely to be reversible once established.

IV thiamine replacement

There is no licensed IV thiamine preparation in the UK. One pair of Pabrinex® IV high-potency (vitamin B and C injection BPC) ampoules contain 250mg of thiamine. IV Pabrinex® should be given initially to those with severe withdrawal symptoms.

Dose

One pair of ampoules should be added to 100mL sodium chloride 0.9% solution or glucose 5% solution and administered IV over at least 10min once daily for 3 days or until the patient can take oral thiamine. In established Wernicke's encephalopathy higher doses are needed (consult product literature).

Oral thiamine replacement

If symptoms of withdrawal are not severe the following regimen is recommended:

- Oral thiamine 100mg should be given four times daily until withdrawal is complete. Then reduce the dose to 100mg twice daily.

Other vitamins

- Locally approved multivitamin product.
- Folic acid 5mg once daily (if folate deficient).

At discharge

Oral supplements should be continued at discharge in patients who are malnourished or have inadequate diets. Thiamine should be continued long term if there is cognitive impairment or peripheral neuropathy (100mg twice daily).

Consideration should also be given to the setting in which withdrawal occurs. Careful monitoring of withdrawal severity is essential in all cases, and more severe withdrawal requires in-patient care. Specialist alcohol treatment services and most hospitals can provide charts to be used in the monitoring of symptom severity.

Recommendations on the prevention of relapse in alcohol dependence

Acamprosate and supervised oral disulfiram are treatment options recommended as adjuncts to psychosocial interventions.

The opioid system modulator nalmefene is the first pharmacological therapy to be approved in the EU to reduce alcohol consumption in adults with alcohol dependence and a high drinking risk level. Oral nalmefene was generally well tolerated in patients with alcohol dependence. Thus, as-needed nalmefene provides an important new option for use in the treatment of alcohol dependence.

Further reading

NICE (2011). 'Alcohol-use disorders: diagnosis, assessment and management of harmful drinking and alcohol dependence [CG115]', ℘ www.nice.org.uk/Guidance/cg115

Perry EC (2014). Inpatient management of acute alcohol withdrawal syndrome. *CNS Drugs* 28(5): 401–10.

Dealing with poisoning enquiries

Poisoning incidents can be caused by the following means:
- Accidental poisoning—e.g. small children eating tablets or berries.
- Non-accidental—e.g. Munchausen's syndrome by proxy (in this syndrome one person creates symptoms in another by, for example, administering drugs).
- Deliberate self-poisoning—e.g. tablets or chemicals are ingested intentionally, sometimes to manipulate family or friends and, rarely, with the intention of (successful) suicide.

Any enquiry regarding a possible acute poisoning incident should be treated as potentially serious and urgent. Questioning can quickly establish if there is little possibility of harm, but if there is any doubt the patient should be referred to the nearest A&E department and/or a poisons information centre should be contacted for advice.

Some misconceptions

Members of the public might not be aware of the following:
- Alcohol poisoning can be potentially fatal, especially in children and adolescents. In children, if there are any signs of intoxication the patient should be referred to an A&E department.
- Some forms of poisoning might not cause symptoms initially—e.g. paracetamol overdose, or ingestion of sustained-release tablets and capsules. This can create the impression that there is no intoxication. Referral to an A&E department should be made if sufficient tablets have been taken, even in the absence of symptoms.

Be aware that some over-the-counter preparations might have similar brand names, e.g. Piriton® and Piriteze®, and Anadin® and Anadin®-paracetamol. Ensure that you and other healthcare professionals are clear what product is involved.

Sources of information

TICTAC

TICTAC is a computerized visual tablet, capsule, and (some) patches identification system; it includes prescription and over-the-counter medicines, as well as illicit substances mainly from the UK. TICTAC is used by regional medicines information centres, poisons information centres and some A&E departments and police forces. Information required to identify a tablet, capsule, or patch using TICTAC includes:
- shape—straight, rounded, or bevelled edge for tablets
- colour—cap, body, and contents for capsules
- markings or texts—including whether half or quarter scored
- coating—film, sugar, or uncoated
- length and width (in millimetres)—at longest/widest point
- weight.

TOXBASE®

TOXBASE®[2] is a UK online clinical toxicology database, provided by the National Poisons Information Service (NPIS), which covers drugs (prescription, over-the-counter medication and illicit), plants, household, industrial and agricultural chemicals, snake and insect bites, and exposure in pregnancy where known. Details of potential hazardous doses, toxicity, features of poisoning, and appropriate management are provided, which is continually updated daily. TOXBASE® is a free service to registered health professionals and is password protected. Medicines information and poisons information centres have access to TOXBASE®, and NHS pharmacy departments can apply for a password through the website.[2]

Poisons information centres

The NPIS is a UK wide network of poisons information centres that provides 24h telephone advice. If there is any cause for concern in an acute poisoning incident, a poisons information centre should be contacted immediately. It is inappropriate to cause unnecessary delay in what might be a life-threatening situation by looking elsewhere for information. The doctor dealing with an acute incident should contact the poisons information centre direct so that first-hand information is given and received. Advise the doctor of the sort of information the poisons information centre might require. For a non-acute or general enquiry, it is appropriate for a pharmacist to contact the centre.

Information required to deal with a poisoning enquiry

Eliciting as much information as possible about a poisoning incident can facilitate speedy management. It is especially important to have the relevant information available when contacting a poisons information centre:

- Identity—brand name and active ingredients, including whether it was a mixed overdose or taken with alcohol.
- Route of exposure – whether it was a tablet, liquid, patch, via inhalation etc.
- Timing—when did the incident occur relative to the time of the enquiry. Was the incident a single acute, staggered or chronic poisoning?
- Quantity—number of tablets or volume of liquid. An estimate is better than no information. Checking the quantity left in a container versus its full contents at least gives an estimate of the maximum quantity ingested.
- If tablets or capsules—are these sustained release?
- Age, weight, and gender of the patient—especially if a child.
- Any relevant PMH—e.g. renal impairment, regular medication.
- Any signs and symptoms observed.
- If the patient has vomited—any sign of the poison (e.g. coloured liquid, undigested plant material, tablet fragments).
- Any treatments or first aid already administered and the outcome.

If attendance at an A&E department is recommended, the enquirer should be advised to take any containers or plant material with them that could help with identification (taking suitable precautions to avoid contamination of skin or clothing with the poison).

First aid for poisoning incidents

- Do not induce vomiting.
- If fully conscious, give sips of water or milk.
- If unconscious, check ABC. As needed, perform the following:
    - Perform cardiopulmonary resuscitation, but not mouth-to-mouth except with a face shield (because of the risk of contaminating the first aider).
    - Place patient in the recovery position.
    - Call emergency services.
- Take the patient to an A&E department or phone the emergency services.

Further reading

Dines A et al. (2007). Poisoning: an overview of treatment. *Hospital Pharmacist* **14**: 7–9.
Dines A et al. (2007). Poisoning: antidotes and their use. *Hospital Pharmacist* **14**: 10–14.

Reference

2. 'TOXBASE®' website, ⬚ www.toxbase.org

Drug desensitization

Patients with drug hypersensitivity can usually be treated with an alternative agent. However, on rare occasions if there is no suitable alternative, drug desensitization might be appropriate. Drug desensitization is potentially hazardous and should never be attempted in patients who have had a severe allergic reaction, such as bronchospasm, facial swelling, or anaphylaxis. However, it can be attempted in those who have had a mild or moderate rash provided that this was not a severe skin reaction, such as Stevens–Johnson syndrome.

Desensitization schedules using both oral and parenteral administration have been developed for a variety of drugs, but mostly for antibacterials (notably penicillins) and some chemotherapy drugs. Examples of these are listed at the end of this topic as ➲ 'Further reading', p. 665.

Drug desensitization is potentially hazardous because there is always a risk of anaphylaxis. Thus, when attempting the procedure, the following precautions should be observed:

- The patient is informed of the potential risks (it is advisable that they give written consent to the procedure).
- The patient must be reasonably well (i.e. no active disease other than the current infection).
- The patient's drug history should be reviewed and any drugs known to exacerbate allergic reactions stopped—notably β-blockers and NSAIDs.
- Desensitization should be carried out as an in-patient or closely monitored day-case procedure.
- A doctor or appropriately trained nurse with authority to administer emergency drugs should be present throughout.
- Drugs and equipment required for treatment of anaphylaxis should be available (see ➲ 'Treatment of anaphylaxis', pp. 29–31).
- The patient should have an IV cannula placed for administration of emergency drugs before starting the procedure.
- Prophylactic antihistamines, adrenaline (epinephrine), or steroids should not usually be given as these can mask a reaction.
- Patient monitoring should be carried out before each dose and every 30min (if the dose interval is longer), and should include:
  - temperature, pulse, and BP
  - respiratory signs, including peak flow measurement
  - observation and direct questioning of the patient for signs and symptoms of allergic reaction (e.g. skin flushing, rash, itching, wheeze, shortness of breath, and tingling lips or tongue).
- Patients should continue to be monitored for at least 1h after the final dose of the desensitization schedule.
- Observations and details of drug administration should be documented in the patient's medical notes.

It is important to ensure that the desensitization schedule is followed as rigorously as possible:

- Measure doses accurately—e.g. using an oral syringe. If very small volumes are involved, rinse the syringe with water after the dose has been given and ask the patient to also take this.
- The patient should rinse their mouth with water and swallow after small volume oral doses.
- Doses should be administered at exactly the specified time intervals.

Because of the requirement for direct medical observation throughout the procedure, most schedules involve rapid desensitization. However, some longer schedules have been used, in which case the procedure may be carried out on an out-patient basis. The patient's GP should be informed that out-patient desensitization is planned.

It is important that patients performing drug desensitization at home are carefully selected and that the patient agrees to the following:

- Undertakes never to be on their own throughout the procedure.
- Understands the risks and what action to take if a reaction occurs. Ideally, another responsible person in the home should also be informed.
- Should have access to a telephone and contact numbers for the physician supervising the procedure.
- Has access to suitable transport so that they can attend the hospital in the event of a minor reaction (the patient should call emergency services if there is a major reaction).
- Lives reasonably close to the hospital, and certainly not in a remote area with difficult access.

After the schedule is complete and treatment doses of the drug are being administered without adverse effects, a treatment course of the drug can be given. Desensitization is usually lost within 1–2 days of stopping the drug. If it is probable that further courses of the drug will be needed, low doses should be administered until the next course is required. It is important that patients understand that drug desensitization is only temporary.

Further reading

Examples of drug desensitization schedules

Confino-Cohen R, Fishman A, Altaras M, *et al.* (2005). Successful carboplatin desensitisation in patients with proven carboplatin allergy. *Cancer* 104: 640–3.

Eapen SS, Page RL 2nd, Zolty R (2005). A successful rapid desensitisation protocol in a loop diuretic allergic patient. *Journal of Cardiac Failure* 11: 481.

Kalanadhabhatta V, Muppidi D, Sahni H, *et al.* (2004). Successful oral desensitisation to trimethoprimsulpha-methoxazole in acquired immune deficiency syndrome. *Ann Allergy Asthma Immunol* 92: 409–13.

Sullivan TJ, Yecies LD, Shatz GS, *et al.* (1982). Desensitisation of patients allergic to penicillin using orally administered beta-lactam antibiotics. *J Allergy Immunol* 69: 275–82.

Drug interference with laboratory tests

Drugs can interfere with laboratory tests through a pharmacological, toxic effect or through actual chemical interference with the testing process.

A pharmacological or toxic effect on the laboratory value is often expected and reflects what is happening within the body—e.g. steroids causing hyperglycaemia or diuretics affecting electrolyte concentrations. An example of the toxic effect is elevated LFTs (e.g. elevated transaminase, bilirubin levels, and clotting factors) subsequent to paracetamol overdose.

An analytical interference differs in that the true laboratory value is not measured accurately. The result is inaccurate because of a problem with an *in vitro* laboratory test procedure, or occurs when a substance or process falsely alters an assay result. This may lead to inappropriate further tests, incorrect diagnoses, and treatments with potentially unfavourable outcomes for the patient.

Drug interference may be (1) chemical where the parent drug, metabolites, or additives cross-react; (2) where drugs or additives act as accelerators or inhibitors of the assay; or (3) photometric where the parent drug, metabolites, or additives may have similar absorption peaks to that of the measured chromogen.

Table 27.1 is in no way intended to be comprehensive but to highlight to practitioners examples of analytical interference from drugs or their metabolites.

Table 27.1 Drug–laboratory interferences are usually overlooked

Laboratory test	Increased by	Decreased by
Blood, serum, plasma		
Albumin		Aspirin, phenylbutazone
Calcium	Calcium containing antacids	Diuretics (↑ renal excretion)
Creatinine	Ascorbic acid, dopamine, flucytosine, furosemide, levodopa, methyldopa, nitrofurantoin	Acetylcysteine, amikacin, dopamine, methyldopa
Glucose	Cefotaxime, dextran, diclofenac, dextran, mercaptopurine methyldopa, metronidazole	Hydralazine, isoniazid, levodopa, metronidazole
Iron	Citrate salts, ferrous salts, rifampicin	Heparin, desferrioxamine
Magnesium	Calcium salts, cefotaxime	Cefotaxime, phosphate salts
Potassium	Iodine salts	
Thyroxine	Heparin	Danazol, heparin
Uric acid	Paracetamol, caffeine, hydralazine, isoniazid, theophylline	Levodopa, methyldopa, ascorbic acid, rasburicase
Drug assay		
Serum lithium levels	Inadvertent use of lithium–heparin collection tube leads to spuriously high serum lithium determination	
Digoxin assay	Spironolactone	Interferes with certain specific digoxin assays. Refer to biochemistry department for type of assay used locally
Plasma cortisol levels (Synacthen® test)	Metabolites of spironolactone fluoresce, which interferes when fluorometric analysis is used for tests. Erroneously ↑ cortisol levels	
Urine		
Ketones	Ifosfamide, levodopa, mesna, aspirin	
Protein test (bromophenol blue reagent, sulfosalicylic acid)	Carbonic anhydrase inhibitors (IV). False positive	

Therapeutic drug monitoring (TDM) in adults

Dosage requirements of certain drugs in individual patients can vary significantly, particularly if the drug has a narrow therapeutic window. Although an estimate of the apparent volume of distribution and clearance of a drug can be made from population values, these should only be used as a guide when commencing treatment. Measured plasma/blood levels will enable a more accurate idea of the pharmacokinetic values in specific patients. This will result in a reduction in the risk of toxicity and/or optimization of the effectiveness of the drug regimen.

Sample collection

Drug concentrations can be measured in blood, plasma, saliva, CNS fluid, and urine. The timing of the sample (relative to the previous dose and method of administration) influences the interpretation of a drug concentration measurement. For most drugs there is a relationship between response and concentration which is based on steady-state samples taken at specific times after the dose.

Trough concentrations taken at the end of the dose interval are commonly used for anticonvulsant drugs. Peak concentration measurements are useful for some antimicrobials, though troughs are used more often for antimicrobials although a relationship between concentration by time over a threshold value (e.g. MIC) is sometimes determined. Responses to some anticancer drugs and immunosuppressants have been related to the overall exposure to a drug, as measured by the area under the concentration–time curve (AUC).

Patient/drug characteristics

The appropriate use of therapeutic drug monitoring (TDM) requires more than simply measuring the concentration of a drug and comparing it with a target range. It starts at the point when the drug is first prescribed and involves determining an initial dosage regimen that is appropriate for the clinical condition being treated, the patient's clinical characteristics, and the drug's characteristics:

- Age, weight, gender, nicotine exposure, renal function, concomitant drug therapy
- Clinical issues that might affect bioavailability of oral drug forms—e.g. diarrhoea, short gut anomalies
- Dosage form, administration rate, first-pass metabolism, protein binding, volume of distribution, loading dose.

When interpreting concentration measurements, the following factors need consideration:

- The sampling time in relation to the dose
- Dosage history (whether or not the result represents steady state)
- Patient's response and desired clinical targets
- Missed doses.

This information provides an assessment of the drug concentration that will assist in achieving rapid, safe, and optimum treatment.

TDM is generally of value in the following situations:
- Good correlation between blood concentration and effect
- Wide variations in metabolism
- High risk of side effects
- Narrow therapeutic index.

Routine measurements might be warranted, for example, in determining adequate concentrations after organ transplantation or more commonly ordered to add evidence to a specific clinical problem—e.g. investigate handling a patient with concurrent disease or confirm excessive dosing correlating with signs of toxicity. Table 27.2 covers common drugs and Table 27.3 covers antimicrobials. However, other drugs, such as those used to treat HIV, might also benefit from TDM.
- For antimicrobials assays, doses should ideally be timed for convenience (e.g. 10.00am). For pre-dose levels, a sample should be taken and the dose administered.
- For dosage adjustment, sampling at steady state is essential, except for suspicion of toxic concentrations.
- Sampling is taken at an appropriate time during a dose interval. You must coordinate when, or if, your pathology department can undertake the test or coordinate with another centre.
- Concentrations can be affected by various factors, such as age, drug interactions, protein binding, metabolism, and organ dysfunction.
- The pharmacist has a very important role in interpreting results from TDM:
  - Advice on what to do if there is an unexpectedly high/low result—e.g. check that dose was given, timing of sample in relation to dose or sampling technique.
  - Advice on whether or not another dose should be given if awaiting result.
  - Dose adjustment—most drugs follow linear kinetics (i.e. doubling the dose will double the level), but certain drugs (e.g. phenytoin) exhibit non-linear kinetics and require small incremental dose adjustments.
  - Timing of sampling if there is a suspicion of drug interaction from the introduction of new therapies.

Table 27.2 Common drugs

Drug	Therapeutic range	Ideal sampling time	Indication for drug monitoring	Type of sample required
Carbamazepine	4–10mg/L 17–42micromol/L	Trough measurement before dose	Initiation of therapy: 3wks (induces own metabolism). Change of dose: 3–5 days, before maximal auto-induction 1–3wks Loss of seizure control: immediately Assess toxicity or compliance: immediately Introduction or withdrawal of a potentially interacting drug: 1–2wks later	Serum or plasma—SST (orange) or PST heparin (green)
Ciclosporin	Varies with indication Generally 100–200 micrograms/L	Trough measurement before dose	Transplant surgery: initially every 2 days until therapeutic level achieved Graft vs host disease: immediately Change in the route of administration: 2–3 days later Change in dose: 2 days later Assess toxicity or compliance: immediately Introduction or withdrawal of a potentially interacting drug: 2–3 days later	Whole blood—EDTA (lavender)
Digoxin	0.8–2 micrograms/L Reference range is valid for specimens taken 6–8h post-dose Adults, 1.0–2.6nmol/L	Sampling 8–24h after last dose	Initiation of dose: 8 days (if renal function normal) Assess toxicity or compliance: immediately Introduction or withdrawal of a potentially interacting drug: 8 days later Changing renal function: immediately	Serum or plasma—SST (orange) or PST heparin (green)

Drug	Therapeutic range	Sampling time	Indications	Sample type
Lithium	Minimum effective concentration in mania prophylaxis is 0.5–1.2mmol/L Toxic conc. >1.5mmol/L Not in lithium heparin tube Please measure maintenance range 12h after last dose	12h post-dose	Initiation of therapy: 7 days Subsequent levels weekly until stabilized and then every 3 months Change in dose: 7 days Assess toxicity or compliance: immediately Introduction or withdrawal of a potentially interacting drug: 7 days later Change in sodium of fluid intake: 12h after previous dose	Serum—SST (orange)
Phenytoin	10–20mg/L 40–80micromol/L	Trough measurement before dose	Initiation of therapy: 2–4wks Change of dose or oral formulation: 2–4wks Loss of seizure control: immediately Assess toxicity or compliance: immediately Introduction or withdrawal of a potentially interacting drug: 2–4wks later	Serum or plasma—SST (orange) or PST heparin (green)
Phenobarbital	15–40mg/L 60–160micromol/L	Trough measurement before dose	Initiation of therapy: 3wks Change of dose or oral formulation: 3wks Loss of seizure control: immediately Assess toxicity or compliance: immediately Introduction or withdrawal of a potentially interacting drug: 3wks later	Serum or plasma—SST (orange) or PST heparin (green)
Theophylline/ aminophylline	10–20mg/L 55–110micromol/L	(1) During a continuous infusion, preferably at 6h and 24h (2) SR preparation— pre-dose	Initiation of IV therapy: 6h Subsequent levels for IV therapy every 24h Initiation of oral therapy 2–4 days Assess toxicity: immediately	Serum or plasma—SST (orange) or PST heparin (green)
Tacrolimus	5–15ng/mL	Trough measurement before dose	NA	Blood—EDTA (lavender)

Table 27.3 Antimicrobials

Drug	Therapeutic range (mg/L)	Ideal sampling time	Comments	Type of sample required
Gentamicin, once daily	20	Trough level 18–24h after the first dose (ideal <1.0mg/L)	Most patients only need one dose. Consult microbiologist advice if >1 dose needed	Blood SST (orange)
Gentamicin, conventional dosing	Trough <2 Peak 5–10	Trough Peak—1h post-dose	Peak for endocarditis if having synergistic therapy 3–5mg/L	Blood SST (orange)
Amikacin	Trough <10 Peak 20–30	Trough Peak–1h post administration	Further usually twice weekly pre-dose levels if no dose changes and normal renal function	Blood SST
Vancomycin	Trough 10–20	Pre-dose before fourth dose	Further monitoring usually twice weekly	Blood SST (orange)
Teicoplanin	Trough 10–20	Trough	>20mg/L (<60mg/L) for deep seated infection	Blood SST (orange).
Tobramycin	Trough <2 Peak 5–10	For tobramycin being given in multiple daily doses peak 1h post-administration and trough(immediately before next dose) are useful to determine dose and dose interval	Samples should be taken pre and post fourth dose, depending on renal function	Blood SST

Ophthalmology principles

It is helpful for pharmacists to be familiar with the terminology of the eye structure, which is detailed as follows.

Eye structure

- *Conjunctiva*—transparent membrane covering the sclera and the eyelids.
- *Cornea*—transparent curved layer in front of the iris and pupil, provides protection to the internal ocular structures and refracts light as it enters the eye working with the lens to focus light onto the retina.
- *Iris*—coloured area at the front of the eye surrounding the pupil, controls the amount of light entering the pupil by contacting and relaxing.
- *Lens*—flexible disc sitting behind the iris which focuses light onto the retina. Thickens to focus on nearby objects and thins to focus on those far away.
- *Optic disc*—the part of the optic nerve closest to the eye; the photoreceptors in the retina convert images into electrical impulses which are carried to the brain by the optic nerve.
- *Orbit*—pear-shaped bony cavity containing the eyeball, muscles, nerves, and blood vessels.
- *Pupil*—black dot in the middle of the eye, able to constrict and dilate as the lighting conditions change.
- *Retina*—situated at the back of the eye and contains photoreceptors which are most densely packed in the macula, responsible for converting light into electrical signals. Photoreceptors are either rods or cones, rods are sensitive to dim light and cones are sensitive to colour and enable us to see in daylight.
- *Sclera*—outer white-coloured covering of the eyeball.
- *Anterior segment*—the front section of the eye from the inside of the cornea to the front surface of the lens, filled with aqueous humour.
- *Posterior segment*—the back section of the eye extending from the back of the lens to the retina, filled with vitreous humour which gives the eye its shape and provides nutrients.

There are many ocular conditions that may be seen on general wards or in general practice. Some examples of the most common conditions and their treatment are detailed in this section.

Glaucoma

Glaucoma refers to a group of eye diseases which can lead to optic neuropathy causing visual loss. Damage to the optic nerve is due to ↑ intraocular pressure (IOP). In the Western world, glaucoma is present in 3% of those >70yrs and it is the leading cause of irreversible blindness.

Open-angle glaucoma

Optic nerve neuropathy leads to peripheral vision loss followed by central vision loss. There is usually, but not always, an ↑ in IOP (>21mmHg).

Risk factors
- Age >40yrs
- Ethnicity—more common and often more severe in Afro-Caribbean populations
- Family history—first-degree relative ↑ risk to ~1 in 8
- Steroid use (can ↑ IOP)
- Vascular disease—e.g. diabetes and hypertension.

Treatment (define target for reduction in IOP, e.g. >20%)
Royal College of Ophthalmology guidelines recommend treatment for patients >60yrs with IOP >25mmHg. Treatment should be reviewed 6wks post initiation to consider whether target IOP has been reached and whether the patient has experienced any systemic or local side effects. Thought should also be given to whether the treatment should be continued.

First line—prostaglandin analogues
- Prostaglandin analogues ↑ uveoscleral outflow and subsequently reduce IOP.
- Latanoprost is a prostaglandin analogue, it is available generically and it has few systemic side effects.
- Counselling points—educate patient that prostaglandin analogues may cause brown pigmentation to iris, and lengthening/thickening/darkening of eyelashes.
- If patients are not responding to treatment, their adherence and drop-instillation technique should be checked (including nasolacrimal occlusion).
- If patients are not able to tolerate prostaglandin analogues, consider if the patient is intolerant of the preservative; if so, switch to a preservative-free formulation.

Second line—alpha- or beta-blocker
- If prostaglandin analogues are not appropriate, patients may be switched to an alternative agent—e.g. α-blocker or β-blocker.
- In circumstances where some reduction in IOP has been seen with a prostaglandin analogue, but the target has not been reached, then a combination of topical agents may be needed—e.g. prostaglandin analogue with a β-blocker.
- Combination products are available, but should only be used to improve compliance or adherence.

Third line
- For patients in which pharmacological treatment is inadequate and two or more agents have been tried, surgical or laser intervention may be indicated.

Angle-closure glaucoma

The anterior chamber angle (where the cornea and iris join) in the eye becomes closed or narrowed preventing the drainage of aqueous humour leading to a rapid ↑ in IOP (>50mmHg). Patients can present with a red eye, headache, plus nausea/vomiting. Angle-closure glaucoma is an ocular emergency. The pressure must be lowered urgently to prevent optic nerve damage which can lead to blindness.

Risk factors
- Age >40 years
- Ethnicity—more common in Chinese, south east Asians, and Inuit populations.

Treatment
Aims to control ↑ IOP and reverse angle closure.

Immediate
- Acetazolamide IV 500mg stat then PO 250mg four times a day
- Topical—β-blocker (timolol 0.5%) stat, wait 1min then
  - Sympathomimetic (apraclonidine 1%) stat, wait 1min then
  - Pilocarpine 2% one drop every 15min for two doses, wait 1min after the first dose then
  - Steroid (prednisolone 1%) stat then 0.5–1-hourly.

In addition treat associated symptoms—e.g. pain/nausea with analgesia and antiemetics.

Intermediate
Check IOP hourly. If not improving consider mannitol 20% IV 1–1.5g/kg or glycerol PO 1g/kg.

Definitive
Surgical intervention—e.g. laser peripheral iridotomy to create a small hole in the iris to allow outflow of aqueous humour.

Ocular infections

Conjunctivitis
The direct translation of conjunctivitis is inflammation of conjunctiva, the mucous membrane lining the inside of the eyelids and covering the globe of the eye. Infectious conjunctivitis is usually caused by bacteria but may be viral. Non-infectious conjunctivitis may be caused by an allergic reaction. Bacterial conjunctivitis is typically associated with a thick or coloured discharge. The most common causative organisms include *Staph. epidermidis, Staph. aureus, Strep. pneumoniae*, and *H. influenza*. Allergic or viral conjunctivitis is more associated with a watery discharge. Conjunctivitis is a very common, self-limiting infection; however, topical antibiotic treatment may reduce the duration of symptoms. Patients often present with one or two red and discharging eyes.

When diagnosing, ensure more severe, sight-limiting eye conditions are ruled out first—e.g. acute angle-closure glaucoma or infectious keratitis. Look out for 'red flag' symptoms:
- Reduction in vision
- Ciliary flush (redness more pronounced in a ring)
- Photophobia
- Sensation of a foreign body
- Corneal opacity
- Fixed pupil
- Severe headache ± nausea.

Treatment
- First-line (bacterial) non-contact lens wearers—chloramphenicol 0.5% drops start 1–2-hourly and wean as condition improves. Treat for 7–10 days. Ointment may also be used, but only requires four-times-a-day dosing. Chloramphenicol drops may be used in paediatric patients and neonates; however, more serious ocular infections in neonates may require systemic antibiotics.
- First-line (bacterial) contact lens wearers—fluoroquinolone, e.g. ofloxacin or levofloxacin drops due to the high incidence of pseudomonas infections. Advise patient not to wear lenses until treatment is completed and there has been no discharge from the eye for 24h.
  - In patients not responding to therapy within 1–2 days consider taking conjunctival swabs and sending for MC&S and tailor therapy to results.
- General advice to patients (bacterial and viral cases)—avoid rubbing the eye, avoid sharing towels to prevent spread, and encourage frequent handwashing.
- Viral conjunctivitis often does not require direct treatment, some patients may find symptomatic relief from antihistamines (topical or oral) or topical nasal decongestants.

Bacterial keratitis
Keratitis presents as infection and inflammation of the cornea and is considered an emergency. It can be a sight-threatening condition, however it is usually treatable. Visual loss can occur if treatment is delayed, inappropriate therapy is given, or there is no follow up. Prolonged wear or inappropriate contact lens hygiene can be a causative factor, but keratitis can also be seen in patients with other ocular disorders (e.g. dry eye or nasolacrimal diseases).

Early corneal scrapes should be performed, and if the patient is a contact lens wearer, the lenses, storage pots, and solutions should also be sent for culture.

Treatment
- Stop contact lens wear.
- Intensive topical antibiotics—hourly dual therapy with broad-spectrum antibiotics, e.g. cefuroxime (Gram-positive cover) and levofloxacin (Gram-negative cover). Gentamicin 1.5% may be used in place of levofloxacin. Use preservative-free preparations due to frequency of instillation.
- Consider systemic antibiotics if corneal perforation—e.g. ciprofloxacin 750mg twice a day.
- Cyclopentolate 1% two to three times a day if photophobia or ciliary spasm.
- Oral analgesia if needed.
- Patients require daily monitoring.
- As the eye starts to improve, reduce frequency of topical antibiotics, and consider switching to a preserved formulation.
- Add ocular lubricants to promote healing and consider topical steroids to reduce inflammation.

Viral keratitis

The most common causative organism of viral keratitis is herpes simplex virus which can lead to visual loss due to corneal scarring and opacity. The infection is characterized by infection in the superficial layer of the cornea with the presence of dendritic lesions. The majority of cases are unilateral and can be reoccurring.

Treatment
- Topical antivirals—e.g. aciclovir 3% eye ointment (if unavailable, ganciclovir 0.15% eye gel may be substituted), apply five times a day until healing occurs then continue three times a day for up to 1wk.
- Systemic antivirals—e.g. aciclovir 400mg five times/day may also be used. Oral antivirals have been found to be equally as effective as topical agents in randomized controlled trials and may often be used in preference due to the convenience. However, there has been no reported benefit in using the topical and systemic treatment in conjunction. Aciclovir at lower doses (e.g. 400mg twice a day) may be continued long term as suppressive treatment in those patients particularly at risk of corneal scarring and visual loss, or those who present with frequent episodes.
- Administration of topical steroid treatment without concurrent topical antiviral treatment can lead to worsening of the infection if inflammation is due to active infection rather than immune response to previous infection. Steroid use is contraindicated in the presence of dendritic ulcers.

Acanthamoeba keratitis

Protozoal keratitis caused by *Acanthamoeba* species remains rare; however, the incidence is rising due to ↑ contact lens use. It is often resistant to broad-spectrum, first-line antibiotics.

Risk factors
- Poor contact lens hygiene.
- Swimming or showering with lens *in situ*.
- Corneal trauma with soil contamination.

Treatment
- Stop contact lens wear.
- Topical antiamoeba agents—e.g. polyhexamethylene biguanide 0.02% or chlorhexidine 0.02% hourly plus propamidine isethionate 0.1% hourly.
- Cyclopentolate 1% two or three times a day—prevents photophobia and treats pain associated with ciliary muscle spasm.
- Analgesia.
- Topical steroids to prevent corneal scarring (may be initiated once eye starts to improve, and after at least 2wks of antiamoeba therapy).
- Taper treatment according to clinical response, patients will often need prolonged courses of treatment to fully eradicate the amoeba (upwards of 6 months).

Endophthalmitis

Endophthalmitis is a deeper infection in the eye involving the aqueous and/ or vitreous humours (the liquid part of the eye which provides its shape). Cases may be exogenous, e.g. following trauma, surgery (e.g. cataract, occurs within 6wks) or intravitreal injection to the eye; or endogenous with no preceding insult to the eye which may be also associated with bacteraemia or endocarditis. In cases of endogenous endophthalmitis, blood cultures should be taken prior to starting antibiotic therapy. Acute endophthalmitis is vision-threatening and should be treated as an emergency, including referral to ID/micro and ophthalmology.

Diagnosis
- Aqueous or vitreous biopsy.
- Send for MC&S, the most common causative organism is coagulase-negative staphylococci.

Treatment
- Intravitreal antibiotics—vancomycin 2mg in 0.1mL plus ceftazidime 2mg in 0.1mL or amikacin 0.4mg in 0.1mL (amphotericin 0.01mg in 0.1mL may be added if fungi are suspected). These may be repeated after 48h if inflammation/vision is not improving.
- Systemic antibiotics—usually quinolone, e.g. moxifloxacin 400mg once a day or ciprofloxacin 500–750mg twice a day.
- Surgical intervention—e.g. vitrectomy to debride the affected vitreous.
- Tailor antibiotic therapy to sensitivity test result from biopsy once known.
- All cases of exogenous endophthalmitis following surgical intervention or intravitreal injection are investigated with a root cause analysis in line with infection control procedures.

Supplementary data

Sodium content of parenteral drugs

The sodium content of drugs

A number of parenteral and enteral formulations contain a significant amount of sodium ions (Table A1). At maximum daily doses of some preparations, the amount of sodium ingested could exceed the maximum recommended daily amount (for adults: ~100mmol). This sodium load is unlikely to be important in most patients, other than potentially contributing to total daily intake being higher than the recommended level. However, in patients who have conditions exacerbated by high sodium levels (e.g. hypertension, heart failure, liver or renal impairment), or in neonates, this could be clinically significant. Occasionally, the sodium load from drug therapy will be the cause of, or contribute to, a high serum sodium level.

Intravenous medicines

Several factors should be taken into account when assessing the sodium content of IV medicines:

- Use the summary of product characteristics (SPC) for the correct brand of product to check how much sodium is in the product; this is usually listed in the 'qualitative and quantitative composition section' or 'list of excipients'.
- If the SPC does not give enough information, consider checking the National Injectable Medicines Guide (MEDUSA[1]) or contacting the manufacturer directly.
- Check whether the drug is further diluted for administration, each additional 100mL of sodium chloride 0.9% increases the sodium load by 15mmol.

Oral medicines

Similar principles apply to oral medicines as to IV medicines:

- Use the SPC and *BNF* to check for the sodium content of oral medicines.
- Soluble, effervescent, or dispersible tablets often have a high sodium content.
- Some antacids contain high amounts of sodium; the *BNF* annotates antacids with a low sodium as 'low Na'.
- Orodispersible preparations usually do not contain significant amounts of sodium.

If a reduction in sodium load is required, consider:

- Is the medicine really necessary?
- Can it be given by an alternative route (e.g. switch from IV to oral or NG)?
- Can the infusion volume be safely reduced (e.g. give undiluted via a central line)?
- For infusions, can a diluent other than sodium chloride 0.9% be used?
- For oral preparations, can an alternative form be used (e.g. suspension instead of soluble tablet)?
- Does the drug increase serum sodium by its pharmacological effect?

Other sources that quote the sodium content of parenteral formulations

Barber N, Wilson A (2006). *Clinical Pharmacy* (2nd ed). Edinburgh: Churchill Livingstone.

Pharmacy Department, University College London Hospitals (2010). *UCL Hospitals Injectable Drug Administration Guide* (3rd ed). Chichester: John Wiley and Son.

electronic Medicines Compendium (eMC). 'Summaries of Product Characteristics' ℗ www.emc. medicines.org.uk

Table A1 Sodium content of parenteral drugs

Name	Vial/ampoule size	Sodium content per vial (mmol)
Acetylcysteine	2g	12.78
Aciclovir	250mg	1
Addiphos®	20mL	30
Amoxicillin	250mg	0.7
Amphotericin lipid complex (Abelcet®)	100mg	3.13
Amphotericin liposomal (AmBisome®)	50mg	<0.5
Ampicillin	250mg	0.7
Atenolol	5mg	1.3–1.8
Benzylpenicillin	600mg	1.68
Cefotaxime	500mg	1.1
Ceftazidime	500mg	1.2
Ceftriaxone	1g	3.6
Cefuroxime	50mg	1.8
Chloramphenicol sodium succinate	1g	3.14
Ciprofloxacin	200mg	15.4
Clomethiazole	500mL	15–16
Co-amoxiclav	600mg	1.6
Co-trimoxazole	480mg	1.7
Desmopressin	4 micrograms	0.15
Diazoxide	300mg	15
Disodium hydrogen phosphate	10mL	12
Ertapenem	1g	6
Flucloxacillin	250mg	0.5
Fluconazole	200mg	15

(Continued)

Table A1 (*Contd.*)

Name	Vial/ampoule size	Sodium content per vial (mmol)
Flucytosine	2.5g	34.44
Folinic acid	15mg	0.2
Foscarnet	1g	15.6
Furosemide	250mg	1
Ganciclovir	500mg	2
Granisetron	3mg	1.17
Heparin	25000IU/mL	0.625–0.8
Human albumin solution (all concentrations)	100mL	100–160 (check label for exact amount)
Hydrocortisone:		
Sodium phosphate	100mg	0.66
Sodium succinate	100mg	0.37
Imipenem	500mg	1.72
Levofloxacin	500mg	15.4
Meropenem	1g	3.9
Metoclopramide	10mg	0.27
Metronidazole	500mg	13–14.55
Ofloxacin	200mg	15.4
Pamidronate:		
Dry powder	15mg	0.1
	30mg	0.2
	90mg	0.3
Solution	15mg	1.1
	30mg	1.1
Phenytoin	250mg	1.1
Piperacillin + tazobactam	4.5g	9.4
Rifampicin	300mg	<0.5
	600mg	<0.5
Sodium bicarbonate	1.26%	150/L
	4.2%	500/L
	8.4%	1000/L
Sodium chloride	0.9%	150/L
Sodium nitroprusside	50mg	0.34
Sodium valproate	400mg	2.41
Sotalol	40mg	0.5

Table A1 (*Contd.*)

Name	Vial/ampoule size	Sodium content per vial (mmol)
Teicoplanin	200mg	<0.5
	400mg	<0.5
Terbutaline	500 micrograms	0.15
Thiopental sodium	500mg	23.26
Ticarcillin + clavulanic acid	3.2g	16
Verapamil	5mg	0.3
Vitamins B and C:		
Pabrinex® high-potency IV	1+2 ampoules	2.95
Pabrinex® high-potency IM	1+2 ampoules	2.92

Reference

1.'MEDUSA', website, www.medusa.wales.nhs.uk

Pathology ranges and interpretation

See Table A2.

Table A2 Pathology ranges and interpretation

	Levels ↑ by	Levels ↓ by	Comments
Sodium (Na⁺) 135–145mmol/L	Water depletion, nephrogenic diabetes insipidus, (e.g. lithium toxicity), mineralocorticoid excess (e.g. Cushing's syndrome), corticosteroids. Secondary aldosteronism (e.g. CCF), nephritic syndrome, hepatic cirrhosis, and uraemia *Symptoms:* dry skin, postural hypotension, oliguria. Cerebral dehydration → thirst, confusion, and eventually coma	Water excess, mineralocorticoid deficiency (e.g. Addison's, thyroid deficiency), thiazide and loop diuretics, burns, SIADH, excess sweating, diarrhoea, vomiting, aspiration, atypical pneumonia, haemodilution caused by cardiac, hepatic or renal failure, oedema, infection, and carcinoma *Symptoms:* headache, nausea. hypertension, cardiac failure, cramps, confusion, convulsions, and overhydration	Regulated by aldosterone (ADH)
Potassium (K⁺) 3.5–5.0mmol/L	Mineralocorticoid deficiency (e.g. Addison's thyroid deficiency) ACE inhibitors, K⁺-sparing diuretics, renal failure, severe tissue damage (e.g. burns), hypoaldosteronism, diabetic ketoacidosis, excess K⁺ therapy, NSAIDs, β-blockers, heparin infusions, and sodium depletion (very rare) *Symptoms:* muscle weakness and abnormal cardiac conduction (e.g. ventricular fibrillation, and asystole)	Thiazide and loop diuretics, vomiting, diarrhoea, ileostomy, fistula, steroids, glucose and insulin therapy, mineralocorticoid excess (e.g. Cushing's syndrome), β-agonists, aspiration and metabolic alkalosis *Symptoms:* hypotonia, cardiac arrhythmias, muscle weakness, and paralytic ileus	Regulated by aldosterone, insulin/glucose. For hypokalaemia, if on diuretics, then ↑ bicarbonate is the best indication that hypokalaemia is likely to be longstanding. Magnesium might be low and hypokalaemia is often difficult to correct until magnesium is normalized

Chloride (Cl⁻) 95–105mol/L	Excess ingestion and dehydration *Symptoms*: non-specific	Vomiting, diarrhoea, diuretics, dehydration and nephropathy *Symptoms*: non-specific	Cl⁻ follows Na⁺ movement
Bicarbonate (HCO₃⁻) 24–30mmol/L	Excessive antacid use, thiazide and loop diuretics, metabolic alkalosis, bicarbonate, hypokalaemia, vomiting, and Cushing's syndrome *Symptoms*: vomiting	Diarrhoea, renal failure, diabetes mellitus, metabolic acidosis, respiratory alkalosis, and hyperventilation *Symptoms*: headache, drowsiness, and coma in severe acicosis	Reflects renal, metabolic, and respiratory functions
Glucose 3.0–8.0mmol/L	Diabetes mellitus, severe stress, occasionally after CVA, corticosteroids, thiazides, relative insulin deficiency caused by ↑ growth hormone, ↑ glucocorticoids or placental lactogen during pregnancy (glucagonaemia) *Symptoms*: polyuria, polydipsia and ketoacidosis	Insulin overdose, sulphonylureas especially in the elderly, insulinoma, alcohol, and hepatic failure *Symptoms*: dizziness, lethargy, sweating, tachycardia, agitation, and coma	
Magnesium (Mg²⁺) 0.70–1.10mmol/L	Renal failure and excessive antacids *Symptoms*: loss of muscle tone, lethargy and respiratory depression	Severe diarrhoea, fistula, alcohol abuse, diuretics, diabetes mellitus, TPN, hyper-aldosteronism, hepatic cirrhosis, and malabsorption *Symptoms*: tetany, paraesthesiae, cramps, arrhythmias, neuromuscular excitability, and hypoparathyroidism	Deficiency can exacerbate digitalis toxicity and Mg²⁺ is excreted by the kidneys
Zinc (Zn²⁺) 11–24µ	Zinc therapy	Cirrhosis, diarrhoea, alcoholism, drugs, parenteral nutrition, inadequate diet, steroids, diuretics, malabsorption syndrome, and rarely genetic *Symptoms*: poor wound healing and growth, alopecia, infertility, and poor resistance to infection	

(Continued)

Table A2 (Contd.)

	Levels ↑ by	Levels ↓ by	Comments
Calcium (Ca^{2+}) 2.20–2.60mmol/L (Determine corrected calcium level in hypoal-buminaemia and hyperalbuminaemia)	Paget's disease, vitamin A overdose, hyper-parathyroidism, vitamin D overdose, thiazides, oestrogen, lithium, tamoxifen, excess milk ingestion, excess calcium absorption, Hodgkin's disease, and myeloma *Symptoms:* nausea, vomiting, constipation, abdominal pain, renal stones, cardiac arrhythmias, headache, depression, mental fatigue, and psychosis	Thyroid surgery, hypoparathyroidism, alkalosis, renal failure, osteomalacia, vitamin D deficiency and acute pancreatitis *Symptoms:* ↑ nervous excitability, tetany, convulsions, muscle cramps, spasms, tingling, numbness of fingers, and ECG changes	Apparent hypocalcaemia might be caused by hypoalbuminaemia. Regulated by parathyroid hormone calcitonin (1.25-dihydroxychole-calc iferol)
Phosphate (PO_4^{3-}) 0.8–1.4mmol/L	Renal failure, hypoparathyroidism, diabetic ketoacidosis, and ↑ vitamin D	Osteomalacia (starvation), hyperparathyroidism, alcohol abuse, ↓ vitamin D, $Al(OH)_3$ therapy, and septicaemia	Ca^{2+} and PO_4^{3-} metabolism closely linked
Urea 2.5–7.0mmol/L	Renal failure, elderly (caused by ↓ renal function), urinary tract obstruction, CCF, dehydration, corticosteroids, high-protein diet, ↑ catabolism (e.g. starvation), sepsis, and GI bleed	↑ GFR, pregnancy, excessive IV infusion, low protein intake, anabolic states or synthesis, liver failure, diabetes insipidus, diuresis, and overhydration.	Derived from amino-acid metabolism in the liver; indicator of kidney function
Creatinine 20–110µmol/L (Cr/ Cl 80–139mL/min (not considered impaired unless <50mL/min))	Dehydration, renal failure, ↓ GFR, urinary tract obstruction, and ↑ meat/vitamin C	Pregnancy and chronic muscle wasting	Derived from muscle mass, determined by lean body mass, and indication of glomerular insufficiency

Alkaline phosphatase <125IU/L	Renal failure, cholestasis, liver cell damage, osteomalacia and bone disease, hyper-parathyroidism (e.g. Paget's disease) and metastases. Also during third trimester of pregnancy, post menopause, carcinoma of liver/prostrate, and drug-induced (e.g. chlorpromazine)	Hypothyroidism and growth retardation	~50% bone-related, ~50% hepatic fraction, and ~2–3% intestinal fraction
Creatine kinase 32–184IU/L	MI, skeletal muscle damage (even IM injection), muscular dystrophy, acute psychotic episodes, head injury, surgery, hypothyroidism, alcoholism, and neonates		Found in heart, skeletal and smooth muscle, and brain
Haemoglobin ♂: 135–180g/L ♀: 115–160g/L	Polycythaemia and dehydration	Sickle cell disease, thalassaemia, GI bleed, haemorrhage (acute/chronic) deficient RBC production, iron deficiency, bone marrow depression, renal failure, ↓ haemolysis and chronic liver disease	
White cell count 4.0–11.0 × 10⁹/L	Drugs (e.g. steroids), infection, septicaemia, malignancy, sulphonamides, bacterial infection, alcohol hepatitis, and cholecystitis	Drugs, bacterial infections, HIV, hypersensitivity reactions, surgery, trauma, burns, haemorrhage, leukaemia, radiation, cytotoxics, ↓ vitamin B_{12} and ↓ folate	Produced in bone marrow and stimulated by GSF
Haematocrit or packed cell volume ♂: 0.4–5.0L/L ♀: 0.37–0.47L/L	Addison's thyroid deficiency, dehydration, polycythaemia and pregnancy	Anaemia and haemorrhage	Relative measure of cells in blood and packed cell volume

(Continued)

Table A2 (*Contd.*)

	Levels ↑ by	Levels ↓ by	Comments
Platelets 150–400 × 10⁹/L	Inflammatory disorders, bleeding, malignancy, splenectomy, and polycythaemia	↓ production: bone-marrow failure/ suppression, leukaemia, drugs (notably cytotoxic drugs), megaloblastic anaemia, SLE, heparin. ↑ consumption: DIC, splenomegaly, furosemide, gold, idiopathic thrombocytopenia.	Derived from megakaryocytes in bone marrow and destroyed in spleen
Prothrombin time 10–14s INR~0.8–1.2	Severe liver damage, cholestasis causing malabsorption of vitamin K and warfarin		Used to monitor anticoagulant therapy (not DOACs) and assess liver function
Thrombin time 12–15s	Heparin and DIC		
APPT	Heparin, haemophilia, and liver failure		Used to monitor heparin therapy
Fibrinogen 1.7–4.1g/L	Nephrotic syndrome, Hodgkin's, and PE	DIC and massive blood transfusion	
Total protein 60–80g/L	Mineralocorticoid deficiency (e.g. Addison's thyroid deficiency) and myeloma	Catabolic states (e.g. septicaemia)	
Albumin 35–50g/L t½ =20–26 days	Dehydration and shock	Lost through skin (e.g. burns and psoriasis) liver disease, mal-nutrition, septicaemia, nephrotic syndrome, and late pregnancy *Symptoms:* oedema and toxic effects of drugs normally bound to albumin (e.g. calcium, bilirubin, and phenytoin)	

Bilirubin—total <17μmol/L Bilirubin—conjugated (bound to albumin) <4μmol/L	Hepatocellular damage (e.g. viral hepatitis—inability to conjugate bilirubin), cholestasis (e.g. by phenothiazines and flucloxacillin) gallstones, inflammation, malignancy, Gilbert's syndrome, haemolysis, methyldopa, GI bleed, extensive bruising, and sulphonamides (displace bilirubin from albumin)	Derives from breakdown of RBCs by monocyte macrophage system
	Symptoms: jaundice	
γ-glutamyl transpeptidase ♂: 11–51IU/L ♀: 7–33IU/L	Cholestasis (e.g. carcinoma of pancreas or biliary tract), liver cell damage (e.g. hepatitis and cirrhosis). Enzyme inducers (e.g. alcohol, phenytoin, and phenobarbital) and alcoholism	Found in liver, kidneys, pancreas and prostate; released by tissue damage
Aspartate transaminase 5–35IU/L	Hepatocellular damage, cirrhosis, viral hepatitis, severe haemolytic anaemia, myocardial injury (e.g. MI), cholestasis, trauma, or surgery	Found in liver, heart, kidneys, skeletal muscle, and erythrocytes
Amylase <180U/dL random urine <650IU/L	Acute pancreatitis, abdominal trauma, diabetic ketoacidosis, chronic renal failure, cholecystitis, intestinal obstruction, mumps, ruptured ectopic pregnancy, post-MI ruptured DU, and morphine	Found in parotid glands and pancreas. Smaller amounts in ovaries, intestine, and skeletal muscle
Fibrin degradation products <10 micrograms/mL	DIC and adult respiratory distress syndrome	
		Renal failure and vitamin B deficiency
		Hepatitis and pancreatic insufficiency

(Continued)

Table A2 (*Contd.*)

	Levels ↑ by	Levels ↓ by	Comments
Cholesterol 3.9–6mmol/L	Diabetes mellitus, familial hypercholesterolaemia excess alcohol, hypothyroidism, and hepatic and renal diseases	Severe illness, severe weight loss, and MI (during first 2wks)	Treatment will depend on other risk factors
pH 7.35–7.45	Vomiting, K^+ loss, burns, hyperventilation, stroke, SAH, anxiety, hyperthyroidism, excess antacids, aspirin overdose, fever, and uncompensated alkalosis	Respiratory failure, hypoventilation, diarrhoea, renal failure, ketoacidosis, trauma, shock, high plasma lactate (e.g. liver failure), hypoxia, anaemia, and uncompensated acidosis	Reflects ratio of acid to base and not absolute concentration. Therefore it might mask a defect for which the body has compensated
PaO_2 >10.6kPa	Artificial over-ventilation with O_2	COAD, respiratory failure, ARDS, and cardiogenic pulmonary oedema	
$PaCO_2$ 4.7–6.0kPa Total CO_2 24–30mmol	COAD, hypoventilation, respiratory acidosis and ARDS-compensated metabolic alkalosis	Hyperventilation, respiratory alkalosis, CVA, anxiety, aspirin overdose, compensated metabolic acidosis, pulmonary embolism, and non-cardiogenic ARDS	Indicator of respiratory function

Normal ranges

See Table A3.

Table A3 Normal ranges

Sodium	135–145mmol/L	White cell count	4.0–11 × 10⁹/L
Potassium	3.5–5.0mmol/L	PCV/haematocrit	♂=0.4–0.54L/L
Chloride	95–105mmol/L	PCV/haematocrit	♀=0.37–0.47L/L
Bicarbonate	24–30mmol/L	Platelets	150–400 × 10⁹/L
Glucose (fasting)	3.5–5.5mmol/L	INR	0.8–1.2
Magnesium	0.75–1.05mmol/L	KCR	0.8–1.2
Phosphate	0.8–1.4mmol/L	Thrombin time	Ratio <1.2
Zinc	11–24µmol/L	Fibrinogen	1.7–4.1g/L
Calcium	2.12–2.65mmol/L	Albumin	35–50g/L
FDP	<10 micrograms/mL	Total protein	60–80g/L
Urea	2.5–6.7mmol/L	Bilirubin (total)	3–17µmol/L
Creatinine	70–150µmol/L	Bilirubin (conjugated)	<4µmol/L
Cr/Cl	80–139mL/min	GGT	♂: 11–40IU/L ♀: 7–33IU/L
Alk phos	<150IU/L	AST	5–35IU/L
Creatine kinase	♂: 25–195IU/L ♀: 25–170IU/L		
Haemoglobin	♂=135–180g/L	Amylase	<180IU/L
Haemoglobin	♀=115–160g/L	Amylase (random urine)	<650IU/L
Cholesterol	3.9–6mmol/L	PaO₂	>10.6kPa
pH	7.35–7.45	PaCO₂	4.7–6.0kPa

Paediatric normal laboratory values

The values given in Tables A4–A10 are a guide; local laboratories may differ. Check normal values with the laboratory you use. You will find here tables on biochemistry (Table A4), haematology (Table A5), respiratory rate (Table A6), blood pressure (Table A7), urinary output (Table A8), hypoglycaemia (Table A9), and electrolyte requirements (Table A10).

Table A4 Biochemistry

Alanine aminotransferase	Newborn–1 month		≤70IU/L
	Infants and children		15–55IU/L
Albumin	Preterm		25–45g/L
	Newborn (term)		25–50g/L
	1–3 months		30–42g/L
	3–12 months		27–50g/L
	1–15yrs		32–50g/L
Alkaline phosphatase	Newborn		150–600U/L
	6 months–9yrs		250–800U/L
Amylase			70–300IU/L
Aspartate amino-transferase			<45IU/L
Bilirubin	Full term	Day 1	<65µmol/L
		Day 2	<115µmol/L
		Days 3–5	<155µmol/L
		>1 month	<10µmol/L
Calcium	Preterm		1.5–2.5mmol/L
	Infants		2.25–2.75mmol/L
	>1yr		2.25–2.6mmol/L
Chloride			95–105mmol/L
Creatine kinase	Newborn		<600IU/L
	1 month		<400IU/L
	1yr		<30IU/L
	Children	♂	<190IU/L
		♀	<130IU/L
Creatinine	0–2yrs		20–50µmol/L
	2–6yrs		25–60µmol/L
	6–12yrs		30–80µmol/L
	>12yrs	♂	65–120µmol/L
		♀	50–110µmol/L
Creatinine clearance	<37wks' gestation		<15mL/min/m²
	Neonate		10–20mL/min/m²
	1–2wks		20–35mL/min/m²
	2–4 months		35–45mL/min/m²
	6–125 months		45–60mL/min/m²
	12 months to adult		50–85mL/min/m²

Table A4 (*Contd.*)

C-reactive protein		<20mg/L
γ-glutaryl transferase	Newborn	<200IU/L
	1 month–1yr	<150IU/L
	>1yr	<30IU/L
Glucose	Newborn–3 days	2–5mmol/L
	>1wk	2.5–5mmol/L
Lactate		0.7–1.8mmol/L
Magnesium	Newborn	0.7–1.2mmol/L
	Child	0.7–1mmol/L
Phosphate	Pre-term first month	1.4–3.4mmol/L
	Full-term newborn	1.2–2.9mmol/L
	1yr	1.2–2.2mmol/L
	2–10yrs	1–1.8mmol/L
	>10yrs	0.7–1.6mmol/L
Potassium	0–2wks	3.7–6mmol/L
	2wks–3 months	3.7–5.7mmol/L
	>3 months	3.5–5mmol/L
Protein (total)	1 month	50–70g/L
	1yr	60–80g/L
	1–9yrs	60–81g/L
Sodium		135–145mmol/L
Urea	0–1yr	2.5–7.5mmol/L
	1–7yrs	3.3–6.5mmol/L
	7–16yrs ♂	2.6–6.7mmol/L
	♀	2.5–6mmol/L

Table A5 Haematology

Age	Hb (g/L) Mean (range)		MCV (fL) Mean (range)		WBC (× 10⁹/L) range	Reticulocyte (%) range
Birth	185	(145–215)	108	(95–116)	5–26	3–7
1 month	140	(100–165)	104	(85–108)	6–15	0–1
6 months	110	(850–135)	88	(80–96)	6–15	0–1
1yr	120	(105–135)	78	(70–86)	6–15	0–1
6yrs	125	(115–140)	81	(75–88)	6–15	0–1
12yrs	135	(115–145)	86	(77–94)	5–15	0–1

Note: an artefactual high neonate WBC may be reported because automatic cell counters may wrongly include in the WBC the many normoblasts (red cell precursors) in the neonate.

Table A6 Respiratory rate

Newborn	30–60 breaths/min	Heart rate is usually four
6 months	30–45 breaths/min	times the respiratory rate
1–2yrs	25–35 breaths/min	
3–6yrs	20–30 breaths/min	
>7yrs	20–25 breaths/min	

Table A7 Blood pressure

	Mean (mmHg)	
	Systolic BP	Diastolic BP
Newborn to 2yrs	95	55
3–6yrs	100	65
7–10yrs	105	70
11–15yrs	115	70

Table A8 Urinary output

	mL/day
Infant	250–600
Child	500–1000
Adolescent	500–1500
Adult	500–2000

Table A9 Hypoglycaemia

	Serum glucose (mmol/L)
Pre-term	<1.4
Term	<2.0
Child	<2.5

Table A10 Electrolyte requirements

Na^+	2–4mmol/kg body weight/24h
K^+	1–3mmol/kg body weight/24h
Cl^-	3–5mmol/kg body weight/24h
Ca^{2+}	1mmol/kg body weight/24h
Mg^{2+}	0.15mmol/kg body weight/24h

Useful websites

See Table A11.

Table A11 Useful websites

Description	→ Web address (URL)
American Society of Clinical Oncology (ASCO)	http://www.asco.org
American Society of Hematology (ASH)	http://www.hematology.org
American Society of Health-System Pharmacists	http://www.ashp.org
Annals of Internal Medicine	http://www.annals.org
Australian Therapeutic Goods Administration	http://www.tga.gov.au
BNF	http://www.bnf.org
British Committee for Standards in Haematology (BCSH) guidelines	http://www.bcshguidelines.com
British Medical Journal (*BMJ*)	http://www.bmj.com
British Oncology Pharmacy Association (BOPA)	http://www.bopawebsite.org
British Society for Haematology (BSH)	http://www.b-s-h.org.uk
Canadian Health Technology Assessment Programme	http://www.nlm.nih.gov/hsrinfo/evidence_based_practice.html
Cancer Improvement	http://www.improvement.nhs.uk/cancer
Cancer Research UK	http://www.cancerresearchuk.org
COREC	http://www.corec.org.uk
Counterfeit drugs	http://www.pharmacistscombatcounterfeiting.org
CPD for Pharmacists	http://www.uptodate.org.uk
Cytotoxic guidelines	http://www.marchguidelines.com
Department of Health	http://www.dh.gov.uk
Drugs in breast milk	http://www.ukmicentral.nhs.uk
Electronic Medicines Compendium	http://www.medicines.org.uk/emc
European Society for Medical Oncology (ESMO)	http://www.esmo.org
Evidence in Health and Social Care	http://www.evidence.nhs.uk
Gene Therapy Advisory Committee (GTAC)	http://www.dh.gov.uk/ab/GTAC/index.htm?ssSourceSiteId=en

(Continued)

Table A11 (*Contd.*)

Description	➔ Web address (URL)
General Pharmaceutical Council	http://www.pharmacyregulation.org
Health and Safety Executive (HSE)	http://www.hse.gov.uk/
Herbal medicines—includes evidence for efficacy, ADRs and drug interactions	http://www.herbmed.org
International Society of Oncology Pharmacy Practitioners (ISOPP)	http://www.isopp.org
Journal of Clinical Oncology (JCO)	http://www.jco.org
Journal of the American Medical Association (JAMA)	http://www.jama.ama-assn.org
Lancet	http://www.thelancet.com
Macmillan Cancer Information	http://www.macmillan.org.uk
Malaria advice (no prophylaxis advice)	http://www.malariahotspots.co.uk
Medicines and Healthcare products Regulatory Agency (MHRA)	http://www.mhra.gov.uk
Medicines information	http://www.ukmi.nhs.uk
Medicines management and pharmaceutical care	http://www.pharmalife.co.uk
Merck manual full-text online	http://www.merck.com/mmpe/index.html
National Electronic Library for Health	http://www.library.nhs.uk
National Institute for Health and Care Excellence (NICE)	http://www.nice.org.uk
National Prescribing Centre	http://www.npc.co.uk
National Treatment Centre for Substance Misuse	http://www.nta.nhs.uk
New England Journal of Medicine	http://www.nejm.org
Oxford Handbook of Clinical Medicine	http://ohcm.oxfordmedicine.com
Palliative care	http://www.palliativedrugs.com
Paracetamol Information Centre (includes guidelines on treatment of overdose)	http://www.pharmweb.net/paracetamol.html
Patient-group directions	http://www.nelm.nhs.uk/en/Communities/NeLM/PGDs
Pharmaceutical Journal	http://www.pjonline.com
Renal Association	http://www.renal.org/home.aspx
RPSGB	http://www.rpharms.com
Scottish Intercollegiate Guideline Network (SIGN)	http://www.sign.ac.uk

(*Continued*)

Table A11 (*Contd.*)

Description	➜ Web address (URL)
TB information in various languages	http://www.dh.gov.uk/en/Publicationsandstatistics/Publications/PublicationsPolicyAndGuidance/DH_116689
Travel advice, specific to destination—includes vaccinations and malaria prop	http://www.fitfortravel.scot.nhs.uk
Travel shop, includes travel health information and medical supplies	http://www.nomadtravel.co.uk
Travel—health information (subscription required, free NHS Scotland)	http://www.travax.scot.nhs.uk
WHO Action Programme on Essential Drugs	http://www.who.int/dap

In vitro activity of antibacterials

See Table A12

Table A12 In vitro activity of antibacterials

√ = usually sensitive   ? = variable sensitivity   X = usually resistant or inappropriate therapy

Note: These are generalizations. There are major differences between countries, areas, and hospitals. Check local Public Health or Microbiology laboratories for local sensitivity patterns. Antibacterials may not be licensed to treat the bacteria for which they are active.

	Gram positives								Anaerobes			Gram negatives									Atypicals		
	Staphylococcus aureus MSSA	Staphylococcus aureus MRSA	Staphylococcus epidermidis	Haemolytic streptococci (Strep A, C, G and Strep B)	Enterococcus faecalis	Enterococcus faecium	Streptococcus pneumoniae	Listeria monocytogenes	Clostridium perfringens	Clostridium difficile	Bacteroides fragilis	Neisseria meningitidis	Neisseria gonorrhoeae	Haemophilus influenzae	Escherichia coli	Klebsiella spp	Proteus mirabilis	Proteus vulgaris	Pseudomonas aeruginosa	Moraxella catarrhalis	Legionella spp	Mycoplasma pneumoniae	Chlamydia spp
Penicillins																							
Phenoxymethylpenicillin	×	×	×	✓	✓	?	✓	×	✓	×	×	✓	?	×	×	×	×	×	×	×	×	×	×
Benzylpenicillin	×	×	×	✓	?	?	✓	✓	✓	×	×	✓	?	×	×	×	×	×	×	×	×	×	×
Ampicillin / Amoxicillin	×	×	×	✓	✓	?	✓	✓	✓	×	×	✓	?	?	?	×	✓	✓	×	×	×	×	×
Co-amoxiclav	✓	×	?	✓	✓	×	✓	✓	✓	×	✓	✓	×	✓	?	?	✓	✓	×	✓	×	×	×
Flucloxacillin	✓	×	?	✓	×	×	✓	×	✓	×	×	✓	×	×	×	×	×	×	×	×	×	×	×
Pip+tazobactam	✓	×	?	✓	✓	?	✓	×	✓	×	✓	✓	×	✓	✓	✓	✓	✓	✓	✓	×	×	×
Cephalosporins																							
Cefradine/Cefalexin	✓	×	?	✓	×	×	✓	×	✓	×	×	×	×	?	✓	✓	✓	?	×	✓	×	×	×

(Continued)

	Gram positives								Anaerobes			Gram negatives									Atypicals		
	Staphylococcus aureus MSSA	Staphylococcus aureus MRSA	Staphylococcus epidermidis	Haemolytic streptococci (Strep A, C, G and Strep B)	Enterococcus faecalis	Enterococcus faecium	Streptococcus pneumoniae	Listeria monocytogenes	Clostridium perfringens	Clostridium difficile	Bacteroides fragilis	Neisseria meningitidis	Neisseria gonorrhoeae	Haemophilus influenzae	Escherichia coli	Klebsiella spp	Proteus mirabilis	Proteus vulgaris	Pseudomonas aeruginosa	Moraxella catarrhalis	Legionella spp	Mycoplasma pneumoniae	Chlamydia spp
Cefotaxime	✓	×	~	✓	×	×	✓	×	×	×	×	✓	~	✓	✓	✓	✓	✓	~	✓	×	×	×
Cefuroxime	✓	×	~	✓	×	×	✓	×	×	×	×	×	~	✓	✓	✓	✓	✓	×	✓	×	×	×
Ceftriaxone	✓	×	~	✓	×	×	✓	×	×	×	×	✓	✓	✓	✓	✓	✓	✓	~	✓	×	×	×
Ceftazidime	~	×	~	✓	×	×	~	×	×	×	×	~	~	✓	✓	✓	✓	✓	✓	✓	×	×	×
Carbapenems																							
Ertapenem	✓	×	✓	✓	~	×	✓	~	✓	×	✓	✓	✓	✓	✓	✓	✓	✓	×	✓	×	×	×
Meropenem/Imipenem	✓	×	✓	✓	~	~	✓	×	✓	×	✓	✓	✓	~	✓	✓	✓	✓	✓	✓	×	×	×
Macrolides/Lincosamides																							
Azithromycin	✓	×	×	✓	×	×	✓	~	×	×	×	✓	~	✓	×	×	×	×	×	✓	✓	✓	✓
Erythromycin	✓	×	~	✓	×	×	✓	×	×	×	×	✓	~	~	×	×	×	×	×	✓	✓	✓	✓
Clarithromycin	✓	×	×	✓	×	×	✓	×	×	×	×	×	~	✓	×	×	×	×	×	✓	✓	✓	✓
Clindamycin	✓	×	×	✓	×	×	~	×	✓	×	✓	×	×	×	×	×	×	×	×	×	×	×	×
Aminoglycosides																							
Amikacin	✓	✓	~	×	✓¹	×	×	✓¹	×	×	×	✓	×	✓	✓	✓	✓	✓	✓	✓	✓	×	×
Gentamicin	✓	✓	~	×	✓¹	✓¹	×	✓¹	×	×	×	✓	×	~	✓	✓	✓	✓	✓	✓	✓	×	×
Diaminopyrimidines and sulphonamides																							
Co-trimoxazole	✓	~	~	✓	✓	~	~	×	×	×	×	✓	~	✓	✓	✓	✓	✓	×	✓	×	×	✓
Trimethoprim	~	~	~	~	~	×	~	×	×	×	×	~	~	~	✓	✓	✓	✓	×	✓	✓	~	~

Table A12 (Contd.)

	Staphylococcus aureus MSSA	Staphylococcus aureus MRSA	Staphylococcus epidermidis	Haemolytic streptococci (Strep A, C, G and Strep B)	Enterococcus faecalis	Enterococcus faecium	Streptococcus pneumoniae	Listeria monocytogenes	Clostridium perfringens	Clostridium difficile	Bacteroides fragilis	Neisseria meningitidis	Neisseria gonorrhoeae	Haemophilus influenzae	Escherichia coli	Klebsiella spp	Proteus mirabilis	Proteus vulgaris	Pseudomonas aeruginosa	Moraxella catarrhalis	Legionella spp	Mycoplasma pneumoniae	Chlamydia spp
	Gram positives								Anaerobes			Gram negatives									Atypicals		
Quinolones																							
Ciprofloxacin	✓	×	×	×	×	×	×	×	✓	?	×	✓	✓	✓	✓	✓	✓	✓	✓	✓	✓	✓	✓
Levofloxacin	✓	×	×	?	✓	×	✓	×	✓	×	?	✓	✓	✓	✓	✓	✓	✓	~	✓	✓	✓	✓
Moxifloxacin	✓	×	✓	✓	✓	~	✓	×	✓	×	✓	✓	✓	✓	✓	✓	✓	✓	~	✓	✓	✓	✓
Glycopeptides																							
Vancomycin (IV)	✓	✓	✓	✓	✓	~	✓	✓	✓	×[2]	×	×	×	×	×	×	×	×	×	×	×	×	×
Teicoplanin	✓	✓	~	✓	✓	~	✓	✓	✓	✓	✓	×	×	×	×	×	×	×	×	×	×	×	×
Nitromidazoles																							
Metronidazole	×	×	×	×	×	×	×	×	✓	✓	✓	×	×	×	×	×	×	×	×	×	×	×	×
Oxazolidinones																							
Linezolid	✓	✓	✓	✓	✓	✓	✓	✓	✓	?	~	×	×	?	×	×	×	×	×	×	✓	×	×
Tetracyclines																							
Doxycycline	✓	?	✓	✓	~	×	✓	✓	✓	×	~	✓	×	~	×	×	×	×	×	✓	✓	✓	✓
Miscellaneous																							
Chloramphenicol	?	×	×	✓	?	✓	✓	✓	?	×	~	✓	×	✓	✓	✓	?	?	×	✓	✓	✓	✓
Quinupristin/dalfopristin (Synercid®)	✓	✓	✓	✓	×	✓	✓	×	✓	?	✓	×	×	×	×	×	×	×	×	✓	✓	✓	✓

[1] Sensitive if used synergistically with penicillins/glycopeptides.

[2] IV vancomycin ineffective for Clostridium difficile.

Index